SYSTEMIC DRUGS FOR SKIN DISEASES

Stephen E. Wolverton, M.D.

Assistant Professor, Department of
  Dermatology
Indiana University
School of Medicine
Indianapolis, Indiana
Formerly Assistant Professor
Division of Dermatology
The Ohio State University
School of Medicine
Columbus, Ohio

Jonathan K. Wilkin, M.D.

Professor, Departments of Medicine
  and Pharmacology
Director, Division of Dermatology
The Ohio State University
School of Medicine
Columbus, Ohio

W.B. SAUNDERS COMPANY
A Division of Harcourt Brace & Company
Philadelphia London Toronto
Montreal Sydney Tokyo

W.B. SAUNDERS COMPANY
A Division of
Harcourt Brace & Company

The Curtis Center
Independence Square West
Philadelphia, Pennsylvania 19106

Library of Congress Cataloging-in-Publication Data

Systemic Drugs for Skin Diseases / [edited by] Stephen E. Wolverton, Jonathan K. Wilkin.

   p.   cm.

ISBN 0-7216-2987-3

1. Dermatologic agents.   I. Wolverton, Stephen E.
  II. Wilkin, Jonathan K.

[DNLM: 1. Dermatologic Agents—therapeutic use. 2. Skin—drug effects.   QV 60 D794]

RM303.D78 1991

615'.778—dc20

DNLM/DLC   90-8921

Editor: W. B. Saunders Staff
Designer: Susan Hess Blaker
Production Manager: Bill Preston
Manuscript Editor: Anne Ostroff
Illustration Coordinator: Brett MacNaughton
Indexer: Julie Figures

Systemic Drugs for Skin Diseases   ISBN 0-7216-2987-3

Copyright © 1991 by W. B. Saunders Company

All rights reserved. No part of this publication may be reproduced or transmitted in any form or by any means, electronic or mechanical, including photocopy, recording, or any information storage and retrieval system, without permission in writing from the publisher.

Printed in the United States of America

Last digit is the print number: 9   8   7   6   5   4   3

*This book is dedicated
to our sons
Jay Edward and Justin David Wolverton
and
Christopher Keith and Nathaniel Kevin Wilkin*

Contributors

Wilma F. Bergfeld, M.D. • Professor, Cleveland Clinic Educational Foundation; Clinical Assistant Professor, Department of Dermatology, Case Western Reserve Medical School; Head, Clinical Research, Department of Dermatology, and Head, Dermatopathology, Department of Pathology, Cleveland Clinic Foundation, Cleveland, Ohio • *Antiandrogens*

Brian Berman, M.D., Ph.D. • Associate Professor and Vice-Chairman, Department of Dermatology, University of California, Davis, School of Medicine, Davis; Chief, Dermatology Service, Veterans Affairs Medical Center, Martinez, California • *Antiviral Agents*

Suzanne Bruce, M.D. • Assistant Professor of Dermatology, Baylor College of Medicine; Staff, The Methodist Hospital, Ben Taub General Hospital, Veterans Administration Medical Center, St. Luke's Episcopal Hospital, and Texas Children's Hospital, Houston, Texas • *Antibacterial Agents*

Jeffrey P. Callen, M.D., F.A.C.P. • Professor of Medicine and Director, Division of Dermatology, Department of Medicine, University of Louisville School of Medicine, Louisville, Kentucky • *Methotrexate*

Charles Camisa, M.D. • Head, Section of Clinical Dermatology, and Director, Dermatology Residency Program, Cleveland Clinic Foundation, Cleveland, Ohio • *Antimalarials*

Loretta Smrtnik Davis, M.D. • Assistant Professor of Medicine, Division of Dermatology, Department of Internal Medicine, Ohio State University, Columbus, Ohio • *New Uses for Old Drugs*

James Q. Del Rosso, D.O. • Clinical Assistant Professor, Division of Dermatology, Ohio State University; Volunteer Clinical Faculty, Ohio University College of Osteopathic Medicine, Department of Medical Specialties; Fellow, Mohs Micrographic Surgery and Dermatologic Surgery, Department of Otolaryngology, Ohio State University, Columbus, Ohio • *Antihistamines*

Kenneth E. Greer, M.D. • Professor of Dermatology and Vice-Chairman, Department of Dermatology, University of Virginia School of Medicine, Charlottesville, Virginia • *Dapsone and Sulfapyridine*

Lyn Guenther, M.D., F.R.C.P.C. • Clinical Assistant Professor, The University of Western Ontario; Staff, St. Joseph's Hospital and University Hospital, London, Ontario, Canada • *Cyclosporine*

Robert E. Jordon, M.D. • Professor and Chairman, Department of Dermatology, University of Texas Medical School; Chief of Dermatology, Hermann Hospital; Consultant, M. D. Anderson Cancer Center and St. Luke's Hospital, Houston, Texas • *Cytotoxic Agents*

Contributors

Marshall B. Kapp, J.D., M.P.H. • Professor, Department of Community Health, Wright State University, Dayton, Ohio • *Informed Consent for Systemic Drugs Used in Dermatology*

Suzanne L. Kilmer, M.D. • Chief, Dermatology Residents, University of California, Sacramento, California • *Antiviral Agents*

Carol L. Kulp-Shorten, M.D. • Clinical Instructor of Medicine (Dermatology), University of Louisville; Active Staff, Humana Hospital University, Methodist Evangelical Hospital, Norton-Kosair Hospital, and Veterans Administration Medical Center; Courtesy Staff, Jewish Hospital and Humana Hospital Audubon, Louisville, Kentucky • *Methotrexate*

Larry E. Millikan, M.D. • Professor and Chairman, Tulane University Medical School; Staff, Tulane Medical Center Hospital; Consultant, Charity Hospital, Tulane Dermatology Affiliates, and Tulane Covington Clinic, New Orleans, Louisiana • *Antifungal Agents*

Ronald P. Rapini, M.D. • Associate Professor of Dermatology and Pathology, University of Texas Medical School at Houston, Houston, Texas; Staff, Hermann Hospital, and the University of Texas M. D. Anderson Cancer Center, Houston, Texas • *Cytotoxic Agents*

Geoffrey Redmond, M.D. • President, Foundation for Developmental Endocrinology, Inc.; Attending Physician, Mount Sinai Medical Center, Cleveland, Ohio • *Antiandrogens*

Joseph P. Shrum, M.D. • Assistant Professor of Dermatology, Tulane University; Staff, Tulane Medical Center, New Orleans, Louisiana • *Antifungal Agents*

Robert B. Skinner, Jr., M.D. • Associate Professor, Department of Medicine (Dermatology), University of Tennessee at Memphis; Staff, William F. Bowld Hospital, Regional Medical Center, Baptist Memorial Hospital, Le Bonheur Children's Medical Center, St. Jude Children's Research Hospital, and Veterans Administration Medical Center, Memphis, Tennessee • *Psoralens*

Jonathan K. Wilkin, M.D. • Professor, Departments of Medicine and Pharmacology, Ohio State University; Director, Division of Dermatology, Ohio State University Hospitals; and Columbus Children's Hospital (privileges), Columbus, Ohio • *Vasoactive and Antiplatelet Agents*

John E. Wolf, M.D. • Professor and Chairman, Department of Dermatology, Baylor College of Medicine; Chief of Dermatology Service, The Methodist Hospital, Houston, Texas • *Antibacterial Agents*

Stephen E. Wolverton, M.D. • Assistant Professor, Department of Dermatology, Indiana University School of Medicine, Indianapolis, Indiana; formerly Assistant Professor, Division of Dermatology, Ohio State University College of Medicine, Columbus, Ohio; Staff, University Hospitals, Wishard Hospital, and Richard Roudebush Veterans Administration Medical Center, Indianapolis, Indiana • *Glucocorticosteroids; Cytotoxic Agents; Retinoids; An Approach to Monitoring for Adverse Effects; Informed Consent for Systemic Drugs Used in Dermatology*

Preface

This text represents an attempt to increase the clinician's skill and comfort, while minimizing the anxiety that commonly accompanies the use of systemic agents for dermatologic problems. The focus of the book is clearly on "how to use" and "how to use safely" the spectrum of systemic drugs prescribed by the dermatologist. The indications tables and related text sections contain numerous pertinent therapeutic references, which along with the therapeutic guidelines sections address the "how to use" issue. Detailed and well-organized discussions on important adverse effects are accompanied in most chapters by tables that list monitoring guidelines for detecting these adverse effects. The guidelines simplify the "how to use safely" issue. Concise descriptions on important drug interactions accompany each chapter.

There are multiple additional organizational features to assist the clinician in rapid information retrieval. The indications tables are grouped by disease categories, discriminating indications approved by the U.S. Food and Drug Administration from other dermatologic uses for the drugs discussed. Systemic agents that are most commonly used in clinical practice are discussed first in each chapter, receiving detailed emphasis on key areas of pharmacologic and clinical information. Briefer discussions on less commonly used drugs conclude the respective chapters. Tremendous effort has been focused on including thorough and up-to-date reference lists on the practical aspects of "how to use" and "how to use safely." All chapters discussing specific drugs or drug categories contain a bibliography of "Key Reviews/Chapters" to assist the reader in pursuit of additional current background information. Dermatologic conditions are highlighted with boldface type to allow easy cross-referencing when the clinician seeks therapeutic options for a specific disease.

Three truly unique chapters conclude the book. Chapter 15, "New Uses for Old Drugs," addresses newer dermatologic indications for nine unrelated drugs or drug categories originally developed for nondermatologic indications. Chapter 16, "An Approach to Monitoring for Adverse Effects," presents an overview of principles central to surveillance for potential adverse effects, complementing the individual chapter discussions on the various systemic agents. Chapter 17, "Informed Consent for Systemic Drugs Used in Dermatology," addresses the complicated subject of informed consent as it applies to the use of medications that entail a risk of significant adverse effects.

It is our hope that the reader will find this book a practical, understandable, and well-organized reference text. Clinicians in dermatology, as well as those in various primary care specialties, will benefit greatly by keeping this book easily accessible to their patient care setting. The many distinguished authors of these 17 chapters have responded in an excellent fashion to the unique organizational challenges described above.

Acknowledgments

We would like to express our gratitude to a number of dedicated individuals. Tracy Tucker was the W. B. Saunders editor who initiated the concepts that led to the development of this book. Bill Lamsback, and subsequently Lisette Bralow, both were editors instrumental in the completion of this challenging project. The Ohio State University Division of Dermatology secretaries Jeannette Painter and Lucille Ankrom ably worked with numerous letters to contributing authors and financial matters related to the production of this book. Laura Duren and Matt Carmean skillfully performed numerous literature searches that were central to the aggressive editorial review used throughout the book development. Both Ellen Smith and Timothy Mazik utilized their mastery of the WordPerfect 5.0 word processing software used throughout the editing process. Of all these individuals, the organizational skills, efficiency, and perseverance of Timothy Mazik were most critical to the successful completion of *Systemic Drugs for Skin Diseases*.

Contents

Drugs for Infectious Diseases

1   Antiviral Agents   1
Brian Berman
Suzanne L. Kilmer

2   Antifungal Agents   25
Larry E. Millikan
Joseph P. Shrum

3   Antibacterial Agents   47
Suzanne Bruce
John E. Wolf, Jr.

Immunomodulatory and Antiproliferative Agents

4   Glucocorticosteroids   86
Stephen E. Wolverton

5   Cytotoxic Agents   125
Ronald P. Rapini
Robert E. Jordon
Stephen E. Wolverton

6   Methotrexate   152
Jeffrey P. Callen
Carol L. Kulp-Shorten

7   Cyclosporine   167
Lyn Guenther

8   Retinoids   187
Stephen E. Wolverton

xii   Contents

Other Systemic Dermatologic Agents

9 Psoralens   219
   Robert B. Skinner, Jr.

10 Dapsone and Sulfapyridine   247
   Kenneth E. Greer

11 Antimalarials   265
   Charles Camisa

12 Antihistamines   285
   James Q. Del Rosso

13 Antiandrogens   327
   Wilma F. Bergfeld
   Geoffrey Redmond

14 Vasoactive and Antiplatelet Drugs   347
   Jonathan K. Wilkin

15 New Uses for Old Drugs   364
   Loretta Smrtnik Davis

Special Topics

16 An Approach to Monitoring for Adverse Effects   385
   Stephen E. Wolverton

17 Informed Consent for Systemic Drugs Used
   in Dermatology   400
   Stephen E. Wolverton
   Marshall B. Kapp

Appendix I   Sample Patient Handout: Prednisone
           Patient Information Summary   411

Appendix II   Example of a Laboratory Flow Sheet   415

Index   417

1 Antiviral Agents

Brian Berman, M.D., Ph.D.
Suzanne L. Kilmer, M.D.

ACYCLOVIR (ZOVIRAX)

During the 1970s and 1980s, the field of antiviral agents evolved tremendously. In particular, the advent of acyclovir has greatly enhanced the management and outcome of herpesvirus infections and paved the way for further promising antiviral agents. Although newer drugs such as ganciclovir, foscarnet, and deoxyacyclovir are in experimental use, acyclovir remains the first-line agent for therapy of herpesvirus infections.

Acyclovir was first discovered by Shaeffer and colleagues in 1974[1] during an intensive screening by Burroughs Wellcome for compounds with antiviral activity. By 1977, clinical trials were under way, and in 1982 acyclovir became available in a topical form; systemic preparations followed soon after.[1]

Pharmacology

Structure

Acyclovir (9-[2-hydroxyethoxymethyl] guanine) is a guanosine analog lacking carbon atoms at the 2' and 3' positions. The resulting acyclic side chain distinguishes it from guanine.

Absorption/Distribution

Only 20% of orally administered acyclovir is absorbed through the gastrointestinal tract; food does not affect absorption. Acyclovir is widely distributed throughout the body, including the central nervous system, where the concentration is 30%–50% of the serum concentration. Acyclovir crosses the placenta and is present in breast milk in a greater concentration than in the maternal plasma, which suggests that it is actively secreted.[2–4]

Metabolism/Excretion

Fortunately, metabolism of acyclovir is minimal, enabling oral doses to be therapeutically beneficial. More than 90% of the drug is excreted unchanged by the kidney. Elimination is primarily through glomerular filtration with a smaller component of tubular secretion, which results in a serum half-life of 2½–3 hours. Therefore, renally impaired patients with a creatinine clearance rate less than 10 ml/min require a dosage adjustment. Acyclovir is efficiently removed by hemodialysis.[3, 5–7] Of note, Hintz and colleagues[8] found no significant difference between adult and neonatal pharmacokinetics.

Mechanism of Action

Acyclovir is an ideal antiviral agent in that it essentially destroys only virally infected cells, leaving normal cells intact. Acyclovir is inactive until phosphorylated within cells infected with the herpesvirus. Phosphorylation to the monophosphate form occurs much more efficiently by virally induced thymidine kinase than by cellular thymidine kinase. Host cellular kinases then phosphorylate the monophosphate form to the diphosphate and triphosphate forms. Acyclovir triphosphate competes for viral DNA polymerases, and once incorporated into the growing DNA chain, it binds tightly leading to chain termination, thereby inactivating the viral DNA polymerase.[6, 7]

Acyclovir's activity is greatest against herpes simplex virus (HSV). HSV type I is more sensitive than type II; its growth is inhibited by the lowest drug concentration.[1, 9] The herpesvirus responsible for varicella-zoster is relatively resistant; at least a two- to fourfold increase in dose is required to inhibit viral growth. Epstein-Barr virus (EBV) is slightly more resistant, and cytomegalovirus is essentially unaffected by acyclovir. Both of these viruses lack thymidine kinases. In spite of this, acyclovir has proved to be therapeutically useful for EBV infection, as the EBV DNA polymerase is highly sensitive to acyclovir triphosphate, and the levels attained in normal host cells, albeit low, inhibit growth of EBV.[10]

Clinical Use (Table 1–1)

Approved Indications

HERPES SIMPLEX VIRUS INFECTIONS. Therapy for genital herpes has come a long way since the advent of acyclovir. Primary herpes infections are more severe and last longer than subsequent recurrences. However, the U.S. Food and Drug Administration (FDA) has approved acyclovir for both primary and frequently recurrent genital herpes, as well as for mucocutaneous HSV infections in immunocompromised patients.[5]

Intravenous administration of acyclovir is indicated for immunocom-

Table 1–1. Acyclovir Indications/Contraindications

FDA-Approved Dermatologic Indications

Genital Herpes Simplex Virus Infections
   Initial episode[11, 12]*
   Recurrent episodes (frequent, severe, or both)[14-18]*

Mucocutaneous HSV Infections in Immunocompromised Host*

Other Dermatologic Uses

Herpex Simplex Virus Infections
   Labialis[19, 20]
   Recurrent erythema multiforme[20-22]
   Eczema herpeticum[21, 23, 24]*
   Sun- or wind-triggered outbreaks[13, 25]
   Immunosuppression-triggered outbreaks[13, 26]*
   Reports of use in pregnancy[27-29]

Varicella in Immunocompromised Host[30-35]*

Herpes Zoster [26, 36]
   Ophthalmicus[37]
   Disseminated[34, 38]
   Prevention of post-herpetic neuralgia[36, 39, 40]

AIDS Management—Augment Zidovudine Effect[41]

Contraindication

Hypersensitivity to acyclovir formulations

   *Acyclovir is generally considered the drug of choice.

promised patients with initial and recurrent mucocutaneous HSV infections and for nonimmunocompromised patients with severe initial episodes of herpes genitalis.[5] A dosage of 5 mg/kg intravenously every 8 hours for 5 days substantially decreases the duration of viral shedding, length of the acute illness, and wound healing time, especially when administered early in the course of the outbreak.[11, 12] For immunocompromised patients it is recommended to extend treatment to 7 days.[5]

Oral acyclovir also decreases viral shedding and healing time and is sufficient for most cases of primary genital herpes. A dosage of 200 mg five times a day for 10 days is recommended and should be started within 3–5 days of the onset of lesions for maximal benefit.[5]

In addition, recurrent attacks can be controlled with chronic administration of oral acyclovir. Dosages of 40 mg twice a day and 200 mg three times a day are equally efficacious at suppressing outbreaks of HSV infection. Even though the current recommendation is to discontinue therapy after 12 months, Mertz[13] suggested that suppressive treatment is safe and effective for periods of up to 2 years. Unfortunately, recurrences usually resume at pretreatment frequency and severity after discontinuation of acyclovir. The initial recurrence after discontinuation of long-term acyclovir may rebound to a greater severity than that of pretreatment episodes. However, long-term suppressive treatment does not appear to lead to acyclovir-resistant HSV infections.[6, 13]

An alternative regimen is to use intermittent short-term treatment, which is especially beneficial for infrequently recurring (fewer than six episodes/year), moderately severe outbreaks. In this case, the patient initiates treatment with acyclovir, upon the earliest sign or symptom of recurrence, at a dosage of 200 mg five times a day for 5 days.[14] Two large trials[15, 16] compared these two regimens (400 twice a day chronically versus 200 mg five times daily for 5 days) and found significantly fewer recurrences with chronic suppressive therapy than with intermittent therapy; the number of recurrences with the latter did not differ significantly from pretreatment recurrence rates. In addition, 800 mg twice a day is as efficacious as 200 mg five times a day for 5 days for acute attacks.[16] Mostow and associates[17] found that a single dose of 800 mg daily was effective for chronic suppression. Further studies exploring the efficacy of lower dosages and intermittent chronic therapy (e.g., every weekend) are under way.

Higher dosages of acyclovir (400 mg five times per day) are recommended for acute HSV infections in acquired immunodeficiency syndrome (AIDS) patients. Once the eruption has cleared, acyclovir is tapered down to 400 mg three times a day for 1–2 months and, if the patient is symptom-free, then decreased to 400 mg twice per day chronically.[18]

Acyclovir is not indicated for every case of genital herpes. Patients with the more severe and frequently recurrent cases of herpes derive the greatest benefit. Mild cases, even though recurrent, do not warrant chronic suppressive therapy.

Other Dermatologic Uses

HERPES SIMPLEX VIRUS INFECTIONS. Treatment of herpes labialis with 200 mg of oral acyclovir five times per day in a controlled study demonstrated an antiviral effect, but no difference was found in duration of pain, time to heal, or lesion area even though the treatment was initiated within 1 hour of prodromal symptoms.[19] Although good data are lacking, severe cases of herpes labialis may warrant a 5-day course of acyclovir with the 200-mg dosage; studies with higher dosages are under way.[20]

Other manifestations of herpes simplex virus infection include recurrent erythema multiforme[20-22] and eczema herpeticum (Kaposi's varicelliform eruption).[21, 23, 24] Both are appropriately treated with 200 mg of acyclovir orally five times a day for a minimum of 5 days; parenteral use is confined to severe cases. Recurrent cases of erythema multiforme may warrant chronic suppressive therapy (200 mg three to five times per day for 6 months) if frequent or severe, and this therapy will aid in elimination of erythema multiforme triggered by subclinical HSV infection.[20-22]

Prophylactic use of acyclovir before sun or wind exposure helps to prevent herpesvirus infections in patients susceptible to these triggering factors.[25] Dosages of 400 mg twice a day 1 day before through 2–3 days after exposure are currently recommended.[13] Acyclovir has also been used prophylactically in patients undergoing an immunosuppressive event, such as bone marrow transplantation, to prevent herpes simplex and zoster outbreaks.[26] The oral route is preferred, but parenteral acyclovir may be indicated for those unable to tolerate oral medications.[13]

Although the use of acyclovir during pregnancy has not been fully studied, many women have been treated successfully with acyclovir for genital herpes[27,28] and herpetic whitlow[27,29] without detrimental effects on the fetus. Unfortunately, we still are unsure whether acyclovir is safe to use during early pregnancy or even whether use in later pregnancy will prevent perinatal HSV transmission.[27] Antiviral prophylaxis of neonates born to mothers with active genital lesions is generally not warranted unless other risk factors are present.[6]

VARICELLA (CHICKENPOX). Chickenpox in otherwise healthy children is not severe enough to warrant treatment. However, in previously healthy adults as well as immunocompromised children[30,31] and adults,[32] varicella is best treated with systemic acyclovir, replacing vidarabine as the drug of choice.[33] The recommended dosage is 10 mg/kg intravenously every 8 hours for at least 7 days in immunocompromised patients of all ages and in normal hosts with pneumonia.[34] The oral route is not an appropriate substitute for prevention or treatment of the serious complications of varicella.[35]

HERPES ZOSTER. Herpes zoster also responds well to oral acyclovir if given within the first 48–72 hours. An oral dosage of 800 mg five times daily for 10 days is superior to 400 mg five times daily and will significantly promote healing and decrease pain.[36] This higher dose will also reduce ocular complications in herpes zoster ophthalmicus.[37] In contrast, the intravenous route is preferred for disseminated herpes zoster, especially in immunocompromised patients.[34,38]

A major disappointment with acyclovir has been its inability to reliably decrease post-herpetic neuralgia.[39] Huff and colleagues found the higher dosage of 800 mg five times daily to significantly ameliorate this problem.[36] Further studies are needed to confirm these findings. The addition of corticosteroids may decrease the incidence and severity of post-herpetic neuralgia, especially in the elderly; however, an analysis of the literature revealed minimal long-term benefit.[40]

AIDS MANAGEMENT. Acyclovir has also been shown to act synergistically with zidovudine in the treatment of AIDS patients. Although it has no intrinsic antiretroviral activity, preliminary reports show that acyclovir apparently augments the antiretroviral effect of zidovudine. In a pilot study, Surbone and colleagues[41] found that 100 mg of zidovudine given with 800 mg of acyclovir every 4 hours was therapeutically beneficial. The pharmacokinetics of acyclovir and zidovudine are independent of each other, and thus the drugs can be safely administered concomitantly without increased toxicity.[41]

Adverse Effects

In general, acyclovir is a remarkably safe antiviral agent. In the studies cited previously, no significant toxic effects were noted. Toxic effects from overdosage have not occurred with oral acyclovir; however, renal and neurologic sequelae have developed with parenteral doses, as noted in the following discussion.

RENAL TOXICITY. Of greatest concern, impaired renal function has been reported in 10% of patients who receive rapid (less than 10 minutes) intravenous (IV) infusions and in 5% of patients who receive slow (over 1 hour) IV infusion of acyclovir.[3] Acyclovir precipitates in the renal tubules, which leads to an obstructive nephropathy when high doses are given rapidly intravenously. Elevated blood urea nitrogen or serum creatinine returns to pretreatment levels with appropriate dosage adjustment (based on creatinine clearance), discontinuation of the drug, or correction of fluid and electrolyte abnormalities. In rare cases, however, acute renal failure occurs.[3, 5, 42]

OTHER ADVERSE EFFECTS. Nausea or vomiting (8%) and diarrhea (9%) are encountered frequently with oral administration of acyclovir but rarely with parenteral use. In contrast, parenteral acyclovir is most frequently associated with inflammation or phlebitis at infiltrated IV sites, and 1% of patients develop encephalopathic changes (lethargy, tremors, confusion, and seizures). Headaches, also a common side effect, are seen mostly with chronic suppressive therapy (13%) and less so with short-term therapy. Vertigo, dizziness, fatigue, and anorexia are rarely reported. Cutaneous side effects include occasional rashes and urticaria, and one case of an erythematous rash associated with vasculitis has been reported.[3, 5, 42]

VIRAL RESISTANCE. Resistance to acyclovir has been noted, particularly in patients with human immunodeficiency virus (HIV) infection who require chronic administration of acyclovir for HSV infections. In these immunocompromised patients, the resistant HSV strains have not been particularly virulent. Foscarnet has proved beneficial for several of these patients.[43, 44]

ACYCLOVIR MONITORING GUIDELINES

Laboratory evaluation should include baseline and follow-up urinalysis, blood urea nitrogen analysis, and creatinine analysis in patients receiving IV or high oral doses of acyclovir.[3] For episodic or long-term suppressive treatment with standard oral doses, no laboratory surveillance is required.

Drug Interactions

Concomitant use of probenecid will decrease urinary excretion of acyclovir, presumably by competitive inhibition of tubular secretion, and thereby increase the plasma half-life of acyclovir.[3] Amphotericin B, ketoconazole, and interferon have been shown to be synergistic with acyclovir in vitro, enhancing its antiviral activity. Parenteral acyclovir should be used with caution in patients who have had neurologic reactions to cytotoxic drugs and to intrathecal methotrexate or interferon.[45] Finally, severe lethargy and fatigue was noted in an AIDS patient receiving zidovudine, or azidothymidine (AZT) when acyclovir was added to treatment for a herpes infection.[46]

ZIDOVUDINE (AZT; RETROVIR)

Since the recognition of AIDS and its etiologic agent, HIV, there has been a concerted effort to find effective antiretroviral agents. Zidovudine, an anticancer agent synthesized in 1964, was shown in 1974 to inhibit the replication of type C murine retroviruses. The clinical significance of this became apparent in early 1985, when activity against HIV was demonstrated in vitro.[47] The flurry of studies that followed confirmed the ability of zidovudine (previously known as azidothymidine or AZT) to decrease morbidity and mortality in AIDS patients.[48] The escalating nature of the AIDS epidemic has allowed rapid accumulation of data on the effects of zidovudine. First approved in March 1987, it remains the only currently FDA-approved drug for treatment of HIV-infected persons. Several newer antiretroviral agents now in experimental use include dideoxyinosine (ddI), dideoxyadenosine (ddA; rapidly converted to ddI), and dideoxycytidine (ddC; use limited by neurotoxicity).[47, 49, 50]

Pharmacology

Structure

Zidovudine is produced by substituting an azido group for the 3-OH group in thymidine. This thymidine analog is then phosphorylated by cellular kinases to 3'-azido-3'-dideoxythymidine.

Absorption/Distribution

More than 90% of orally administered zidovudine and its major metabolite can be recovered in the urine, and thus it has excellent oral absorption.[51] Peak blood levels are reached at 1 hour. It is well distributed throughout all body cavities, including the cerebrospinal fluid, in which levels at steady state are about 50% of the serum levels.[51, 52] Zidovudine crosses the placenta and is found in the breast milk of mice, but its levels in human breast milk still await further documentation.[3]

Metabolism/Excretion

Zidovudine is rapidly metabolized by hepatic glucuronide conjugation.[51] This significant first-pass effect results in a bioavailability of 65%. The major metabolite and the remainder of the unaltered drug are cleared by glomerular filtration and active tubular secretion in the kidneys. This gives rise to the short half-life of 1 hour, necessitating a dosing interval of 4 hours to maintain adequate blood levels for inhibition of viral replication.[5] As with acyclovir, the pharmacokinetics of intravenously and orally administered zidovudine are similar in adults and in children.[53]

Mechanism of Action

Like acyclovir, zidovudine triphosphate is incorporated into a growing chain of proviral DNA by viral reverse transcriptase, inhibiting further 5'-3' phosphodiester linkages. Its affinity for viral reverse transcriptase is much greater than its affinity for human DNA polymerases; thus viral DNA chain synthesis is aborted.[9] Unfortunately, only an actively dividing virus is affected by zidovudine. Latent virus in macrophages/monocytes will survive and may later become activated.

Clinical Use (Table 1–2)

Approved Indications

    AIDS MANAGEMENT. Official FDA indications for zidovudine are limited to HIV-infected persons with a cytologically confirmed diagnosis of

Table 1–2. Zidovudine Indications/Contraindications

FDA-Approved Dermatologic Indications

AIDS Management
  Pneumocystis carinii infection history or CD4 lymphocyte count less than 200 per cubic millimeter[3, 5]*

Other Dermatologic Uses

AIDS-Associated Dermatoses
  Candida albicans infection[54]
  Psoriasis[55-57]
  Oral Kaposi's sarcoma[58]
  Generalized granuloma annulare[59]

Combination With Acyclovir/Interferon
  Kaposi's sarcoma[60, 61]
  Oral hairy leukoplakia[62]
  Chronic herpes simplex[63]

Contraindication

Hypersensitivity (severe) to any component of zidovudine formulation

*Zidovudine is generally considered the drug of choice.

Pneumocystis carinii pneumonia (PCP) and symptomatic patients with CD4 (T-helper) lymphocyte counts less than 200/cu mm. It is generally agreed, however, that zidovudine is indicated for any patient carrying the diagnosis of AIDS, including AIDS patients with other opportunistic infections, Kaposi's sarcoma, dementia, and "wasting disease."[3, 5] Studies are currently under way to determine whether treatment extended to asymptomatic persons with HIV infection can slow the rate of disease progression and decrease the infectivity of the carrier.

Other Dermatologic Uses

AIDS-ASSOCIATED DERMATOSES. Anecdotal reports by many investigators using zidovudine have unveiled several possible uses for mucocutaneous disorders. Coldiron and Bergstresser[54] noted that none of the AIDS patients receiving zidovudine had Candida albicans infections, whereas 23% of matched patients on oral ketoconazole did have persistent candidiasis. Psoriasis, noted to flare up in HIV-infected patients, also responds quite favorably to zidovudine.[55-57] Langford and colleagues[58] reported regression of oral Kaposi's sarcoma. Finally, generalized granuloma annulare rapidly resolved once treatment with zidovudine was initiated for an AIDS-related illness.[59] In most cases, the dosage of zidovudine used was 200 mg orally every 4 hours, although adverse effects may necessitate a lower dosage.

Combination therapies are also being investigated. Brockmeyer and colleagues[60] demonstrated regression of Kaposi's sarcoma in 5 patients treated with zidovudine and interferon; their findings support a similar observation in an in vitro preparation.[61] The same researchers also noted rapid resolution of oral hairy leukoplakia in 6 AIDS patients receiving zidovudine when acyclovir (800 mg four times daily) was added to the regimen.[62] EBV was detected in tongue epithelial cells of all 6 patients. Discontinuation of acyclovir led to a recurrence of the hairy leukoplakia. In addition, one AIDS patient's large chronic herpetic lesions, which were highly resistant to parenteral acyclovir alone, cleared with concomitant administration of zidovudine.[63]

Adverse Effects

Because zidovudine has been studied in limited numbers of seriously ill HIV-infected persons, it is difficult to ascertain which adverse affects are solely attributed to zidovudine and which are secondary to the disease itself.

HEMATOLOGIC EFFECTS. Bone marrow suppression is the most frequent and dreaded complication that, fortunately, is reversible upon discontinuation of the drug. In one study, pretreatment CD4 (T-helper) lymphocyte and granulocyte counts, as well as dose and duration of treatment, were inversely related to hematologic toxicity. Anemia (hematocrit <25%) was seen in 38% of zidovudine-treated patients, a threefold increase above its occurrence in the placebo group. Many patients become transfusion-dependent in the effort to continue the medication. Granulocytopenia was noted even more frequently, which required dosage reduction or discontinuation of the drug.[64] In contrast, megakaryocytes were not suppressed, and Finaud and colleagues[65] and Oksenhendler and colleagues[66] demonstrated reversal of HIV-related thrombocytopenia with the use of zidovudine.

In an effort to minimize bone marrow toxicity, studies are under way to assess concomitant use of acyclovir, interferon, or dideoxycytidine (ddC) for a possible zidovudine-sparing effect.[49] In addition, studies have shown ddI to be an effective agent against HIV with minimal bone marrow suppression.[67]

OTHER ADVERSE EFFECTS. Other frequent but less serious side effects include headache, nausea, myalgias, and insomnia.[64] Less commonly reported are seizures,[5] Wernicke's encephalopathy,[68] myopathy,[69] irreversible bone marrow suppression with pancytopenia,[70] progressive bluish discoloration of the nails,[71,72] diffuse hyperpigmented macules mimicking primary adrenal insufficiency,[73] and heightened cutaneous response to mosquito bites.[74]

> **ZIDOVUDINE MONITORING GUIDELINES**
>
> Appropriate laboratory evaluation includes frequent (at least every 2 weeks) complete blood counts. Zidovudine should be used with extreme caution for patients with a granulocyte count of less than 100/cu mm or hemoglobin level of less than 9.5 g/dl.[3,5]

Drug Interactions

Interference with the glucuronyl transferase system by competitive inhibition is seen with drugs such as nonsteroidal anti-inflammatory agents, narcotic analgesics, and sulfonamide antibiotics. These agents reduce metabolism of zidovudine, thereby increasing its toxicity. Poor renal or hepatic function or concomitant use of drugs that inhibit renal excretion may also increase plasma half-life and blood concentration to toxic levels. Probenicid inhibits both hepatic glucuronidation and renal excretion, significantly reducing the elimination of zidovudine.[3,5,75]

INTERFERON (ROFERON-A, INTRON A, ALFERON-N)

Interferons are a family of secretory glycoproteins produced by most eukaryotic cells in response to a variety of viral and nonviral inducers. All interferons display antiviral activity but also modulate other cellular functions. Interferon was originally described as a product of the interaction of heat-inactivated influenza virus and isolate pieces of chick chorioallantoic membrane, which was capable of inducing interference with virus growth in fresh tissue.[76] In early studies on the antiviral action of interferon, it was shown that interferon did not inactivate virus directly but rendered cells resistant to virus[77,78] and, in most cases, displayed "species" specificity.[79] Soon afterward, Ho and Enders[80] demonstrated that interferon production by human primary cell cultures was induced by live polio virus.

Depending upon cellular source and mode of induction, human cells produce three antigenically distinct forms of human interferon: leukocyte (alpha), fibroblast (beta), and immune (gamma). This chapter identifies interferons (IFNs) as IFN-alpha, IFN-beta, or IFN-gamma because a single cell type can produce more than one type of interferon.[81] Use of recombinant DNA technology has led to the production of large quantities of highly purified human interferons[82] by *Escherichia coli*. At present, only three forms of human IFN-alpha have been approved by the FDA for clinical use. Therefore, we focus our comments on IFN-alpha.

Pharmacology

Structure

There are more than 30 species of IFN-alpha that have a molecular weight of around 20,000 daltons with very similar sequences of 165–172 amino acids. Two of the marketed forms, IFN-alpha 2_a and IFN-alpha 2_b, differ in a single amino acid and are produced by *E. coli* with recombinant DNA biotechnology. IFN-alpha n3 (human leukocyte–derived) is a formulation of purified, natural, human IFN-alpha proteins that comprises approximately 166 amino acids. It is manufactured from pooled units of human leukocytes induced by incomplete infection by Sendai virus.

Absorption/Distribution

Injection of 5 million international units (IU) per sq m of IFN-alpha 2_b intramuscularly (IM) or subcutaneously (SC) results in similar peak serum levels reached in 6–8 hours after injection, with undetectable levels after 24 hours. Calculated absorption and elimination half-lives are 3–4 and 6–7 hours, respectively. At the end of a 30-minute IV infusion, peak serum interferon levels are three times those achieved after IM or SC administration. The IFN-alpha becomes undetectable beyond 4 hours and has an elimination half-life of 48 minutes.

Metabolism/Excretion

Human interferons do not appear to cross the placental barrier. It is not known whether human interferons are excreted into breast milk, but mouse interferons are. IFN-alpha 2_b has not been detected in human urine samples after IM, SC, or IV administration. Proteolytic inactivation of interferon is likely. The primary site of such inactivation is unknown.

Mechanism of Action

Interferon requires binding to specific receptors on the surface of target cells in order to be active. IFN-alpha and IFN-beta share the same receptor, encoded on chromosome 21, and IFN-gamma binds to an unrelated receptor encoded on chromosome 6. The intracellular events following receptor binding leading to gene expression are unclear. The antiviral activity of interferon can be explained, in part, by its ability to induce the expression of oligo-adenylate synthetase (2'-5'A synthetase). This enzyme polymerizes adenosine triphosphate into 2'-5'-linked oligomers, some of which are capable of activating a latent cellular endonuclease that degrades both viral and cellular RNA.[83] Ribonuclease L is also induced by interferons, is activated by trimers of 2'-5'-linked polyA oligomers, and degrades single-stranded viral RNA.[84] Protein kinase P1, also induced by interferons, phosphorylates serine and threonine moieties of the alpha subunit of elongation factor 2,[85] resulting in inhibition of tRNA binding to ribosomes and inhibition of the normal translation of viral mRNA.[86]

With respect to the antiproliferative effects of interferon, interferons affect all phases of the cell cycle. The mechanisms of such inhibition may involve interferon inductions of 2'-5'A synthetase with its products inhibiting mitosis, its inhibition of growth factors, and its down-regulation of c-myc, c-fos, and certain c-ras oncogenes.

IFN-alpha and IFN-beta are generally less potent stimulators of major histocompatibility complex antigens required for cellular immune reactions than is IFN-gamma. However, they are capable of enhancing/inducing the expression of class I and II antigens on immunocompetent cells,[87] as well as other normal and tumor cells. Increases in natural killer cell numbers and activity occur after exposure to interferon, also leading to an enhanced immune status.

Clinical Use (Table 1–3)

Approved Indications

CONDYLOMATA ACUMINATA (GENITAL WARTS). Condylomata acuminata are benign tumors commonly due to sexually transmitted human papillomavirus infections, usually types 6 and 11. In light of the antiviral, antiproliferative, and immunomodulatory activities of interferon, a multicenter, double-blind, placebo-controlled study was undertaken, and it revealed intralesional IFN-alpha 2_b to be safe and effective in the treatment of condylomata acuminata on the external surfaces of the genital and perianal areas.[88] In three such studies, a total of 487 lesions were injected intralesionally with 0.1 ml, containing 1 million IU of IFN-alpha 2_b per wart, three times weekly for 3 weeks, and 539 lesions were intralesionally injected with placebo. By 17 weeks after treatment, 52% of interferon-treated warts completely cleared, in comparison with 24% of placebo-treated lesions. Of those interferon-treated patients whose lesions cleared and were followed up, 81% remained lesion-free for a period of 9–33 months.

Furthermore, in one study,[89] 1 week after the completion of therapy, interferon produced a 62.4% decrease in mean wart area, which was a significantly ($p < 0.001$) greater reduction than the 1.2% increase in area in the placebo group. Thirteen weeks after the completion of therapy, the mean wart area was still 39.9% smaller than baseline in the interferon

Table 1–3. Interferon Indications/Contraindications

FDA-Approved Dermatologic Indications

Condylomata Acuminata[88, 89]

AIDS-Associated Kaposi's Sarcoma[90]*

Other Dermatologic Uses

Neoplastic
  Basal cell carcinoma[91]
  Squamous cell carcinoma[92-94]
  Melanoma—metastatic[95]
  Mycosis fungoides[96, 97]
  Actinic keratoses[98]
  Keloids[99]

Viral Infections
  Verruca vulgaris[100, 101]
  Herpes zoster[102, 103]
  Varicella[98, 104]
  Herpes simplex[105]

Contraindication

Hypersensitivity to IFN-alpha (2_a or 2_b) formulations or to mouse immunoglobulin.

*IFN-alpha is generally considered the drug of choice.

---

group, whereas it increased by 46% in the placebo group ($p < 0.001$). Reduction in wart area may allow for other therapeutic modalities, such as surgical excision, to be used subsequently, and results of combining interferon treatment of condylomata with cryosurgery or podophyllin resin have been promising.

AIDS-ASSOCIATED KAPOSI'S SARCOMA. The FDA has approved the use of IFN-alpha 2_a and IFN-alpha 2_b in the treatment of Kaposi's sarcoma in patients with AIDS (KS/AIDS) due to HIV. Those who responded to interferon therapy tended to develop fewer opportunistic infections and appeared to have a distinct survival advantage over the nonresponders.[90]

The overall objective response rates with interferon equaled or surpassed those achieved with conventional cytotoxic chemotherapy. However, interferon provides only a palliative approach to KS/AIDS. Even in patients in whom complete Kaposi's sarcoma tumor regression was achieved, the underlying immunodeficiency was not reversed. The beneficial cosmetic effects of interferon in the treatment of KS/AIDS were evident and had a dramatic impact on the patients' quality of life. The recommended dosages of IFN-alpha 2_a and IFN-alpha 2_b are 36 and 30 million IU, respectively, administered SC daily. As a single agent, IFN-alpha induces approximately a 75% response rate in those patients with more than 400 CD4 cells/cu mm, whereas only 13% of patients with fewer than 200 CD4 cells/cu mm respond. The combination of zidovudine (100 mg every 4 hours) and IFN-alpha 2_b (4–6 million IU daily) appears to increase tumor regression to 50% in those patients with fewer than 200 CD4 cells/cu mm. Therapy is continued until no remaining tumor is evident, unless severe adverse effects develop (in which case the dose is reduced by 50% or therapy is discontinued for a week) or if evidence of opportunistic organisms is detected (in which case therapy is discontinued).

Other Dermatologic Uses

BASAL CELL CARCINOMA. Basal cell carcinoma is the most common form of skin cancer and accounts for about about ⅛ of all cancers diagnosed in the United States. Results of a multicenter, placebo-controlled, randomized study of 172 patients with biopsy-proven basal cell carcinoma confirmed the findings of earlier pilot studies that the optimal intralesional dose of IFN-alpha 2_b is 1.5 million IU administered three times weekly for 3 weeks. This interferon regimen resulted in an 86% complete response rate, including normal biopsy results, in comparison with a 29% rate in the placebo group ($p < 0.0001$). One year after initiation of therapy, 81% of IFN-alpha 2_b recipients and 20% of those given the placebo remained tumor free.[91]

SQUAMOUS CELL CARCINOMA. Squamous cell carcinoma of the skin accounts for 10%–25% of nonmelanoma skin cancers. In an ongoing pilot study, 39 patients had a biopsy-proven squamous cell carcinoma in sun-exposed areas of the skin treated intralesionally with 1.5 million IU IFN alpha 2_b three times weekly for 3 weeks. At the end of the 21-week study, the treated area was excised and examined histologically for residual squamous cell carcinoma. Of 39 patients, 37 had a complete response clinically and histologically, an observed cure rate of 95%.[92] In addition, human papillomavirus infections with malignant transformation to squamous cell carcinoma in patients with epidermodysplasia verruciformis appear to respond to interferon therapy.[93, 94]

MALIGNANT MELANOMA. IFN-alpha as a single agent in doses as high as 100 million IU daily intravenously results in a response rate (complete and partial responses) of 4%–29%, depending upon the individual study. In a randomized, prospective study,[95] dacarbazine 250 mg per sq m IV for 5 days every 28 days resulted in a 16% response rate but, when combined with interferon-alpha 2_b (15 million IU per sq m IV for 5 days for 3 weeks as induction and 10 million IU per sq m SC three times weekly as maintenance), resulted in a 39% response rate. The added benefit from this combination over dacarbazine alone was not found in previous reports and needs to be confirmed.

MYCOSIS FUNGOIDES. Cutaneous T cell lymphoma (of which mycosis fungoides is a subtype) is a malignant proliferation of T lymphocytes, typically helper/inducer, with initial presentation in the skin. Olsen and colleagues[96] treated 22 patients with stage Ia to IVa (without visceral involvement) histologically confirmed cutaneous T cell lymphoma with a daily 3- to 36-million IU IFN-alpha 2_a escalating IM induction dose for 10 weeks, followed by a maintenance dose dependent upon the response at the end of induction. Of the 22 patients, 13 had a complete[3] or partial[10] response; remissions lasted 4–27.5 months. The overall complete response rate with further treatment was 27%, the majority of complete responses being those with extensive plaque stage mycosis fungoides. These results suggest that IFN-alpha 2_a provides effective single-agent therapy for both early and advanced cutaneous T cell lymphoma.

Intralesional injection of plaques of mycosis fungoides with IFN-alpha 2_b (1 million IU three times a week for 4 weeks) produced substantial localized clinical and histologic improvement in 10 of 12 patients; complete regression was localized to the interferon-injected sites.[97]

ACTINIC KERATOSES. Up to 93% of actinic keratoses completely cleared after intralesional injection of 0.5 million IU of IFN-alpha 2_b three times weekly for 2–3 weeks.[98] There was no clearing in the placebo-injected group. Because of practical considerations and the availability of other effective treatments, the clinical usefulness of this modality for treatment of actinic keratoses is quite limited.

KELOIDS. In light of the in vitro evidence of the ability of interferons to normalize the phenotype of activated scleroderma fibroblasts with respect to collagen and glycosaminoglycan production, Berman and Duncan[99] injected a keloid intralesionally with 1.5 million IU of IFN-alpha 2_b (0.15 ml) twice over 4 days. The area of the keloid was reduced by approximately 50% by day 9. In vitro testing of the patient's keloid fibroblasts before and after the two injections of interferon revealed that the original excessive production of both collagen and glycosaminoglycan was normalized, approaching that of the patient's own normal fibroblasts. Furthermore, the reduced collagenase activity elaborated by the keloidal fibroblasts was also normalized after the in vivo treatment. This study furthers the rationale for using interferons in the treatment of fibrotic disorders.

VERRUCA VULGARIS. Niimura[100] reported a "good response" in 81% of common warts treated with nonrecombinant IFN-beta, in comparison with 17% in nontreated warts. Berman and colleagues[101] reported an 86% improvement in common warts treated with 0.1 million IU of IFN-alpha 2_b, in comparison with a 38% improvement in warts treated by placebo.

HERPES ZOSTER. The multiplication of varicella-zoster virus within infected cells in tissue culture is inhibited by human interferon, and although little or no circulating interferon could be demonstrated in varicella-zoster infections, high titers are detected in resolving vesicle fluid.[102] The development of detectable interferon in vesicular fluid is delayed in those patients with dissemination beyond the primary dermatome. These findings suggest that interferon might be involved in the recovery process from varicella-zoster infection. The most comprehensive study was performed by Merigan and co-workers,[103] who treated 90 patients with malignancies and herpes zoster in a single dermatome with either placebo (45 patients) or nonrecombinant human IFN-alpha in a dose of 0.48–5.1×10^5 U/kg per day (in two divided doses for 4–8 days) in double-blind fashion. They found a significant decrease ($p < 0.01$) in cutaneous dissemination in patients receiving interferon, and no dissemination occurred in those receiving the highest dosage. The number of days of new vesicle formation within the primary dermatome was decreased in the latter group to a mean of 2.3 days ($p < 0.05$). Early treatment was required to show the therapeutic effect of IFN on new lesion formation, owing to the short overall duration of treatment for the placebo recipients. Treated patients tended to experience less severe pain, and at higher dosages the severity of post-herpetic neuralgia was significantly ($p < 0.05$) diminished. Interestingly, no difference was observed in the time to complete healing between the IFN-treated group (50 ± 7 days) and the placebo recipients (49 ± 8 days). Six visceral complications—meningoencephalitis, post-herpetic segmental paresis, keratitis, and hemorrhagic vesicles with consumption coagulopathy—occurred in placebo recipients, whereas only one such complication occurred in the IFN-treated group ($p < 0.05$).

VARICELLA. Arvin and co-authors[104] treated children who had malignancy and early varicella with nonrecombinant IFN-alpha (4.2×10^4 to 2.55×10^5 U/kg every 12 hours for an average of 6.4 days) or with placebo in a double-blind trial. Six of 9 placebo-treated patients, in comparison with 2 of 9 IFN-treated patients, developed serious complications. The development of fever was a prominent side effect of the IFN treatment. Two placebo-treated patients and 1 patient receiving IFN died.

HERPES SIMPLEX VIRUS INFECTIONS. Frequently after surgical treatment of trigeminal neuralgia, reactivation of herpes labialis occurs in patients with a history of such lesions. Pazin and co-workers[105] recognized this and initiated a double-blind, placebo-controlled prospective study of 37 patients with a history of herpes labialis who were to undergo surgical treatment of trigeminal neuralgia. Starting 1 day before surgery, 19 patients received either nonrecombinant IFN-alpha (7×10^4 U/kg/day in divided doses every 12 hours for 5 days) or placebo. Five of 19 interferon-treated patients, in comparison with 10 of 18 placebo-treated patients, had reactivation of herpes labialis. In addition, a statistically significant reduction in both frequency and duration of oropharyngeal HSV shedding was detected in the interferon-treated group.

Adverse Effects

The adverse effects of IFN-alpha are dose-dependent and generally remit either during continued therapy (tolerance) or after dose reduction and are usually rapidly reversible upon cessation of therapy. Of 352 patients receiving IFN-alpha 2_b for condylomata, 311 (88%) reported an adverse reaction some time during treatment. Of the 40 receiving 5 million IU three times weekly for 5 weeks, all reported an adverse reaction. Most reactions were mild to moderate, transient, and rapidly reversible and did not interfere with therapy (see Intron A package insert).

CARDIOVASCULAR EFFECTS. Significant hypotension, arrhythmia, or tachycardia (150 beats per minute or more) was observed in approximately 3% of patients studied who had various malignancies and were treated at doses higher than those for condylomata acuminata. Cardiac dysfunction that is reversible after discontinuance of IFN therapy has been reported.[106] Incidence of these complications in patients with pre-existing heart disease is unknown. Hypotension may occur during administration or for up to 2 days posttherapy and may require supportive therapy, including fluid replacement to maintain intravascular volume. Supraventricular arrhythmias occur rarely and appear to be correlated with pre-existing conditions and prior therapy with cardiotoxic agents. These adverse experiences are controlled by modifying dosage or discontinuing treatment, but they may require specific additional therapy. Patients with a recent history of myocardial infarction or previous or current arrhythmic disorder should be closely monitored (see Intron A package insert).

OTHER ADVERSE EFFECTS. Use of high dosages of interferon in the treatment of KS/AIDS results in an increase in the severity of the adverse effects, the most disturbing possibly being depression (28%). Patients receiving IFN-alpha 2_a and IFN-alpha 2_b can develop neutralizing antibodies that appear to be specific to the recombinant interferon and not to natural interferon. In the case of long-term use of IFN-alpha 2_a, the development of neutralizing antibodies in hairy-cell leukemia patients was correlated with the development of resistance to IFN-alpha 2_a and disease progression.[107] These patients responded to subsequent treatment with natural IFN-alpha.

Warnings

Moderate to severe adverse experiences may require modification of the patient's dosage regimen or, in some cases, termination of therapy with IFN-alpha. Because of the fever and other flu-like symptoms associated with IFN-alpha administration, IFN should be used cautiously in patients with debilitating medical conditions, such as those with a history of cardiovascular disease (e.g., unstable angina, uncontrolled congestive heart failure), pulmonary disease (e.g., chronic obstructive pulmonary disease), or diabetes mellitus prone to ketoacidosis. Caution should also be observed in patients with coagulation disorders (e.g., thrombophlebitis or pulmonary embolism) or severe myelosuppression. Interferon should be administered SC and not IM to patients with platelet counts lower than 50,000/cu mm.

The use of IFN-alpha in adolescents has not been studied. IFN-alpha has been shown to affect the menstrual cycle and decrease serum estradiol and progesterone levels. At doses higher than those used in humans, IFN-alpha has abortifacient activity in animals. Consideration should be given as to whether the pregnant or adolescent patient should be treated.

INTERFERON MONITORING GUIDELINES

In addition to tests normally required for monitoring AIDS patients, the following tests are recommended for all patients on interferon therapy before beginning treatment and periodically thereafter:

Standard hematologic tests with complete blood counts and differential tests, platelet counts, blood chemistries, electrolytes, and liver function tests. Patients with pre-existing cardiac abnormalities or in advanced stages of cancer should have electrocardiograms taken before and during treatment.

Drug Interactions

In one study, a single IM injection of IFN-alpha 2_a significantly reduced the clearance of aminophylline by 33%–81% in 8 of 9 subjects, probably as a result of inhibition of the cytochrome P-450 enzyme system.

BIBLIOGRAPHY: Key Reviews/Chapters

Thiers BH: Antiretroviral therapy. J Am Acad Dermatol 1989; 21:443–454.
Rachlis AR: Antiviral therapy. Clin Dermatol 1989; 7(3):69–79.

Stadler R, Mayer-da-Silva A, Bratzke B, et al.: Interferons in dermatology. J Am Acad Dermatol 1989; 20:650–656.
Crowe S, Mills J: The future of antiviral chemotherapy. Dermatol Clin 1988; 6:521–537.
Felserstein D, Hirsch MS: Antiviral agents. In Fitzpatrick TB, Eisen AZ, Wolfe K, et al. (eds): Dermatology in General Medicine. New York: McGraw-Hill, 1987, 2609–2616.
O'Brien JJ, Campoli-Richards DM: Acyclovir: An updated review of its antiviral activity, pharmacokinetic properties and therapeutic efficacy. Drugs 1989; 37:233–309.
Dorsky DI, Crumpacker CS: Drugs five years later: Acyclovir. Ann Intern Med 1987; 107:859–874.

REFERENCES

1. King AH: History, pharmacokinetics and pharmacology of acyclovir. J Am Acad Dermatol 1988; 1(pt 2):176–179.
2. Furman PA, Spector T, Fyfe JA: Acyclovir: Mechanism of action. In Lopez C, Roizman B (eds): Human Herpesvirus Infection. New York: Raven Press, 1986, 129–140.
3. McEvoy GK (ed): AHFS Drug Information. Bethesda, MD: American Society of Hospital Pharmacology Inc, 1989:352–358, 371–376.
4. Meyer LJ, deMiranda P, Sheth NI, et al: Acyclovir in human breast milk. Am J Obstet Gynecol 1989; 158:586–588.
5. Physicians Desk Reference, 43rd ed. Oradell, NJ: Medical Economics, 1989:793–795, 808–812.
6. O'Brien JJ, Campoli-Richards DM: Acyclovir: An updated review of its antiviral activity, pharmacokinetic properties and therapeutic efficacy. Drugs 1989; 37:233–309.
7. Dorsky DI, Crumpacker CS: Drugs five years later: Acyclovir. Ann Intern Med 1987; 107:859–874.
8. Hintz M, Connor JD, Spector SA, et al: Neonatal acyclovir pharmacokinetics in patients with herpes virus infections. Am J Med 1982; 73:210–214.
9. Thiers B: Dermatologic therapy in the 1980s. Dermatol Clin 1988; 6:609–622.
10. Crowe S, Mills J: The future of antiviral therapy. Dermatol Clin 1988; 6(4):521–537.
11. Corey L, Fife KH, Benedetti JK, et al: Intravenous acyclovir for the treatment of primary genital herpes. Ann Intern Med 1983; 98:914–921.
12. Peacock JE, Kaplowitz LG, Sparling PF, et al: Intravenous acyclovir therapy of first episodes of genital herpes: A multicenter double-blind, placebo-controlled trial. Am J Med 1988; 85:301–306.
13. Mertz GJ: Diagnosis and treatment of genital herpes infections. Infect Dis Clin North Am 1987; 1:341–365.
14. Kruzinski PA: Treatment of mucocutaneous herpes simplex infections with acyclovir. J Am Acad Dermatol 1988; 18:179–181.
15. Mertz GJ, Eron L, Kaufman R, et al: Prolonged continuous versus intermittent oral acyclovir treatment in normal adults with frequently recurring genital herpes simplex virus infection. Am J Med 1988; 85(Suppl 2A):14–19.
16. Mattison HR, Reichman RC, Benedetti J, et al: Double-blind, placebo-controlled trial comparing long-term suppressive with short-term oral acyclovir therapy for management of recurrent genital herpes. Am J Med 1988; 85(Suppl 2A):20–25.
17. Mostow SR, Mayfield JL, Marr JJ: Suppression of recurrent genital herpes by single daily dosages of acyclovir. Am J Med 1988; 85(Suppl 2A):30–33.
18. Conant MA: Prophylactic and suppressive treatment with acyclovir and the management of herpes in patients with acquired immunodeficiency syndrome. J Am Acad Dermatol 1988; 18:186–193.
19. Raborn GW, McGaw WT, Creace M, et al: Oral acyclovir and herpes labialis: A randomized double blind placebo controlled study. J Am Dent Assoc 1987; 115:38–42.

20. Huff JC: Acyclovir for recurrent erythema multiforme caused by herpes simplex. J Am Acad Dermatol 1988; 18:197–198.
21. Leigh IM: Management of non-genital herpes simplex virus infections in immunocompetent patients. Am J Med 1988; 85(Suppl 2A):34–38.
22. Molin L: Oral acyclovir prevents herpes simplex virus-associated erythema multiforme. Br J Dermatol 1987; 116:109–111.
23. Niimura M, Nishikawa T: Treatment of eczema herpeticum with oral acyclovir. Am J Med 1988; 85(Suppl 2A):49–52.
24. Bork K, Brauninger W: Increasing incidence of eczema herpeticum: Analysis of seventy-five cases. J Am Acad Dermatol 1988; 19:1024–1029.
25. Spruance SL: Cutaneous herpes simplex virus lesions induced by ultraviolet radiation: A review of model systems and prophylactic therapy with oral acyclovir. Am J Med 1988; 85(Suppl 2A):43–45.
26. Perrin TJ, Powles RL, Easton D, et al: Prevention of herpes zoster in patients by long-term oral acyclovir after allogeneic bone marrow transplantation. Am J Med 1988; 85(Suppl 2A):99–101.
27. Strauss SE: Oral acyclovir for recurrent herpes virus infection. In Lopez C, Roizman B (eds): Human Herpesvirus Infection. New York: Raven Press, 1986, 165–175.
28. Andrews EB, Tilson HHH, Hurn BAL, et al: Acyclovir in pregnancy registry: An observational epidemiologic approach. Am J Med 1988; 85(Suppl 2A):123–128.
29. Tschen EH, Baack B: Treatment of herpetic whitlow in pregnancy with acyclovir. J Am Acad Dermatol 1987; 17:1059.
30. Feldman S, Lott L: Varicella in children with cancer: Impact of antiviral therapy and prophylaxis. Pediatrics 1987; 80:465–472.
31. Prober CG, Kirk LE, Keeney KE: Acyclovir therapy of chickenpox in immunosuppressed children—A collaborative study. J Pediatr 1982; 101:622–625.
32. Balfour HH: Varicella zoster virus infections in immunocompromised hosts. Am J Med 1988; 85(Suppl):68–73.
33. Shepp DH, Dandliker PS, Meyers JD: Current therapy of varicella zoster virus in immunocompromosed patients: A comparison of acyclovir and vidarabine. Am J Med 1988; 85(Suppl 2A):96–98.
34. Balfour HH, Bean B, Laskin OL, et al: Acyclovir halts progression of herpes zoster in immunocompromised patients. N Engl J Med 1983; 308:1448–1453.
35. Strauss SE: The management of varicella and zoster infections. Infect Dis Clin North Am 1987; 1(2):367–382.
36. Huff JC, Bean B, Balfour HH, et al: Therapy of herpes zoster with oral acyclovir. Am J Med 1988; 85(Suppl 2A):84–89.
37. Cobo M: Reduction of ocular complications of herpes zoster ophthalmicus by oral acyclovir. Am J Med 1988; 85(Suppl 2A):90–95.
38. Cohen PR, Beltrani VP, Grossman ME: Disseminated herpes zoster in patients with human immunodeficiency virus infection. Am J Med 1988; 84:1076–1080.
39. McKendrick MW, McGill JI, Wood MJ: Lack of effect of acyclovir on post-herpetic neuralgia. Br Med J 1989; 298:431.
40. Schmader KE, Studenski S: Are current therapies useful for the prevention of post-herpetic neuralgia? J Gen Intern Med 1989; 4:83–89.
41. Surbone A, Yarchoan R, McAtee N, et al: Treatment of the acquired immunodeficiency syndrome (AIDS) and AIDS-related complex with a regimen of 3'-azido-2',3'-dideoxythymidine (azidothymidine or zidovudine) and acyclovir: A pilot study. Ann Intern Med 1988; 108:534–540.
42. Arndt KA: Adverse reactions to acyclovir: Topical, oral and intravenous. J Am Acad Dermatol 1988; 18:188–190.
43. Erlich KS, Jacobson MA, Koehler JF, et al: Foscarnet therapy for severe acyclovir-resistant herpes simplex virus infections in patients with acquired immunodeficiency syndrome (AIDS). Ann Intern Med 1989; 110:710–713.

44. Chatis PA, Miller CH, Schrager LE, et al: Successful treatment with foscarnet of an acyclovir-resistant mucocutaneous infection with herpes simplex virus in a patient with acquired immunodeficiency syndrome. N Engl J Med 1989; 320:297–299.
45. Wade JC, Meyers JD: Neurologic symptoms associated with parenteral acyclovir treatment after marrow transplantation. Am J Med 1983; 98:921–925.
46. Bach MC: Possible drug interactions during therapy with azidothymidine and acyclovir for AIDS [letter]. N Engl J Med 1987; 316:547.
47. Mitsuya H, Weinhold KJ, Furman PA, et al: 3'-azido-3'-deoxythymidine (BW A509U): An antiviral agent that inhibits the infectivity and cytopathic effect of human T-lymphotropic virus type III/lymphadenopathy-associated virus in vitro. Proc Natl Acad Sci USA 1985; 82:7096–7100.
48. Fischl MA, Richman DD, Greico MH, et al: The efficacy of azidothymidine (AZT) in the treatment of patients with AIDS and AIDS-related complex. N Engl J Med 1987; 317:185–191.
49. Yarchoan R, Mitsuya H, Broder S: Clinical and basic advances in the antiretroviral therapy of human immunodeficiency virus infection: a review. Am J Med 1989; 87:191–200.
50. Thiers B: Antiretroviral therapy. J Am Acad Dermatol 1989; 21:443–454.
51. Blum MR, Liao SHT, Good SS, et al: Pharmacokinetics and bioavailability of zidovudine in humans. Am J Med 1988; 85:189–194.
52. Klecker RW, Collins JM, Yarchoan R, et al: Plasma and cerebrospinal fluid pharmacokinetics of 3'-azido-3'-deoxythymidine: A novel pyrimidine analog with potential application for the treatment of patients with AIDS and related diseases. Clin Pharmacol Ther 1987; 41:407–412.
53. Balis FM, Pizzo PA, Eddy J, et al: Pharmacokinetics of zidovudine administered intravenously and orally in children with human immunodeficiency virus infection. J Pediatr 1989; 114:880–884.
54. Coldiron BM, Bergstresser PR: Prevalence and clinical spectrum of skin disease in patients infected with human immunodeficiency virus. Arch Dermatol 1989; 125:357–361.
55. Duvic M, Rios A, Brewton GW: Remission of AIDS-associated psoriasis with zidovudine. Lancet 1987; 2:627.
56. Duvic M, Johnson TM, Rapini RP, et al: Acquired immunodeficiency syndrome-associated psoriasis and Reiter's syndrome. Arch Dermatol 1987; 123:1622–1632.
57. Kaplan MH, Sadick NS, Wieder J, et al: Antipsoriatic effects of zidovudine in human immunodeficiency virus-associated psoriasis. J Am Acad Dermatol 1989; 20:76–82.
58. Langford A, Ruf B, Kunze R, et al: Regression of oral Kaposi's sarcoma in a case of AIDS on zidovudine (AZT). Br J Dermatol 1989; 120:709–713.
59. Leenutaphong V, Hölzle E, Erckenbrecht J, et al: Remission of human immunodeficiency virus-associated granuloma annulare under zidovudine therapy [letter]. J Am Acad Dermatol 1988; 19:1126–1127.
60. Brockmeyer NH, Mertins L, Daecke C, et al: Regression of Kaposi's sarcoma and improvement of performance status by a combined interferon beta and zidovudine therapy in AIDS patients [letter]. J Invest Dermatol 1989; 92:776.
61. Hartshorn KL, Vogt MW, Chou TC, et al: Synergistic inhibition of human immunodeficiency virus in vitro by azidothymidine and recombinant alpha A interferon. Antimicrob Agents Chemother 1987; 31:168–172.
62. Brockmeyer NH, Kreuzfelder E, Mertins L, et al: Zidovudine therapy of asymptomatic HIV1-infected patients and combined zidovudine-acyclovir therapy of HIV1-infected patients with oral hairy-leukoplakia [letter]. J Invest Dermatol 1989; 92:647.
63. Coldiron BM, Orcutt VL: Resolution of resistant chronic herpetic lesions with zidovudine in patient with acquired immunodeficiency syndrome. Arch Dermatol 1988; 124:1571–1572.

64. Richman DD, Fischl MA, Greico MH, et al: The toxicity of azidothymidine (AZT) in the treatment of AIDS and AIDS-related complex. N Engl J Med 1987; 317:192–197.
65. Finaud M, Gallais H, Gastaut JA, et al: Thrombocytopenia HIV mediated is reversible with AZT therapy [abstract 3636]. Paper presented at the Fourth International Conference on AIDS, Stockholm, Sweden, 1988.
66. Oksenhendler E, Bierling P, Ferchal F, et al: Zidovudine for thrombocytopenic purpura related to human immunodeficiency virus (HIV) infection. Ann Intern Med 1989; 110:365–368.
67. Yarchoan R, Mitsuya H, Thomas RV, et al: In vivo activity against HIV and favorable toxicity profile of 2′,3′-dideoxyinosine. Science 1989; 245:412–415.
68. Davtyan D, Vintners H: Wernicke's encephalopathy in AIDS patients treated with zidovudine. Lancet 1987; 1:919–920.
69. Gertner E, Thurn JR, Williams DN, et al: Zidovudine-associated myopathy. Am J Med 1989; 86:814–818.
70. Gill PS, Rarick M, Brynes RK, et al: Azidothymidine associated with bone marrow failure in the acquired immune deficiency syndrome (AIDS). Ann Intern Med 1987; 107:502–505.
71. Azon-Masoliver A, Mallolas J, Gatell J, et al: Zidovudine-induced nail pigmentation. Arch Dermatol 1989; 124:1570–1571.
72. Furth PA, Kazakis AM: Nail pigmentation changes associated with azidothymidine (zidovudine). Ann Intern Med 1987; 107:350.
73. Merenick JA, Hannon RN, Gentry RH, et al: Azidothymidine-induced hyperpigmentation mimicking primary adrenal insufficiency. Am J Med 1989; 86:469–470.
74. Diven DG, Newton RC, Ramsey KM: Heightened cutaneous reactions to mosquito bites in patients with acquired immunodeficiency syndrome receiving zidovudine. Arch Intern Med 1988; 148:2296.
75. Yarchoan R, Mitsuya H, Myers C, et al: Clinical pharmacology of 3′-azido-2′,3′-dideoxythymidine (zidovudine) and related dideoxynucleosides. N Engl J Med 1989; 321:726–738.
76. Isaacs A, Lindenmann J: Virus interference. I. The interferons. Proc R Soc Lond (Biol) 1957; 147:258–267.
77. Isaacs A, Lindenmann J, Valentine RC: Virus interference. II. Some properties of interferon. Proc Soc Lond [Biol] 1957; 147:268–273.
78. Lindenmann J, Burke D, Isaacs A: Studies on the production, mode of action and properties of interferon. Br J Exp Pathol 1957; 38:551–552.
79. Vilcek J: The Action of Interferon: Interferon. New York: Springer-Verlag, 1969, 72–73.
80. Ho M, Enders JF: An inhibitor of viral activity appearing in infected cell cultures. Proc Natl Acad Sci USA 1959; 45:385.
81. Havell EA, Berman B, Ogburn CA, et al: Two antigenically distinct species of human interferon. Proc Natl Acad Sci USA 1975; 72:2185–2187.
82. Streuli M, Nagata S, Weissman C: At least three human type interferons: Structure of two. Science 1980; 209:1343–1346.
83. Chebath J, Benech P, Hovanessian A, et al: Four different forms of interferon-induced 1′,5′-oligo(A) synthetase identified by immunoblotting in human cells. J Biol Chem 1987; 262:3852–3857.
84. Ratner L, Sen GC, Brown GE, et al: Interferon, double-stranded RNA and RNA degradation: Characteristics of an endonuclease activity. Eur J Biochem 1977; 79:565–577.
85. Lebleu B, Sen GC, Shaila S, et al: Interferon, double-stranded RNA, and protein phosphorylation. Proc Natl Acad Sci USA 1976; 73:3107–3111.
86. Sen GC: Biochemical pathways in interferon action. Pharmacol Ther 1984; 24:235–257.
87. Rhodes J, Ivanyi J, Cozens P: Antigen presentation by human monocytes: Effects of modifying major histocompatibility complex class II antigen expression and interleu-

kin 1 production by using recombinant interferons and corticosteroids. Eur J Immunol 1986; 16:370–375.
88. Vance JC, Brit BJ, Hassen RC, et al: Intralesional recombinant alpha-2 interferon for the treatment of patients with condyloma accuminatum or verruca plantaris. Arch Dermatol 1986; 122:272–277.
89. Eron LJ, Judson F, Tucker S, et al: Interferon therapy for condylomata acuminata. N Engl J Med 1986; 315:1059–1064.
90. Abrams DI, Volberding PA: Alpha interferon therapy in AIDS-associated Kaposi's sarcoma. Semin Oncol 1987; 14:43–47.
91. Cornell RC, Greenway HT, Tucker SB, et al: Intralesional interferon therapy for basal cell carcinoma. J Am Acad Dermatol 1990; 23:694–700.
92. Berman B, Whiting DA, Edwards L, et al: Efficacy of interferon alfa-2_b treatment of cutaneous squamous cell carcinoma [abstract]. J Invest Dermatol 1989; 93:541.
93. Andophy EJ, Dvoretzky I, Malaish AE, et al: Response of warts in epidermodysplasia verruciformis to treatment with systemic and intralesional interferon. J Am Acad Dermatol 1984; 11:197–202.
94. Blanchet-Bardon C, Puissant A, Lutzner M, et al: Interferon treatment of skin cancer in patients with epidermodysplasia verruciformis [letter]. Lancet 1981; 1:274.
95. Vorobiof DA, Falkson G, Voges CW: DTIC vs DTIC and recombinant interferon alfa 2_b in the treatment of patients with advanced malignant melanoma. Proc Annu Meet ASCO 1989; 8:A1105.
96. Olsen EA, Rosen ST, Vollmer RT, et al: Interferon alfa-2a in the treatment of cutaneous T cell lymphoma. J Am Acad Dermatol 1989; 20:395–407.
97. Vonderheid EC, Thompson R, Smiles KA, et al: Recombinant interferon alfa-2b in plaque-phase mycosis fungoides: Intralesional and low-dose intramuscular therapy. Arch Dermatol 1987; 123:757–763.
98. Edwards L, Levine N, Weidner M, et al: Effect of intralesional alpha interferon in actinic keratoses. Arch Dermatol 1986; 122:779–782.
99. Berman B, Duncan MR: Short-term keloid treatment in vivo with human interferon-alpha 2_b results in a selective and persistent normalization of keloidal fibroblast collagen, glycosaminoglycan and collagenase production in vitro. J Am Acad Derm 1989; 21:694–706.
100. Niimura M: Intralesional human fibroblast interferon in common warts. J Dermatol (Tokyo) 1983; 10:217–220.
101. Berman B, Davis-Reed L, Silverstein L, et al: Treatment of verrucae vulgaris with alpha-2 interferon. J Infect Dis 1986; 154:328–330.
102. Stevens DA, Merigan TC: Interferon, antibody, and other host factors in herpes zoster. J Clin Invest 1972; 51:1170–1176.
103. Merigan TC, Rand KH, Pollard RB: Human leukocyte interferon for the treatment of herpes zoster in patients with cancer. N Engl J Med 1978; 298:981–987.
104. Arvin AM, Kushner JH, Feldman S, et al: Human leukocyte interferon for the treatment of varicella in children with cancer. N Engl J Med 1982; 306:761–765.
105. Pazin GJ, Armstrong SA, Lam MT, et al: Prevention of reactivated herpes simplex infection by human leukocyte interferon after operation on the trigeminal root. N Engl J Med 1979; 301:225–230.
106. Deyton LR, Walker RE, Kovac JA, et al: Reversible cardiac dysfunction associated with interferon alfa therapy in AIDS patients with Kaposi's sarcoma. N Engl J Med 1989; 321:1246–1249.
107. Steis RG, Smith JW, Urba WJ, et al: Resistance to recombinant interferon alfa-2a in hairy-cell leukemia associated with neutralizing anti-interferon antibodies. N Engl J Med 1988; 318:1409–1413.

2 | Antifungal Agents

Larry E. Millikan, M.D.
Joseph P. Shrum, M.D.

GRISEOFULVIN

Griseofulvin is an antibiotic derived from several different species of the Penicillium mold. Griseofulvin was initially investigated for its potential as an antifungal for protection of plants and was later shown to cure certain dermatophyte infections in animals.[1] In 1959, it was demonstrated to be effective in the oral treatment of superficial fungal infections in humans.[2] Griseofulvin is fungistatic against species of Microsporum, Epidermophyton, and Trichophyton, common causes of fungal infections of the skin, hair, and nails.[2]

Pharmacology

Structure

The structure consists of three connected carbon rings, one of which is a benzene ring. Attached to this benzene ring is a chloride atom.

Absorption/Distribution

Griseofulvin is insoluble in the aqueous medium of the upper gastrointestinal tract and is therefore poorly absorbed on an empty stomach. However, ingestion of griseofulvin after a meal, especially a fatty one, results in a steeper rise to greater serum levels of griseofulvin.[3] The efficiency of gastrointestinal absorption of the ultramicrocrystalline formulation is approximately 1.5 times that of conventional microsized griseofulvin. After absorption, griseofulvin is primarily bound to serum albumin. Tissue distribution is determined by the plasma free drug concentration. After absorption, there is diffusion of griseofulvin from both extracellular fluid and sweat in the epidermal cell layers into the stratum corneum.[4]

Metabolism/Excretion

Griseofulvin is metabolized in the liver. Hepatic demethylation reduces griseofulvin to inactive compounds, including the major metabolite, 6-demethyl griseofulvin. These compounds are then excreted primarily by the kidneys.[5, 6]

Mechanism of Action

The exact mechanism of action of griseofulvin is unclear. Once griseofulvin reaches the stratum corneum, however, fungal RNA, DNA, microtubular assembly, and cell wall synthesis are inhibited. Normal development of terminal hyphae is impaired, which leads to their distortion, thickening, and curling.[7]

The drug is tightly bound to newly developed keratin, which becomes highly resistant to fungal invasion. Previously infected cells eventually desquamate (in skin) or contain fungal elements until growing out (in nails, hair).

Clinical Use (Table 2–1)

Approved Indications

Griseofulvin is indicated for dermatophyte infections of the skin, hair, and nails. It has no effect on bacteria, viruses, yeast, molds, or deep mycotic infections. The successful use of griseofulvin has been reported

Table 2–1. Griseofulvin Indications/Contraindications

FDA-Approved Dermatologic Indications

Dermatophyte Infections—Hair, Nails, Skin

> Tinea capitis[2, 8, 9]*
> Tinea unguium[10–14]*
> Tinea corporis, CRURIS, PEDIS, manuum, and other cutaneous surfaces.[2, 15–17] (* if widespread, resistant to topical therapy)

Other Dermatologic Use

Lichen planus[18–20]

Contraindications[21]

Hypersensitivity to griseofulvin
Porphyria
Hepatocellular failure
Pregnancy

*Griseofulvin is generally considered the drug of choice.

for diseases as varied as gout, peripheral vascular disease, monilethrix, scleroderma, and leprosy.[21] Minimal data support these claims.

After the diagnosis of a dermatophyte infection is established, a wide variety of microsize (microcrystalline) and ultramicrosize (ultramicrocrystalline) formulations can be administered. In general, cutaneous dermatophyte infections require a daily dose of 500 mg microsize (250–330 mg/day ultramicrosize) for adults. Hair and nail infections require a daily dose of 1000 mg microsize (500–660 mg/day ultramicrosize). Children require 5–10 mg/kg/day microsize for cutaneous infections and 15–20 mg/kg/day for adequate efficacy in hair and nail infections. Although some dermatophyte resistance has been reported,[22] this occurs so rarely that routine sensitivity studies are not indicated.

TINEA CAPITIS. Tinea capitis can be characterized by erythema and scale, "black dot" type of alopecia, or an inflammatory kerion. Most infections today are due to *Trichophyton tonsurans*, which replaced several *Microsporum* species that predominated in the 1950s. Most tinea capitis occurs in children, requiring 15–20 mg/kg/day of griseofulvin microsize. This is available in liquid formulation with 125 mg/5 ml concentration. Total length of therapy is usually 6–8 weeks or until all the infected hair is replaced. Selenium sulfide shampoo, as adjunctive therapy, may shorten the duration required for the scalp fungal culture to become negative.[8] In cases of kerion celsi, a brief course of systemic steroids may lower the chance of permanent scarring.[9]

TINEA UNGUIUM. Tinea unguium is generally due to *Trichophyton rubrum*; a smaller percentage of cases is due to *T. mentagrophytes*, among other dermatophytes.[10] Anderson reviewed the existing studies in 1965, reporting a cure rate of 57% for fingernails and 17% for toenails.[11] Minimal lengths of treatment of 4 and 6 months, respectively, were required for successful therapy. In reality, most toenail cases require 12–18 months of continuous griseofulvin, and fingernails require up to 9 months. Treating cases of recent onset of tinea unguium involving a limited number of nails may improve the success rate.

In one series, 82% of cases resistant to griseofulvin either failed to improve with ketoconazole or quickly relapsed after ketoconazole therapy.[12] Thus Davies and colleagues suggested using only chronic griseofulvin for severe, painful tinea unguium.[10] Compliance may limit success, given the long treatment period required. Almost 50% of patients fail to take the proper dosage, generally reducing the dosage below the recommended amount.[13] One can monitor therapy by marking the junction of involved and uninvolved nail with a scalpel blade nick. In adequately treated cases, this junction should grow out at least 2 mm per month after the first few months.[14]

CUTANEOUS DERMATOPHYTE INFECTIONS. Griseofulvin can be used for dermatophytes at any location. However, tinea pedis is the site that most commonly requires oral antifungal therapy. Only 4–6 weeks of therapy are required in most cases, although cases that relapse may require maintenance therapy. Moist, inflammatory vesicular plantar and interdigital cases often require short-term griseofulvin along with soaks for débridement and drying effect.[15] Adding topical clotrimazole will improve the griseofulvin success rate in intertriginous cases, but will give no added benefit in the dry, moccasin type of tinea pedis.[16] Adjunctive topical keratolytic therapy, such as Whitfield's ointment, can hasten the resolution in the moccasin distribution cases.[17]

Dermatophyte infections at other body sites typically respond well to 4–6 weeks or less of griseofulvin therapy. Ideally, follow-up potassium hydroxide preparations or fungal cultures are used to demonstrate adequate response to therapy. An exception to the 4- to 6-week duration may occur in Majocchi's granuloma. For these patients, 3–5 months of griseofulvin may be required.[15] Total length of treatment in all cases should be based on clinical response and, if readily obtainable, follow-up potassium hydroxide or fungal cultures.

Other Dermatologic Uses

LICHEN PLANUS. At least three significant series have evaluated griseofulvin therapy in lichen planus.[18–20] Sehgal and colleagues reported clearing in more than 80% of patients treated with 500 mg/day microsize.[19] Massa and Rogers noted clearing in only 20% of patients.[20] Low-dose maintenance therapy may be required. Cases of erosive oral lichen planus are probably more responsive than cutaneous varieties. The mechanism of action for griseofulvin in lichen planus is unknown.

Adverse Effects

Griseofulvin has been used for decades in a large number of patients and has resulted in a relatively small number of complications. Nevertheless, adverse reactions to griseofulvin have been reported.

Early animal studies with griseofulvin revealed cessation of mitotic activity in cells of normally rapidly dividing tissue, such as intestines and bone marrow.[23] Subsequently, reactions noted in humans include cutaneous eruptions such as urticaria, fixed drug eruption, drug phototoxicity, and exfoliative erythroderma. Additional adverse effects include flare-up of pre-existing lupus erythematosus, anaphylactoid reactions, nausea, vomiting, diarrhea, dizziness and headache, and, in rare instances, hepatic toxicity, proteinuria, and leukopenia.

Some of these side effects may resolve spontaneously even with continued drug administration or when the dosage of griseofulvin is first reduced and then slowly increased.[21] In spite of the aforementioned possible side effects, griseofulvin is a remarkably safe medication. There has never been a death clearly caused by griseofulvin administration.[24]

GRISEOFULVIN MONITORING GUIDELINES

Unless medical history suggests a specific problem, pretreatment status of hepatic, renal, and hematopoietic function need not be determined for short (4- to 6-week) courses of therapy. When treating tinea unguium or other sites requiring maintenance griseofulvin therapy, one should draw periodic complete blood count and liver function tests.[15, 25] A reasonable surveillance program would be for laboratory studies to be obtained at baseline, after 1 month, and then every 3 months in long-term therapy. Significant hematologic or hepatic toxicity is quite uncommon, though.

Drug Interactions

Griseofulvin has been shown to interact with several other medications. The effect of warfarin-type anticoagulants may be inhibited by griseofulvin.[26] In addition, phenobarbital may decrease absorption of griseofulvin.[27] Monitoring laboratory and clinical responses in patients taking these medications may necessitate adjustment in drug dosage. In addition, griseofulvin may affect the enzymes involved in steroid metabolism, but its role is not well established as a cause of contraceptive failure.[28]

KETOCONAZOLE (NIZORAL)

Oral ketoconazole represented a major step forward in antimycotic therapy. It was the first, easily administered oral imidazole. Of more importance was that it represented the first orally effective antimycotic agent of broad spectrum. Previous therapy required intravenous therapy (amphotericin or miconazole) or had a limited spectrum (nystatin for yeasts and griseofulvin for dermatophytes). The clinical experience with this drug is now substantial.

The imidazole category of antifungals includes a large number of drugs, the first of which were clotrimazole, econazole, and miconazole. Other substituted derivatives have also appeared; virtually all of them are topicals. The two systemic imidazoles were miconazole (by intravenous route only) and ketoconazole, the first of the imidazole group to be orally available. Only ketoconazole will be discussed further in this section. Oral ketoconazole is effective against candidiasis, pityrosporosis, dermatophytosis, blastomycosis, coccidioidomycosis, cryptococcosis, and histoplasmosis.

Pharmacology

Structure

Ketoconazole is an imidazole drug. Many modifications of the standard imidazole molecule have led to multiple antifungals. Each substitution provided some different physical characteristics. The structure of ketoconazole represented an agent that was effective orally, providing there was a sufficiently low gastrointestinal pH (see the following section).

Absorption/Distribution

The absorption of ketoconazole is related to gastric pH. Because ketoconazole is a weakly dibasic imidazole derivative, optimal solubility in water requires a pH lower than 3. Patients with achlorhydria absorb the drug erratically and poorly.[29, 30] This has become an increasing problem in patients with acquired immunodeficiency syndrome (AIDS). Acquired achlorhydria is being seen with increasing frequency in these patients. The availability of serum ketoconazole levels is important for patients when there is a question of adequate absorption. For the patient with established achlorhydria, one can substitute therapy with itraconazole (next section). The use of an acidified liquid ingested with the morning capsule seems to provide an alternative means for optimal absorption of the drug. The issue of optimal gastric pH must be considered for patients receiving antacids, anticholinergics, antiparkinsonian agents, and H_2 receptor antagonists. One can usually circumvent these problems by giving ketoconazole first and the other therapeutic agents approximately 2 hours later. With these caveats in mind, absorption is usually a minimal problem. Plasma concentration peaks about 2 hours after the drug is taken and declines rapidly thereafter (2–4 mg/l peak decreasing to 0.1 mg/l after 12 hours).[31] Because of the drug's water solubility, there is no accumulation even with prolonged therapy. At the higher dosages necessary to treat deep fungi (400–600 mg per day), higher serum levels are achieved (5.5–6.5 mg/l declining to 0.3–0.4 mg/l after 12 hours).[32]

A two-compartment model for the drug has been proposed;[33] the more rapid phase shows a half-life of 1–2 hours.[34] There is a wide distribution in urine, saliva, sebum, eccrine sweat, cerebrum, cerebral spinal fluid, joint fluid, and many other tissues.[29] At the concentration of 1 mg/l in plasma, 1% of the drug remains free. The rest is bound to plasma proteins, and of this 99%, 84% is bound to plasma proteins and 15% to blood cells.[31]

Metabolism/Excretion

Ketoconazole is primarily metabolized through oxidation and degradation of the piperazine rings and the imidazole ring, oxidative degradation, and aromatic hydroxylation.[29, 32] These metabolites are largely excreted by the biliary system and excreted in feces, 0.7% per hour.[30]

Excretion is primarily by the liver, and a minor part occurs through urinary excretion. The half-life of the drug is variable. The half-life is also dosage-dependent over the therapeutic range. At the usual dose of 200 mg, the half-life is between 7 and 8 hours. A few studies demonstrated a 2- to 4-hour half-life with higher dosages.

Renal insufficiency has only a minor effect on drug metabolism. In renal failure there is a reduction in ketoconazole protein binding, accompanied by an approximately twofold increase in free drug in the plasma.

Pre-existing liver disease is an area of concern. Given the inherent risk of liver toxicity from ketoconazole, all patients receiving therapy at least 1–2 weeks require careful laboratory monitoring. Preliminary studies do not show drug accumulation, even with impaired liver function.

Mechanism of Action

The primary mechanism of action for all the imidazoles is inhibition of sterol metabolism. Interference in human steroid metabolism, at higher dosage levels, occurs in both the corticosteroid and the androgen synthetic pathways. Several reviewers[30, 35] discuss the mechanisms. A primary mechanism relates to the interference with the 14-alpha methyl group of the precursors of ergosterol and lanosterol.[36] The C14-methyl sterol resulting from this interference is unable to replace cholesterol or ergosterol. It has been suggested that this occurs through inhibition of the cytochrome P450-dependent lanosterol, 14-alpha demethylase activity. The effect of the drug against the cytochrome P450 system may have additional important long-term clinical implications. Significant inhibition of androgen synthesis at high drug levels can result in gynecomastia and impotence.

The effect on ergosterol formation in the cells of fungi is much greater than the effect on cholesterol formation in mammalian cells. This is the basis for the differential toxicity in fungi and humans.

Clinical Use (Table 2–2)

Approved Indications

A broad spectrum of organisms has been shown to be susceptible to ketoconazole. Those organisms and disease states for which ketoconazole currently has been approved are shown in Table 2–2. All dermatophytes and dimorphic fungi (including *Histoplasma duboisii* and *Paracocci-*

Table 2–2. Ketoconazole Indications/Contraindications

FDA-Approved Dermatologic Indications

Candidiasis
   Chronic mucocutaneous candidiasis[37–40]*
   Oral thrush[37, 38]

Blastomycosis (localized cutaneous cases)[34]
Chromomycosis[34]
Severe Recalcitrant Dermatophyte Infections[14, 41, 42]
   (Other indications of dermatologic interest: coccidioidomycosis, paracoccidioidomycosis, histoplasmosis)

Other Dermatologic Uses

Fungal/Yeast Infections
   Candidiasis (purely cutaneous,[34] onychomycosis[34, 43–46])
   Tinea versicolor[34, 47]
   Pityrosporum folliculitis[48]
   Sporotrichosis[34]

Papulosquamous/Dermatitis
   Seborrheic dermatitis[49, 50]
   Psoriasis of scalp[49]

Contraindication

Hypersensitivity to ketoconazole

*Ketoconazole is generally considered the drug of choice.

---

dioides) have shown responsiveness. Many of the phycomycetes also respond. The actinomycetes and most yeasts (other *Candida* species, *Torulopsis*, *Rhodotorula*, *Trichosporon*, and others) show variable susceptibility.[51] Heel and colleagues[31] reviewed the microbial spectrum of potential clinical effectiveness.

CHRONIC MUCOCUTANEOUS CANDIDIASIS (CMCC). Ketoconazole is the drug of choice for CMCC.[37–40] Oral thrush is eradicated within 1 week, although clotrimazole troches may be required for maintaining eradication.[37] Complete response for cutaneous (3 weeks) and nail (3 months) involvement is commonly seen.[37] Ketoconazole is required at a dose of 200–400 mg/day. Most patients are adequately treated with 200 mg/day. Maintenance therapy with ketoconazole is commonly required for nail and skin involvement.[38]

ORAL THRUSH. Severe oral *Candida* involvement in syndromes such as CMCC[37, 38] or in human immunodeficiency virus (HIV) infections may require ketoconazole. Maintenance therapy with clotrimazole troches is preferable to long-term use of ketoconazole once an adequate response has been obtained.

BLASTOMYCOSIS/CHROMOMYCOSIS. Jones extensively reviewed ketoconazole use in a variety of uncommon cutaneous and systemic fungal infections.[34] Blastomycosis and chromomycosis are official indications for ketoconazole. Ketoconazole in doses of 400 mg/day for 6 months may be effective in localized cutaneous cases of blastomycosis. Flucytosine is the drug of choice for chromomycosis, although the addition of ketoconazole may be synergistic.

SEVERE RECALCITRANT DERMATOPHYTE INFECTIONS. The U.S. Food and Drug Administration (FDA) added this indication for ketoconazole. The recommended dose is 200 mg/day for 2 weeks. The majority of cutaneous dermatophytes unresponsive to griseofulvin are responsive to ketoconazole.[41, 42] Relapse after completion of therapy occurs in at least half of successfully treated patients.[12, 41, 42] To avoid chronic ketoconazole therapy, topical antifungal therapy prophylaxis is instituted before the oral therapy is discontinued.

Other Dermatologic Uses

ONYCHOMYCOSIS. Ketoconazole has proved efficacious for both dermatophyte and *Candida* nail infections.[43–46] Torok and colleagues reported that 200 mg/day led to eradication of *Candida* in 18 of 26 cases of onychomycosis, with a mean duration of therapy of 7 months.[43] Botter and Nuigen reported a similar success rate, noting that onychomycosis was due to *Candida* in 40% of fingernail infections and 10% of toenail infections.[44] Ketoconazole is less likely to be successful in nails infected with dermatophytes.[45]

The relatively high incidence of ketoconazole-induced hepatotoxicity in long-term therapy of onychomycosis is of particular importance.[52, 53] Older women seem to be at particular risk for hepatotoxicity, and several deaths among older women have been associated with long-term ketoconazole therapy. With properly selected cases and careful laboratory surveillance, ketoconazole can provide gratifying results in *Candida* and dermatophyte nail infections.

CUTANEOUS CANDIDIASIS. Reviews by Jones[34] and by Symoens and colleagues[46] serve as a useful guide to ketoconazole use in selected cases of cutaneous candidiasis. Severe or refractory perlèche, intertrigo, and paronychia cases can be treated generally with 200 mg/day for 2–4 weeks.

TINEA VERSICOLOR. Several options for systemic ketoconazole use in treating tinea versicolor have been recommended.[34, 47] Savin reported a 97% complete response rate with 200 mg/day for 4 weeks.[47] All patients were clear of fungus at 8 weeks, and 64% were clear after 1 year. In 1984, Jones reviewed the existing studies on ketoconazole use for tinea versicolor. Overall, there was 90% efficacy.[34] Fewer relapses were noted with oral ketoconazole than for topical therapy for tinea versicolor.

Maintenance therapy with 200 mg given 3 days each month and 400 mg given once each month were both successful options.[34] Another approach involves a 400-mg dosage followed by exercise 60–90 minutes later. This dosage is repeated 1 week later, and maintenance therapy is continued with selenium sulfide topically. This approach utilizes the significant ketoconazole excretion into eccrine sweat.

Clearly, most cases of tinea versicolor require only topical measure such as selenium sulfide. For selected patients, brief courses of ketoconazole therapy can be safe and successful.[34]

PITYROSPORUM FOLLICULITIS. Although *Pityrosporum*-induced folliculitis can be detected in immune-competent patients, it is increasingly diagnosed in HIV-infected patients. Ketoconazole administered at a dosage of 200 mg/day for 28 days has led to resolution of more than 75% of cases in one series.[48] Relapse is common after the drug is discontinued. Selenium sulfide used topically for maintenance therapy is a reasonable alternative to long-term ketoconazole therapy.

SPOROTRICHOSIS. Therapy with ketoconazole has been disappointing in cases of cutaneous sporotrichosis.[34] Roughly a third of patients will respond; this makes the drug a secondary choice after saturated solution of potassium iodide.

SEBORRHEIC DERMATITIS. Several researchers have evaluated ketoconazole in seborrheic dermatitis.[49, 50] Ford and colleagues found that 33 of 37 patients demonstrated a good response when given 200 mg/day for 4 weeks.[50] Seborrheic dermatitis in HIV-infected patients is significantly less responsive.[50] Given the efficacy of topical steroids, topical ketoconazole, or both, in most seborrheic dermatitis, ketoconazole should be given orally only in unusually severe or refractory cases.

Adverse Effects

HEPATOTOXICITY. Ketoconazole-induced hepatotoxicity is believed to be due to a metabolic idiosyncrasy in susceptible persons.[52] Original estimates for serious hepatic injury were 1 in 10,000 to 1 in 15,000 exposed persons.[52, 53] Janssen Pharmaceutica estimated the current incidence to be 1 in 50,000 exposed persons (personal communication, September 1988: G. Huebner, Janssen Pharmaceutica Medical Director, and S. E. Wolverton, Editor). Presenting symptoms include anorexia, malaise, nausea, and vomiting in one third of cases.[52] Jaundice occurs in more than 80% of affected persons; it appears between days 11 and 168 of ketoconazole therapy. Liver function tests demonstrate a hepatocellular injury pattern in the majority of patients; cholestatic injury or a mixed pattern occurs less frequently. Asymptomatic and completely reversible serum transaminase elevations occur in up to 14% of patients.[34] Many cases of symptomatic hepatotoxicity occur by the 4th week of therapy, and 75% present by 3 months.[34]

Patients at greatest risk appear to be women over 40 years old on chronic therapy with ketoconazole. Overall, of cases with hepatotoxicity, 61.3% were being treated for onychomycosis and 16.8% for chronic recalcitrant dermatophytosis (see package insert). Several deaths have occurred from severe hepatic necrosis in which recognition of that condition was delayed and follow-up was inadequate.[34]

In general, the risk of hepatotoxicity is minimal when treatment duration is less than 2 weeks. Several activities improve the safety in chronic ketoconazole therapy: patient education; emphasizing key symptoms to report; proper laboratory surveillance; and cessation of therapy when serum transaminase values exceed two to three times the upper normal value.

KETACONAZOLE MONITORING GUIDELINES[34]

Baseline

- Complete blood count with differential
- Liver function tests: aspartate aminotransferase or AST (serum glutamate oxaloacetic transaminase or SGOT), alanine aminotransferase or ALT (serum glutamate pyruvate transaminase or SGPT), alkaline phosphatase, lactate dehydrogenase, bilirubin

Follow-up

- Complete blood count with differential every 2 weeks for 2 months, then monthly
- Liver function tests every 2 weeks for 3 months, then monthly

Note: More frequent surveillance needed if laboratory values are abnormal or with high-risk patients.

STEROID SYNTHESIS. Effects on sterol and steroid metabolism can be expected with doses of 800 mg/day and can occur at 600 mg/day.[34, 55, 56] Only transient (8- to 24-hour) effects on adrenal corticosteroid synthesis occur in the dosage range (200–400 mg/day) of ketoconazole for dermatologic purposes.[34] By giving the entire day's dose in the morning, one avoids clinically important suppression of corticosteroid synthesis. Gynecomastia due to impaired testicular androgen synthesis has been reported from high doses of ketoconazole.[55] This antiandrogen effect is under investigation as adjunctive therapy for prostatic carcinoma.

Drug Interactions

First, coumarin-like drugs show enhanced anticoagulant effect when both they and ketoconazole are given concomitantly. Ketoconazole increases the blood level of cyclosporine. This is important in patients on cyclosporine who often need ketoconazole therapy for secondary yeast or fungal infections.[56]

Concurrent administration with rifampin or isoniazid (INH), or both, will result in decreased ketoconazole concentrations. Altered levels of both ketoconazole and phenytoin are seen when these drugs are given together. The package insert for Nizoral recommends that both drugs be monitored carefully when given together.

ITRACONAZOLE (SPORONOX)

The next generation in oral antimycotic therapy includes the newest of the triazoles, itraconazole, a dioxolane triazole derivative that is highly lipophilic.[51] Itraconazole appears to have most of the antifungal spectrum of ketoconazole and, thus far, few of the potential hepatic and endocrine side effects.

Pharmacology

Structure

The drug has a triazole structure with a long lipophilic tail. This lipophilic characteristic gives it a distribution similar to that of ketoconazole, although the latter is slightly more hydrophilic.

Absorption/Distribution

As with the other azoles, pH is a significant factor in drug solubility. It is virtually nonionized at physiologic pHs. This lack of solubility in water and in weak acidic solutions has impeded development of oral preparations. More recently, a special vehicle incorporating acidified polyethylene glycol has allowed oral administration that gives consistent blood levels. The lipophilic characteristics play an important role in absorption and distribution of the drug. Heykants and colleagues demonstrated a prolonged level of the drug in tissue, even when plasma levels rapidly fell.[57] Persistent high levels were demonstrated in beard, back, and hands.

Healthy patients given 100 mg/day for 28 days demonstrated a rapid decrease in serum levels (T½ = 1.4 days) with undetectable serum levels by 36 days. In contrast, drug levels in both beard clippings and stratum corneum on the hand remained almost the same, with only a slight decline in the tissue levels from the back.[58] This highlights the drug's potential benefit in the treatment of fungal infections of skin, hair, and nails. Reduction in itraconazole dosage schedules is usually not necessary for patients with renal disease or cirrhosis.[58] In contrast to ketoconazole, the plasma protein binding of itraconazole is not significantly altered in patients with renal disease.

Metabolism/Excretion

Itraconazole has several possible metabolic pathways.[57] More than 20 urinary metabolites have been reported in different species. Several identified catabolic reactions include oxidation, separation of the triazole portion, dioxolane scission, dealkylation at several steps on the lipophilic tail, and oxidation of the piperazine nucleus. The hydroxylation of several of the aromatic metabolites also occurs. Aliphatic limb oxidation can occur, as well as oxidative nitrogen dealkylation.[57] In general, a greater diversity of metabolic degradation pathways occurs with itraconazole than with ketoconazole. The stability of the triazole ring is important in the more prolonged elimination half-life of itraconazole and its persistence in tissue. Heykants and colleagues summarized the excretion of itraconazole in their review[57] and pointed out that excretion through the urinary pathway amounts to 7.2% of the dose. The remainder is eliminated through the feces by biliary excretion.

Mechanism of Action

The mechanism of action for itraconazole is believed to be identical to that for ketoconazole (discussed earlier).

Clinical Use

Although there are many reports of a broad spectrum of antifungal activity,[59, 60] further extension of this spectrum in clinical usage will occur before and after the drug is approved for marketing. Preliminary studies have not identified significant contraindications or adverse effects, but a greater number of studies will broaden our understanding of potential problems in therapy. Similarly, potential drug interactions have not been clearly defined.

Itraconazole will find a ready acceptance because of the apparent paucity of the hepatic problems seen with the imidazoles. Patients at high risk for ketoconazole hepatotoxicity (elderly women with chronic onychomycosis) will constitute an important test population for itraconazole. A somewhat broader spectrum, including efficacy against Aspergillus species, will be an advantage for itraconazole. Also, preliminary work suggests that itraconazole possesses a greater specificity for sterol synthesis of fungi with less inhibitory effect on mammalian steroid synthesis. This should decrease the potential for the androgen suppression that still limits the use of high-dose ketoconazole in conditions such as coccidioidomycosis infections and should permit more aggressive use for other deep fungal infections.

TERBINAFINE (LAMASIL)

The newest group of antimycotic agents are the allylamines. The first available agent in this group was naftifine, which is available only in topical form. The first oral allylamine to be released should be terbinafine. The allylamines have a mode of action similar to that of the thiocarbamate antifungals (tolnaftate and others). The allylamines represent a major new therapeutic addition, because they act at a different site in sterol synthesis (the squalene epoxidase step) than other currently available antifungal agents.[61]

Pharmacology

Structure

Modification of the allylamine prototype by addition of a triple-bond side chain and increased branching of the alkyl group[62] has increased the antifungal activity.[63]

Absorption/Distribution

Absorption is nearly complete after all doses in the clinical range, with peak plasma concentrations at about 2 hours after administration. The significant distribution into the pilosebaceous areas and superficial stratum corneum is explained by the high lipid solubility of terbinafine.

Metabolism/Excretion

The primary metabolism of terbinafine occurs in the liver. The degradation of the drug involves three catabolic targets. There is separation at the central nitrogen atom, oxidation of the alkyl side chain at any of the three methyl groups, and an aromatic oxidation following action by epoxide hydrolase, resulting in a dihydrodiol metabolite. Ultimately, these metabolic events result in oxidation to the corresponding carboxylic acids, conjugation in the liver, and excretion in the urine.

Roughly 70% of the drug is found in the liver. After a single dose with radioactive tracers, 85% is excreted within 72 hours of administration. Excretion is primarily urinary (70%), and much of the remainder is excreted in the feces. The slow elimination in humans is due to the lipophilic nature of the drug. After oral administration of 250 mg, maximal plasma concentrations range between 0.8 and 1.5 mcg/ml.[64]

Mechanism of Action

Terbinafine was initially investigated as SF 86–327. Its effect on ergosterol synthesis is greater than that on cholesterol synthesis, which ensures a lesser toxicity in mammalian systems.[61]

Terbinafine is highly effective in vitro with a 50% inhibition concentration (IC_{50}) for dermatophytes of 2 mcg/ml and for yeasts of 8 mcg/ml.[65] It shows a broad range of activities against *Aspergillus, Sporothrix*, *Candida* blastospores, and *Candida* mycelial phase. It also acts against *Cryptococcus, Torulopsis*, some dematiaceous fungi (including chromoblastomycosis), *Curvularia*, and *Alternaria*.[66, 67] In addition, terbinafine has demonstrated antiprotozoal activity against promastigote and amastigote stages of *Leishmania*.[68]

The toxicological profile of terbinafine is most encouraging. Terbinafine has no effect on the cytochrome P-450 system, an important metabolic target of the imidazoles leading to adverse effects. Ketoconazole-induced drug interactions and suppression of adrenal and testicular androgen production involve the cytochrome P-450 system. Also, no problems with hepatotoxicity have thus far been ascribed to terbinafine.[69]

Clinical Use

Indications

Because terbinafine has not received FDA approval, official indications are not established. Clinical research has shown effectiveness in treating a broad variety of organisms. These include *Candida* in its mycelial phase, as well as dermatophyte-induced tinea corporis,[69] tinea pedis,[70] and onychomycosis.[71, 72] Preliminary reports show effectiveness in these diseases with doses of 250 mg/day, usually given in a divided dose of 125 mg twice a day. In preliminary studies the drug has been ineffective against tinea vericolor when given orally, yet it has been effective when applied topically. Uses for the systemic mycoses seem very likely.

Contraindications

The initial studies have shown few systemic adverse effects, and no definite contraindications have been established.

Adverse Effects

Because of the problems with imidazole-induced hepatotoxicity, liver-related problems have been searched for carefully. There has been no evidence to date that establishes a significant risk of hepatotoxicity. As with any other uncommon drug reaction, only widespread clinical use provides accurate data regarding the true risk of hepatotoxicity.

Studies on patients with compromised renal or liver functions suggest the need for dose reductions, but no significant problems have been identified. There is a low potential for acute or chronic toxicity, for impaired fertility or reproduction, or for change of immunity.

Drug Interactions

The potential for drug interactions related to the cytochrome P-450–dependent mechanism seems unlikely. Although no significant drug interactions have been identified, such interaction is unlikely to be detected, given the necessity of monotherapy in clinical trials. At least, terbinafine neither inhibits nor induces metabolism of antipyrine.[67]

FLUCYTOSINE (ANCOBON)

Flucytosine (5-fluorocytosine; 5FC) is a synthetic, oral antimycotic agent developed in the late 1950s by Duschinsky and colleagues.[73] Although very effective in treating some systemic mycoses, this drug has a rather limited clinical role in the treatment of systemic fungal infections.

Pharmacology

Flucytosine is a structural analog of the pyrimidine cytosine. This medication is rapidly and thoroughly absorbed from the gastrointestinal tract after ingestion. There is virtually complete penetration of flucytosine into the cerebrospinal fluid and other body fluids and tissues. Virtually all of the oral dose is excreted, almost totally unchanged, in the urine.[74]

The fungistatic mode of action of this cytosine analog is based on inhibition of fungal nucleic acid synthesis. Flucytosine is converted into 5-fluorouracil by organisms possessing the enzyme cytosine deaminase. Furthermore, enzymatic conversions lead to the production of 5-fluorodeoxyuridylic acid monophosphate, which inhibits fungal DNA synthesis;[75] 5-fluorouracil then replaces uracil in fungal RNA, which results in defective fungal proteins.

Clinical Use

Monotherapy with flucytosine as an antifungal agent is accompanied by a relatively high incidence of fungal resistance. This resistance can develop during treatment, as well as exist before therapy. Sensitivity studies should be obtained before treatment with flucytosine is begun.[76] These studies should be repeated during therapy if clinically indicated.

Flucytosine is approved only for treatment of serious infections caused by *Candida* or *Cryptococcus*. Flucytosine has also been shown to be effective in plantar chromomycotic skin infections and, in combination with amphotericin B, in cryptococcal, candidal, and *Aspergillus* infections.[77, 78] Combination therapy increases medication efficacy while limiting fungal resistance.

Adverse reactions associated with the use of flucytosine are usually mild and reversible upon cessation of therapy. As with dermatophytes, mammalian bone marrow has the ability to convert flucytosine into its metabolites. As a result, leukocytopenia and thrombocytopenia may occur, especially in patients with serum flucytosine levels higher than 100 mcg/ml. Other reported toxicities include hepatic dysfunction, nausea, vomiting, enterocolitis, urticaria, and photosensitivity.[79]

The kidneys are the primary route of excretion for flucytosine. Although no renal toxicity has been reported with flucytosine, renal function should be followed. In addition, hepatic and hematopoietic function should be examined before and during therapy. If renal dysfunction exists, dosage should be adjusted in order to maintain serum levels between 50 and 100 mcg/ml.[80]

Flucytosine is prescribed in dosages of 150 mg/kg/day in divided doses at 6-hour intervals. This dosage schedule is continued for approximately 6–12 weeks, depending on clinical and laboratory response.

NYSTATIN

Nystatin, first isolated in 1949 at a dairy farm in Virginia, is a polyene antibiotic derived from the actinomycete *Streptomyces noursei*.[81] The name "nystatin" is derived from the New York State laboratory at which the drug was developed.

Pharmacology

Nystatin possesses four methyl groups and contains four conjugated double bonds. The mode of action of nystatin is based on its affinity to bind to the major fungal cell membrane sterol, ergosterol. There is resultant leakage of cellular constituents and ultimate lysis and cell death.[82] Simple inhibition of membrane function provides fungistatic activity, but alteration of membrane permeability can result in lysis and cell death. Thus nystatin is both fungistatic and fungicidal.

Clinical Use

Topical nystatin is useful for cutaneous and mucous membrane candidiasis. Its efficacy is comparable with that of clotrimazole.[83]

The absorption of oral nystatin from the gastrointestinal tract is negligible, which has resulted in limited systemic use. Nystatin may be administered orally to treat intestinal candidiasis. In addition, the oral form can be given to suppress *Candida* growth in the gastrointestinal tract in order to limit "seeding" of neighboring skin and vaginal mucosa. Candidiasis of the groin in infants and adults has been correlated with the presence of intestinal candidiasis.[84, 85] More recently, use of oral nystatin has been employed as adjunctive therapy in various seborrheic and psoriatic disorders.[86] Even improvement in acne vulgaris after treatment with oral nystatin has been reported in one patient.[87]

Adverse reactions to oral nystatin are limited to gastrointestinal complaints, such as nausea, vomiting, and diarrhea.

Oral dosage of nystatin usually is 500,000 units to 1,000,000 units three or four times daily until there is clinical improvement.

BIBLIOGRAPHY: Key Reviews/Chapters

Lesher JL Jr, Smith JG Jr: Antifungal agents in dermatology. J Am Acad Dermatol 1987; 17:383–394.

Graybill JR, Craven PC: Antifungal agents used in systemic mycoses: Activity and therapeutic use. Drugs 1983; 25:41–62.

Heel RC, Brogden RN, Carmine A, et al: Ketoconazole: A review of its therapeutic efficacy in superficial and systemic fungal infections. Drugs 1982; 23:1–36.

Cohen J: Antifungal chemotherapy. Lancet 1982; 2:532–537.

Jones HE: Therapy of superficial fungal infections. Med Clin North Am 1982; 66:873–893.

Jones HE: Ketoconazole. In Fleischmajer R (ed): Progress in Diseases of the Skin, Vol. 2. New York: Grune & Stratton, 1984, 217–249.

REFERENCES

1. Brian PW: Control of fungal diseases of plants with griseofulvin. Trans St John's Hosp Dermatol Soc 1960; 45:4–6.
2. Blank H, Roth FJ Jr, Smith JG Jr, et al: The treatment of dermatomycoses with orally administered griseofulvin. Arch Dermatol 1959; 79:259–266.
3. Crounse RG: Human pharmacology of griseofulvin: The effect of fat intake on gastrointestinal absorption. J Invest Dermatol 1961; 529–532.
4. Epstein WL, Shah VP, Riegelman S: Griseofulvin levels in stratum corneum: Study after oral administration in man. Arch Dermatol 1972; 106:344–348.
5. Lesher JL Jr, Smith JG Jr: Antifungal agents in dermatology. J Am Acad Dermatol 1987; 17:383–394.
6. Davies RR: Griseofulvin. In Speller DCE (ed.): Antifungal Chemotherapy. Chichester: Wiley, 1980:149–182.
7. Brian PW, Curtis PJ, Hemming HG, et al: A substance causing abnormal development

of fungal hyphae produced by *Penicillium janozewskii:* I. Biological assay, production and isolation of curing factor. Trans Br Mycol Soc 1946; 29:173–187.
8. Allen HB, Honig PJ, Leyden JJ, et al: Selenium sulfide: Adjunctive therapy for tinea capitis. Pediatrics 1982; 69:81–83.
9. Foged EK, Jepsen LV: Hair loss following kerion celsi: A follow-up examination. Mykosen 1984; 27:411–414.
10. Davies RR, Everdall JD, Hamilton E: Mycological and clinical evaluation of griseofulvin for chronic onychomycosis. Br Med J 1967; 3:464–468.
11. Anderson DW: Griseofulvin: Biology and clinical usefulness. Ann Allergy 1965; 23:103–110.
12. Hay RJ, Clayton YM: Treatment of chronic dermatophyte infections: The use of ketoconazole in griseofulvin treatment failures. Clin Exp Dermatol 1982; 2:611–617.
13. Meinhof W, Girardi RM, Stracke A: Patient noncompliance in dermatomycosis: Results of a survey among dermatologists and general practitioners and patients. Dermatologica 1984; 169(Suppl 1):57–66.
14. Zaias N, Drachman D: A method for the determination of drug effectiveness: Trials with ketoconazole and griseofulvin ultramicrosize. J Am Acad Dermatol 1983; 9:912–919.
15. Jones HE: Therapy of superficial fungal infections. Med Clin North Am 1982; 66:873–893.
16. Zaias N, Battistin E, Gomez-Urcoyo F, et al: Treatment of tinea pedis with griseofulvin and topical antifungal cream. Cutis 1978; 22:196–199.
17. Prazak G, Ferguson JS, Comer JE, et al: Treatment of tinea pedis with griseofulvin. Arch Dermatol 1960; 81:821–826.
18. Sehgal VN, Abraham G, Gauri-Bazaz M: Griseofulvin therapy in lichen planus: A double-blind controlled study. Br J Dermatol 1972; 87:383–385.
19. Sehgal VN, Bikhchandani R, Koranne RV, et al: Histopathologic evaluation of griseofulvin therapy in lichen planus: A double-blind controlled study. Dermatologica 1980; 61:22–27.
20. Massa MC, Rogers RS III: Griseofulvin therapy of lichen planus. Acta Derm Venereol (Stockh) 1981; 61:547–550.
21. Blank H: Commentary: Treatment of dermatomycoses with griseofulvin. Arch Dermatol 1982; 118:835–836.
22. Greenberg JR: Griseofulvin resistance. Int J Dermatol 1979; 18:701.
23. Paget GE, Walpole AL: Some cytological effects of griseofulvin. Nature 1958; 182:1320.
24. Lyell A: A review of toxic epidermal necrolysis in Britain. Br J Dermatol 1967; 79:662–671.
25. Gris-PEG product information. In Physicians' Desk Reference (44th ed). Oradell, NJ: Medical Economics, 1990, 1038.
26. Cullen SI, Catalano PM: Griseofulvin-warfarin antagonism. JAMA 1967; 199:582–583.
27. Riegelman S, Rowland M, Epstein WL: Griseofulvin phenobarbital interaction in man. JAMA 1970; 213:426–431.
28. Van Dijke CPH, Weber JCP: Interaction between oral contraceptives and griseofulvin. Br Med J 1984; 288:1125–1126.
29. Daneshmend TK, Warnock DW: Clinical pharmacokinetics of systemic antifungal drugs. Clin Pharmacokinet 1983; 8:17–42.
30. Van Tyle JHV: Ketoconazole. Pharmacotherapy 1984; 4:343–373.
31. Heel RC, Brogden RN, Carmine A, et al: Ketoconazole: A review of its therapeutic efficacy in superficial and systemic fungal infections. Drugs 1982; 23:1–36.
32. Daneshmend TK, Warnock EL, Turner A, et al: Pharmacokinetics of ketoconazole in normal subjects. J Antimicrob Chemother 1981; 8:299–304.
33. Huang YC, Colaizzi JL, Bierman RH, et al: Pharmacokinetics and dose proportionality of ketoconazole in normal volunteers. Antimicrob Agents Chemother 1986; 30:206–210.

34. Jones HE: Ketoconazole. In Fleischmajer R (ed): Progress in Diseases of the Skin, Vol. 2. New York: Grune & Stratton, 1984, 217–249.
35. Borgers M: Structural changes in Candida albicans after ketoconazole treatment. In Eliot BW (ed): Oral Therapy in Vaginal Candidosis. Oxford: The Medicine Publishing Foundation, 1984, 43–49.
36. Borgers M, Van Cutsem J: Ketoconazole-induced morphological changes in yeasts and dermatophytes. In Meinhof W (ed): Oral Therapy in Dermatomycosis: A Step Forward. Oxford: The Medicine Publishing Foundation, 1985, 51–60.
37. Horsburgh CR Jr, Kirkpatrick CH: Long-term therapy of chronic mucocutaneous candidiasis with ketoconazole: Experience with twenty-one patients. Am J Med 1983; 74(1B):23–29.
38. Petersen EA, Alling DW, Kirkpatrick CH: Treatment of chronic mucocutaneous candidiasis with ketoconazole: A controlled clinical trial. Ann Intern Med 1980; 93:791–795.
39. Hay RJ, Clayton YM: The treatment of patients with chronic mucocutaneous candidiasis and Candida onychomycosis with ketoconazole. Clin Exp Dermatol 1982; 7:155–162.
40. Graybill JR, Herndon JH, Kniker WT, et al: Ketoconazole treatment of mucocutaneous candidiasis. Arch Dermatol 1980; 116:1137–1141.
41. Cox FW, Stiller RL, South DA, et al: Oral ketoconazole for dermatophyte infections. J Am Acad Dermatol 1982; 6:455–462.
42. Laurberg G: Ketoconazole in trichophyton rubrum. Acta Derm Venereol (Stockh) 1982; 62:273–274.
43. Török I, Simon G, Pap M: An evaluation of two years of clinical experience with ketoconazole. Mykosen 1982; 25:136–142.
44. Botter AA, Nuigen STM: Further experiences with ketoconazole in the treatment of onychomycosis. Mykosen 1981; 24:156–166.
45. Robertson MH, Rich P, Parker F, et al: Ketoconazole in griseofulvin-resistant dermatophytosis. J Am Acad Dermatol 1982; 6:224–229.
46. Symoens J, Moens M, Dom J, et al: An evaluation of two years of clinical experience with ketoconazole. Rev Infect Dis 1980; 2:674–687.
47. Savin RC: Systemic ketoconazole in tinea versicolor: A double-blind evaluation and 1 year follow-up. J Am Acad Dermatol 1984; 10:824–830.
48. Ford GP, Ive FA, Midgley G: Pityrosporum folliculitis and ketoconazole. Br J Dermatol 1982; 107:691–695.
49. Wishner AJ, Teplitz ED, Goodman PS: Pityrosporum, ketoconazole, and seborrheic dermatitis. J Am Acad Dermatol 1987; 12:140–141.
50. Ford GP, Farr PM, Ive FA, et al: The response of seborrheic dermatitis to oral ketoconazole. Br J Dermatol 1984; 111:603–607.
51. Van Cutsem J, Janssen PAJ: Antifungal activity of new azoles, recent advances in chemotherapy antimicrobial (Section 3). In Ishigume J (ed): Proceedings of the 14th International Congress of Chemotherapy Kyoto. Tokyo: University of Tokyo Press, 1985, 1942–1943.
52. Lewis JH, Zimmerman HJ, Benson GD, et al: Hepatic injury associated with ketoconazole therapy: Analysis of 33 cases. Gastroenterology 1984; 86:503–513.
53. Janssen PAJ, Symoens JE: Hepatic reactions during ketoconazole treatment. Am J Med 1983; 74(1B):80–85.
54. Pont A, Williams PL, Loose DJ, et al: Ketoconazole blocks adrenal steroid synthesis. Ann Intern Med 1982; 97:370–372.
55. Pont A, Williams PL, Azhar S: Ketoconazole blocks testosterone synthesis. Ann Intern Med 1982; 97:370–372.
56. Gupta AK, Brown MD, Ellis CN, et al: Cyclosporine in dermatology. J Am Acad Dermatol 1989; 21:1245–1256.
57. Heykants J, Michaels M, Meuldermans W, et al: The pharmacokinetics of itraconazole in animals and in man: An overview. In Fromling RA (ed): Recent Trends in the

Discoveries, Development, and Evaluation of Antifungal Agents. Barcelona: Prous Science Publishers SA 1987:57–83.
58. Cauwenbergh G, Degreef H, Heykants J, et al: Pharmacokinetic profile of orally administered itraconazole in human skin. J Am Acad Dermatol 1988; 19:263.
59. Degreef H, Borghijs A, Dupre KM, et al: Reduction of treatment length with itraconazole in common dermatophytoses. Oral azole antifungals: Present and future. Paper presented at the 17th World Congress on Dermatology, Berlin, 1987, 24–29.
60. Van Cutsem J, Van Gerven F, Janssen PAJ: Activity of orally, topically, and parenterally administered itraconazole in the treatment of superficial and deep mycoses: Animal models. Rev Infect Dis 1987; 9(Suppl 1):S15–S32.
61. Ryder NS: Selective inhibition squalene epoxidation by allylamine antimycotic agents. In Nombela C (ed): Microbial Cell Wall Synthesis and Autolysis. New York: Elsevier Science Publishers, 1985:313–321.
62. Stutz A, Petranyi G: Synthesis and antifungal activity of (E)-N-(6,6-dimethyl-2-hepten-4-ynyl)-N-methyl-1-napththalenemethanamine (SF 86–327) and related allylamine derivatives with enhanced oral activity. J Med Chem 1984; 27:1539–1543.
63. Ryder NS: Specific inhibition of fungal sterol biosynthesis by SF 86–327, a new allylamine antimycotic agent. Antimicrob Agents Chemother 1985; 27:252–256.
64. Goad LJ, Hole GG, Reach DH: Effect of the allylamine antifungal drug SF 86–327 on the growth and sterol synthesis of *Leishmania mexicana* promastigotes. Biochem Pharmacol 1985; 34:3785–3788.
65. Ryder ND: The mechanism of action of terbinafine. Clin Exp Dermatol 1989; 14:98–100.
66. Mieth IT, Retranyi G: Preclinical evaluation of terbinafine in vivo. Clin Exp Dermatol 1989; 14:104–107.
67. Shadomy S, Espinel-Ingroff A, Gebhart RJ: In-vitro studies with SF 86–327, a new orally active allylamine derivative. Sabouraudia 1985; 23:125–132.
68. Jensen JC: Clinical pharmacokinetics of terbinafine (Lamasil). Clin Exp Dermatol 1989; 14:110–113.
69. Villars V, Jones TC: Clinical efficacy and tolerability of terbinafine (Lamasil). Clin Exp Dermatol 1989; 14:124–127.
70. Savin R: Successful treatment of chronic tinea pedis (moccasin type) with terbinafine (Lamasil). Clin Exp Dermatol 1989; 14:116–119.
71. Zaias N, Serrano L: The successful treatment of finger trichophyton rubrum onychomycosis with oral terbinafine. Clin Exp Dermatol 1989; 14:120–123.
72. Kagawa S: Clinical efficacy of terbinafine in 629 Japanese patients with dermatomycosis. Clin Exp Dermatol 1989; 14:114–115.
73. Duschinsky R, Pleven E, Heidelberger C: The synthesis of 5-fluoro-pyrimidines. J Am Chem Soc 1957; 79:4559–4560.
74. Medoff G, Kobayashi GS: Strategies in the treatment of systemic fungal infections. N Engl J Med 1980; 302:145–155.
75. Cohen J: Antifungal chemotherapy. Lancet 1982; 2:532–537.
76. Vandevelde AG, Mauceri AA, Johnson JE III: 5-fluorocytosine in the treatment of mycotic infections. Ann Intern Med 1972; 77:43–51.
77. Mauceri AA, Cullen SI, Vandevelde AG, et al: Flucytosine: An effective oral treatment for chromomycosis. Arch Dermatol 1974; 109:873–876.
78. Fass RJ, Perkins RL: 5-fluorocytosine in the treatment of cryptococcal and *Candida* mycoses. Ann Intern Med 1971; 74:535–539.
79. Graybill JR, Craven PC: Antifungal agents used in systemic mycoses: Activity and therapeutic use. Drugs 1983; 25:41–62.
80. Roberts DT: The current status of systemic antifungal agents. Br J Dermatol 1982; 106:597–602.
81. Rippon JW: A new era in antimycotic agents [editorial]. Arch Dermatol 1986; 122:399–402.

82. Hamilton-Miller JM: Fungal sterols and the mode of action of the polyene antibiotics. Adv Appl Microbiol 1974; 17:109–134.
83. Clayton YM, Connor BL: Comparison of clotrimazole cream, Whitfield's ointment and nystatin ointment for the topical treatment of ringworm infections, pityriasis versicolor, erythrasma and candidiasis. Br J Dermatol 1973; 89:297–303.
84. Taschdjian CL, Kozinn PJ: Laboratory and clinical studies on candidiasis in the newborn infant. J Pediatr 1957; 50:426–433.
85. Lynch PJ, Minkin W, Smith EB: Ecology of Candida albicans in candidiasis of the groin. Arch Dermatol 1969; 99:154–160.
86. Crutcher N, Rosenberg EW, Belew PW, et al: Oral nystatin in the treatment of psoriasis [letter]. Arch Dermatol 1984; 120:435–436.
87. Newbold HL: Nystatin for treatment of acne vulgaris [letter]. J Am Acad Dermatol 1989; 20:861.

3 | Antibacterial Agents

Suzanne Bruce, M.D.
John E. Wolf, Jr., M.D.

Antibiotics are among the oral medications most frequently prescribed by dermatologists. In addition to short courses of therapy for acute cutaneous infections such as impetigo, folliculitis, furunculosis, and wound infections, dermatologists use long-term antibiotic therapy for the treatment of diseases such as acne vulgaris, acne rosacea, and perioral dermatitis. This chapter is a review of the clinical pharmacology of the antimicrobial agents most commonly prescribed by dermatologists. The focus is primarily on oral agents, but selected parenteral agents (clindamycin, vancomycin, aztreonam) are discussed. Drugs or drug groups discussed include tetracyclines, erythromycin, penicillins, cephalosporins, amoxicillin-potassium clavulanate, trimethoprim-sulfamethoxazole, rifampin, ciprofloxacin, and metronidazole. A brief section of common clinical scenarios concludes the chapter.

TETRACYCLINES

The tetracycline antibiotics were the first broad-spectrum antibiotics effective against a broad range of gram-positive and gram-negative organisms. They were discovered after large scale screening of soil samples for antibiotic-producing organisms.[1] Chlortetracycline was isolated from *Streptomyces aureofaciens* in 1948.

The other first-generation tetracyclines and their dates of development were oxytetracycline in 1950, tetracycline in 1953, demethylchlortetracycline in 1957, and methacycline in 1965. The second generation tetracyclines were semisynthetic congeners with longer half-lives, enhanced antibacterial activity, and lower toxicity. Doxycycline first appeared in 1967, and minocycline was introduced in 1972.[2]

Tetracyclines are less widely used in nondermatologic fields today than when they were first introduced. This is the result of the development of antimicrobial resistance and the advent of newer and more effective antibiotic agents.[3] Nevertheless, the central role of tetracyclines in dermatology remains.

Pharmacology

Structure

The tetracyclines are a group of antibiotics characterized by a four-ring carbocyclic structure. They differ in the substituents in the ring.[4]

Absorption/Distribution

All the tetracyclines are absorbed well from the gastrointestinal tract, especially in the fasting state. Heavy-metal ions such as calcium, magnesium, aluminum, and iron form chelates with the tetracyclines.[5-7] Thus antibiotics of this group should not be taken concurrently with milk, antacids, or iron preparations. A comparison of the absorption of minocycline and tetracycline revealed that tetracycline's absorption was significantly more inhibited by food and milk than was minocycline's absorption. Iron, in the form of ferrous sulfate, produced a dramatic decrease in absorption of both drugs.[8]

After oral ingestion of 500 mg of tetracycline, peak serum levels of approximately 3–4 mcg/ml occur after about 1–3 hours, falling to about 2 mcg/ml after 8 hours. Two hours after a 200-mg dose of doxycycline or minocycline, peak serum levels are around 2.5 mcg/ml. The half-life of tetracycline is 10 hours, in comparison with 15 hours for minocycline and 18 hours for doxycycline.[3]

Tetracyclines are widely distributed within the body with an apparent volume of distribution of 1.5 l/kl.[9] Because of their lipophilic nature, especially that of minocycline and doxycycline, tetracyclines are highly diffusible and penetrate even hard-to-reach areas such as prostate, eye, and brain tissues. They penetrate into sebum and are excreted in eccrine sweat, which probably accounts for their efficacy in combating acne. Tetracyclines cross the placenta and are also excreted in breast milk.[3]

Metabolism/Excretion

Tetracyclines are metabolized by the liver and concentrated in bile, but their metabolism has not been well defined.[1] The main route of excretion is urinary and, to a lesser extent, fecal.[3] Thus the tetracyclines should be avoided or administered in adjusted dosage to patients with renal insufficiency. An exception is doxycycline, which is excreted primarily in the feces and is the tetracycline of choice for a patient with renal failure.[1]

Mechanism of Action

The mechanism of action of tetracyclines is inhibiting protein synthesis by binding to the 30S ribosomal-mRNA unit. This blocks the binding of aminoacyl tRNA to the 30S ribosome and prevents the addition of new amino acids to the growing peptide chain.[3] Tetracyclines are bacteriostatic drugs; thus they should not be used by patients with bacterial endocarditis or granulocytopenia.[2]

Clinical Use

Indications

GENERAL INDICATIONS. Although tetracyclines are rarely the drugs of first choice for common bacterial infections, they are indicated in the treatment of a wide variety of uncommon infections, such as those caused by chlamydiae, rickettsiae, spirochetes, mycoplasma, protozoa, and some fungal species.[2] Tetracycline is the drug of choice for the treatment of chlamydial infections, rickettsial infections, and the cutaneous manifestations of Lyme disease (erythema chronicum migrans). *Chlamydia trachomatis* is an important pathogen in a number of genital infections, including urethritis, epididymitis, pelvic inflammatory disease, and lymphogranuloma venereum. Rickettsial infections for which tetracycline is the first-line drug include Rocky Mountain spotted fever, Q fever, scrub typhus, typhus, and rickettsial pox. In early Lyme disease, administration of oral tetracycline 250 mg four times a day for 10–21 days has been shown to reduce the duration of the rash and to prevent the sequelae of arthritis, carditis, and meningitis.[3] Tetracyclines are also useful as first-line agents in brucellosis, granuloma inguinale, melioidosis, and relapsing fever.

Infections for which tetracyclines may be an alternative therapy include anthrax, tularemia, chancroid, Vincent's infection, rat bite fever, *Pasteurella multocida*, plague, syphilis, yaws, leptospirosis, *Actinomyces israelii*, *Chlamydia* conjunctivitis, *Mycobacterium marinum*, *Nocardia*, and *Vibrio vulnificus*.

DERMATOLOGIC INDICATIONS. The most common dermatologic uses of tetracyclines are in the treatment of acne vulgaris, rosacea, and perioral dermatitis. The mechanism of action of the tetracyclines in these facial inflammatory disorders is speculative. It is known that large doses of tetracycline (1 g/day) influence acne by reducing the number of *Propionibacterium acnes*. Small dosages (500 mg/day) work by reducing the formation of bioactive substances that mediate inflammation without any major change in bacterial colony count.[10] Tetracycline may also exert an anti-inflammatory effect by inhibiting leukocyte chemotaxis.[11] Tetracycline for acne is commonly prescribed initially in dosages of 1 g/day. After control is achieved, the dosage can often be reduced to 250–500 mg/day for maintenance therapy.[12]

In addition to the common use of tetracyclines for acne and related conditions, there have been anecdotal reports on the successful use of tetracyclines for a variety of other noninfectious cutaneous diseases. Bullous pemphigoid,[13] intestinal bypass dermatitis,[14] pityriasis lichenoides,[15] pyoderma gangrenosum,[16,17] and even mycosis fungoides[18] have all been reported to improve after tetracycline or minocycline is administered. Of these possible indications, bullous pemphigoid appears to show the most promising response. Tetracycline at 1–1.5 g/day can provide a steroid-sparing effect and, in milder cases, possibly be used as monotherapy.

Contraindications

Tetracyclines are contraindicated in pregnant women and children under the age of 8. Bony anomalies may, in the fetus, result from the use of tetracyclines during pregnancy. The highest risk of dental staining and enamel dysgenesis occurs with tetracycline exposure between the 4th and 6th months of intrauterine life.[3] Tetracycline administration during the first trimester of pregnancy is unlikely to cause teeth discoloration or teratogenic effects in the fetus; nevertheless, it is contraindicated during all trimesters of pregnancy.[19]

Adverse Effects

GASTROINTESTINAL EFFECTS. In addition to the effects on developing teeth and bones, tetracyclines can cause a wide variety of adverse reactions. Because of their acidic pH in solution, tetracyclines can irritate the esophageal and gastric mucosa, resulting in epigastric burning, abdominal discomfort, nausea, vomiting, esophagitis, and esophageal ulceration. Diarrhea can result from irritation of the bowel mucosa or from bacterial superinfection.[1,3] Pseudomembranous colitis due to *Clostridium difficile* has been reported with tetracycline. Overgrowth of *Candida albicans* may occur in the oral mucosa, vagina, and bowel.

CUTANEOUS EFFECTS. A variety of cutaneous reactions to tetracyclines have been reported. Hypersensitivity reactions, ranging from morbilliform rashes to urticaria and anaphylaxis, occur rarely. More common are phototoxic dermatitis and photo-onycholysis, which are seen especially with doxycycline and demethylchlortetracycline. Phototoxicity is less common with tetracycline and has not been reported with minocycline. Ultraviolet A wavelengths of 320–400 nm are responsible for the photoreaction. Fixed drug eruptions have been caused by both tetracycline and minocycline.[20]

Long-term administration of minocycline has been associated with the rare occurrence of abnormal pigmentation. At least two types of minocycline-induced pigmentation can be distinguished on the basis of clinical and histologic features. The first type consists of dark bluish-black macules arising in areas of inflammation, such as acne scars. This type shows staining properties of hemosiderin histologically. The second type is characterized by a more generalized brown or blue-gray pigmentation, with accentuation on sun-exposed skin. Histologically, the pigment appears to stain like melanin.[21] In addition to cutaneous pigmentation, minocycline has also been associated with grayish discoloration of the teeth, black thyroid glands, and black galactorrhea.[20]

OTHER ADVERSE EFFECTS. Other reported effects include renal, hepatic, and neurologic toxicities. Hepatotoxicity has been reported in patients receiving high dosages of intravenous tetracycline.[1] Pregnant and postpartum women with renal disease are especially vulnerable.[22] Tetracyclines (with the exception of doxycycline) exacerbate azotemia in patients with pre-existing renal disease. Benign intracranial hypertension (pseudotumor cerebri) has been associated with tetracyclines.[23] Minocycline administration may cause dizziness, vertigo, and ataxia, especially in women. The symptoms begin soon after the patient starts taking the drug, are dose-related, and are reversible when therapy is discontinued.[24]

Drug Interactions

Drug interactions with tetracyclines, other than interference with absorption by concomitant therapy, relate primarily to hepatic metabolism. Thus they are seen most commonly with doxycycline. The serum half-life of doxycycline is decreased by drugs such as barbiturates, phenytoin, and carbamazepine, which induce enzymes that control the rate of hepatic metabolism of tetracyclines. The half-life is increased by cimetidine and ketoconazole, which inhibit hepatic metabolism of tetracyclines.[25] The general anesthetic methoxyflurane has been reported to cause renal failure in patients receiving tetracycline.[26]

A variety of drugs, foods, and some dairy products may interfere with the gastrointestinal absorption of tetracycline; they include liquid antacids, cimetidine, iron salts, and sodium bicarbonate. Tetracyclines may rarely increase the serum levels of digoxin and may increase or decrease lithium levels. Tetracyclines may decrease insulin requirements and may increase the hypothrombinemic effects of concurrent anticoagulants. Bacteriostatic drugs such as tetracycline may interfere with the bactericidal action of penicillins.

The putative interaction between oral contraceptives and antibiotics is of concern. Possible mechanisms of this alleged interaction include increased liver degradation of sex steroids, decreased enterohepatic circulation of sex steroids, and increased excretion of the contraceptive hormones. The information, to date, is insufficient for one to conclude whether the risk of pregnancy is increased, decreased, or not affected.[27] It is prudent to discuss with a female patient the possibility of such an interaction before she starts any antibiotic therapy.[27]

ERYTHROMYCIN

Erythromycin was derived in 1952 from a strain of Streptomyces erythreus, an actinomycete isolated from soil collected in the Philippines. McGuire and associates introduced the drug into clinical medicine in the same year.[28]

Pharmacology

Structure

Erythromycin is the most important member of the class of antibiotics known as macrolides ("large ring"). Other members of this group include spiramycin, trioleandomycin, oleandomycin, albocycline, megalomycin, josamycin, and rosaramicin.[29] The structure of erythromycin consists of a macrocyclic lactone ring attached to sugar moieties. Four oral preparations are available: erythromycin base, stearate, estolate, and ethylsuccinate.[30] The free base is the form that has antimicrobial activity, and the other three forms are hydrolyzed to the active base in the body.

Absorption/Distribution

Erythromycin base and stearate are inactivated by acid. Thus they are usually administered in an enteric-coated form that dissolves in the duodenum. Higher serum levels are achieved when the drug is administered when the stomach is empty. Erythromycin estolate is acid-stable, and its absorption is not diminished by food intake. The ethylsuccinate form of erythromycin is absorbed as both the intact ester and the free base after hydrolysis in the intestine. Its absorption is decreased somewhat by food intake, but less so than is the base. In spite of their differences, all oral preparations attain adequate serum levels of free base, and no one preparation appears to be more clinically efficacious than the others.[28, 31] Erythromycin penetrates well throughout tissues and body fluids, except for brain cerebrospinal fluid. It crosses the placenta and is also present in breast milk.[31]

Metabolism/Excretion

Only 4% of an oral dose and 15% of a parenteral dose of erythromycin are excreted unchanged in the urine.[28] The liver concentrates the drug and excretes it into bile in high concentrations. Metabolism of the drug occurs in the liver by demethylation. The serum half-life of the drug is approximately 1.5 hours in normal patients. This increases to about 5 hours in anuric patients. A dosage reduction is generally not necessary in renal failure because the route of elimination is primarily hepatic.[32]

Mechanism of Action

The mechanism of action of erythromycin is based on its binding to the 50S subunit of 70S ribosomes of susceptible bacteria. This causes blockage of transpeptidation or of translocation reactions, which in turn results in the inhibition of RNA-dependent protein synthesis.[28, 31]

Clinical Use

Indications

The dermatologic indications approved by the U.S. Food and Drug Administration (FDA) for the use of erythromycin include skin and soft tissue infections of mild to moderate severity caused by Streptococcus pyogenes or Staphylococcus aureus, Chlamydia trachomatis urethritis, and erythrasma. It is an alternative choice of treatment of syphilis and gonorrhea.[33]

STAPHYLOCOCCAL/STREPTOCOCCAL INFECTIONS. Erythromycin may be used to treat a variety of skin infections caused by S. pyogenes, such as erysipelas, cellulitis, lymphangitis, impetigo, and ecthyma. The cure rate with erythromycin of these infections is almost equal to that obtained with penicillins.[34] The drug is an acceptable alternative in minor skin infections due to S. aureus such as folliculitis, furunculosis, and infected dermatitis.[35] However, because of the emergence of erythromycin-resistant strains of S. aureus, the drug should not be used in serious staphylococcal infections.[28] The usual dosage for cutaneous infections is 1 g/day. Sensitivity testing should be performed if the therapeutic response to erythromycin is not prompt.

OTHER CUTANEOUS INFECTIONS. Other, non–FDA-approved indications for infectious diseases with cutaneous manifestations in which erythromycin is effective include Lyme borreliosis,[36] anthrax,[37] actinomycosis,[38] chancroid,[39] and granuloma inguinale.[40]

OTHER DERMATOLOGIC INDICATIONS. Because erythromycin has an excellent safety profile, its use as an alternative to tetracycline in the treatment of acne vulgaris, rosacea, and perioral dermatitis has become widespread. Like tetracycline, erythromycin appears to have anti-inflammatory properties in addition to its antibacterial action.[41] Other noninfectious, cutaneous diseases that have been reported to respond to erythromycin therapy include pseudofolliculitis barbae,[42] eosinophilic pustular folliculitis,[43] bullous pemphigoid,[44] and pityriasis lichenoides.[45, 46]

Contraindications

Erythromycin is contraindicated in the rare patient with hypersensitivity to the drug. The estolate form of erythromycin should not be given to patients 12 years of age or older or to pregnant patients because it is associated with an increased risk for cholestatic jaundice in these patient groups.

Adverse Effects

Erythromycin is one of the safest antibiotics in use today. The most common adverse reactions associated with erythromycin are dose-related gastrointestinal disturbances: nausea, vomiting, epigastric distress, and diarrhea. The syndrome of erythromycin estolate–induced cholestatic jaundice just mentioned is the most serious adverse effect associated with erythromycin. The clinical presentation includes fever, abdominal pain, nausea, vomiting, eosinophilia, and elevated serum bilirubin and transaminases.[30] Rare instances of reversible hearing loss after the use of high doses of the drug have been reported, particularly in elderly patients with renal insufficiency.[28] Pseudomembranous colitis caused by overgrowth of *Clostridium difficile* has been reported in association with the use of oral erythromycin.[47] The drug may interfere with the fluorometric determination of urinary catecholamines and with aspartate aminotransferase or AST (serum glutamate oxaloacetic transaminase or SGOT) determinations.

Drug Interactions

Drugs that interact with erythromycin include theophylline, cyclosporine, carbamazepine, warfarin, digitalis, ergotamine, and methylprednisolone.[48] Theophylline toxicity can result from competitive inhibition by erythromycin for the binding site of the cytochrome P450 oxidase system. Thus by inhibiting these drugs' hepatic metabolism, erythromycin may lead to increases in blood levels of these drugs and consequent toxicity.[29]

PENICILLINS

In 1928, Alexander Fleming discovered that a substance from the mold *Penicillium notatum*, which he named penicillin, inhibited the growth of *Staphylococcus aureus*. Florey and colleagues characterized the structure and properties of the compound, and they began successful clinical trials in 1941. The new drug was used extensively in World War II to treat soldiers with gangrene and sepsis.[49] Further research subsequently yielded modifications of the penicillin molecule; these modifications changed the activity spectrum.

Penicillin G and the semisynthetic penicillinase-resistant penicillins are considered to be the first generation. The isoxazolyl penicillins are a subgroup of the latter that includes oxacillin, cloxacillin, and dicloxacillin. The second-generation agents are the aminopenicillins, ampicillin, and amoxicillin, which have some activity against gram-negative bacteria. Ticarcillin and carbenicillin are third-generation penicillins, distinguished by their activity against *Pseudomonas aeruginosa*. The fourth generation penicillins are piperacillin, azlocillin, and mezlocillin. Their activity spectrum is similar to that of the third generation but broader.[50] The following discussion emphasizes the first- and second-generation penicillins, which can be given orally (unlike the third- and fourth-generation drugs).

Pharmacology

Structure

The penicillin nucleus is composed of three basic parts: a thiazolidine ring, a beta-lactam ring, and a side chain. The pharmacologic characteristics and antibacterial spectrum of a particular penicillin are determined by its side chain. For example, the penicillinase-resistant penicillins have bulky substituents around the side chain linkage that interfere with the attachment of penicillinase.[51]

Absorption/Distribution

Oral absorption varies markedly among the penicillins. Penicillin G is readily destroyed by gastric acid and therefore is not given orally. Penicillin V is well absorbed orally, even when ingested with food. Methicillin, nafcillin, and the third- and fourth-generation penicillins

Antibacterial Agents

require parenteral administration because of their poor absorption when they are given by mouth. The isoxazolyl penicillins (cloxacillin and dicloxacillin) are acid stable and can be administered orally; peak serum levels occur at 1–1.5 hours after administration. The presence of food in the stomach delays absorption and causes peak serum levels to be lower. Thus the isoxazolyl penicillins are best given on an empty stomach. Oral absorption of dicloxacillin is superior to that of cloxacillin. Ampicillin and amoxicillin are both acid stable and can be administered orally. Amoxicillin has superior absorption (90%), and, unlike that of ampicillin, its peak serum concentration is not altered by food ingestion.[49, 51]

Penicillins distribute widely in most body fluids and tissues, including those of the lungs, the liver, the kidneys, the bones, the muscles, and the placenta. In the absence of inflammation, the penicillins have poor distribution to the eye, the brain, cerebrospinal fluid, and the prostate. The penicillinase-resistant penicillins are reversibly bound to serum albumin to varying degrees, with the highest being that of dicloxacillin (97%). Although protein-bound drug is inactive, the binding is reversible and has little effect on the therapeutic activity of the penicillins.[52]

Metabolism/Excretion

The penicillins are excreted unchanged into the urine by both glomerular filtration and renal tubular secretion. The percentage of the administered dose that is excreted unchanged varies with the type of penicillin. Probenecid competitively inhibits the tubular secretion of the penicillins, thus increasing serum concentrations. Metabolism of the penicillins occurs to a minor degree. Approximately 10% of a dosage of ampicillin, amoxicillin, or dicloxacillin is metabolized in the body, primarily in the liver. Most penicillins, including penicillin G, amoxicillin, and nafcillin, are actively secreted into bile, yielding serum levels that are 10–100 times the serum level.[53]

Mechanism of Action

Penicillins inhibit bacterial cell wall synthesis or maintenance. Penicillins were originally thought to inhibit cell wall synthesis by inhibiting transpeptidase, the enzyme necessary for cross-linking of peptide strands in the growing peptidoglycan. Subsequent research has shown that penicillins inhibit a number of enzymes, known as penicillin-binding proteins, that are involved in the synthesis of the bacterial cell wall.[54]

Clinical Use

Indications

PENICILLIN V/G. Penicillin G is not used in oral form because it is destroyed quickly by gastric acid. Repository forms of penicillin G such as procaine penicillin or benzathine penicillin are given by the intramuscular route. Procaine penicillin G is effective in the treatment of susceptible strains of gonorrhea, and benzathine penicillin G is the preferred drug for syphilis. Penicillin V has excellent in vitro activity against group A streptococci, but because of its ineffectiveness against beta-lactamase–producing strains of S. aureus, it is rarely used as the initial drug in the treatment of pyoderma.[55] The drug is a suitable treatment for erysipeloid and is an alternative to tetracycline for the early stages of Lyme disease. The usual adult dosage is 250–500 mg every 6 hours.

ISOXAZOLYL PENICILLINS. The main indication of the isoxazolyl penicillins is the treatment of suspected or proven staphylococcal infections that are due to beta-lactamase–producing strains. Because these agents are also effective against most streptococci and non–beta-lactamase–producing S. aureus, they provide empiric coverage for most cases of pyoderma until the causative organism is identified by the laboratory. Some strains of S. aureus are resistant to methicillin and the other antistaphylococcal penicillins. Although encountered primarily in the hospital setting, the strains are being seen more frequently in the community as well.[53,55] Methicillin-resistant strains of S. aureus are resistant to all other beta-lactam antibiotics. The usual adult dosage of dicloxacillin is 250–500 mg every 6 hours; 1 g/day is sufficient for most dermatologic uses.

AMINOPENICILLINS. The aminopenicillins, ampicillin and amoxicillin, have side chains that permit better penetration into the lipophilic outer envelope of gram-negative bacteria. This also provides activity against some strains of Haemophilus influenzae and other gram-negative organisms. In addition, the aminopenicillins are active against enterococci, group A streptococcus, and Neisseria gonorrhoeae. Beta-lactamase–producing organisms hydrolyze amoxicillin and ampicillin. Thus aminopenicillins are not effective against most S. aureus and H. influenza and some strains of gonococci. Although the two drugs are comparable in efficacy, amoxicillin has several advantages over ampicillin, including better absorption and production of less diarrhea.[56] The usual dosage of ampicillin is 250–500 mg every 6 hours, and that of amoxicillin is 250–500 mg every 8 hours.

When given as single oral-dose treatments concomitantly with 1 g of probenecid, both aminopenicillins are effective against sensitive strains of gonorrhea. The dosages are 3.5 g for ampicillin and 3 g for amoxicillin. Ampicillin, in doses of 1 g/day, has been reported to be useful in the treatment of acne vulgaris, rosacea, and gram-negative folliculitis.[57,58]

Contraindications

Hypersensitivity is the only contraindication to the use of penicillin. Allergy to one penicillin means probable allergy to all other penicillins. The possibility of cross-reaction in patients with hypersensitivity to another beta-lactam antibiotic, such as the cephalosporins, must be considered.

Adverse Effects

HYPERSENSITIVITY. The majority of adverse reactions to penicillins are hypersensitivity reactions. These range in severity from a mild rash to anaphylaxis and, rarely, death. In addition to immunoglobulin E–mediated immediate hypersensitivity, penicillins have been associated with delayed hypersensitivity, cytotoxic antibody responses, and immune complex disease.[53] Morbilliform drug eruptions, exfoliative dermatitis, serum sickness, and Stevens-Johnson syndrome have been reported in association with penicillins. The oral route of administration is much less likely to cause serious cutaneous reactions than is the parenteral route.

Ampicillin and amoxicillin have a higher incidence of rash than do the other penicillins. These drugs cause a nonallergic maculopapular eruption in approximately 5%–10% of patients. The risk of a rash is increased in patients receiving allopurinol and in those with infectious mononucleosis, acquired immunodeficiency syndrome (AIDS), renal failure, or chronic lymphocytic leukemia.[51, 59]

OTHER ADVERSE EFFECTS. Other less commonly associated adverse reactions include gastrointestinal disturbances, hematologic complications (such as leukopenia), neurotoxicity, nephrotoxicity, and elevation of hepatic enzymes.[51, 53] All these adverse reactions are only rarely associated with dicloxacillin and cloxacillin. Antibiotic-induced pseudomembranous colitis and *Candida* vaginitis may result from the use of the penicillins.[51, 55]

Drug Interactions

Administration of allopurinol concurrently with ampicillin may increase the risk of ampicillin-induced skin rash. Concomitant use of bacteriostatic antibiotics, such as erythromycin and tetracycline, with penicillins may reduce the bactericidal effects of the penicillins.

The use of beta-blockers with penicillin may increase the risk and severity of anaphylactic reactions. Concurrent use of penicillins may reduce the efficacy of the oral contraceptives. Probenecid prolongs blood levels of penicillin by blocking its renal tubular secretion. Ampicillin may cause false-positive urine glucose reactions with the use of Clinitest, Benedict's solution, or Fehling's solution.[60]

CEPHALOSPORINS

In 1945, Brotzu isolated a fungus, *Cephalosporium acremonium*, which inhibited the growth of a variety of gram-negative and gram-positive bacteria. An antibiotic fraction called cephalosporin C was subsequently isolated from cultures of the organism. This was the parent compound from which the first cephalosporins were derived.[61]

Since the introduction of cephalothin in 1962, numerous other broad-spectrum antibiotics of this class have been released. The parenteral cephalosporins are generally divided into first-, second-, and third-generation agents. The first-generation drugs include cephalothin (Keflin, Seffin), cephapirin (Cefadyl), cefazolin (Ancef, Kefzol), and cephradine (Anspor, Velosef). These drugs possess excellent coverage for staphylococcal infections, in addition to their efficacy in treating gram-negative organisms such as *Escherichia coli* or *Proteus*.[62]

The second-generation cephalosporins are cefoxitin (Mefoxin), cefamandole (Mandol), cefonicid (Monocid), ceforanide (Precef), and cefuroxime (Zinacef). Third-generation agents include cefotaxime (Claforan), ceftizoxime (Cefizox), moxalactam (Moxam), ceftriaxone (Rocephin), cefoperazone (Cefobid), cefmenoxime (Cefmax), cefsulodin (Cefomonid), and ceftazidime (Fortaz, Tazidime, Tazicef). The second- and third-generation agents are generally less active against gram-positive organisms, but more active against certain gram-negatives and anaerobes, than the first-generation agents.[63]

The orally administered cephalosporins include cephalexin (Keflex), cephradine (Anspor, Velosef), cefadroxil (Duricef, Ultracef), cefaclor (Ceclor), and cefixime (Suprax). All of them are considered first-generation, except for second-generation cefaclor and third-generation cefixime. The emphasis of this discussion will be on the oral cephalosporins and on selected parenteral agents that have potential uses in dermatologic practice, such as ceftriaxone.

Pharmacology

Structure

The basic structure of the cephalosporins resembles that of the penicillins, inasmuch as both are beta-lactams. They differ as to which ring is fused to the beta-lactam portion. Cephalosporins have a six-membered dihydrothiazine ring, and the penicillins have a five-membered thiazolidine ring.[61]

Absorption/Distribution

All the oral cephalosporins are rapidly absorbed from the gastrointestinal tract, achieving peak serum levels in 1–2 hours. The presence of food in the stomach delays absorption but does not affect the extent of absorption. The serum half-life of cefadroxil is almost twice that of cephalexin (90 minutes and 50 minutes, respectively); thus, it can be administered every 12 or 24 hours rather than every 6 hours.[64] The oral cephalosporins are distributed widely in body fluids and tissues, except for spinal fluid and the aqueous humor.[63]

Metabolism/Excretion

The antibiotics in this group are eliminated unchanged primarily by renal excretion. Cephalexin, cephradine, and cefadroxil accumulate in patients with renal insufficiency. Dosage adjustments are necessary for patients whose creatinine clearance is less than 25 ml/minute. Cefaclor does not accumulate in patients with impaired renal function because of its instability in biologic fluids.[63]

Ceftriaxone is a third-generation cephalosporin that can be administered either intravenously or intramuscularly. The long serum half-life of this agent (5.8–8.7 hours) allows for once-daily dosing. Ceftriaxone has a high hepatic excretion rate in comparison with other cephalosporins, but 33%–67% of the drug is still excreted unchanged in the urine. Dosage adjustments are seldom necessary for patients with either renal impairment or hepatic dysfunction.

Mechanism of Action

All beta-lactam antibiotics, including cephalosporins and penicillins, act by inhibiting enzymatic reactions necessary for synthesis and for maintenance of a stable bacterial cell wall. Beta-lactamase enzymes produced by "resistant" bacteria inactivate the cephalosporins.[62]

Clinical Use

Indications

ORAL AGENTS. The oral cephalosporins, with the exception of cefixime, are FDA-approved for the treatment of skin infections caused by S. aureus and group A beta-hemolytic streptococci. The usual adult dosage of cephalexin and cephradine is 250 mg every 6 hours or 500 mg every 12 hours. Cefadroxil has the advantage of once- or twice-daily dosing, either 500 mg every 12 hours or 1 g/day in a single dose. Cefaclor is administered in dosages of 250 mg every 8 hours. Cefaclor and cefixime are both active against *Haemophilus influenzae* and could be used to treat cellulitis due to that organism, although they are not FDA-approved for that indication.

PARENTERAL AGENTS. The parenteral agent ceftriaxone is FDA-approved for the treatment of skin and soft-tissue infections caused by susceptible strains of S. aureus, Staphylococcus epidermidis, Streptococcus species (excluding enterococci), Enterobacter cloacae, Klebsiella species, Proteus mirabilis, and Pseudomonas aeruginosa. A single 250 mg intramuscular dose of ceftriaxone is effective in uncomplicated gonorrhea, including both penicillinase- and non–penicillinase-producing strains. Preliminary studies indicate that ceftriaxone may be more effective than penicillin in the treatment of late Lyme borreliosis.[36]

Contraindications

Cephalosporins are contraindicated for patients who have either a history of allergy to these drugs or a history of anaphylaxis or severe immediate reactions to penicillin. Penicillin-allergic patients may exhibit cross-allergenicity to cephalosporins at a rate of 5%–10%.[61] Patients who have only a history of a nonurticarial, penicillin-induced drug eruption generally can safely tolerate the cephalosporins. If their reaction is of the immediate type (anaphylaxis, angioedema, or urticaria), cephalosporins should not be used.[62]

Adverse Effects

The cephalosporins have an excellent safety profile. The most common adverse systemic effects are hypersensitivity reactions, such as maculopapular rash, eosinophilia, and drug fever. Immediate hypersensitivity reactions such as anaphylaxis, urticaria, and bronchospasm occur less commonly. Gastrointestinal disturbances may occur but are usually mild and transient.[64]

Drug Interactions

Bacteriostatic agents, such as tetracyclines and chloramphenicol, may interfere with the bactericidal action of cephalosporins. Concurrent administration of probenicid with cephalosporins competitively inhibits renal tubular secretion, thus increasing and prolonging plasma levels of the cephalosporin. False-positive reactions for urine glucose may occur with Clinitest tablets, Benedict's solution, or Fehling's solution in patients taking cephalosporins.[60]

AMOXICILLIN–POTASSIUM CLAVULANATE (AUGMENTIN)

Clavulanic acid is a naturally occurring beta-lactam isolated from a strain of *Streptomyces clavuligerus*. The combination of amoxicillin and the potassium salt of clavulanic acid was developed as a new antimicrobial preparation by Beecham Laboratories. It was approved for marketing in the United States as Augmentin in 1984.

Pharmacology

Structure

Clavulanic acid is a naturally occurring beta-lactam that is structurally similar to the penicillin nucleus. This similarity accounts for the affinity between clavulanic acid and beta-lactamases.[65]

The combination drug is available in 4:1 and 2:1 dosage forms. Tablets contain 500 or 250 mg of amoxicillin with a constant 125 mg of clavulanic acid. Two formulations of the oral suspension are available: 125 mg of amoxicillin and 31.25 mg of clavulanic acid per 5 ml or 250 mg of amoxicillin and 62.5 mg of clavulanic acid per 5 ml.

Absorption/Distribution

Both amoxicillin and clavulanic acid are well absorbed from the gastrointestinal tract, and their absorption is not affected by concomitant intake of food, milk, or antacids.[66] The serum half-life of both is approximately 60 minutes. Both drugs penetrate well into body fluids and tissues, except for respiratory tract secretions and the central nervous system.[66]

Metabolism/Excretion

Amoxicillin and clavulanic acid are excreted primarily through the urinary tract. Within 6 hours after an oral dose, approximately 75% of the amoxicillin and 57% of the clavulanic acid are found unchanged in the urine.[67] Clavulanic acid undergoes greater metabolism in the body than does amoxicillin. Both drugs accumulate in patients with renal insufficiency.[68]

Mechanism of Action

Beta-lactam antibiotics such as amoxicillin act by inhibiting cross-linking of the bacterial cell wall, which results in the death of the organism. Bacteria that produce beta-lactamases may be resistant to penicillins and cephalosporins. Clavulanic acid is a potent inhibitor of the beta-lactamases of staphylococcal and many gram-negative organisms. Clavulanic acid has only weak antibacterial activity by itself; in combination with amoxicillin, however, it produces a synergistic antibacterial effect.[65] The combination drug is active against a wide range of pathogenic bacteria.[65]

Clinical Use

Indications

CUTANEOUS INFECTIONS. The only FDA-approved dermatologic indications for amoxicillin–clavulanic acid are the treatment of skin and soft-tissue infections. The drug is highly effective against the primary causes of such infections: S. aureus and streptococci, including group A. Gram-negative infections, such as with E. coli, Klebsiella, or Bacteroides, frequently respond to amoxicillin–clavulanic acid, although with lower success rates than do staphylococcal and streptococcal infections. Amoxicillin–clavulanic acid could be a useful drug in mild cases of facial cellulitis in children. Here the possible pathogens include Haemophilus influenzae and streptococci.[66] Methicillin-resistant strains of S. aureus and S. epidermidis are not susceptible to the drug.[65, 66] The usual adult dosage for cutaneous infections is 250 mg amoxicillin/125 mg clavulanate every 8 hours. For severe infections, 500 mg amoxicillin/125 mg clavulanate every 8 hours is recommended. The pediatric dose is 20–40 mg/kg/day of amoxicillin in three divided doses.

SEXUALLY TRANSMITTED DISEASES. Sexually transmitted diseases are another area of potential use of this agent. Chancroid appears to have an excellent cure rate with amoxicillin–clavulanic acid, but the drug's role in gonorrhea therapy is not clear. Failure rates for single high-dose treatment of amoxicillin-resistant gonorrhea may be unacceptably high.[66, 69, 70] Chancroid is effectively treated with either 500 mg amoxicillin/125 mg clavulanate or 500 mg amoxicillin/250 mg clavulanate three times daily for 7 days.[71]

Contraindications

The only contraindication to amoxicillin–clavulanic acid is allergy to either component of the preparation.

Adverse Effects

The most common adverse effects of amoxicillin–clavulanic acid are gastrointestinal disturbances, such as nausea, vomiting, and diarrhea. The incidence of these side effects may decrease, if the drug is taken with food. Women may develop Candida vulvovaginitis, as with other antibiotics. Side effects reported less often include dizziness, drowsiness, urticaria, rash, and fever. Occasionally, patients have developed mild elevations of serum transaminases, blood urea nitrogen, or serum creatinine; however, no consistent changes in hematologic or biochemical parameters have been associated with amoxicillin–clavulanic acid.[65, 66] The drug may cause false-positive results when urine is tested for glucose with Clinitest tablets, Benedict's solution, or Fehling's solution.[68]

Drug Interactions

Simultaneous administration of probenecid with the drug delays the renal excretion of amoxicillin, but not clavulanic acid.[68]

TRIMETHOPRIM-SULFAMETHOXAZOLE
(BACTRIM, SEPTRA)

German chemists synthesized sulfonamide-containing compounds in the early 1900s for use as dyes. In the 1930s, it was discovered that one of the dyes, Prontosil, had antibacterial action in streptococci-infected mice. Many sulfonamide compounds were then synthesized and developed for use as antibiotics.[72]

The development of trimethoprim originated from basic research on bacterial and mammalian folate reductases. Trimethoprim is a more potent inhibitor of the bacterial dihydrofolate reductase than of the mammalian enzyme. It is one of several compounds that were synthesized to exploit this difference.[72] Further investigations with trimethoprim eventually led to the development of a fixed-proportion combination of trimethoprim (TMP) and sulfamethoxazole (SMX) in 1968.[73] After several years of successful use in Europe and England, trimethoprim-sulfamethoxazole (TMP-SMX) was approved for use in the U.S. in 1973 as Septra and Bactrim.[74]

Pharmacology

Structure

Trimethoprim is a 2,4-diamino–5-(3′,4′,5′-trimethoxybenzyl) pyrimidine, and sulfamethoxazole is 5-methyl–3-sulfanilamidoisoxazole. The combination drug TMP-SMX contains the two agents in a ratio of 1:5 (TMP to SMX). It is available in the U.S. in tablets containing 80 mg of TMP and 400 mg of SMX and in double strength tablets of 160 mg of TMP and 800 mg of SMX. A pediatric suspension contains 40 mg of TMP and 200 mg of SMX per 5 ml.

Absorption/Distribution

Both TMP and SMX are well absorbed from the upper intestinal tract without any delay in absorption by food in the stomach.[75] A single dose of TMP-SMX (1:5 ratio) results in peak serum concentrations of TMP to SMX in a 1:20 ratio, which is the proportion with optimal synergistic effect against most susceptible bacterial species.[74] Peak serum levels for both drugs are achieved in about 1–2 hours, and the serum half-lives for both are approximately 8–10 hours.[76] TMP is much more lipid-soluble than SMX. Thus, the concentration of TMP in body tissues is higher than its serum concentration. The reverse is true for SMX.[74]

Metabolism/Excretion

SMX is metabolized more extensively than is TMP. Approximately 70% of SMX is inactivated, mainly by acetylation, whereas 30% is excreted unchanged in the urine.[74] Only 10%–20% of TMP is metabolized. Approximately 60% of a dose of TMP is excreted in the urine in 24 hours.[72] Because both compounds are excreted primarily by the kidney, the dosage should be decreased in cases of significant renal insufficiency.

Mechanism of Action

Both TMP and SMX act on the folic acid biosynthesis pathway of bacteria, a process which is crucial to the formation of purines and ultimately of DNA. Early in the folate pathway, SMX competitively inhibits the conversion of para-aminobenzoic acid into folic acid by the enzyme dihydropteroate synthetase. At a later stage in the pathway, TMP competitively inhibits the enzyme dihydrofolate reductase and thus interferes with the conversion of dihydrofolic acid to tetrahydrofolic acid. Separately, each drug is bacteriostatic, but their synergistic effect is considered to be bactericidal.[73]

Clinical Use

Indications

Although TMP-SMX does not have FDA approval for the treatment of cutaneous infections, there are several important, non–FDA-approved uses of the drug for dermatologic diseases.

SEXUALLY TRANSMITTED DISEASES. Sexually transmitted diseases are one area of use for TMP-SMX. A number of different regimens have been found effective in the treatment of uncomplicated gonorrhea with cure rates of 90%–100%, depending on the dosage regimen.[73, 77, 78] TMP-SMX produced a cure rate of 68% in the treatment of nongonococcal urethritis due to *Chlamydia trachomatis*, which is substantially lower than the rate for the drug of choice, tetracycline (cure rate 85%).[73] The combination drug has been shown to be highly effective for the treatment of simultaneous *Neisseria gonorrhoeae* and *C. trachomatis* infections.[79] TMP–SMX is an effective alternative to tetracycline in the treatment of chancroid and lymphogranuloma venereum. Syphilis does not respond to TMP-SMX.

CUTANEOUS INFECTIONS. Other infections with dermatologic manifestations that may respond to TMP-SMX are *Nocardia asteroides* infections, *Mycobacterium marinum* infections, brucellosis, and melioidosis.[74] The drug may be useful in treating impetigo, folliculitis, and other common skin infections, particularly in penicillin-allergic patients. Several studies have shown TMP-SMX to be effective in acne vulgaris, but it is not generally considered a first-line drug.[41, 80] Likewise, the drug has a secondary role in hidradenitis suppurativa. The usual adult dose is one double-strength tablet twice a day.

Contraindications

Contraindications to the use of TMP-SMX include a history of hypersensitivity to either trimethoprim or sulfonamides or to the combination of the two. Use of the drug should be avoided for patients with severe liver or hematologic disease, glucose–6-phosphate dehydrogenase deficiency, and folate deficiency. Pregnant patients and neonates should not be treated with TMP-SMX. Patients with renal failure whose creatinine clearance is less than 15 ml/minute should be treated with the drug only if they are receiving dialysis, and blood levels of SMX should be closely monitored.[73] If the creatinine clearance is between 15 and 30 ml/minute, the maintenance dosage of TMP-SMX should be half the usual dosage after a full loading dosage is administered.[81]

Adverse Reactions

GASTROINTESTINAL EFFECTS. Adverse reactions to TMP-SMX are primarily gastrointestinal, cutaneous, and hematologic. Upper gastrointestinal upset, manifested most commonly by nausea and vomiting, occurs in approximately 4% of patients. Diarrhea is an infrequent side effect.[82]

CUTANEOUS EFFECTS. Cutaneous reactions, usually erythematous macular eruptions, urticaria, or pruritus, occurred in 3.3% of patients in one large series.[82] Severe skin reactions such as Stevens-Johnson syndrome and toxic epidermal necrolysis have been associated with TMP-SMX but are rare. Lawson and Paice estimated that approximately 1 of 100,000 TMP–SMX recipients develops a serious cutaneous adverse reaction.[83]

Antibacterial Agents   67

The apparent relative frequency of these serious cutaneous reactions from sulfonamides is a function of the very common use of these drugs.

HEMATOLOGIC EFFECTS. Hematologic side effects reported include thrombocytopenia, leukopenia, and hemolytic anemia.[84] Patients who have been receiving the drug for more than three months should have regular blood counts performed to monitor for laboratory evidence of folate impairment. If folate deficient patients, such as alcoholic or malnourished persons, must be treated with TMP-SMX, supplementation with folinic acid (Leucovorin) or folic acid should be considered.[73] AIDS patients have a much higher frequency of adverse reactions than does the general population.[85]

Drug Interactions

A number of drug interactions with TMP-SMX have been reported. The drug may potentiate the antifolate effect of pyrimethamine, which results in megaloblastic anemia. SMX displaces warfarin from plasma albumin-binding sites and could potentially cause hypoprothrombinemia. TMP-SMX prolongs the half-life of phenytoin and sulfonylurea drugs and could result in toxicity.[73] Sulfonamides can displace methotrexate from plasma protein-binding sites, which results in increased free methotrexate concentrations and possible bone marrow suppression. Concomitant use of TMP-SMX and thiazide diuretics is associated with an increased incidence of thrombocytopenic purpura, especially in elderly patients. Trimethoprim may cause a decrease in the therapeutic effect of cyclosporine and an increased risk of nephrotoxicity.[60]

RIFAMPIN (RIFADIN, RIMACTANE)

Rifamycin B, the parent compound of rifampin, was first isolated in 1957 from a culture of the soil microorganism *Nocardia mediterranei*. The Dow-Lepetit Research Laboratories in Milan, Italy, searched to find a derivative of the rifamycin molecule that had antibacterial activity when administered orally. After successful clinical trials, rifampin was introduced into clinical use in Italy in 1968. The U.S. FDA approved the drug for use in pulmonary tuberculosis and meningococcal carriage in 1971. During the 1980s, the clinical use of rifampin expanded into the treatment of nontuberculous infections. A consensus regarding its exact place in the chemotherapeutic armamentarium is still evolving.[86]

Pharmacology

Structure

Rifampin (rifampicin in Europe) is 3-([[4-methyl-1-piperazinyl]imino] methyl) rifamycin. It is a zwitterion that is soluble in organic solvents and in water at low pH.[87]

Absorption/Distribution

Rifampin is almost completely absorbed from the stomach and duodenum, achieving peak serum concentrations of approximately 7 mcg/ml (the range is 4–32 mcg/ml) within 1–4 hours after an oral dose of 600 mg. Food and para-aminosalicylic acid cause a delay in absorption of the drug and a lowering of peak blood levels.[88, 89] Because of its lipophilic properties, rifampin has excellent penetration in body fluids and tissues, including hard-to-reach areas such as the central nervous system, bones, and abscess cavities.[87]

Metabolism/Excretion

Metabolism of rifampin occurs in the liver by deacetylation to an active metabolite. Deacetyl-rifampin is excreted into bile, but reabsorption of the drug by the enterohepatic route does occur. Approximately 16% of a rifampin dosage is excreted unchanged into the urine. The half-life is 1.5–5 hours at the onset of therapy, but this decreases by 40% with continued treatment, as a result of enhanced biliary excretion. Hepatic insufficiency prolongs the half-life of rifampin, and the drug should be avoided or used in reduced dosages by these patients. The half-life is unaffected by renal failure, and therefore dosage adjustment is unnecessary.[87, 88]

Mechanism of Action

Rifampin exerts its bactericidal action by inhibiting DNA-dependent RNA polymerase at the beta-subunit, stopping chain initiation but not elongation. This unique mechanism of action prevents bacterial cross-resistance with other classes of antibiotics. Bacterial resistance to rifampin may develop rapidly as a result of mutations leading to alterations in the structure of the beta-subunit of RNA polymerase. This resistance develops more frequently during monotherapy with rifampin than with combination antimicrobial chemotherapy.[88]

Clinical Use

Indications

STAPHYLOCOCCAL INFECTIONS. In addition to its FDA-approved use in the treatment of tuberculosis, rifampin has a number of non–FDA-approved uses in skin disorders. Because of its excellent antimicrobial activity against both methicillin-sensitive and methicillin-resistant *S. aureus* and *S. epidermidis* and its superior tissue penetration, rifampin is effective in a variety of staphylococcal infections. Rifampin (300 mg twice a day) in combination with cloxacillin has been shown to be effective in the treatment of patients with recurrent furunculosis (including those who are also nasal carriers of *S. aureus*).[88] Methicillin-resistant *S. aureus* colonization has been successfully eradicated with the combination of rifampin and a variety of other antimicrobial agents such as erythromycin or trimethoprim-sulfamethoxazole.[90-94]

OTHER CUTANEOUS INFECTIONS. Other reported uses of rifampin include the treatment of patients with chronic granulomatous disease who are infected with staphylococci and other sensitive organisms.[95] Rifampin has been used successfully in leprosy, brucellosis, chancroid, lymphogranuloma venereum, gonorrhea, and chlamydial urethritis.[88,96] Rosenberg and associates used rifampin in combination with penicillin or erythromycin to treat streptococcal-associated psoriasis.[97]

Contraindications

Contraindications to the use of rifampin include pregnancy (except for patients with severe tuberculosis infection) and known hypersensitivity to the drug. The drug should be avoided by patients with jaundice or impaired liver function, especially if other potentially hepatotoxic drugs are taken concomitantly.

Adverse Effects

The adverse effects encountered with the use of rifampin are related to the dosage and duration of therapy. Patients who receive short courses of the drug experience very few side effects, primarily red discoloration of urine and tears (the latter may cause permanent staining of contact lenses). Treatment regimens entailing intermittent administration of rifampin are associated with an increased incidence of hypersensitivity reactions, particularly a flu-like syndrome.[88]

HEPATIC EFFECTS. Hepatic toxicity occurs in 5%–14% of patients and is usually manifested by a mild transient elevation of serum bilirubin, alkaline phosphatase, and aminotransferases. Rifampin appears to increase the possibility of the hepatotoxic effects of isoniazid and other potentially hepatotoxic drugs.[98,99]

CUTANEOUS EFFECTS. Cutaneous adverse effects occur in up to 5% of patients. These include urticaria, pruritus, maculopapular eruptions, and drug-induced pemphigus. Acute rifampin overdose causes an orange-red discoloration of the skin, termed "red man" syndrome.[98]

OTHER ADVERSE EFFECTS. Other uncommon adverse effects associated with rifampin include anorexia, nausea, pseudomembranous colitis, dizziness, drowsiness, headache, and visual disturbance. In addition to the flu-like syndrome mentioned earlier, other hypersensitivity reactions include immune thrombocytopenic purpura, hemolytic anemia, and acute renal failure.[98]

Drug Interactions

Rifampin is associated with a number of drug interactions. Three drugs that have been reported to decrease serum rifampin levels are para-aminosalicylic acid, probenecid, and ketoconazole. Rifampin is a potent inducer of hepatic microsomal enzymes. This results in enhanced hepatic metabolism and a decreased half-life of various drugs, including corticosteroids, digitoxin, metoprolol, propranolol, chloramphenicol, clofibrate, progestins, oral contraceptives, oral sulfonylureas, quinidine, verapamil, heroin, methadone, warfarin, and dapsone.[98] There have been some reports of synergistic hepatotoxicity in patients treated with rifampin and isoniazid.[60]

CIPROFLOXACIN (CIPRO)

Nalidixic acid, the forerunner of the quinolone antimicrobials, was discovered serendipitously during chloroquine synthesis in the early 1960s. Although effective against gram-negative urinary tract infections, nalidixic acid was not found to be useful in treating other systemic infections. The quinolones that were introduced in the 1970s, such as cinoxacin and oxolinic acid, were not much more effective than nalidixic acid.[100]

The addition of fluorine into the basic nucleus extended greatly the antibacterial spectrum of the quinolones. These third-generation quinolones (fluoroquinolones) include norfloxacin, ciprofloxacin, enoxacin, ofloxacin, pefloxacin, temafloxacin, and others.[101] Norfloxacin and ciprofloxacin were the first to be approved for use in the U.S.

Pharmacology

Structure

Ciprofloxacin, like the other third-generation quinolones, is a 6-fluoro, 7-piperazinyl substituted fluoroquinolone.

Absorption/Distribution

Ciprofloxacin is rapidly absorbed after oral administration. Peak serum concentrations of 1–3 mcg/ml are obtained within 1–3 hours after a standard oral dose of 500 mg. Concomitant administration of aluminum- and magnesium-containing antacids reduces absorption,[100] and food intake slows absorption.[102] Because ciprofloxacin is a small molecular substance with low serum protein binding, it is distributed widely in body tissues and penetrates blister fluid readily.[101, 103] The serum half-life of the drug is 3–4 hours.[103]

Metabolism/Excretion

Ciprofloxacin undergoes some degree of hepatic metabolism. Metabolites constitute from 15%–30% of the drug recoverable in the urine. The drug may accumulate in patients with hepatic insufficiency.[100] Renal excretion of ciprofloxacin occurs by both glomerular filtration and tubular secretion. Significantly decreased renal function prolongs the serum half-life of the drug and requires a dosage adjustment.[100]

Mechanism of Action

The mechanism of action of quinolone antibiotics is based on their inhibition of bacterial DNA gyrase. The functions of this enzyme are to maintain the bacterial chromosome in its supercoiled state and to repair nicks in DNA that occur during the process of transcription. Inhibition of this enzyme accounts for the bactericidal activity of the quinolones.[104]

Clinical Use

Indications

Ciprofloxacin is FDA-approved for the treatment of skin infections caused by E. coli, Klebsiella pneumoniae, Enterobacter cloacae, Proteus mirabilis, Proteus vulgaris, Providencia stuartii, Morganella morganii, Citrobacter freundii, Pseudomonas aeruginosa, S. aureus, S. epidermidis, and Streptococcus pyogenes.

CUTANEOUS INFECTIONS. Various clinical trials of ciprofloxacin in skin and soft-tissue infections have shown cure rates of 70%–100%.[105–109] In a large, controlled trial, the effectiveness of oral ciprofloxacin was shown to be equivalent to that of intravenous cefotaxime in the treatment of skin infections caused primarily by S. aureus or gram-negative bacilli.[108] Ciprofloxacin is not a first-line drug for most mild to moderate skin infections due to staphylococci and streptococci. These can be treated as effectively and more economically with beta-lactam agents such as dicloxacillin. Ciprofloxacin does hold an important place in the treatment of certain problematic skin infections such as diabetic foot ulcers, infected decubitus ulcers, lower limb infections, and perianal cellulitis, because of its efficacy against *P. aeruginosa* and other gram-negative organisms. Ciprofloxacin is one of the few oral agents effective against methicillin-resistant *S. aureus*.[110]

SEXUALLY TRANSMITTED DISEASES. Another area in which ciprofloxacin is playing an increasingly important role is the treatment of sexually transmitted diseases. The quinolones are active against both penicillinase-producing and chromosomally mediated resistant *Neisseria gonorrhoeae*. A single oral dose of 250 mg of ciprofloxacin has been shown to be curative in 98.7% of men with uncomplicated urethral gonorrhea. The drug is generally not effective in the treatment of chlamydial and nongonococcal infections.[111] *Haemophilus ducreyi* is particularly susceptible to ciprofloxacin. A single 500-mg dose and a 3-day regimen of 500 mg of ciprofloxacin twice a day have both been shown to be highly effective against chancroid. The 3-day regimen produced slightly better results.[112] Although there are few clinical data available, it appears that the quinolones will not be useful in the treatment of syphilis or bacterial vaginosis.[111]

Contraindications

Ciprofloxacin should not be used by children, adolescents, or pregnant or nursing women. Persons with a history of hypersensitivity to quinolone antibiotics should also avoid the drug. The contraindication in patients younger than 18 years of age is based on animal studies that showed that the drug caused cartilage lesions in weight-bearing joints when it was administered to immature dogs (see Cipro package insert). Cross-allergenicity with penicillins and cephalosporins has not been reported.

Adverse Effects

The quinolones usually cause few side effects. The most frequent complaint (by 5.2% of patients) during the use of ciprofloxacin is of nausea. Other adverse reactions such as diarrhea, vomiting, and headache are mild and occur in 2% of patients or fewer. Laboratory abnormalities that occur in fewer than 2% of patients who are taking ciprofloxacin include elevation of liver enzymes, eosinophilia, and crystalluria.[113]

Drug Interactions

The primary drug interaction of concern with ciprofloxacin is that with theophylline. Concurrent administration of the two drugs may lead to elevated plasma levels of theophylline and result in theophylline-related adverse reactions. By the same mechanism (interference with hepatic metabolism), serum concentrations of warfarin may be elevated in patients taking ciprofloxacin. Probenecid interferes with renal tubular secretion of ciprofloxacin, thereby increasing serum levels of the latter. Concomitant use of cyclosporine and quinolones may increase the nephrotoxic effect of cyclosporine. Antacids interfere with gastrointestinal absorption of ciprofloxacin.[60]

METRONIDAZOLE (FLAGYL, PROTOSTAT)

Metronidazole is the first of the nitroimidazole group of antibiotics. It is the only one approved for use in the U.S. It was discovered in 1956 by the Rhone-Poulenc Laboratories in France after an intensive search for a drug effective against *Trichomonas vaginalis*. [114]

Pharmacology

Structure

Metronidazole is a low molecular weight 5-nitroimidazole with the chemical name 1-(beta-hydroxyethyl)-2-methyl-5-nitroimidazole.[115] Other members of this class of drugs include tinidazole and ornidazole.

Absorption/Distribution

Oral metronidazole is well absorbed from the gastrointestinal tract, with 80% absorption within 1 hour after administration.[116] Peak serum concentrations of approximately 6.0 mcg/ml are achieved within 1–3 hours after a single 250-mg dose. Concomitant food ingestion delays absorption but does not decrease the peak serum levels obtained. Serum half-life varies from 7.0 to 8.7 hours. The drug diffuses well into all tissues, including bones, the gallbladder, cerebrospinal fluid, and hepatic and brain abscesses.[115]

Metabolism/Excretion

The drug is metabolized in the liver into acid and hydroxyl metabolites, which are excreted in the urine. Approximately 14% and 15% of an oral dose of the drug are excreted unchanged in the feces and urine, respectively.[115] The dosage does not have to be altered for patients with renal insufficiency, but it should be reduced for patients with hepatic insufficiency, and serum drug levels should in addition be monitored.[117]

Mechanism of Action

The mechanism of action of metronidazole is only partially understood. The nitro group at position 5 of metronidazole undergoes electrochemical reduction within the cells of organisms that possess nitroreductase. During this process, highly cytotoxic, but labile, intermediates of the parent compound that are lethal to bacterial DNA are formed. Because of this unique mode of action, the activity spectrum of metronidazole is primarily restricted to obligate anaerobes that can reduce the drug.[114]

Clinical Use

Indications

Metronidazole is FDA-approved for the treatment of cutaneous infections due to *Bacteroides species*, including the *B. fragilis* group, *Clostridium* species, *Peptococcus* species, and *Fusobacterium* species.

Metronidazole is as effective as tetracycline in the treatment of rosacea, but it is not generally used for this purpose because of safety concerns in long-term use.[118] Topical metronidazole has been released for use in rosacea. One report described a case of perianal and vulval Crohn's disease that cleared completely during a 4-month course of metronidazole.[119]

Contraindications

Contraindications to the use of metronidazole include a serious hypersensitivity reaction to the drug, which is rare. Patients with hepatic disease or a history of seizures should be carefully monitored while taking the drug.[114] Although no direct evidence of teratogenicity exists, it is prudent to avoid use of metronidazole during pregnancy, especially during the first trimester.[115]

Adverse Effects

The most common side effects of metronidazole, occurring in 5%–10% of patients, are gastrointestinal symptoms such as anorexia, metallic taste, nausea, vomiting, and diarrhea. The most serious adverse reactions are neurologic symptoms and include peripheral neuropathy, ataxia, headaches, convulsions, and encephalopathy. These effects usually occur after prolonged administration with high doses or in patients with hepatic failure.[120] Use of the drug for longer than 3 months should be avoided because of the risk of sensory peripheral neuropathy.[121] Pseudomembranous colitis has been reported after metronidazole administration.[122]

The urine of patients on metronidazole may be red-brown because of the presence of an azo metabolite of the drug.[115] The serum aspartate aminotransferase or AST (serum glutamate oxaloacetic transaminase or SGOT) of patients taking metronidazole may be falsely decreased because of interference with the standard laboratory assay.[123]

Various animal studies have shown carcinogenic effects of metronidazole. Other animal studies have been negative. Although there is no evidence of carcinogenicity in humans thus far, the question is not settled.[124]

Drug Interactions

Drug interactions with metronidazole include a disulfiram-like reaction that occurs in approximately 10% of patients who consume ethanol while taking the drug.[125] Patients should be warned to avoid alcoholic beverages and pharmaceutical preparations containing alcohol throughout metronidazole therapy and for 48 hours after discontinuing the drug.[114] Alcoholic patients taking disulfiram may experience an acute psychotic state from concurrent ingestion of metronidazole.[126] Metronidazole increases the plasma half-life of racemic sodium warfarin, which results in a hypoprothrombinemic effect.[127] Simultaneous administration of cimetidine decreases the plasma clearance and prolongs the half-life of metronidazole.[128] Increased metabolism, and shorter half-life, of metronidazole may occur when the drug is given concurrently with phenobarbital or phenytoin.[60]

CLINDAMYCIN (CLEOCIN)

Clindamycin, a derivative of lincomycin, binds to the 50s subunit of bacterial ribosomes and inhibits protein synthesis. It is FDA-approved for the treatment of serious cutaneous infections caused by susceptible anaerobes, S. aureus, and S. pyogenes. Pseudomembranous colitis has been estimated to occur in 0.01%–10% of patients on oral clindamycin.[129] With this risk accounted for, the drug is indicated primarily for serious infections in which a less toxic alternative is not available. One possible use for oral clindamycin is in antibiotic-resistant nodulocystic acne in which isotretinoin is contraindicated. The patient should be instructed to discontinue the drug at the first sign of diarrhea. The drug can be administered by the oral, intramuscular, or intravenous routes.[130, 131]

VANCOMYCIN (VANCOCIN)

Vancomycin, a glycopeptide antibiotic, was introduced for clinical use in 1958. Its current clinical uses are primarily the treatment of staphylococcal infections due to antibiotic-resistant strains and the treatment of antibiotic-associated colitis. Vancomycin is not well absorbed after oral administration. It is usually administered intravenously to treat systemic infections, but it is used orally for antibiotic-associated colitis.

AZTREONAM (AZACTAM)

Aztreonam is a member of the monobactams, a new class of beta-lactam antibiotics synthesized by bacteria. The antibacterial spectrum of activity of aztreonam is almost entirely against gram-negative aerobic rods such as *Pseudomonas aeruginosa* and *Enterobacteriaceae*. It is not effective against gram-positive bacteria and anaerobes. Clinical uses of the drug include gram-negative infections such as septicemia, respiratory tract infection, osteomyelitis, urinary tract infection, and intra-abdominal infections. Aztreonam is not well absorbed by the oral route and is usually administered parenterally.[62]

COMMON CLINICAL SCENARIOS

STAPHYLOCOCCAL INFECTIONS. Staphylococcal skin infections can present in a variety of guises, such as folliculitis, furuncles, carbuncles, bullous impetigo, and cellulitis. S. aureus is the most common cause of secondary infections of primary skin conditions such as atopic eczema, contact dermatitis, burns, surgical wounds, and epidermal inclusion cysts. The treatment of choice for S. aureus cutaneous infections is a penicillinase-resistant semisynthetic penicillin such as dicloxacillin. For penicillin-allergic patients, there are a wide variety of alternative agents from which to choose, including oral cephalosporins, erythromycin, amoxicillin-clavulanate, clindamycin, trimethoprim-sulfamethoxazole, and ciprofloxacin. Antibiotic selection may be influenced by a variety of factors, such as cost, dosage, and drug interactions. For example, a busy patient who can afford the extra cost might prefer the convenience of once-a-day dosing with cefadroxil. An asthmatic patient taking theophylline and who is penicillin-allergic should not be prescribed erythromycin or ciprofloxacin because of a potential drug interaction that could result in theophylline toxicity. In this circumstance, an oral cephalosporin would be a better choice; one should, however, keep in mind the 10% rate of cross-reaction in penicillin-allergic patients. Another factor to consider is changing rates of resistance to various antibiotics. In some populations, a high percentage of patients with S. aureus show resistance to erythromycin, which makes that drug a poor choice for empirical therapy of skin infections.[132, 133] However, because erythromycin is much less expensive than dicloxacillin, it is still a reasonable choice as a first-line agent for mild to moderate skin infections in penicillin-allergic patients.

Patients with recurrent furunculosis due to nasal carriage of S. aureus may be treated with long-term systemic antibiotics, such as dicloxacillin, erythromycin, clindamycin, or ciprofloxacin. Rifampin, in combination with other antistaphylococcal agents such as dicloxacillin or TMP–SMX, is also an effective therapy. These oral agents may be used in conjunction with topical measures such as bathing with antibacterial soap and applying topical antibiotics in the nose. The topical measures may be tried alone initially.

STREPTOCOCCAL INFECTIONS. Streptococcal skin infections can take the form of impetigo contagiosa, ecthyma, erysipelas, cellulitis, and blistering distal dactylitis. Although in group A beta-hemolytic streptococcus was in the past the primary pathogen causing impetigo contagiosa, more recent studies have shown a shift to a predominance of S. aureus.[132, 134] This transition in the bacteria responsible for superficial skin infections has resulted in a change in patterns of antibiotic usage. Oral penicillin is no longer the treatment of choice for the empirical treatment of impetigo. It has been replaced by penicillinase-resistant penicillins or erythromycin, which provide better coverage of S. aureus. The streptococcal carrier state may be eliminated by combination therapy with rifampin and penicillin.[135, 136]

PSEUDOMONAS INFECTIONS. P. aeruginosa may be the pathogen in a variety of cutaneous infections, including subungual infections, otitis externa, toe web intertrigo, infected diabetic foot ulcers, and infected decubitus ulcers. Ciprofloxacin provides good oral therapy on an outpatient basis for selected patients with these infections, which otherwise might require parenteral therapy. Hot tub folliculitis, which is also caused by P. aeruginosa, resolves spontaneously without antibiotic therapy. However, in our experience, the signs and symptoms of this condition resolve faster when treated with ciprofloxacin.

GRAM-NEGATIVE FOLLICULITIS. Gram-negative folliculitis is a complication of antibiotic therapy for acne vulgaris in which the patient develops either superficial pustules or deep nodules and cysts. Culture of the lesions grows gram-negative organisms such as *Proteus mirabilis*, *Klebsiella species*, or *Enterobacter* species. Reports in the literature describe successful therapy for gram-negative folliculitis with ampicillin and isotretinoin.[58, 137] Although the choice of antibiotics should be guided by the results of sensitivities, two other antibiotics that are likely to be effective in this setting are amoxicillin-clavulanate and ciprofloxacin.

LYME BORRELIOSIS. Erythema chronicum migrans is one of the cutaneous manifestations of Lyme borreliosis. Treatment recommendations have continued to change as more research on this tick-borne infection is conducted. One problem in evaluating therapeutic modalities is the lack of reliable microbiologic or immunologic criteria for diagnosis or cure of this infection. Although both penicillin and tetracycline have been shown to be efficacious, they are not uniformly effective. In a review article, Luft and colleagues recommended a more aggressive approach than the standard therapy of 1 g of tetracycline a day for the early stages of the disease.[36] Their best treatment options for early-stage Lyme disease are 100 mg of doxycycline two or three times a day for 21 days, 100 mg of minocycline twice a day for 21 days, or 500–1000 mg of amoxicillin three times a day for 21 days plus 500 mg of probenecid three times a day for 21 days. An alternative therapy is 250 mg of erythromycin four times a day for 10–21 days, but this regimen may be less effective. If tetracycline is to be used, Luft and colleagues recommend a dosage of 500 mg four times a day.[36] Jarisch-Herxheimer reactions have been reported to occur in some erythema chronicum migrans patients after treatment.

ANAEROBIC INFECTIONS. Skin and soft-tissue infections involving anaerobic bacteria range from the commonplace (infected epidermal cysts) to the serious and life-threatening (necrotizing fasciitis). Other infections in the latter group include synergistic necrotizing cellulitis, anaerobic cellulitis, bite wounds, and infected vascular gangrene. The antibiotic regimen chosen should be active against both coliforms and anaerobes. This includes agents such as an aminoglycoside plus either clindamycin, metronidazole, chloramphenicol, cefoxitin, or an antipseudomonal penicillin. Surgical débridement is also important.[138] In one series of infected epidermal cysts, anaerobic bacteria, either alone or in mixed infections with aerobes, were recovered in 56% of 231 specimens. Anaerobes were isolated more frequently in cyst abscesses in the perirectal, valvovaginal, and head areas.[139] Surgical drainage is the treatment of choice for cyst abscesses; however, in certain severe cases or in immunocompromised patients, systemic antibiotics may be indicated. Regimens that are active against S. aureus, as well as against anaerobic bacteria, include cefoxitin, clindamycin, imipenem-cilastin, and the combination of beta-lactamase inhibitors and penicillin. An alternative is the combination of metronidazole and a penicillinase-resistant penicillin.[139]

ANTIBIOTICS IN PREGNANCY. Because dermatologists often prescribe long-term oral antibiotics to young women for acne, the topic of antibiotics in pregnancy is particularly relevant to dermatologists. Tetracycline should not be used during pregnancy because of the increased risk of developing fatty liver, the risk of tooth staining in the fetus, the possible effects on bone growth, and other possible teratogenic effects.

On the other hand, if a woman inadvertently takes tetracycline during the first few weeks of pregnancy, it is extremely unlikely to be teratogenic.[19] Erythromycin and erythromycin ethylsuccinate are generally considered to be safe for both the pregnant woman and her fetus when administered for only a few weeks. There are no studies evaluating the long-term use of erythromycin in pregnancy.[19] When faced with short-term antibiotic use for cutaneous infections, penicillins are generally considered safe in pregnancy. Most newer antibiotics have not had sufficient sporadic use in pregnancy to be regarded even as "probably safe" for use in pregnancy.

In general, avoidance of any systemic drug during the first trimester is prudent. After that time, informed consent by the patient and concurrence by the delivering physician with regard to specific drug use are appropriate steps to take.

BIBLIOGRAPHY: Key Reviews/Chapters

Reboldi AC, Delbene VE. Oral antibiotic therapy of dermatologic conditions. Dermatol Clin 1988; 6:497–520.
Feingold DS, Wagner RF. Antibacterial therapy. J Am Acad Dermatol 1986; 14:535–548.
Rothman KF, Pochi PE: Use of oral and topical agents for acne in pregnancy. J Am Acad Dermatol 1988; 19:431–442.
1985 STD treatment guidelines. J Am Acad Dermatol 1986; 14:707–726.

REFERENCES

Tetracyclines

1. Pratt WB, Fekety R: Bacteriostatic inhibitors of protein synthesis [Tetracycline]. In The Antimicrobial Drugs. New York: Oxford University Press, 1986, 205–228.
2. Jonas M, Comer JB, Cunha BA: Tetracyclines. In Ristuccia AM, Cunha BA (eds): Antimicrobial Therapy. New York: Raven Press, 1984, 219–234.
3. Williams DN: Tetracyclines. In Peterson PK, Verhoef J (eds): The Antimicrobial Agents Annual 3. Amsterdam: Elsevier, 1988, 218–228.
4. Chopra I, Howe TGB, Linton AH, et al: The tetracyclines: Prospects at the beginning of the 1980s. J Antimicrob Chemother 1981; 8:5–21.
5. Kakemi K, Sezaki H, Ogata H, et al: Absorption and excretion of drugs. XXXVI. Effect of Ca2+ on the absorption of tetracycline from the small intestine. Chem Pharm Bull (Tokyo) 1968; 16:2200–2205.
6. Neuvonen PJ: Interactions with the absorption of tetracyclines. Drugs 1976; 11:45–54.
7. Neuvonen PJ, Gothoni G, Hackman R, et al: Interference of iron with the absorption of tetracyclines in man. Br Med J (Clin Res) 1970; 4:532–534.
8. Leyden JJ: Absorption of minocycline hydrochloride and tetracycline hydrochloride: Effect of food, milk, and iron. J Am Acad Dermatol 1985; 12:308–312.
9. Kunin CM, Finland M: Clinical pharmacology of the tetracycline antibiotics. Clin Pharmacol Ther 1961; 2:51–69.
10. Cunliffe WJ: The conventional treatment of acne. Sem Dermatol 1983; 2(2):138–144.

11. Esterly NB, Furey NL, Flanagan LE: The effect of antimicrobial agents on leukocyte chemotaxis. J Invest Dermatol 1978; 70:51–55.
12. Hubbell CG, Hobbs ER, Rist T, et al: Efficacy of minocycline compared with tetracycline in treatment of acne vulgaris. Arch Dermatol 1982; 118:984992.
13. Thornfeldt CR, Menkes AW: Bullous pemphigoid controlled by tetracycline. J Am Acad Dermatol 1987; 16:305–310.
14. Stein HB, Schlappner OLA, Boyko W, et al: The intestinal bypass: Arthritis–dermatitis syndrome. Arthritis Rheum 1981; 24:684–690.
15. Piamphongsant T: Tetracycline for the treatment of pityriasis lichenoides. Br J Dermatol 1974; 91:319–322.
16. Lynch WS, Bergfeld WF: Pyoderma gangrenosum responsive to minocycline hydrochloride. Cutis 1978; 21:535–538.
17. Davies MG, Piper S: Pyoderma gangrenosum: Successful treatment with minocycline. Clin Exp Dermatol 1981; 6:219–223.
18. Thomsen K: Mycosis fungoides responding to tetracycline and griseofulvin [letter]. Br J Dermatol 1981; 105:483–484.
19. Rothman KF, Pochi PE: Use of oral and topical agents for acne in pregnancy. J Am Acad Dermatol 1988; 19:431–442.
20. Fellner MJ, Ledesina GN, Miller D: Adverse reactions to antibiotics other than penicillin. Clin Dermatol 1986; 4(1):142–148.
21. Ferguson J, Frain-Bell W: Pigmentary disorders and systemic drug therapy. Clin Dermatol 1989; 7(2):44–54.
22. Schultz JC, Adams JS Jr, Workman WW, et al: Fatal liver disease after intravenous administration of tetracycline in high doses. N Engl J Med 1963; 269:999–1004.
23. Walters BNJ, Gubbay SS: Tetracycline and benign intracranial hypertension: Report of five cases. Br Med J 1981; 282:19–20.
24. Williams DN, Laughlin LW, Lee YH: Minocycline: Possible vestibular side effects. Lancet 1974; 2:744–746.
25. Sande MA, Mandell GL: Antimicrobial agents: Tetracyclines, chloramphenicol, erythromycin and miscellaneous antibacterial agents. In Gilman AG, Goodman LS, Rall TW, et al (eds): Goodman and Gilman's The Pharmacological Basis of Therapeutics (7th ed). New York: Macmillan, 1985, 1170–1189.
26. Kuzucu EY: Methoxyflurane, tetracycline, and renal failure. JAMA 1977; 211:712–717.
27. Fleischer AB Jr, Resnick SD: The effect of antibiotics on the efficacy of oral contraceptives: A controversy revisited. Arch Dermatol 1989; 125:1562–1564.

Erythromycin

28. Chow AW: Erythromycin. In Ristuccia AM, Cunha BA (eds): Antimicrobial Therapy. New York: Raven Press, 1984, 209–218.
29. Auckenthaler RW, Zwahlen A, Waldvogel FA: Macrolides. In Peterson PK, Verhoef J (eds): The Antimicrobial Agents Annual 3. Amsterdam: Elsevier, 1988, 122–137.
30. Steigbigel NH. Erythromycin, lincomycin, and clindamycin. In Mandell GL, Douglas RG Jr, Bennett JE (eds): Anti-Infective Therapy. New York: John Wiley, 1985, 197–218.
31. Washington JA II, Wilson WR: Erythromycin: A microbial and clinical perspective after 30 years of clinical use (1). Mayo Clin Proc 1985; 60:189–203.
32. Pratt WB, Fekety R: Bacteriostatic inhibitors of protein synthesis [Erythromycin]. In The Antimicrobial Drugs. New York: Oxford University Press, 1986, 195–200.
33. Washington JA II, Wilson WR: Erythromycin: A microbial and clinical perspective after 30 years of clinical use (2). Mayo Clin Proc 1985; 60:271–278.

34. Modai J: The clinical use of macrolides. J Antimicrob Chemother 1988; 22(Suppl B):145–153.
35. Ginsburg CM, Eichenwald HF: Erythromycin: A review of its use in pediatric practice. J Pediatr 1986; 89:872–884.
36. Luft BJ, Gorevic PD, Halperin JJ, et al: A perspective on the treatment of Lyme borreliosis. Rev Infect Dis 1989; 11(Suppl 6):S1518-S1525.
37. Dutz W, Kohout-Dutz E: Anthrax. Int J Dermatol 1981; 20:203–206.
38. Richtsmeier WJ, Johns ME: Actinomycosis of the head and neck. Crit Rev Clin Lab Sci 1979; 11:175–202.
39. Fiumara NJ, Rothman K, Tang S: The diagnosis and treatment of chancroid. J Am Acad Dermatol 1986; 15:939–943.
40. Sehgal VN, Prasad ALS: Donovanosis: Current concepts. Int J Dermatol 1986; 25:8–16.
41. Eady EA, Holland KT, Cunliffe WJ: The use of antibiotics in acne therapy: Oral or topical administration? J Antimicrob Chemother 1982; 10:89–115.
42. Brown LA: Pathogenesis and treatment of pseudofolliculitis barbae. Cutis 1983; 32:373–375.
43. Cutler TP: Eosinophilic pustular folliculitis. Clin Exp Dermatol 1981; 6:327–332.
44. Fox BJ, Odom RB, Findlay RF: Erythromycin therapy in bullous pemphigoid: Possible anti-inflammatory effects. J Am Acad Dermatol 1982; 7:504–510.
45. Shavin JS, Jones TM, Aton JK, et al: Mucha-Habermann's disease in children: Treatment with erythromycin. Arch Dermatol 1978; 114:1679–1680.
46. Truhan AP, Hebert AA, Esterly NB: Pityriasis lichenoides in children: Therapeutic response to erythromycin. J Am Acad Dermatol 1986; 15:66–70.
47. Gantz NM, Zawacki JK, Dickerson J, et al: Pseudomembranous colitis associated with erythromycin. Ann Intern Med 1979; 91:866–867.
48. Ginsburg CM: Macrolide antibiotics. In Koren G, Prober CG, Gold R (eds): Antimicrobial Therapy in Infants and Children. New York: Marcel Dekker, 1988, 339–354.

Penicillins

49. Neu HC: Penicillins. In Mandell GL, Douglas RG Jr, Bennett JE (eds): Anti-Infective Therapy. New York: John Wiley, 1985, 37–75.
50. Eng RHK: New antibiotics: New hopes and new problems. Int J Dermatol 1984; 23:153–165.
51. Lisby SM, Nahata MC: Penicillins. In Koren G, Prober CG, Gold R (eds): Antimicrobial Therapy in Infants and Children. New York: Marcel Dekker, 1988, 117–152.
52. Molavi A, LeFrock JL: Antistaphylococcal penicillins. In Ristuccia AM, Cunha BA (eds): Antimicrobial Therapy. New York: Raven Press, 1984, 183–195.
53. Neu HC: Antistaphylococcal penicillins. Med Clin North Am 1982; 66:51–60.
54. Georgopapadakou NH: Penicillin-binding proteins. In Peterson PK, Verhoef J (eds): The Antimicrobial Agents Annual 3. Amsterdam: Elsevier, 1988, 409–431.
55. Feingold DS, Wagner RF Jr: Antibacterial therapy. J Am Acad Dermatol 1986; 14:535–548.
56. Rehm SJ, McHenry MC: Oral antimicrobial drugs. Med Clin North Am 1983; 67:57–98.
57. Shore RN: Usefulness of ampicillin in treatment of acne vulgaris. J Am Acad Dermatol 1983; 9:604–605.
58. Leyden JJ, Marples RR, Mills OH Jr, et al: Gram-negative folliculitis—A complication of antibiotic therapy in acne vulgaris. Br J Dermatol 1973; 8:533–538.
59. Pratt WB, Fekety R: The inhibitors of cell wall synthesis, II. In The Antimicrobial Drugs. New York: Oxford University Press, 1986, 113–152.
60. Olin BR: Facts and Comparisons: Drug Information. St. Louis: J.B. Lippincott, 1989.

Cephalosporins

61. Mandell GL: Cephalosporins. In Mandell GL, Douglas RG Jr, Bennett JE, (eds): Anti-Infective Therapy. New York: John Wiley, 1985, 76–94.
62. Thompson RL: Cephalosporins, carbapenem, and monobactam antibiotics. Mayo Clin Proc 1987; 62:821–834.
63. Quintiliani R, Nightingale CH, Rossi JG, et al: Cephalosporins: An overview. In Ristuccia AM, Cunha BA (eds): Antimicrobial Therapy. New York: Raven Press, 1984: 289–303.
64. Tanrisever B, Santella PJ. Cefadroxil: A review of its antibacterial, pharmacokinetic and therapeutic properties in comparison with cephalexin and cephradine. Drugs 1986; 32(Suppl 3):1–16.

Amoxicillin–Potassium Clavulanate

65. Stein GE, Gurwith MJ: Amoxicillin–potassium clavulanate, a beta-lactamase-resistant antibiotic combination. Clin Pharm 1984; 3:591–599.
66. Weber DJ, Tolkoff-Rubin NE, Rubin R: Amoxicillin and potassium clavulanate: An antibiotic combination. Pharmacotherapy 1984; 4:122–136.
67. Adam D, Visser ID, Koeppe P: Pharmacokinetics of amoxicillin and clavulanic acid administered alone and in combination. Antimicrob Agents Chemother 1982; 22:353–357.
68. Anonymous: Amoxicillin–clavulanic acid (Augmentin). Med Lett Drugs Ther 1984; 26:99–100.
69. DeKoning GAJ, Tio D, Coster JF, et al: The combination of clavulanic acid and amoxicillin (Augmentin) in the treatment of patients infected with penicillinase-producing gonococci. J Antimicrob Chemother 1981; 8:81–82.
70. Lim VKE, Bakar R, Hussin Z: Single dose oral amoxicillin and clavulanic acid in the treatment of gonococcal urethritis in males. Med J Malaysia 1982; 37:235–238.
71. Fast MV, Nsanze H, D'Costa LJ, et al: Treatment of chancroid by clavulanic acid with amoxicillin in patients with beta-lactamase positive *Haemophilus ducreyi* infection. Lancet 1982; 2:509–511.

Trimethoprim-Sulfamethoxazole

72. Pratt WB, Fekety R: The antimetabolites. In The Antimicrobial Drugs. New York: Oxford University Press, 1986, 229–251.
73. Salter AJ: Trimethoprim-sulfamethoxazole: An assessment of more than 12 years of use. Rev Infect Dis 1982; 4:196–236.
74. Smith LG, Sensakovic J: Trimethoprim–sulfamethoxazole. Med Clin North Am 1982; 66:143–156.
75. Brumfitt W, Faiers MC, Pursell RE, et al: Bacteriological, pharmacological and clinical studies with trimethoprim-sulfonamide combinations. Postgrad Med J 1969; 45(Nov Suppl):56–61.
76. Brumfitt W, Hamilton-Miller JMT: Trimethoprim-sulfamethoxazole. In Ristuccia AM, Cunha BA (eds): Antimicrobial Therapy. New York: Raven Press, 1984, 277–288.
77. Svindland HB: Treatment of gonorrhea with sulphamethoxazole-trimethoprim: Lack of effect on concomitant syphilis. Br J Vener Dis 1973; 49:50–53.
78. Lawrence A, Phillips I, Nicol C: Various regimens of trimethoprim-sulfamethoxazole used in the treatment of gonorrhea. J Infect Dis 1973; 128(Suppl):S673–S678.
79. Stamm WE, Guinan ME, Johnson C, et al: Effect of treatment regimens for *Neisseria gonorrhoea* on simultaneous infection with *Chlamydia trachomatis*. N Engl J Med 1984; 310:545–549.
80. Nordin K, Hallander H, Fredriksson T, et al: A clinical and bacteriological evaluation

of the effect of sulphamethoxazole-trimethoprim in acne vulgaris, resistant to prior therapy with tetracyclines. Dermatologica 1978; 157:245–253.
81. Craig WA, Kunin CM: Trimethoprim-sulfamethoxazole: Pharmacodynamic effects of urinary pH and impaired renal function: Studies in humans. Ann Intern Med 1973; 78:491–497.
82. Jick H: Adverse reactions to trimethoprim-sulfamethoxazole in hospitalized patients. Rev Infect Dis 1982; 4:426–428.
83. Lawson DH, Paice BJ: Adverse reactions to trimethoprim-sulfamethoxazole. Rev Infect Dis 1982; 4:429–433.
84. Cockerill FR III, Edson RS: Trimethoprim-sulfamethoxazole. Mayo Clin Proc 1987; 69:921–929.
85. Jaffe HS, Abrams DI, Ammann AJ, et al: Complications of co-trimoxazole in treatment of AIDS-associated *Pneumocystis carinii* pneumonia in homosexual men. Lancet 1983; 2:1109–1111.

Rifampin

86. Sensi P: History of the development of rifampin. Rev Infect Dis 1983; 5(Suppl 3):S402–S406.
87. Kapusnik JE, Sande MA: Rifampin. *In* Peterson PK, Verhoef J (eds): The Antimicrobial Agents Annual 3. Amsterdam: Elsevier, 1988, 203–217.
88. Farr B, Mandell GL: Rifampin. *In* Mandell GL, Douglas RG Jr, Bennett JE (eds): Anti-Infective Therapy. New York: Wiley, 1985, 175–184.
89. Yoshikawa TT, Norman DC: Rifampin. *In* Ristuccia AM, Cunha BA (eds): Antimicrobial Therapy. New York: Raven Press, 1984, 335–337.
90. Ellison RT III, Judson FN, Peterson LC, et al: Oral rifampin and trimethoprim/sulfamethoxazole therapy in asymptomatic carriers of methicillin-resistant *Staphylococcus aureus* infections. West J Med 1984; 140:735–740.
91. Finley RS, Schimpff SC, Fortner CL, et al: Rifampin and cloxacillin in the reduction of staphylococcal colonization. Clin Pharmacol 1982; 1:370–372.
92. Dixson S, Brumfitt W, Hamilton-Miller JMT: Activity of rifampicin against staphylococci, with special reference to multi-resistant strains. J Antimicrob Chemother 1984; 13(Suppl C):7–16.
93. Ward TT, Winn RE, Harstein AI, et al: Observations relating to an interhospital outbreak of methicillin-resistant *Staphylococcus aureus*: Role of antimicrobial therapy in infection control. Infect Control 1981; 2:453–455.
94. Walsh TJ, Auger FA, Tatem BA, et al: Novobiocin and rifampin in combination against methicillin-resistant *Staphylococcus aureus*: An in-vitro comparison with vancomycin plus rifampin. J Antimicrob Chemother 1986; 17:75–82.
95. Lorber B: Rifampin in chronic granulomatous disease. N Engl J Med 1980; 303:111.
96. Bullock WE: Rifampin in the treatment of leprosy. Rev Infect Dis 1983; 5(Suppl 3):S606–S613.
97. Rosenberg EW, Noah PW, Zanolli MD, et al: Use of rifampin with penicillin and erythromycin in the treatment of psoriasis. J Am Acad Dermatol 1986; 14:761–764.
98. Shalit I. Rifampin. *In* Koren G, Prober CG, Gold R (eds): Antimicrobial Therapy in Infants and Children. New York: Marcel Dekker, 1988, 373–403.
99. Grosset J, Leventis S: Adverse effects of rifampin. Rev Infect Dis 1983; 5(Suppl 3):S440–S446.

Ciprofloxacin

100. Norris S, Mandell GL: The quinolones: History and overview. *In* Andriole VT (ed): The Quinolones. London: Academic Press, 1988, 1–22.

101. Bergan T. Quinolones. *In* Peterson PK, Verhoef J (eds): The Antimicrobial Agents Annual 3. Amsterdam: Elsevier, 1988, 177–202.
102. Ledergerber B, Better JD, Joos B, et al: Effect of standard breakfast on drug absorption and multiple-dose pharmacokinetics of ciprofloxacin. Antimicrob Agents Chemother 1985; 27:350–352.
103. Hooper DC, Wolfson JS: The fluoroquinolones: Pharmacology, clinical uses, and toxicities in humans. Antimicrob Agents Chemother 1985; 28:716–721.
104. Walker RC, Wright AJ: The quinolones. Mayo Clin Proc 1987; 62:1007–1012.
105. Eron LJ: Therapy of skin and skin structure infections with ciprofloxacin: An overview. Am J Med 1987; 82(Suppl 4A):224–226.
106. Parish LC, Asper R: Systemic treatment of cutaneous infections: A comparative study of ciprofloxacin and cetotaxime. Am J Med 1987; 82(Suppl 4A):227–229.
107. Valainis GT, Pankey GA, Katner HP, et al: Ciprofloxacin in the treatment of bacterial skin infections. Am J Med 1987; 82(Suppl 4A):230–232.
108. Arcieri G, Griffith E, Gruenwaldt, et al: Ciprofloxacin: An update on clinical experience. Am J Med 1987; 82(Suppl 4A):381–386.
109. Fass RJ: Treatment of skin and soft tissue infections with oral ciprofloxacin. J Antimicrob Chemother 1986; 18(Suppl D):153–157.
110. Fong IW: The role of fluoroquinolones in the management of skin, soft tissue, and bone infections. Clin Inves Med 1989; 12(1):44–49.
111. Megran DW: Quinolones in the treatment of sexually transmitted diseases. Clin Inves Med 1989; 12(1):50–60.
112. Naamara W: Treatment of chancroid with ciprofloxacin: A prospective, randomized clinical trial. Am J Med 1987; 82(Suppl 4A):317–320.
113. Data on file, Miles Inc., Pharmaceutical Division.

Metronidazole

114. Ralph ED: Nitroimidazoles. *In* Koren G, Prober CG, Gold R (eds): Antimicrobial Therapy in Infants and Children. New York: Marcel Dekker, 1988, 729–745.
115. Molavi A, LeFrock JL, Prince RA: Metronidazole. Med Clin North Am 1982; 66:121–133.
116. McGilveray IJ, Midha KK, Loo JC, et al: The bioavailability of commercial metronidazole formulations. Int J Clin Pharmacol Biopharm 1978; 16:110–115.
117. Rosenblatt JE, Edson RS: Metronidazole. Mayo Clin Proc 1987; 62:1013–1017.
118. Saihan EM, Burton JL: A double-blind trial of metronidazole versus oxytetracycline therapy for rosacea. Br J Dermatol 1980; 102:443–445.
119. Duhra P, Paul CJ: Metastatic Crohn's disease responding to metronidazole. Br J Dermatol 1988; 119:87–91.
120. Gerding DN: Metronidazole. *In* Peterson PK, Verhoef J (eds): The Antimicrobial Agents Annual 3. Amsterdam: Elsevier, 1988, 138–143.
121. Burton JL, Saihan EM: Rosacea, metronidazole, and pregnancy. Br J Dermatol 1980; 103:585–586.
122. Thomson G, Clark AH, Hare K, et al: Pseudomembranous colitis after treatment with metronidazole. Br Med J 1981; 282:864–865.
123. Rissing JP, Newman C, Moore WL Jr: Artifactual depression of serum glutamic oxaloacetic transaminase by metronidazole. Antimicrob Agents Chemother 1978; 14:636–638.
124. Noble JI, Tally FP: Metronidazole. *In* Ristuccia AM, Cunha BA (eds): Antimicrobial Therapy. New York: Raven Press, 1984, 255–263.
125. Alexander I: "Alcohol-antabuse" syndrome in patients receiving metronidazole during gynecological treatment. Br J Clin Pract 1985; 39:292–293.
126. Rothstein E, Clancy DD: Toxicity of disulfiram combined with metronidazole. N Engl J Med 1969; 280:1006–1007.

127. O'Reilly RA: The stereoselective interaction of warfarin and metronidazole in man. N Engl J Med 1976; 295:354–357.
128. Gugler R, Jensen JC: Interaction between cimetidine and metronidazole. N Engl J Med 1983; 309:1518–1519.

Clindamycin

129. Bartlett JG: Antimicrobial agents implicated in *Clostridium difficile* toxin-associated diarrhea of colitis. Johns Hopkins Med J 1981; 149:6–9.
130. Wilson WR, Cockerill FR III: Tetracyclines, chloramphenicol, erythromycin, and clindamycin. Mayo Clin Proc 1987; 62:906–915.
131. Klainer AS: Clindamycin. Med Clin North Am 1987; 71(6):1168–1175.

Common Clinical Scenarios

132. Coskey RJ, Coskey LA: Diagnosis and treatment of impetigo. J Am Acad Dermatol 1987; 17:62–63.
133. Tunnessen W: Practical aspects of bacterial skin infections in children. Pediatr Dermatol 1985; 2:255–265.
134. Schachner L, Taplin D, Scott G, et al: A therapeutic update of superficial skin infections. Pediatr Clin North Am 1983; 30:397–403.
135. Schulman ST, Tanz R, Willert C, et al: Rifampin treatment for group A streptococcal carriers. In Kimura Y, Kotami S, Shiokawa Y (eds): Recent Advances in Streptococci and Streptococcal Disease. London: Reedbooks Ltd, 1984, 302–303.
136. Chaudhary S, Billinsky SA, Hennessy JL, et al: Penicillin V and rifampin for the treatment of group A streptococcal pharyngitis: A randomized trial of 10 days penicillin vs. 10 days penicillin with rifampin during the final 4 days of therapy. J Pediatr 1985; 106:481–486.
137. Plewig G, Nikolowski J, Wolff HH: Action of isotretinoin in acne rosacea and gram-negative folliculitis. J Am Acad Dermatol 1982; 6:766–785.
138. Anonymous: Drugs for anaerobic infections. Med Lett Drugs Ther 1984; 26:87–89.
139. Brook I: Microbiology of infected epidermal cysts. Arch Dermatol 1989; 125:1658–1661.

4 Glucocorticosteroids

Stephen E. Wolverton, M.D.

Kendell described compound E (cortisone) in 1935.[1] A Mayo clinic group first described the use of cortisone and adrenocorticotropic hormone (ACTH) in patients with rheumatoid arthritis in 1948.[1] In 1950, Hench and colleagues presented the first report on the basic effects and toxicities of glucocorticosteroids (GCS).[2]

Sulzberger and colleagues' 1951 report described the use of cortisone and ACTH in a variety of inflammatory dermatoses.[3] This report on GCS radically changed the therapeutic approach of dermatologists. As the list of steroid-responsive dermatoses grew, so did the list of potential adverse effects. In 1961, Reichling and Kligman suggested alternate-day GCS use.[4] This was an important step toward decreasing adverse effects and yet maintaining anti-inflammatory effect over the 48-hour period between doses.

Two major advances in GCS therapy occurred during the 1970s and 1980s. Adjunctive therapy with immunosuppressive drugs, such as azathioprine and cyclophosphamide, has been used increasingly for "steroid-sparing" effect. These drugs allow lower GCS doses to be used, which lessens the risk of serious adverse effects while maintaining adequate immunosuppressive effect. High-dose, pulse intravenous methylprednisolone therapy has also been increasingly utilized. Quicker remission with lower risk from therapy is the goal of this method of GCS administration. Pemphigus vulgaris, bullous pemphigoid, and pyoderma gangrenosum patients have all benefited from pulse therapy.[5-7]

This chapter covers the pharmacology and clinical use of systemic GCS. Particular attention is given to the risks of systemic GCS, especially focusing on measures to prevent, detect, and manage these important complications. The physician who is thoroughly familiar with these measures will more comfortably and intelligently use these drugs to the benefit of many grateful patients.

This chapter includes sections covering the following areas: normal hypothalamic-pituitary-adrenal (HPA axis) function; intramuscular GCS administration; pulse intravenous GCS administration; HPA axis suppression; and therapeutic guidelines.

Pharmacology

Structure

The basic structure of all GCS consists of three hexane rings and one pentane ring.[1,8] The combined ring structure is known as the cyclopentenoperhydrophenanthrene nucleus. The rings are designated by letters A, B, C, and D, and each carbon is assigned a number from 1 to 21 (Figure 4–1). The designations alpha (away from the GCS receptor) and beta (toward the GCS receptor) refer to the position of any added molecules in reference to the stereochemical plane.

Cortisone and hydrocortisone both possess a 4,5 double bond and a ketone (carbonyl) group at the 3 position.[9-11] Cortisone, which is an inactive form, has a ketone at the 11 position. The active form, hydrocortisone (cortisol), is formed through hepatic conversion of the 11-ketone to an 11-hydroxyl group. The addition of a 1,2 double bond results in increased glucocorticoid activity and decreased rate of degra-

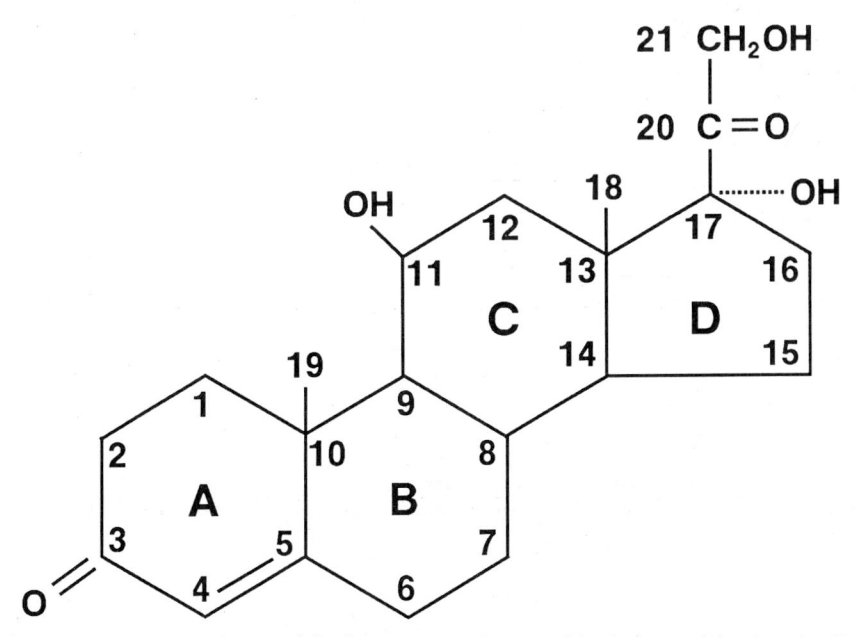

Figure 4–1. Structure of cortisol (hydrocortisone). Structural basis for modifications leading to all other glucocorticosteroids.

dation. This results in prednisone (with an 11-ketone group), and through 11-hydroxylation, the active analog, prednisolone, is formed. Methylprednisolone is formed through the addition of a 6-methyl group to prednisolone, which leads to slightly increased glucocorticoid potency.

The addition of fluorine to hydrocortisone at the 9-alpha position leads to increased glucorticoid but excessive mineralocorticoid activity.[9,11] The resulting compound is 9-alpha fluorohydrocortisone (fludrocortisone, Florinef). This compound is the basic structure of most fluorinated topical steroids. In general, the mineralocorticoid effect is decreased in topical steroids by the masking of the 16- or 17-hydroxyl group with various esters (e.g., acetonide, valerate, propionate).

With systemic GCS, 9-alpha fluorohydrocortisone with an added 1,2 double bond is also modified further.[9,11] By adding a 16-alpha hydroxyl group (triamcinolone), a 16-alpha methyl group (dexamethasone), or a 16-beta methyl group (betamethasone), one can form three compounds with high glucocorticoid and low mineralocorticoid effects. Because all have an 11-hydroxyl group, these three are active forms. All GCS have a hydroxyl group at the 17 position (17-hydroxycorticosteroids). Androgenic steroid compounds have a 17-ketone group and a 19-carbon basic ring structure (17-ketosteroids).

Absorption/Distribution

Exogenous GCS are absorbed in the upper jejunum.[1] More than 50% of prednisone is absorbed. Food delays but does not decrease the amount absorbed. Peak plasma levels are reached 30–100 minutes after the drug is taken.

The primary endogenous carrier protein is cortisol-binding globulin (CBG, transcortin).[1,10] Eighty to 90% of endogenous cortisol is bound; the free fraction represents the active form. CBG is a low-capacity, high-affinity binding system. Albumin (corticosteroid-binding albumin) represents a low-affinity, high-capacity binding reserve. The avidity with which synthetic GCS bind to these carrier proteins is less than the avidity with endogenous cortisol. Thus a greater free fraction is available. Prednisolone is reported to bind with greater affinity than other synthetic forms, with resultant displacement of endogenous cortisol from the protein-binding sites.

CBG is decreased by hypothyroidism, liver disease, renal disease, and obesity, all of which may result in increased amount of the free fraction.[12] CBG is increased by estrogen therapy, pregnancy, and hyperthyroidism.

High-dose therapy results in a greater proportion of free GCS in the body. Likewise, prolonged GCS treatment increases the free fraction.

Overall, GCS are widely distributed to most body tissues. All endogenous and synthetic GCS are well distributed into fetal tissue with the exception of prednisone.[13]

Metabolism/Excretion

All the biologically active GCS and their synthetic congeners have a double bond in the 4,5 position and a ketone group at the 3 position.[10, 11] Reduction at the 4,5 double bond can occur at both hepatic and extrahepatic sites, yielding an inactive substance. Reduction of the 3-ketone substituent to a 3-hydroxyl group to form tetrahydrocortisol has been demonstrated only in the liver. Most of the aforementioned metabolites are conjugated at the 3-hydroxyl site with sulfate or glucuronic acid to form water-soluble metabolites, which are excreted by the kidney.

Of importance is that the action of 11-beta hydroxydehydrogenase in the liver is necessary to convert cortisone to hydrocortisone and prednisone to prednisolone.[10, 11] Only hydrocortisone and prednisolone are biologically active. Severe liver disease may impair this conversion. Thus the administration of prednisolone rather than prednisone to patients with that condition would be appropriate. In addition, liver disease may result in decreased albumin, which would increase the free fraction of GCS.

The plasma half-lives of the various synthetic GCS do not correlate well with the duration of biologic activity[1] (Table 4–1). A much more important measure of duration of activity is the duration of ACTH

Table 4–1. Pharmacology of Glucocorticosteroids

Drug	*Equivalent Dose**	*MC Effect†*	*Duration‡*	*Plasma t½§*
Short-acting				
Cortisone	25	2+	8–12	30–90
Hydrocortisone (Cortisol)	20	2+	8–12	60–120
Intermediate-acting				
Prednisone	5	1+	24–36	60
Prednisolone	5	1+	24–36	200
Methylprednisolone	4	0	24–36	180
Triamcinolone	4	0	24–36	300
Long-acting				
Dexamethasone	0.75	0	36–54	100–300
Betamethasone	0.60	0	36–54	100–300

Adapted from Fauci AS, Dale DC, Balow JE: Glucocorticosteroid therapy: Mechanism of action and clinical considerations. Ann Intern Med 1976; 84:304–315; Claman HN: Glucocorticosteroids II: The clinical responses. Hosp Pract 1983; 18(7):143–151; and Axelrod L: Glucocorticoid therapy. Medicine 1976; 55:39–65.
  *Equivalent dose for glucocorticoid and anti-inflammatory (AI) effects; in mg.
  †Mineralocorticoid (MC) effect: relative potency.
  ‡Duration of AI effect and HPA axis suppression after a single dose; in hours.
  §In minutes.

suppression after the administration of a single dose of a given GCS. This duration of activity correlates well with glucocorticoid and anti-inflammatory effects.[14–16] There is an inverse correlation between the duration of action and the mineralocorticoid effect.

Mechanism of Action

NORMAL HPA AXIS FUNCTION.
It is important to understand the normal function of the HPA axis in order to better understand the potential for HPA axis suppression by synthetic GCS. For further background information, several reviews are particularly helpful.[10, 11, 17]

The primary stimulus for release of endogenous hydrocortisone (cortisol) originates in the hypothalamus. The tropic hormone is known as corticotropin-releasing factor (CRF). ACTH is subsequently released by the anterior pituitary. ACTH is produced from the prohormone pro-ACTH/endorphin. There are approximately 10 bursts of ACTH release throughout the day. The greatest frequency of these bursts occurs in the early morning hours during a normal sleep cycle. The zona fasciculata of the adrenal cortex is then stimulated to produce and release hydrocortisone. ACTH has a role in stimulating adrenal androgen synthesis. However, it is not significantly involved in the release of the mineralocorticoid aldosterone.

At a basal level, the body produces 20–30 mg/day of hydrocortisone. Under maximal physical stress, this amount can increase to up to 300 mg/day, a tenfold elevation.

There are three main controls of endogenous cortisol production.[17] The first control is the negative feedback provided by endogenous cortisol, which inhibits CRF release from the hypothalamus. The second control, the circadian (diurnal) cycle, results in the greatest production of cortisol in the 6:00–8:00 A.M. time period; the lowest levels occur in the late afternoon. This diurnal variation is due to the related diurnal variation of CRF and subsequent ACTH production. Should a person's occupation require working after midnight, the diurnal cycle will reset, so that peak cortisol production occurs just before the person awakens. The third control is the stress response to various physical stressors, which include infections, surgery, major trauma, or significant illnesses such as myocardial infarction. In addition to CRF, hormones such as vasopressin and catecholamines are believed to stimulate ACTH production in response to these stressors. Acetylcholine and serotonin are involved in both the circadian- and the stress-related production of GCS.

At the molecular level, GCS have specific cytosolic and nuclear receptors.[1, 10] The net result is DNA-triggered messenger RNA production of specific proteins. Lipomodulin is an example of a specific protein that carries out the GCS inhibition of phospholipase A_2-induced prostaglandin synthesis.[1, 9]

GLUCOCORTICOID EFFECTS. GCS play an important teleologic role in maintaining adequate blood glucose levels for brain function.[10] Gluconeogenesis generates glucose at the expense of amino acids derived from endogenous proteins. GCS also produce peripheral insulin resistance, which impedes glucose absorption by various body tissues. In addition, glycogen storage in the liver is enhanced. Lipid stores are stimulated to undergo lipolysis, generating increased amounts of triglycerides from which to derive energy.

The net effect is a catabolic state that produces carbohydrates at the expense of protein and fat stores.[10, 11] Through gluconeogenesis, proteins from muscle, trabecular bone (especially vertebral and hip), dermal connective tissue, and vascular proteins are metabolized. Lipolysis results in triglyceride release with additional fat redistribution to areas that are characteristic of Cushing's syndrome.

WOUND HEALING. The net catabolic effect of GCS inhibits fibroblast production of collagen and ground substance. Angiogenesis and re-epithelialization are also inhibited.[18, 19]

MINERALOCORTICOID EFFECTS. Aldosterone is the primary endogenous mineralocorticoid hormone. The primary effect is sodium absorption and resultant water reabsorption at the proximal tubule site in the kidneys. Sodium is exchanged for potassium, which leads to hypokalemia when there is excessive mineralocorticoid effect. ACTH has no direct control on mineralocorticoid production. The primary mineralocorticoid control mechanisms are through the renin-angiotensin system and serum potassium levels.[12, 17]

CALCIUM METABOLISM. The net GCS effect on endogenous calcium metabolism is to decrease total body stores of calcium. There is impaired gastrointestinal absorption of calcium and increased renal excretion of calcium.[1] In addition, bone osteoclasts are stimulated by the resultant increased levels of parathyroid hormone. Osteoblast function is also inhibited by GCS.

IMMUNOLOGIC EFFECTS. GCS have the overall effect of preventing immunologically competent white blood cell subsets from reaching the sites of inflammation, without affecting the total numbers of these white blood cell subsets.[1] Polymorphonuclear leukocytes (PMNs) are increased in circulation through increased bone marrow release and decreased margination to endothelial cells.[1, 10] There is no change in PMN function. With moderate- to high-dose GCS therapy, the peripheral PMN count is typically 15,000–20,000/cu mm.

GCS have a greater effect on T lymphocytes than on B lymphocytes.[1, 10] Given the greater B cell resistance to GCS, there is little impairment of antibody synthesis. T lymphocytes are primarily redirected to reticuloendothelial sites distant from primary sites of inflammation.

Monocyte function is altered. Macrophages are unavailable for antigen processing because of impaired recruitment to sites of inflammation.[1] The macrophage-like dendritic epidermal cell, the Langerhans cell, has decreased surface markers and impaired antigen-processing function.

Both eosinophils and basophils have GCS-induced decreased numbers, inhibited function, and impaired recruitment to sites of inflammation.[1]

Tissue mast cells have impaired mediator release of histamines and kinins.[1] GCS lead to impaired interleukin-1 and interleukin-2 production by macrophages and T lymphocytes, respectively.[1, 10] In addition, there is decreased gamma-interferon production and a resultant decreased DR positivity of various immunologic cells.

Many of these effects are accomplished through GCS-induced vascular effects.[1] There is significant vasoconstriction and decreased permeability of peripheral capillaries. Various immunologic cells are unable to traverse the endothelial basement membrane to reach sites of inflammation. In addition, immunoglobulins and circulating immune complexes are unable to move across the capillary basement membrane zone.[1] Phospholipase A_2 inhibition decreases the conversion of esterified arachidonic acid to the nonesterified form.[10] The net effect is decreased prostaglandin, leukotriene, and hydroxyeicosatetraenoic acid production and lessened participation of these products in various inflammatory processes.

In vitro, GCS inhibit lysosomal enzyme release.[1] The significance of this inhibition in vivo remains to be clarified.

OTHER GCS EFFECTS. GCS are often used for their antiproliferative and antimitotic effects. These effects are due to the effects on G_1 and G_2 phases of the cell cycle.[1] Growth inhibition is through decreased somatomedin-A effect.[11, 20]

Clinical Use (Table 4–2)

Indications

Several of the dermatoses listed in Table 4–2 are discussed selectively to illustrate various principles of GCS therapy. Conditions such as pemphigus vulgaris, bullous pemphigoid, contact dermatitis, and other conditions in which dermatologists play a central role in the GCS management are examined. Alternative and adjunctive systemic therapies are briefly described.

PEMPHIGUS VULGARIS. The best-studied purely dermatologic indication

Table 4–2. Glucocorticosteroid Indications/Contraindications

Dermatologic Uses

Bullous Dermatoses

    Pemphigus vulgaris/superficial forms[21–31]*†
    Bullous pemphigoid[32–38]*†
    Cicatricial pemphigoid[39–41]†
    Herpes gestationis[42–44]†
    Erythema multiforme minor/major[45–52]*
    Epidermolysis bullosa acquisita[53]
    Linear IgA bullous dermatosis[54, 55]

Connective Tissue Diseases

    Lupus erythematosus (systemic LE*‡)[56–58]
    Dermatomyositis[59–63]*†
    Mixed connective tissue disease[64, 65]†

Vasculitis

    Cutaneous[66, 67]
    Systemic[68, 69]

Neutrophilic Dermatoses

    Pyoderma gangrenosum[7, 70, 71]
    Sweet's syndrome[72, 73]†
    Behçet's disease/aphthous ulcers[30, 74–77]

Dermatitis/Papulosquamous

    Contact dermatitis[78, 79]
    Exfoliative erythroderma[80]
    Lichen planus[81–83]

Other Dermatoses

    Sarcoidosis (pulmonary*)[84]
    Sunburn[85]
    Urticaria (severe*)[86]
    Androgen excess (acne/hirsutism)[87–89]
    Post-herpetic neuralgia[90–95]

Intramuscular Glucocorticosteroids[96–103]
Pulse Intravenous Methylprednisolone[5–7, 70, 104–111]

Contraindications

Absolute

    Systemic fungal infections
    Herpes simplex keratitis
    Hypersensitivity (a problem primarily with ACTH, occasionally noted with intravenous preparations)

Relative§

    Cardiovascular: hypertension, congestive heart failure
    Central nervous system: prior psychosis, severe depression
    Gastrointestinal: active peptic ulcer disease, recent bowel anastomosis
    Infections: active tuberculosis, positive tuberculin skin test
    Metabolic: diabetes mellitus
    Musculoskeletal: osteoporosis
    Ocular: glaucoma, cataracts
    Pregnancy

*FDA-approved indications.
†Glucocorticosteroids systemically are generally considered the drugs of choice (alone or in combination with another immunosuppressive drug).
‡Also for lupus erythematosus.
§The severity of the disease to be treated and the anticipated dose and duration of therapy determine whether relative contraindications prohibit GCS therapy.

for systemic GCS therapy is pemphigus vulgaris. The emphasis here is high-dose GCS therapy with use of adjunctive immunosuppressive therapy. GCS are appropriate for any significant case of pemphigus vulgaris that has no absolute contraindications to their use. An alternative for milder cases includes oral gold therapy. Adjunctive therapy is generally used with a choice of azathioprine, cyclophosphamide, gold, methotrexate, or plasmapheresis.[21,22]

Early reports on oral GCS therapy for pemphigus vulgaris describe doses of 120–240 mg/day of prednisone.[23,24] Disease- and treatment-related deaths occurred in up to 44% of patients. This rate represents significant improvement from the reported 90% disease fatality rate before the availability of GCS therapy.[25] In the 1970s there was further reduction of disease- and treatment-related fatalities to as low as 9.5% from treatment-induced mortality and 24% from combined treatment- and disease-induced mortality.[26,27] Current series report disease- and treatment-fatality rates from 3.8% to just over 10%.[28,29] Earlier diagnosis, lower doses of GCS therapy, improved treatment of secondary infections, and adjunctive azathioprine, cyclophosphamide, or methotrexate therapy are probably responsible for the improved survival statistics.

Current management includes prednisone doses no greater than 2 mg/kg/day in divided doses.[21,22] Disease control is usually attained by 4–6 weeks. At this time the divided dose should be consolidated into a single daily dose and tapered rapidly to the 40-mg/day range. Azathioprine or related immunosuppressive drugs can be added at the time of prednisone tapering in many cases.[21,22] However, the delayed onset of action from azathioprine suggests that in severe cases, early use of azathioprine would be appropriate. Management of oral involvement[29,30] and juvenile pemphigus vulgaris[31] is similar to that just described.

BULLOUS PEMPHIGOID. In patients with bullous pemphigoid, moderate doses of GCS are used. In addition, the GCS course is typically given for a defined duration of time (generally 6–12 months).[32–35] The heterogeneous nature of the disease dictates that the dosage level should be individualized for generalized bullous pemphigoid cases. Dapsone for children and tetracycline or erythromycin for adults are alternative therapies.[35,36] About half of patients require concomitant immunosuppressive therapy with drugs such as azathioprine.[35,37] In addition, plasma exchange has been reported to be successful in treating bullous pemphigoid.[38]

In general, 80 mg/day of prednisone in divided doses is successful in eliminating new blister formation within several weeks' time. Should the patient not respond to this dose or require a high maintenance dose, adjunctive immunosuppressive therapy can be added. In the absence of new blisters over 5–7 days' time, the prednisone dose can be gradually tapered.

CICATRICIAL PEMPHIGOID. In contrast, cicatricial pemphigoid is less responsive to GCS than is bullous pemphigoid. Consultation with an ophthalmologist is necessary in cases with ocular involvement. The disease course is variable; early institution of treatment leads to better results.[39-41] Cyclophosphamide or cyclosporine is usually needed as adjunctive therapy when there is ocular involvement.[39,40] On occasion, dapsone therapy is successful.[41]

In general, 1–1.5 mg/kg/day of prednisone is required for controlling mild cases. Aggressive management is important in ocular cases because of the significant potential for blindness.

ERYTHEMA MULTIFORME MINOR/MAJOR. A controversial indication for systemic GCS is erythema multiforme major (Stevens-Johnson syndrome/toxic epidermal necrolysis). Although proponents of routine GCS therapy exist,[45,46] more recent reports describe the advantages of burn unit care in the absence of GCS therapy.[47-50] There is a higher fatality rate, particularly from sepsis, in GCS-treated patients, than in patients managed in a burn unit without GCS. However, proponents of GCS use suggest that for erythema multiforme major patients, treatment early in the disease course (before significant sloughing of skin), followed by rapid tapering of GCS, may be beneficial.[45,46,51] After widespread sloughing occurs, the risk of infection outweighs the potential GCS benefits. Of importance is that drug and infectious precipitators be sought and eliminated if possible. Should GCS therapy be indicated, doses up to 2 mg/kg/day of intravenous methylprednisolone are generally used.

A more common indication for moderate GCS doses is recurrent oral erythema multiforme minor.[30] Painful oral erosions respond promptly to prednisone in doses up to 1 mg/kg/day, rapidly tapered over 2–3 weeks. For recurrent cases, one should also consider acyclovir on a long-term daily basis, particularly if herpes simplex virus is proved or strongly suspected to be the etiology.

LUPUS ERYTHEMATOSUS. The lupus erythematosus spectrum represents a setting in which GCS therapy is generally indicated only for systemic disease manifestations. Vasculitis and bullous lupus erythematosus, as well as widespread disfiguring discoid lupus erythematosus, are the primary cutaneous indications.[56-58] With vasculitis and bullous findings, there is generally underlying systemic disease. Numerous alternatives to GCS are available. Antimalarial agents, dapsone, retinoids, and gold all are reasonable options for many of the cutaneous findings.[56,57] Most cases can be managed with sunscreens, topical or intralesional GCS, and/or antimalarial therapy. Should systemic GCS be indicated, doses of 20 mg every other day up to 60 mg/day of prednisone may be required.[57,58] The dose should be individualized; low to moderate doses are favored. On the basis of scarring potential, discoid lupus erythematosus is more likely to require prednisone therapy than is subacute cutaneous lupus erythematosus, which has no significant scarring potential.

DERMATOMYOSITIS. Comanagement with either a rheumatologist or a neurologist is appropriate. When indicated, systemic GCS therapy is often successful as monotherapy. Dermatomyositis is a condition in which very slow tapering of treatment is in order.[59-62] Although their efficacy has not been established in controlled trials, systemic GCS are generally accepted as the treatment of choice. Antimalarial agents may improve cutaneous findings as an adjunctive measure. About 90% of patients respond to a prednisone dose of 1–1.5 mg/kg/day. The dose is adjusted on the basis of examination of muscle strength and muscle enzyme levels. Gradual tapering of the dose over 1–2 years or more is appropriate.[60, 61, 63]

VASCULITIS. Vasculitis may be the cutaneous manifestation of a large variety of conditions. Palpable purpura from leukocytoclastic vasculitis and persistent urticarial lesions associated with urticarial vasculitis are the most common presentations. In both settings, drugs such as colchicine, dapsone, indomethacin, and perhaps antihistamines may control the cutaneous findings. Gastrointestinal, renal, and joint involvement may indicate systemic GCS therapy. Patients with chronic cutaneous leukocytoclastic vasculitis with ulcers, infarction, or persistent painful lesions may require 1–1.5 mg/kg/day of prednisone.[66, 67] Rapid tapering to alternate-day dosing is suggested; 20 mg on alternate days is often successful in maintaining the improvement attained by daily doses.[66] For cases of predominantly cutaneous vasculitis, Cupps and colleagues reported less than 50% response to GCS in patients referred to the National Institutes of Health (NIH).[67] Callen and Ekenstam reported a more than 90% response to relatively low-dose GCS therapy in a more traditional tertiary care setting.[66] An approach to systemic vasculitis was outlined in two articles by Fauci.[68, 69] My personal experience dictates that colchicine is a predictably effective alternative to GCS therapy in most cases of chronic cutaneous leukocytoclastic vasculitis.

PYODERMA GANGRENOSUM. Although pulse intravenous methylprednisolone is used for severe cases,[7, 70] "bursts" of moderate-dose oral prednisone may initiate improvement in less severe cases.[71] Alternatively, dapsone is often successful for mild cases of pyoderma gangrenosum. Azathioprine and related immunosuppressive drugs may be required in refractory cases.[71] In general, 40–60 mg/day of prednisone, tapered over 1 month to low-dose alternate-day therapy, is successful. Gradual tapering of doses below 30–40 mg on alternate days is in order.

ACUTE DERMATITIS. Severe acute contact dermatitis due to poison ivy is a classic situation in which a burst of systemic GCS therapy is usually successful at minimal risk.[78] Potential rebound of disease activity due to rapid tapering over less than 10–14 days is important to consider.[78, 79] Cases with widespread cutaneous involvement or significant facial involvement treated early in their course can respond rapidly. Doses up to 1 mg/kg/day (generally 40–60 mg/day of prednisone) tapered over 2–3 weeks yield adequate improvement with minimal risk of rebound flare after cessation of therapy. Acute flares of chronic atopic, nummular, or contact dermatitis can be managed in a similar fashion. Maintenance GCS therapy is best avoided in these settings.

Exfoliative erythroderma management uncommonly requires systemic GCS therapy.[80] Given that psoriasis has been excluded, exfoliative erythroderma refractory to aggressive topical management or to phototherapy may respond to prednisone at 1–1.5 mg/kg/day. This dose is tapered rapidly to low-dose alternate-day therapy.

LICHEN PLANUS. A relatively long burst of systemic GCS may be indicated at times to minimize the disfiguring hyperpigmentation possible from lichen planus. Prednisone given at 40–60 mg/day and tapered over 4–6 weeks consistently eradicates or reduces the intensity of generalized lichen planus.[81, 82] This use is potentially important for blacks or people of other darkly pigmented races in whom pigment incontinence is most notable. Severe oral erosive lichen planus may require judicious low- to moderate-dose GCS therapy. Alternatives such as griseofulvin, psoralens plus ultraviolet A (PUVA), retinoids, and intralesional GCS therapy all should be considered for oral and generalized cases. Because of the chronicity of therapy required, lower doses are indicated for severe oral erosive lichen planus. Lichen planus presenting as desquamative vaginitis is an appropriate indication for even briefer bursts of GCS therapy.[83]

SARCOIDOSIS. Cutaneous findings of sarcoidosis alone rarely justify systemic GCS therapy. However, these lesions predictably respond to such therapy if there is a systemic indication. Ulcerative sarcoidosis or aggressive facial involvement, such as that seen with lupus pernio, may indicate judicious systemic GCS therapy.[84] Alternatives to GCS include antimalarial agents, low-dose methotrexate, and intralesional GCS. Callen recommended starting with 20 mg of prednisone on alternate days and increasing the alternate-day dose if necessary for the aforementioned cutaneous indications.[84]

ANDROGEN EXCESS SYNDROMES. For hirsutism, recalcitrant acne vulgaris, and alopecia due to elevated adrenal androgens, a unique GCS approach is often indicated. In these cases, nighttime suppressive therapy with low-dose (below physiologic replacement levels) dexamethasone therapy is predictably successful. Most cases can be controlled with 0.125–0.375 mg of dexamethasone at bedtime.[87–89] This timing is important to suppress the early morning peak of ACTH, which stimulates adrenal androgen production. For a more complete discussion on androgen excess syndromes, see chapter 13.

POST-HERPETIC NEURALGIA. Another controversial area of systemic GCS therapy is prevention of post-herpetic neuralgia pain. Issues such as proper selection of patients for treatment, overall efficacy, appropriate timing in the disease course, and benefit of adjunctive acyclovir therapy remain to be definitively answered. In reviewing the four controlled studies of GCS for prevention of post-herpetic neuralgia,[90-93] Post and Philbrick concluded that problems with diagnostic criteria, definition of pain, and limited numbers of patients preclude any definitive statements on efficacy.[94] However, Watson determined with a similar review that 60 mg/day of prednisone for 2 weeks early in the disease course in the absence of significant immunosuppression may help selected patients.[95] Particularly good candidates for treatment include patients with facial involvement, patients with severe acute pain during the cutaneous eruption, and patients over 60 years of age. It is logical, although unproved, that concomitant high doses (600–800 mg five times per day) of acyclovir might improve the GCS success rate. Although disseminated herpes zoster from GCS therapy is a concern, this is a distinctly uncommon complication in patients with normal immunity.[94, 95]

INTRAMUSCULAR ADMINISTRATION. Dermatologists have long held widely divergent viewpoints regarding the pros and cons of intramuscular GCS therapy. Proponents of intramuscular administration believe that conditions requiring more than 6 months of systemic GCS therapy may be more amenable to this means of administration.[96] Arnold suggested that diverse conditions such as dermatitis (atopic, contact, exfoliative, nummular), psoriasis, herpes zoster, and lichen planus may benefit from intramuscular GCS. Even more serious conditions such as systemic lupus erythematosus, pemphigus vulgaris, and bullous pemphigoid may respond favorably to intramuscular GCS therapy.[96]

Proponents of intramuscular administration base their arguments on several key points.[96, 97] These arguments include the physician's control over the patient's therapy, a sustained steady level of GCS, and guaranteed compliance. This method may serve as a trial of therapy to determine responsiveness to GCS and is useful even if the patient has nausea and is vomiting.

Opponents of intramuscular GCS administration approach the same issues from a different viewpoint.[97] They note that it is important for patients to be active participants in their own care. The oral administration is more physiologic if given in a single morning dose. The opponents of intramuscular GCS therapy note the somewhat erratic absorption of intramuscular steroids. Even so, this absorption still results in a steady sustained level, as opposed to the body's own diurnal variation. Patient compliance is probably less important when GCS are used for serious or even life-threatening diseases. Precision in tapering is believed to be another advantage of oral GCS, whereas it is impossible to give a short course of intramuscular steroids. Of importance is that oral GCS therapy can be administered by alternate-day dosing. This method significantly decreases most GCS adverse effects; cataracts and osteoporosis are, however, still potential complications.[1, 98] Intramuscular GCS are known to increase the incidence of menstrual irregularity and commonly result in purpura.[96, 97] Specific local complications at the injection site include crystal deposition, atrophy, and cold abscesses.[1]

A pivotal point of debate is the effect of intramuscular GCS on the HPA axis. Kusama and associates detected suppression up to 3–4 weeks after each injection of triamcinolone acetonide as measured by plasma cortisol and urine 17-hydroxycorticosteroids.[99] Mikhail and colleagues studied patients receiving intramuscular triamcinolone acetonide every 6 weeks for 1½–5 years' duration.[100] Roughly half had impaired response to the insulin hypoglycemia test. Mikhail and coauthors noted that the interval between doses is a more important factor in HPA axis suppression than is the dose. Low-dose intramuscular GCS at 2- to 4-week intervals produced greater suppression than did higher doses at 6-week intervals. Using the metyrapone test, Carson and associates found evidence of HPA axis suppression up to 10 months after treatment.[101] Droszcz and colleagues detected abnormal ACTH stimulation in 6 of 48 patients (12%) on every 2- to 6-week intramuscular triamcinolone acetonide.[102] In a related study, Carson and associates evaluated triamcinolone acetonide, 40 mg given every 3 weeks for four doses.[103] This resulted in anovulatory menstrual cycles in women because of decreased gonadotropin levels.

After the arguments and data just given are reviewed, a reasonable neutral viewpoint is as follows. Serious adverse effects are rare with either a single intramuscular GCS injection or a burst of oral prednisone. Rarely do oral bursts, single injections, or long-term use of either form result in adrenal insufficiency of clinical importance.[11, 17] Neither route of administration has an advantage in withdrawal from chronic GCS use. It is important to focus on altering disease precipitators and providing adequately aggressive topical therapy when either oral or intramuscular GCS are given. Should repeated intramuscular GCS therapy be desired, one should use short- to intermediate-acting products such as Celestone and Aristocort. When a long-acting form such as Kenalog is used, a reasonable limit would be 4–6 injections per year. Each clinician has to make up his or her own mind concerning the relative advantages and disadvantages of intramuscular versus oral GCS therapy. As is often the case, the correct answer depends on the clinical situation; neither form has a clear-cut advantage over the other method of administration.

PULSE INTRAVENOUS ADMINISTRATION. Pulse GCS therapy has been proposed as a means to rapidly control life-threatening or serious conditions with minimal toxicity, allowing for less aggressive long-term maintenance therapy. Typically, 500–1000 mg of methylprednisolone is given intravenously over at least 60 minutes' time.[1] This dose is repeated on a daily basis for 5 consecutive days. Pulse methylprednisolone is performed in an inpatient setting with cardiac monitoring mandatory. Alternate-day GCS or a nonsteroidal immunosuppressive drug is used to maintain the improvement from the intravenous GCS.

Systemic vasculitis and systemic lupus erythematosus are indications for pulse GCS therapy that are of peripheral interest to the dermatologist.[104, 105] The initial dermatologic use was in the treatment of pyoderma gangrenosum by Johnson and Lazarus in 1982.[7] In a follow-up report, Prystowsky and colleagues described a total of 8 pyoderma gangrenosum patients treated by this means; 6 responded favorably.[70] Single-case reports have described pulse intravenous GCS use in lichen planus,[106] Sweet's syndrome,[107] and pemphigus vulgaris.[5] The only other significant series of cases with a purely dermatologic indication for pulse intravenous GCS has been for bullous pemphigoid.[6] Eight patients were treated with pulse methylprednisolone therapy, followed by more moderate dose GCS therapy. In 7 of the 8, blistering decreased within 24 hours.

Sudden death of presumed cardiac origin and anaphylaxis are notable complications of intravenous pulse GCS therapy.[108, 109] Acute electrolyte shifts have been postulated to explain the rare cases of sudden cardiac death.[1, 108] Additional problems apparently unique to this mode of GCS administration include seizures and acute electrolyte abnormalities.[110]

The effect on lymphocytes is greater with pulse GCS therapy than with standard doses of oral GCS therapy.[111] In addition, there appears to be a persistent decrease in natural killer cell activity. Other immunologic effects are qualitatively similar to oral administration.

Pulse GCS therapy with intravenous methylprednisolone may gain further acceptance for use in conditions such as refractory pyoderma gangrenosum, pemphigus vulgaris, and bullous pemphigoid. This modality should be used only when the severity of the patient's condition and lack of response to alternative modes of therapy indicate its appropriateness. Pulse intravenous methylprednisolone therapy should be considered experimental and used selectively in an individualized fashion.

Adverse Effects

There is an imposing list of potential adverse effects from the use of systemic GCS. Brief bursts of GCS for 2–3 weeks are surprisingly safe and very useful in self-limiting dermatoses. Lower-dose, long-term regimens at or near replacement (physiologic) levels of GCS also are reasonably safe. With supraphysiologic doses longer than 3–4 weeks, there is an increased risk for more serious complications. The most serious adverse effects come from chronic use at doses well above maintenance (physiologic) levels. Patients with bullous dermatoses, connective tissue diseases, vasculitis, and neutrophilic dermatoses all frequently need such chronic, pharmacologic-level doses of GCS. The following discussion of adverse effects focuses primarily on the risks of long-term use of these drugs.

CARDIOVASCULAR EFFECTS. Sudden death and life-threatening ventricular arrhythmias have primarily occurred with pulse intravenous methylprednisolone regimens.[108] It has been postulated that rapid electrolyte shifts with this mode of therapy are responsible for the ventricular arrhythmias. All patients receiving pulse therapy require cardiac monitoring for the duration of this therapy.

Hypertension due to GCS has several postulated mechanisms.[112–114] Sodium retention, vasoconstriction, and increased renin substrate may be responsible. High-risk groups include patients on pulse GCS therapy, elderly patients, patients receiving therapy for more than one year, and patients receiving GCS with high mineralocorticoid effect.[1, 11, 19] Many patients have pre-existing, borderline hypertension or overt hypertension that is aggravated by GCS therapy. Measures to decrease this risk include sodium restriction and choice of GCS with low mineralocorticoid effect.

Fluid retention can aggravate pre-existing congestive heart failure.[18, 19] Peripheral edema may be a result of this sodium retention that is independent of cardiac, liver, or renal status. Sodium restriction and possibly concurrent diuretics may benefit patients with those conditions.

CENTRAL NERVOUS SYSTEM EFFECTS. The most serious adverse effects involving the central nervous system are psychosis and pseudotumor cerebri. The pathogenesis of GCS-induced psychosis is unknown. However, altered nerve excitability, decreased cortical activity, and electrolyte shifts have all been postulated to be responsible.[115] The risk is greatest in the first few weeks of therapy for patients receiving more than 1 mg/kg/day of prednisone.[116–118] Patients with a prior history of psychiatric disease may be at increased risk. Women are affected more commonly than are men. Overt psychosis is uncommon, although patients commonly experience euphoria and agitation even on short-term therapy.[119] Some patients may have personality changes during therapy. The management of these complications involves tapering the GCS as soon as the disease activity allows.[15] Psychiatric consultation and possibly psychotherapeutic agents may be indicated for selected patients.

Pseudotumor cerebri is an uncommon GCS complication. This has been reported primarily in young women and children.[18, 114] Presenting symptoms include headache, nausea, vomiting, and visual changes.

Papilledema is present on physical examination. This occurs primarily from rapid tapering of the GCS dose.[18] Increasing the GCS dose and tapering more gradually is the primary therapy.

Transient depression is a common event during the tapering phase of GCS therapy.[120] Educating the patient about this possibility and reassuring her or him are the steps generally necessary. Seizures have been reported with pulse GCS therapy.[110]

CUTANEOUS EFFECTS. Skin changes characteristic of Cushing's syndrome commonly develop with chronic GCS therapy. Atrophy, telangiectasias, purpura, and striae are the typical findings.[11]

Patients may develop the androgen-like signs of acne and hirsutism.[11, 114] The acne is characteristically truncal with all the lesions at a similar stage, either papular or pustular. Steroid-induced acne resolves as the dose is tapered.

Wound healing may be impaired by long-term GCS treatment.[18, 19] Decreased fibroblast production of collagen and ground substance along with impaired angiogenesis and re-epithelialization may occur. At doses routinely used in dermatology, this is uncommonly a significant clinical problem.

A telogen effluvium may occur with high-dose GCS therapy even for brief durations.[11] This typically leads to only transient hair loss. Pigmentary alteration is a rare consequence of systemic GCS therapy.

ENDOCRINE EFFECTS. HPA axis suppression is among the most important adverse effects of systemic GCS therapy. This subject is covered completely later.

Impaired growth in children is a very important potential complication that is not often considered. The probable mechanism involved is decreased growth hormone effect that is due to decreased somatomedin-A effect.[20, 121] As long as the epiphyses have not closed, there will be merely a delay in growth. Most studies demonstrate that children treated with high-dose GCS eventually attain their expected height.[20, 122] The risk is lowest with daily morning, low-dose therapy.[20] The risk of growth arrest is lessened further with alternate-day therapy. Children on chronic GCS therapy should have their height plotted on a growth curve at least every 2–3 months.

Menstrual changes are among the most frequent adverse effects from intramuscular GCS therapy.[97, 103] Abnormal menstrual bleeding is uncommon with oral GCS therapy. Decreased sperm counts have been demonstrated on GCS therapy.[11] However, clinically significant impaired fertility does not appear to be a risk.

GASTROINTESTINAL EFFECTS. The most important gastrointestinal adverse effects involve a perforated viscus.[123–126] A surgical bowel anastomosis performed shortly before high-dose GCS therapy has an increased risk of perforating. Perforation of a peptic ulcer may also occur. Of importance is that GCS therapy may mask clinical signs and symptoms of bowel perforation. Pancreatitis, although rare, has led to death in several GCS-treated patients.[127–129] With these risks in mind, new onset of significant abdominal pain deserves significant attention from the dermatologist and liberal referral to the appropriate specialist.

An area of controversy is the risk of peptic ulcer disease from GCS therapy.[130–132] Many diseases treated with GCS inherently have an increased risk of peptic ulcer disease. Putative mechanisms include decreased mucus production, decreased renewal of the mucosa, and increased acid secretion. There does not appear to be a direct irritant effect.[19, 133] High-risk patients include those on concurrent aspirin or nonsteroidal anti-inflammatory drug therapy.[11, 18] In addition, patients at risk include those receiving more than 1 g cumulative of prednisone, psoriasis patients, patients with connective tissue diseases, and patients with a history of peptic ulcer disease. The frequency of peptic ulcer disease in one series was 1.8% of GCS-treated patients versus 0.8% of controls.[130] Mild cases do not preclude the use of prednisone for serious conditions. Treatment with prophylactic antacids for GCS-treated patients is controversial. However, therapy with liquid antacids or oral H_2 antihistamine blockers is appropriate should symptoms of gastritis, esophagitis, or peptic ulcer disease develop. The patient should be made aware of the frequency of minor gastrointestinal symptoms that are common with brief bursts of GCS therapy.

Fatty liver changes have been reported.[11] This uncommonly leads to significant symptoms or altered liver function test results.

IMMUNOLOGIC EFFECTS. An uncommon but important complication is the reactivation of tuberculosis. There are conflicting reports on the magnitude of this risk.[11, 134, 135] Some physicians recommend a baseline chest x-ray on all chronically treated GCS patients. At the minimum, a history for prior tuberculosis or tuberculosis exposure is important. Active tuberculosis is a strong relative contraindication to GCS therapy. Inactive disease, or a positive tuberculin skin test, probably requires isoniazid therapy while a patient is on GCS therapy,[136] although a consensus on this issue is lacking.[11, 137]

The risk of opportunistic infections due to viruses, fungi, parasites, and mycobacteria increases slightly for patients who are taking at least 50 mg/day of prednisone for more than 2 weeks.[15, 18] These infections are much more common in patients who are receiving combination immunotherapy, particularly for organ transplantation purposes. Febrile response to these infections may be blunted by GCS therapy. Alternate-day therapy significantly reduces the risk of opportunistic infection.[138]

Persistent, recurrent, or unusually severe herpesvirus family infections may occur. Concurrent therapy with acyclovir may be necessary.

There is a surprisingly minimal risk of GCS-induced malignancy. Although the immunosuppressive capabilities of GCS rival those of azathioprine, cyclophosphamide, and cyclosporine, there appears to be minimal risk of malignancy induction by GCS monotherapy.[139, 140] Several reports have noted increased risk of Kaposi's sarcoma that may be reversible with cessation of therapy.[141-143]

METABOLIC EFFECTS. Diabetic ketoacidosis and hyperosmolar nonketotic coma are rare complications of GCS therapy.[144, 145] Most patients developing overt diabetes mellitus from GCS therapy have prior abnormal glucose tolerance. Diabetes mellitus developing de novo is uncommon.[146] Most patients revert to their prior glucose tolerance status within several months after discontinuation of therapy.[11, 146] Management includes a proper American Diabetes Association diet. It is prudent to follow blood glucose levels periodically for patients receiving moderate- to high-dose GCS therapy.

Elevated triglyceride levels are a common adverse effect of therapy, although cholesterol elevations are uncommon.[147, 148] Patients with pretreatment elevations of triglyceride levels appear to be at greatest risk. Most patients are asymptomatic unless the triglyceride levels exceed 800 mg/dl, at which level pancreatitis is a risk. Low-calorie diets with low content of saturated fats are important for these patients. Periodic determinations of fasting triglyceride values should be performed for patients with diabetes mellitus, obesity, and hypothyroidism and for patients with a family history of hyperlipidemia. Specific drug therapy is rarely necessary to control these lipid elevations.

Weight gain is a common result both of increased appetite and of fluid retention. This weight gain may occur even with brief bursts of GCS. Patients receiving pharmacologic doses for more than a month generally develop, at least, mild cushingoid facies.[11, 149] Truncal obesity and a "buffalo hump" are noted less frequently. Management includes calorie reduction, exercise, and reassurance regarding the reversibility of these changes with lower GCS doses.

In spite of multiple effects on calcium metabolism, hypocalcemia is uncommon.[150] Neurologic dysfunction due to GCS-induced lipomatosis is a rare but important potential complication.[151, 152] Nerve entrapment may occur because of epidural or peripheral perineural lipid deposits.

MUSCULOSKELETAL EFFECTS. The most important musculoskeletal adverse effect is aseptic bone necrosis (avascular necrosis, osteonecrosis, ischemic bone necrosis). The prevailing theory regarding the mechanism involves microemboli of subchondral endarterioles.[19, 153, 154] Subchondral osteolysis and osteochondritis dissecans may also contribute. Most patients who develop GCS-induced aseptic necrosis have been receiving therapy for longer than 3 months and, typically, for at least 6–12 months.[114, 154, 155] Occasional reports of aseptic necrosis with briefer durations of therapy are of concern. In most such cases, the patients are men in the third through fifth decades of life receiving high-dose, long-term GCS.[114] Alcohol abuse and hyperlipidemia may contribute to the development of the condition. The risk of aseptic necrosis may be inherent to the specific disease treated; prevalence varies significantly within different populations studied.[155–159] The femur is the bone most commonly affected; the humeral head, knee, talus, and capitellum are less frequently involved.[19] Early diagnosis is best obtained through either bone scans or magnetic resonance imaging scans.[155, 160] Abnormalities demonstrated by these techniques may precede radiographic changes by up to 18 months. Plain films show changes only when there is more than 50% demineralization. Early surgical decompression may salvage the affected bone.[161] Careful attention to complaints of persistent focal bone pain is important for surveillance of this important complication.

Osteoporosis is a complication whose incidence is not decreased by alternate-day therapy.[15, 98] Long-term physiologic GCS doses (5 mg/day) probably do not increase the risk of osteoporosis.[162] Areas with high trabecular bone content, such as the spine and ribs, as well as vertebral bodies are at greatest risk. Altered gastrointestinal calcium absorption, increased renal excretion of calcium, and secondary elevation of parathyroid hormone stimulating osteoclast activity all play a role.[1, 18, 163] Elderly, postmenopausal women, particularly those who are immobilized, and rheumatoid arthritis patients are at greatest risk.[19, 164] Osteoporosis is noted in up to 40% of chronic GCS-treated patients; compression fractures develop in 8%–18% of patients on long-term GCS therapy.[1] Management involves calcium in doses of 1–1.5 g/day, exercise, and perhaps vitamin D supplementation of 50,000 units two or three times per week.[165] Careful attention to any focal bone symptomatology is also important in order to diagnose compression fractures.

Steroid myopathy is probably due to decreased glucose and amino acid uptake by the muscles.[166] Fluorinated steroids such as triamcinolone may increase the risk of this complication. Although myopathy often develops with long-term, high-dose GCS therapy, this is not consistently seen.[18, 19, 167] There is no good correlation with the age or sex of the patient. The pelvic muscles are initially involved with progression to the shoulder muscles.[168] These proximal muscle groups demonstrate weakness in the absence of pain. Muscle enzymes, muscle biopsies, and electromyograms are of little help in myopathy diagnosis. A ratio of urinary creatine to urinary creatine plus creatinine that is greater than 1:4 is the standard of diagnosis.[18, 19] Exercise and a more gradual reduction of GCS dose typically aid in the resolution of this problem.[169]

106   *Glucocorticosteroids*

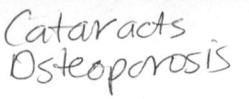

OCULAR EFFECTS. Cataracts are an adverse effect of GCS whose frequency is not decreased by alternate-day therapy.[170] The pathogenesis is uncertain. High-risk patients include those on more than 10 mg/day of prednisone for at least 1 year. Children and rheumatoid arthritis patients may be at increased risk.[19, 171, 172] Most patients present with bilateral posterior subcapsular cataracts and do not have any vision change early on.[173–176] A slit-lamp examination by an ophthalmologist at least every 6–12 months is appropriate for patients on long-term GCS therapy.

Glaucoma induced by systemic GCS therapy is a potential problem.[177, 178] The risk of GCS-induced glaucoma is greater with topical than with systemic therapy.[173] The mechanism is postulated to be an increased aqueous humor production with swelling of the trabecular collagen network.[18, 19, 179] Patients with a family history of glaucoma, with a personal history of myopia, or with diabetes mellitus are at increased risk.[11, 180] Symptoms due to the glaucoma are uncommon. This complication is reversible after discontinuation of therapy.

A rare but dreaded complication of systemic GCS therapy is herpes simplex virus keratitis. Presence of ocular herpes simplex is an absolute contraindication to systemic therapy.[79] Exophthalmos is rarely noted. Although transient myopia may occur, long-term refraction changes due to GCS are uncommon.[11]

HEMATOLOGIC EFFECTS. Venous thrombosis typically presenting as thrombophlebitis is an uncommon but important complication of GCS therapy.[11] The mechanism in part may be due to increased red blood cell content stimulated by GCS. An elevated white blood cell count in the range of 15,000–20,000/cu mm is common and is generally of no concern.[18] A decreased lymphocyte percentage on differential white blood cell count is expected.

RENAL EFFECTS. Increased urinary calcium excretion may lead to urolithiasis.[1] Patients with this condition may be asymptomatic. However, acute flank pain should be evaluated promptly. Hypokalemic alkalosis is an uncommon complication of oral GCS therapy. High-dose pulse regimens present a much greater risk of electrolyte changes.[108, 110]

PREGNANCY RISK. Several studies have demonstrated increased teratogenesis in laboratory animals that is due to GCS therapy. Cleft lip and cleft palate are the most common specific malformations.[13] Multiple studies of patients with GCS-dependent systemic conditions during pregnancy have demonstrated no increased risk of congenital malformations in humans.[13, 181–183] As with any drug in pregnancy, GCS should be used only when the drug is clearly indicated and the potential benefits far exceed the potential risk to the mother and fetus.

Fetal HPA axis suppression is important to consider, particularly when GCS therapy is used near the time of delivery. There may be an increased risk of stillbirth and spontaneous abortion.[11, 13, 19]

OTHER ADVERSE EFFECTS. Hypersensitivity to oral GCS therapy has been rarely reported.[184] Porcine forms of ACTH produce an increased risk of hypersensitivity.[185] Specific risks of intramuscular GCS therapy include abscess formation, crystal deposition, and atrophy if injected into subcutaneous fat.[1] GCS-induced panniculitis has been reported as well.[186, 187]

HPA Axis Suppression

ADRENAL INSUFFICIENCY DEFINITIONS. It is important to have a clear set of definitions for the various types of adrenal insufficiency. There are three types of adrenal insufficiency.[12, 17] The first type is primary adrenal insufficiency, otherwise known as Addison's disease. In order for the patient to present with Addison-like symptoms, more than 90% of the cortisol-producing zona fasciculata must be destroyed. In this condition there is an insufficiency of mineralocorticoid production such that blood pressure and potassium regulation are altered. There is also a secondary increase in ACTH production that results in additional stimulation of melanocytes with the characteristic addisonian pigmentation pattern.

Secondary adrenal insufficiency is divided into endogenous and exogenous types.[12, 17] Secondary endogenous adrenal insufficiency is due to neoplastic lesions of the hypothalamus or pituitary. This leads to decreased or absent ACTH production. In addition, production of other tropic hormones such as the gonadotropins (luteinizing hormone, follicle-stimulating hormone), growth hormone, and thyroid-stimulating hormone is decreased. In this condition, mineralocorticoid production is adequate because the primary regulation of aldosterone is by renin activity and serum potassium level. Because the ACTH level is low, there is no associated hyperpigmentation.

The most important type of adrenal insufficiency for dermatologists to understand is the secondary exogenous type.[12, 17] This type is due to drug therapy, particularly systemic GCS therapy. There is striking individual variability in susceptibility to secondary exogenous adrenal insufficiency. Again, mineralocorticoid production is adequate, making blood pressure and potassium abnormalities unlikely. In addition, ACTH level is not increased, and therefore no pigmentation abnormalities are present.

HPA AXIS SUPPRESSION OVERVIEW. It is important to consider the HPA axis as a unit, rather than simply to focus on the adrenal gland. This is because of the importance of the entire axis in stress responses. The hypothalamus is not only the site most susceptible to drug-induced suppression but is also the quickest to recover after cessation of therapy.[188, 189] This recovery occurs in most clinical scenarios within 14–30 days after cessation of GCS therapy. The adrenal gland is more resistant to suppression and, likewise, is slower to recovery once GCS therapy is stopped.[190] Overall, the hypothalamus is the most important part of the axis in terms of stress responsiveness.[191–194]

The susceptibility to HPA axis suppression is a function of both dose and duration of GCS therapy. Doses significantly exceeding maintenance levels for at least 1 month produce laboratory-detectable HPA axis suppression.[15, 190, 195] Divided-dose regimens and single-dose therapy given at a time other than morning will increase the risk of suppression.[14] Finally, the longer-acting GCS preparations are more likely to produce HPA axis suppression than are short- and intermediate-duration GCS.

Laboratory-detectable suppression may occur within days of moderate- to high-dose therapy.[193, 196–198] This suppression is short-lived and of little clinical importance. Only one study has documented significant HPA axis suppression with physiologic (replacement) amounts of GCS for a prolonged duration.[199] With long-term, high-dose GCS therapy, morning cortisol levels may generally require 6–9 months or more to return to normal limits. Some authors report a period of up to 12–16 months of increased vulnerability to stress, which is based on impaired ACTH stimulation test production of cortisol.[190, 200, 201]

There is only slight blunting of HPA axis function with off-day testing during prolonged alternate-day therapy.[202] Even though alternate-day therapy lessens the risk of HPA axis suppression, it does not speed the recovery once this suppression occurs.[10, 193, 203] Pulsatile administration of corticotropin-releasing factor (CRF) has been shown to speed the rate of recovery from HPA axis suppression.[204]

ALTERNATIVE MEANS OF STRESS RESPONSIVENESS. CRF can be produced by sites other than the hypothalamus.[17] The cerebral cortex and the limbic system contain CRF, which can be released by acetylcholine and serotonin. ACTH release can be triggered by insulin-induced hypoglycemia through catecholamines. Vasopressin can also increase ACTH production.

The GCS effect in producing elevated blood glucose is much slower than the catecholamine response. Both ACTH and cortisol can induce rapid glucose elevation through release of epinephrine.[17]

The mineralocorticoid aldosterone does not play a significant role in the HPA axis stress response. Of importance is that secondary exogenous adrenal insufficiency from GCS therapy leaves mineralocorticoid production intact.[12, 17] Thus the risk of hypotension and electrolyte abnormalities is quite low. In addition, through catecholamine, acetylcholine, and serotonin effects, blood glucose responses remain intact.[17] Finally, the hypothalamus's reponse to stress is rapidly reversibly over 2–4 weeks' time, which makes prolonged supplementation with "stress doses" of GCS unnecessary.[191-194]

HPA AXIS TESTS. It is important to be familiar with the various tests of HPA axis function. In particular, one should know whether a given test reflects function of the entire axis or only one particular organ such as the adrenal gland. In addition, it is important whether the test performed examines basal function versus stress responsiveness. The primary test of basal HPA axis function is that of the morning cortisol level. The normal peak cortisol value occurs around 8:00 A.M., and the trough value is in the late afternoon.[12, 201] Current radioimmunoassay techniques are minimally altered by exogenous prednisone, prednisolone, and dexamethasone therapy.[12] Nevertheless, it is generally recommended to omit the morning GCS dose on the day that the cortisol level is checked. Cortisol levels generally range from 5–30 mcg/dl, with levels up to 60 mcg/dl with stress.[12, 201] With prolonged therapy, cortisol levels below 10 mcg/dl suggest impaired basal HPA axis function.

The ACTH stimulation test is a provocative test assessing only adrenal function. Typically, 250 mcg of synthetic ACTH (Cosyntropin) is administered intramuscularly or intravenously.[12, 201] Basal, 30-, and 60-minute postinjection cortisol levels are measured. Normal responsiveness is determined by a cortisol level rise of 6–7 mcg/dl above baseline or a peak level above 18–20 mcg/dl. An abnormal response suggests subnormal responsiveness of the adrenal gland to physical stress.[12, 201] However, a normal response is not completely reassuring. Many physicians, when presented with a normal ACTH stimulation test, still supplement the patients with "stress doses" of GCS. This practice limits the value of the ACTH test, and the morning cortisol alone may be sufficient to at least ascertain adequate basal HPA axis function.

There are two important tests of the entire HPA axis response to stress.[12, 17, 201] Both tests should be performed only with endocrinologic consultation. They should be performed only after a normal ACTH stimulation is obtained in order to exclude primary adrenal insufficiency. These tests are primarily for detection of secondary adrenal insufficiency of either the endogenous or the exogenous (drug-induced) type. The first test is the metyrapone test. Metyrapone is a potent blocker of 11-beta hydroxylase, inhibiting the production of cortisol from 11-deoxycortisol. The accumulation of 11-deoxycortisol is measured by serum radioimmunoassay or a 24- to 48-hour urine collection. An alternative test for stress responsiveness of the entire HPA axis is the insulin hypoglycemia test. Levels of cortisol before and after insulin injection are measured. The catecholamine response to hypoglycemia will both increase the blood glucose and stimulate cortisol production.

Normal results of metyrapone tests and insulin hypoglycemia tests are not completely reassuring. When indicated, these tests are more reliable for assessing the ability of the hypothalamus to produce increased CRF response to the stress of hypoglycemia or markedly decreased cortisol production.[12, 201]

ADRENAL CRISIS/STEROID WITHDRAWAL SYNDROME. Given the millions of patients who have received systemic GCS therapy since the 1950s, there is a striking paucity of well-documented cases of deaths that were due to acute addisonian crisis.[16, 205–207] Such patients exhibit appropriate symptoms, hypotension, and markedly decreased cortisol levels and show no alternative causes of these findings.[11, 206] In general, momentous stressors are required to produce addisonian vascular collapse. The paucity of cases is largely explained by the preservation of mineralocorticoid function in (drug-induced) secondary exogenous adrenal insufficiency.[12, 17] Alternative nonsteroidal mechanisms of stress response discussed previously will also help explain the paucity of deaths.

Of greater importance to the dermatologist is the entity known as the steroid withdrawal syndrome.[11, 208] In such patients there is no change in the serum cortisol level. However, it is postulated that there may be a sudden decrease in the cellular levels. The condition is precipitated by abrupt GCS tapering. At pharmacologic doses beyond 10 days, it is possible to develop this syndrome.

Presenting signs and symptoms include arthralgias and myalgias, mood swings and headache, fatigue and lethargy, and in severe cases, anorexia, nausea, and vomiting.[11, 208] The return to higher GCS doses with more gradual tapering will prevent these symptoms.

STRESS GCS DOSES. The question of stress GCS doses arises primarily with surgery performed on patients who require prolonged pharmacologic levels of GCS therapy. Through the effects of anesthesia, surgical trauma, or both, most major surgical procedures stimulate a rise in endogenous cortisol production.[17] The regimens are based on the rise of basal cortisol production of 30 mg/day to a maximum of 300 mg/day with stress.[17] Typically, the intravenous form of hydrocortisone (Solu-Cortef) is given. One hundred milligrams is administered the night before surgery, perioperatively, and every 8 hours the day of surgery.[12, 209] The dose is decreased by 50% every day until the GCS dose prior to the stressful event is reached. Although the risk associated with this therapy is low, supplementing patients during major surgery beyond 1 month following cessation of GCS therapy is probably unnecessary.[17] Major infections, trauma, and myocardial infarction may require stress doses, as outlined previously.

Minor physical stresses, such as febrile illnesses, can be supplemented at a dose level two or three times the basal production of endogenous GCS.[201] This amount is rapidly tapered back to the previous dose. This minor stress supplementation is required only for patients taking less than 15–20 mg of prednisone per day.

GLUCOCORTICOSTEROID (GCS) MONITORING GUIDELINES*

Baseline (When Anticipating Long-Term GCS Therapy)

Examination
- Blood pressure, weight
- Height plotted on growth curve in children
- Ophthalmoscopic examination for cataracts

Laboratory
- Tuberculin skin test, chest x-ray (both optional)
- Electrolyte levels, fasting glucose levels, fasting lipid levels (all optional)

Follow-up* (With Long-Term GCS Therapy Above Physiologic Doses)

Examination

At 1 month, then at least every 2–3 months:
- Blood pressure, weight
- Height plotted on growth curve in children
- Thorough history for adverse effects†

At least every 3–6 months initially; at least every 6–12 months long-term:
- Ophthalmologic examination for cataracts, elevated intraocular pressure

Laboratory (at 1 month, then at least every 3–6 months)
- Electrolyte levels
- Glucose levels (fasting)
- Triglyceride levels (fasting)
- Morning cortisol level (only near time of cessation of long-term, pharmacologic dose GCS therapy; see section on "HPA Axis Tests")

Pulse Intravenous Methylprednisolone
- Cardiac monitoring
- Daily electrolyte and glucose levels

Note: More frequent surveillance is needed if laboratory values are abnormal or with high-risk patients.

*There are no well-established guidelines on which to base monitoring for GCS adverse effects. These guidelines are a protocol to follow that is reasonable on the basis of significant GCS adverse effects that do not consistently lead to symptoms.

†Of importance is that many potentially serious central nervous system, gastrointestinal, infectious, musculoskeletal, and ocular adverse effects are detected by careful attention to patients' symptoms, by examination findings, and by well-directed laboratory or radiologic testing. A patients' handout listing important symptoms to report to their physicians would be useful. (See Appendix 1.)

Drug Interactions

Systemic GCS increase renal clearance of acetylsalicylic acid, which results in decreased serum levels.[11, 18] The potential for salicylate toxicity exists with constant acetylsalicylic acid doses when the GCS dose is tapered. There is inhibition of coumarin effect, although there are conflicting data on this GCS effect.[11, 18] Insulin resistance is due to decreased peripheral uptake of glucose. Oral contraceptives may prolong the serum half-life of systemic GCS.[18]

Drugs that increase hepatic metabolism of GCS include phenobarbital, phenytoin, isoniazid, and rifampin.[11, 18] Concomitant use of other GCS with prednisone also decreases the half-life of prednisone. GCS may indirectly lead to digoxin toxicity resulting from GCS-induced hypokalemia.

Therapeutic Guidelines

INDIVIDUALIZED RISK/BENEFIT ANALYSIS. Any decision to use GCS can always be simplified to a risk/benefit ratio. The risks in the equation are specifically the risks of GCS to a particular patient. This includes any contraindications present or factors that put the patient at particularly high risk for a specific adverse effect. The anticipated dose and duration of GCS therapy are most important in determining these risks.

The benefits of GCS therapy are through limiting or eradicating the potential risk of the disease to be treated. The inherent severity and natural history of the disease, as well as the ability of GCS to alter this natural history, are central to the risk/benefit decision. GCS therapy is optimal when the disease can be suppressed quickly with minimal toxicity. Thus the GCS benefits exceed the GCS risks.

In brief, the decision revolves around whether the GCS therapy can be given soon enough, at high enough doses, and for long enough duration to obtain the desired benefits. This is balanced by whether the therapy can be administered with a low enough dose and short enough duration to minimize the risks.

Additional considerations include the availability of additional measures to minimize the risks of GCS therapy. These measures include systemic "steroid-sparing" agents, topical or local adjunctive GCS therapy, and the identification of any reversible precipitators for the condition to be treated.

ACUTE DOSAGE OPTIONS. Most GCS therapy is given as a single oral daily dose in the morning with an intermediate-duration GCS such as prednisone. This method most optimally approximates the body's own diurnal variation of cortisol production. Divided doses, typically given twice a day, are reserved for acute therapy for severe, life-threatening illnesses such as pemphigus vulgaris. Administration four times a day is generally used with intravenous GCS in high-dose (but not pulse) therapy for medical conditions such as status asthmaticus. In divided-dose regimens, the twice a day schedule is consolidated as a single daily dose first, without a change in the daily amount of GCS given. This consolidation is in effect a tapering step; when a constant total daily dose is given, divided-dose regimens have a greater therapeutic benefit than daily-dose regimens.

Although single daily-dose regimens are traditionally given in the morning, on occasion nighttime dosing is appropriate. This method is used when low-dose GCS-induced suppression of the early-morning ACTH peak is desired. This method is used only for low-dose dexamethasone or prednisone suppression of excessive adrenal androgen production.

The briefer the duration for which the GCS therapy exceeds physiologic dosages, the less the risk of significant adverse effects. Brief bursts (2–3 weeks or less), intermediate duration (over 3–4 weeks but not indefinite duration), and chronic therapy are the key options.

Physiologic (replacement) GCS therapy is 5–7.5 mg/day of prednisone or its equivalent. Pharmacologic dosage ranges include high dose (more than 60 mg/day), moderate dose (40–60 mg/day), and low dose (less than 40 mg/day). Aside from life-threatening dermatoses such as pemphigus vulgaris and bullous pemphigoid, most dermatologic conditions can be controlled by moderate- to low-dosage regimens. It is important to determine initially how the disease activity will be followed. Upon achieving a desired outcome, the patient will conclude the acute phase of therapy, and the tapering principles to be described should be followed.

PEDIATRIC DOSAGE RANGE. Pediatric patients rarely require GCS therapy for dermatologic conditions. Conditions such as severe rhus dermatitis will occasionally require 2- to 3-week bursts of GCS. Typically, 1 mg/kg/day is given; the dose is halved every 4–7 days. This regimen has no significant effect on growth and is safe for the pediatric patient without any significant relative contraindications.

GCS FORMULATION CHOICE. Prednisone is generally the GCS of choice for most dermatoses. Prednisone is inexpensive and comes in multiple dosage sizes, which allows easy titration of the dose to obtain maximal therapeutic efficacy. The prednisone doses are well standardized for the various conditions treated. In addition, the duration of action is optimal for allowing daily or alternate-day therapy. In Europe, it is common to use prednisolone instead of prednisone. Prednisolone requires no metabolic conversion to be active; therefore, it has quicker onset of action and has a greater cortisol-binding globulin affinity. Drawbacks to prednisolone use include its greater cost and smaller number of dosage options. Overall, mineralocorticoid effect and duration of action are much more important factors in choice of GCS therapy than is the anti-inflammatory potency of the product. There is equivalent anti-inflammatory efficacy of various preparations at equivalent doses. Prednisone and prednisolone share a reasonable profile of mineralocorticoid effect and duration of action, in comparison with other alternatives. In general, the high-potency products have fewer dosage alternatives. Lower-potency, short-acting GCS, such as hydrocortisone, may not allow for steady day-long control of the disease activity. The mineralocorticoid effect of hydrocortisone is excessive.

ACTH has no particular advantage over oral GCS therapeutic options.[185] Exogenous ACTH is capable of releasing only 100 mg/day of endogenous cortisol. ACTH therapy does not speed up the HPA axis recovery rate. Pain, expense, occasional hypersensitivity, and stimulation of adrenal androgens are all drawbacks of routine ACTH use.

TAPERING PRINCIPLES. There are two issues that affect the decision to taper GCS. The current disease activity and the HPA axis suppression potential are the keys to any tapering decision.

After 2 weeks of therapy, the possibility of steroid withdrawal syndrome must be considered.[8] Any course of therapy that exceeds physiologic doses for 2–3 weeks produces significant laboratory-detectable HPA axis suppression.

Tapering based on the disease activity is performed to avoid undesirable flare-ups of a previously controlled dermatologic condition. Excessively rapid tapering will occasionally allow a marked rebound of disease activity such as that seen with brief (less than 10–14 days) therapy of severe rhus dermatitis. Identification at the outset of key historical, examination, and laboratory parameters of disease activity is important to guide tapering of therapy.

At pharmacologic doses, it is important to periodically attempt GCS tapering to determine the minimal effective dose that a given patient requires. A rough guideline for tapering intermediate- to chronic-duration therapy would be to decrease the dose by 20%–30% every 1–2 weeks as disease activity allows. More serious conditions, such as pemphigus vulgaris, require more gradual tapering at intervals of 3–4 weeks or more.

A reasonable guideline for tapering would be to decrease the prednisone dose in 20-mg decrements from 100 mg down to 60 mg, in 10-mg decrements from 60 mg down to 20–30 mg, and in 5-mg decrements from 20–30 mg down to the physiologic dose range. When long-term pharmacologic doses of prednisone are used, tapering below physiologic doses (5–7.5 mg of prednisone or its equivalent) should proceed cautiously. Decrements of 2.5 mg or less every 4–6 weeks allows gradual recovery of endogenous cortisol production. Basal HPA function can be determined just before cessation of GCS therapy through a morning cortisol level. A cortisol value above 10 mcg/dl ensures adequate basal HPA function, although stress doses of GCS may still be required. The prednisone dose should be increased to the last effective dose level if a significant disease flare-up occurs during the tapering process. When the daily dose exceeds maintenance levels for more than 1 month, one should always consider attempting alternate-day therapy, discussed as follows.

ALTERNATE-DAY GCS THERAPY. Alternate-day therapy was originally reported by Reichling and Kligman in 1961.[4] The basis for alternate-day therapy is that the anti-inflammatory benefits of GCS therapy persist longer than HPA axis suppression when intermediate-duration GCS therapy, such as prednisone, is used. On the off-day, cell-mediated immunity, white blood cell subset levels, and potassium excretion all are normalized.

Alternate-day GCS therapy should be used to maintain disease activity suppression once adequate control has been obtained with daily GCS therapy. Alternate-day therapy is most likely to succeed when the dosage level required to maintain disease control is less than 20–30 mg/day of prednisone. Patients should be aware that complete suppression of disease activity on the off-day may not be possible. However, either small prednisone doses or other nonsteroidal therapeutic measures can be used for the off-day.

There are several options for conversion from daily to alternate-day steroid therapy once disease activity control has been obtained at a relatively low daily dose. The simplest conversion method is to double the previous daily dose for the on-day and to stop therapy altogether on the off-day. Some physicians will increase the on-day dose by 5-mg increments while decreasing the off-day dose by the same amount until GCS therapy is discontinued altogether on the off-day. Both of these methods enable one to maintain a constant dose over the 2-day period while switching to alternate-day therapy. For less serious illnesses, gradually tapering the off-day dose while maintaining a constant on-day dose is an option. In this method, the switch to alternate-day therapy accompanies a decrease in the 2-day total dose. This method is less likely to maintain control of a more serious condition. In both of these methods, the on-day dose can slightly exceed twice the previous daily dose and still be safer than with long-term daily therapy.[15, 203] The risk of cataracts, osteoporosis, and possibly aseptic bone necrosis is not decreased by alternate-day therapy.[15, 98, 170]

Tapering dosages on alternate-day therapy is accomplished by the methods just described. The advantages of alternate-day therapy no longer exist once the dose reaches physiologic levels (10–15 mg of prednisone on alternate days). Tapering this dose may be accomplished with daily prednisone or, more optimal, the short-acting GCS hydrocortisone.[201, 209]

PATIENT INVOLVEMENT. Involvement of the patient and the patient's family is important for intermediate- and chronic-duration GCS therapy. They should be educated about important adverse effects to report, follow-up required, and laboratory tests or special examinations necessary to monitor GCS therapy. They should be informed about conditions that require stress doses of GCS. Measures to decrease adverse effects, such as calcium and vitamin D supplements for prevention of osteoporosis, should be discussed. Medic Alert bracelets or an identification card in the wallet should be carried to notify medical personnel of the patient's high-dose, long-term GCS therapy. Because of the numerous potential adverse effects of GCS therapy, the active participation of the patients and the patient's family is of tremendous importance.

BIBLIOGRAPHY: Key Reviews/Chapters

Lester RS: Corticosteroids. Clin Dermatol 1989; 7(3):80–97.
Spark RF: Systemic corticosteroids. In Fitzpatrick TB, Eisen AZ, Wolff K, et al (eds): Dermatology in General Medicine. Philadelphia: Lippincott, 1987, 2564–2570.
Glick M: Glucocorticosteroid replacement therapy: A literature review and suggested replacement therapy. Oral Surg Oral Med Oral Pathol 1989; 67:614–620.
Truhan AP, Ahmed AR: Corticosteroids: A review with emphasis on complications of prolonged systemic therapy. Ann Allergy 1989; 62:375–391.
Seale JP, Compton MR: Side-effects of corticosteroid agents. Med J Aust 1986; 144:139–142.
Gallant C, Kenny P: Oral glucocorticoids and their complications: A review. J Am Acad Dermatol 1986; 14:161–177.
Davis GF: Adverse effects of corticosteroids: II. Systemic. Clin Dermatol 1986; 4(1):161–169.

REFERENCES

1. Lester RS: Corticosteroids. Clin Dermatol 1989; 7(3):80–97.
2. Hench PS, Kendall EC, Slocumb CH, et al: Effects of cortisone acetate and pituitary ACTH on rheumatoid arthritis, rheumatic fever, and certain other conditions; study in clinical physiology. Arch Intern Med 1950; 85:545–666.
3. Sulzberger MB, Witten VH, Yaffe SN: Cortisone acetate administered orally in dermatologic therapy. Arch Dermatol Syphilol 1951; 64:573–578.
4. Reichling GH, Kligman AM: Alternate-day corticosteroid therapy. Arch Dermatol 1961; 83:980–983.
5. Fine JD, Appell ML, Green LK, et al: Pemphigus vulgaris: Combined therapy with intravenous corticosteroid pulse therapy, plasmapheresis, and azathioprine. Arch Dermatol 1988; 124:236–239.
6. Siegel J, Eaglstein WH: High-dose methylprednisolone in the treatment of bullous pemphigoid. Arch Dermatol 1984; 120:1157–1165.

7. Johnson RB, Lazarus GS: Pulse therapy: Therapeutic efficacy in the treatment of pyoderma gangrenosum. Arch Dermatol 1982; 118:76–84.
8. Spark RF: Systemic corticosteroids. In Fitzpatrick TB, Eisen AZ, Wolff K, et al (eds): Dermatology in General Medicine. Philadelphia: Lippincott, 1987, 2564–2570.
9. Ziment I: Steroids. Clin Chest Med 1986; 7:341–354.
10. Goodman L, Gilman AG: Adrenocortical steroids. In Gilman AG, Goodman LS, Rall TW, et al (eds): Goodman and Gilman's The Pharmacologic Basis of Therapeutics (7th ed). New York: Macmillan, 1985, 1463–1489.
11. Gallant C, Kenny P: Oral glucocorticoids and their complications: A review. J Am Acad Dermatol 1986; 14:161–177.
12. Wand GS, Ney RL: Disorders of the hypothalamic-pituitary-adrenal axis. Clin Endocrinol Metab 1985; 14(1):33–53.
13. Briggs GG, Freeman RK, Yaffe SJ: Drugs in Pregnancy and Lactation. Baltimore: Williams & Wilkins, 1986, 366–367.
14. Fauci AS, Dale DC, Balow JE: Glucocorticosteroid therapy: Mechanism of action and clinical considerations. Ann Intern Med 1976; 84:304–315.
15. Claman HN: Glucocorticosteroids II: The clinical responses. Hosp Pract 1983; 18(7):143–151.
16. Axelrod L: Glucocorticoid therapy. Medicine 1976; 55:39–65.
17. Glick M: Glucocorticosteroid replacement therapy: A literature review and suggested replacement therapy. Oral Surg Oral Med Oral Pathol 1989; 67:614–620.
18. Truhan AP, Ahmed AR: Corticosteroids: A review with emphasis on complications of prolonged systemic therapy. Ann Allergy 1989; 62:375–391.
19. Davis GF: Adverse effects of corticosteroids: II. Systemic Clin Dermatol 1986; 4(1):161–169.
20. Lucky AW: Principles of the use of glucocorticosteroids in the growing child. Pediatr Dermatol 1984; 1:226–235.
21. Bystryn JC: Adjuvant therapy of pemphigus. Arch Dermatol 1984; 120:941–951.
22. Anhalt GJ: Pemphigus. In Provost TT, Farmer ER (eds): Current Therapy in Dermatology—2. Toronto: Decker, 1988, 53–55.
23. Lever WF, White H: Treatment of pemphigus with corticosteroids: Results obtained in 46 patients over a period of 11 years. Arch Dermatol 1963; 87:52–66.
24. Sanders SL, Brodey M, Nelson CT: Corticosteroid treatment of pemphigus: Experience with fifty cases over a period of ten years. Arch Dermatol 1960; 82:717–724.
25. Ryan JG: Pemphigus: A 20-year experience with 70 cases. Arch Dermatol 1971; 104:14–20.
26. Lever WF, Schaumberg-Lever G: Immunosuppressants and prednisone in pemphigus vulgaris: Therapeutic results obtained in 63 patients between 1961 and 1975. Arch Dermatol 1977; 113:1236–1241.
27. Rosenberg FR, Sanders S, Nelson CT: Pemphigus: A 20-year review of 107 patients treated with corticosteroids. Arch Dermatol 1976; 112:962–970.
28. Seidenbaum M, David M, Sandbank M: The course and prognosis of pemphigus: A review of 115 patients. Int J Dermatol 1988; 27:580–584.
29. Mashkilleyson N, Mashkilleyson AL: Mucous membrane manifestations of pemphigus vulgaris. Acta Derm Venereol (Stockh) 1988; 68:413–421.
30. Bean SF: Diagnosis and management of chronic oral mucosal bullous diseases. Dermatol Clin 1987; 5:751–760.
31. David M, Zaidenbaum M, Sandbank M: Juvenile pemphigus vulgaris: A 4- to 19-year follow-up of 4 patients. Dermatologica 1988; 177:165–169.
32. Hadi SM, Barnetson R St C, Gawkrodger OJ, et al: Clinical, histological and immunologic studies in 50 patients with bullous pemphigoid. Dermatologica 1988; 176:6–17.
33. Downham TF, Chapel TA: Bullous pemphigoid in patients with and without diabetes mellitus. Arch Dermatol 1978; 114:1639–1642.

34. Ahmed AR, Maize JC, Provost TT: Bullous pemphigoid: Clinical and immunologic follow-up after successful therapy. Arch Dermatol 1977; 113:1043–1046.
35. Anhalt GJ, Morrison LH: Pemphigoid: Bullous, gestational, and cicatricial. Curr Probl Dermatol 1989; 1:128–156.
36. Marsden RA: Treatment of benign chronic bullous dermatosis of childhood, and dermatitis herpetiformis and bullous pemphigoid beginning in childhood. Clin Exp Dermatol 1982; 7:653–663.
37. Burton JL, Harman RRM, Reachey RDG, et al: Azathioprine plus prednisone in treatment of pemphigoid. Br Med J 1978; 2:1190–1191.
38. Roujeau JC, Morel P, Dalle E, et al: Plasma exchange in bullous pemphigoid. Lancet 1984; 2:468–489.
39. Ahmed AR, Hombal SM: Cicatricial pemphigoid. Int J Dermatol 1986; 25:90–96.
40. Mondino BJ, Brown SI: Immunosuppressive therapy in ocular cicatricial pemphigoid. Am J Ophthalmol 1983; 96:453–459.
41. Hardy KM, Perry HO, Pingree GC, et al: Benign mucous membrane pemphigoid. Arch Dermatol 1971; 104:467–475.
42. Lindemann C, Engstrom WW, Flynn RT: Herpes gestationis: Results of treatment with ACTH and cortisone. Am J Obstet Gynecol 1952; 63:167–170.
43. Hertz KC, Katz SI, Maize J, et al: Herpes gestationis: A clinicopathologic study. Arch Dermatol 1976; 112:1543–1548.
44. Lawley TJ, Stingl G, Katz SI: Fetal and maternal risk factors in herpes gestationis. Arch Dermatol 1978; 114:552–555.
45. Bjornberg A: Fifteen cases of toxic epidermal necrolysis. Acta Derm Venereol (Stockh) 1973; 53:149–152.
46. Chan HL: Observations on drug-induced toxic epidermal necrolysis in Singapore. J Am Acad Dermatol 1984; 10:973–978.
47. Brice SL, Huff JC, Weston WL: Erythema multiforme. Curr Probl Dermatol 1990; 2:5–25.
48. Halebian PH, Madden MR, Findlestein JL, et al: Improved burn center survival of patients with toxic epidermal necrolysis managed with corticosteroids. Ann Surg 1986; 204:504–512.
49. Marvin JA, Heimbach DM, Engrav LH, et al: Improved treatment of the Stevens-Johnson syndrome. Arch Surg 1984; 119:601–605.
50. Ruiz-Maldonado R: Acute disseminated epidermal necrosis types 1, 2, and 3: Study of sixty cases. J Am Acad Dermatol 1985; 13:623–635.
51. Rasmussen JE: Erythema multiforme in children: Response to treatment with systemic corticosteroids. Br J Dermatol 1976; 95:181–186.
52. Rasmussen JE: Toxic epidermal necrolysis: A review of 75 cases in children. Arch Dermatol 1975; 111:1135–1139.
53. Caughman W: Epidermolysis bullosa acquisita. In Provost TT, Farmer ER (eds): Current Therapy in Dermatology—2. Toronto: Decker, 1988, 64–67.
54. Zone JJ: Chronic bullous dermatosis of childhood. In Provost TT, Farmer ER (eds): Current Therapy in Dermatology—2. Toronto: Decker, 1988, 60–62.
55. Mobacken H, Kastrup W, Ljunghall K, et al: Linear IgA dermatosis: A study of ten adult patients. Acta Derm Venereol (Stockh) 1983; 63:123–128.
56. Lee LA, David KM: Cutaneous lupus erythematosus. Curr Probl Dermatol 1989; 1:165–200.
57. Callen JP, Klein J: Subacute cutaneous lupus erythematosus. Arthritis Rheum 1988; 31:1007–1013.
58. Sontheimer RD: Lupus erythematosus. In Provost TT, Farmer ER (eds): Current Therapy in Dermatology—2. Toronto: Decker 1988, 123–128.
59. Plotz PH, Dalakas M, Leff RL: Current concepts in the idiopathic inflammatory myopathies: Polymyositis, dermatomyositis and related disorders. Ann Intern Med 1989; 111:143–157.

60. Henriksson KG, Sandstedt P: Polymyositis—Treatment and prognosis: A study of 107 patients. Acta Neurol Scand 1982; 65:280–300.
61. Bohan A, Peter JB, Bowman RL, et al: A computer-assisted analysis of 153 patients with polymyositis and dermatomyositis. Medicine 1977; 56:255–286.
62. Krain LS: Dermatomyositis in six patients without initial muscle involvement. Arch Dermatol 1975; 111:241–245.
63. Miller G, Zeckmatt JZ, Dubowitz V: Drug treatment of juvenile dermatomyositis. Arch Dis Child 1983; 58:445–450.
64. Barraclough D: The use of corticosteroid agents in connective tissue disorders. Med J Aust 1986; 144:427–432.
65. Hendra TJ: Failure of steroid and immunosuppressant therapy to halt progression of mixed connective tissue disease. Br J Clin Pract 1988; 42:256–257.
66. Callen JP, Ekenstam EA: Cutaneous leukocytoclastic vasculitis: Clinical experience in 44 patients. South Med J 1987; 80:848–851.
67. Cupps TR, Springer RM, Fauci AS: Chronic, recurrent small-vessel cutaneous vasculitis: Clinical experience in 13 patients. JAMA 1982; 247:1994–1998.
68. Fauci AS: Vasculitis. J Allergy Clin Immunol 1983; 72:211–223.
69. Fauci AS: Wegener's granulomatosis: Prospective clinical and therapeutic experience with 85 patients for 21 years. Ann Intern Med 1983; 98:76–85.
70. Prystowsky JH, Kahn SN, Lazarus GS: Present status of pyoderma gangrenosum. Arch Dermatol 1989; 125:57–74.
71. Breathnach SM, Wells GC, Valdimarsson H: Idiopathic pyoderma gangrenosum and impaired lymphocyte function: Failure of azathioprine and corticosteroid therapy. Br J Dermatol 1981; 104:567–573.
72. Gunawardena DA, Gunawardena KA, Ratnayaka RMRS, et al: The clinical spectrum of Sweet's syndrome (acute febrile neutrophilic dermatosis)—A report of 18 cases. Br J Dermatol 1975; 92:363–373.
73. Storer JS, Nesbitt LT, Lalen WK, et al: Sweet's syndrome. Int J Dermatol 1983; 22:8–12.
74. Jorizzo JL: Behçet's disease: An update based on the 1985 international conference in London. Arch Dermatol 1986; 122:556–558.
75. Wong RC, Ellis CN, Diaz LA: Behçet's disease. Int J Dermatol 1984; 23:25–32.
76. Firat T: Results of immunosuppressive treatment in Behçet's disease: Report of 55 cases. Ann Ophthalmol 1978; 10:1421–1423.
77. Chajek T, Fainaru M: Behçet's disease: Report of 41 cases and a review of the literature. Medicine 1975; 54:179–196.
78. Jordan WP: Allergic contact dermatitis. In Provost TT, Farmer ER (eds): Current Therapy in Dermatology–2. Toronto: Decker, 1988, 22–23.
79. Arndt KA: Systemic corticosteroids. In Arndt KA (ed): Manual of Dermatologic Therapeutics (4th ed). Boston: Little, Brown, 1989, 240–246.
80. Mogavero HS: Exfoliative erythroderma. In Provost TT, Farmer ER (eds): Current Therapy in Dermatology—2. Toronto: Decker, 1988, 20–21.
81. Thorn JJ, Holmstrup P, Rindum J, et al: Course of various clinical forms of oral lichen planus. A prospective study of 611 patients. J Oral Pathol 1988; 17:213–218.
82. Conklin RJ, Blasberg B: Oral lichen planus. Dermatol Clin 1987; 5:663–673.
83. Edwards L, Friedrich EG: Desquamative vaginitis: Lichen planus in disguise. Obstet Gynecol 1988; 71:832–836.
84. Callen JP: Sarcoidosis. In Provost TT, Farmer ER (eds): Current Therapy in Dermatology—2. Toronto: Decker, 1988, 42–44.
85. Stone JJ, Elpern DJ: Sunburn. In Provost TT, Farmer ER (eds): Current Therapy in Dermatology—2. Toronto: Decker, 1988, 164.
86. Valentine MD: Chronic urticaria. In Provost TT, Farmer ER (eds): Current Therapy in Dermatology—2. Toronto: Decker, 1988, 115–117.
87. Redmond GP, Gidwani GP, Gupta MK, et al: Treatment of androgenic disorders with

dexamethasone: Dose-response relationship for suppression of dehydroepiandrosterone sulfate. J Am Acad Dermatol 1990; 22:91–93.
88. Marynick SP, Chakmakjian ZH, McCaffree DL, et al: Androgen excess in cystic acne. N Engl J Med 1983; 308:981–986.
89. Saihan EM, Burton JL: Sebaceous gland suppression in female acne patients by combined glucocorticoid-oestrogen therapy. Br J Dermatol 1980; 103:139–142.
90. Clemmensen OJ, Andersen KE: ACTH versus prednisone and placebo in herpes zoster treatment. Clin Exp Dermatol 1984; 9:557–563.
91. Keczkes K, Basheer AM: Do corticosteroids prevent post-herpetic neuralgia? Br J Dermatol 1980; 102:551–555.
92. Eaglstein WH, Katz R, Brown JA: The effects of early corticosteroid therapy of the skin eruption and pain of herpes zoster. JAMA 1970; 211:1681–1683.
93. Esmann V, Kroon S, Peterslund NA, et al: Prednisolone does not prevent post-herpetic neuralgia. Lancet 1987; 1:126–129.
94. Post BT, Philbrick JT: Do corticosteroids prevent post-herpetic neuralgia? J Am Acad Dermatol 1988; 18:605–610.
95. Watson CPN: Post-herpetic neuralgia. Neurol Clin 1989; 7:231–248.
96. Arnold HL: Oral prednisone–An illogical therapy. Int J Dermatol 1987; 26:286–288.
97. Storrs FJ: Intramuscular corticosteroids: A second point of view. J Am Acad Dermatol 1981; 5:600–602. (Replies by Rees RB, Arnold HL, Mikhail GR, pp. 602–606.)
98. Harter JG, Reddy WJ, Thorn GW: Studies on an intermittent corticosteroid dosage regimen. N Engl J Med 1963; 269:591–596.
99. Kusama M, Sakauchi N, Kumaoka S: Studies of plasma levels and urinary excretion after intramuscular injection of triamcinolone acetonide. Metabolism 1971; 20:590–596.
100. Mikhail GR, Sweet LC, Mellinger RC: Parenteral long-acting corticosteroids: Effect on hypothalamic-pituitary-adrenal function. Ann Allergy 1973; 31:337–342.
101. Carson TE, Daane TA, Weinstein RL: Long-term intramuscular administration of triamcinolone acetonide: Effect on the hypothalamic-pituitary-adrenal axis. Arch Dermatol 1975; 111:1585–1587.
102. Droszcz W, Malunowicz E, Lech B, et al: Assessment of adrenocortical function in asthmatic patients on long-term triamcinolone acetonide treatment. Ann Allergy 1979; 42:41–43.
103. Carson TE, Daane TA, Lee PA, et al: Effect of intramuscular triamcinolone acetonide on the human ovulatory cycle. Cutis 1977; 19:633–637.
104. Ballou SP, Khan MA, Kushner I: Intravenous pulse methylprednisolone followed by alternate-day corticosteroid therapy in lupus erythematosus: A prospective evaluation. J Rheumatol 1985; 12:944–948.
105. MacFadyen R, Tron V, Keshmiri M, et al: Allergic angiitis of Churg and Strauss syndrome: Response to pulse methylprednisolone. Chest 1987; 91:629–631.
106. Snyder RA, Schwartz RA, Schneider JS, et al: Intermittent megadose corticosteroid therapy for generalized lichen planus. J Am Acad Dermatol 1982; 6:1089–1090.
107. Case JD, Smith SZ, Callen JP: The use of pulse methylprednisolone and chlorambucil in the treatment of Sweet's syndrome. Cutis 1989; 44:125–129.
108. Bocanegra TS, Castaneda MD, Espinoza LR, et al: Sudden death after methylprednisolone pulse therapy. Ann Intern Med 1981; 95:122.
109. Freedman MD, Shocket AL, Chapel N, et al: Anaphylaxis after intravenous methylprednisolone administration. JAMA 1981; 245:607–608.
110. Wollheim FA: Acute and long-term complications of corticosteroid pulse therapy. Scand J Rheumatol 1984; 54(Suppl):27–32.
111. Kurki P: The effects of "pulse" corticosteroid therapy on the immune system. Scand J Rheumatol 1984; 54(Suppl):13–15.
112. Whitworth JA: Mechanisms of glucocorticoid-induced hypertension [clinical conference]. Kidney Int 1987; 31:1213–1224.

113. Krakoff LR: Glucocorticoid excess syndromes causing hypertension. Cardiol Clin 1988; 6:537–545.
114. Seale JP, Compton MR: Side-effects of corticosteroid agents. Med J Austral 1986; 144:139–142.
115. David DS, Grieco H, Cushman P Jr: Adrenal glucocorticoids after twenty years—A review of their clinically relevant consequences. J Chron Dis 1970; 22:637–711.
116. Hall RCW, Popkin MK, Stickney S, et al: Presentation of the steroid psychoses. J Nerv Ment Dis 1979; 167:229–236.
117. The Boston Collaborative Drug Surveillance Program: Acute adverse reactions to prednisone in relation to dosage. Clin Pharmacol Ther 1972; 13:694–698.
118. Greeves JA: Rapid-onset steroid psychosis with very low dosage of prednisolone. Lancet 1984; 1:1119–1120.
119. Seymour J: Steroid-induced euphoria. Br J Psych 1988; 153:577.
120. Gangat AE, Simpson MA, Naidoo LR: Medication as a potential cause of depression. S Afr Med J 1986; 70:224–226.
121. Hughes IA: Steroids and growth. Br Med J 1987; 295:683–684.
122. Loeb JN: Corticosteroids and growth. N Engl J Med 1976; 295:547–552.
123. Lauber JS, Abrams HL, Ray MC: Silent bowel perforation occurring during corticosteroid treatment for pemphigus vulgaris. Cutis 1989; 43:27–28.
124. Webb PK, Conant MA, Maibach HI: Perforation of the colon in high-dose corticosteroid therapy of pemphigus. J Am Acad Dermatol 1982; 6:1040–1041.
125. Dayton MT, Kreckner SC, Brown DK: Peptic ulcer perforation associated with steroid use. Arch Surg 1987; 122:376–380.
126. Henry DA, Johnston A, Dobson A, et al: Fatal peptic ulcer complications and the use of non-steroidal anti-inflammatory drugs, aspirin, and corticosteroids. Br Med J 1987; 295:1227–1229.
127. Keefe M, Munro F: Acute pancreatitis: A fatal complication of treatment of bullous pemphigoid with systemic corticosteroids. Dermatologica 1989; 179:73–75.
128. Oppenheimer EH, Boitnott JK: Pancreatitis in children following adrenal corticosteroid therapy. Bull Johns Hopkins 1960; 107:297–306.
129. Nelp W: Acute pancreatitis associated with steroid therapy. Arch Intern Med 1961; 108:702–710.
130. Messer J, Reitman D, Sacks HS, et al: Association of adrenocorticosteroid therapy and peptic ulcer disease. N Engl J Med 1983; 309:21–24.
131. Conn HO, Blitzer BL: Nonassociation of adrenocorticosteroid therapy and peptic ulcer. N Engl J Med 1976; 294:473–479.
132. Spiro HM: Is the steroid ulcer a myth? N Engl J Med 1983; 309:45–47.
133. Smith AT, Mason R, Oberhelman H Jr: The acute local effects of prednisone on the gastric mucosa. Am J Dig Dis 1968; 13:79–85.
134. Lieberman P, Patterson R, Kunske R: Complications of long-term steroid therapy for asthma. J Allergy Clin Immunol 1972; 49:329–336.
135. Staples PJ, Gerding DN, Decker JL, et al: Incidence of infection in systemic lupus erythematosus. Arthritis Rheum 1974; 17:1–10.
136. American Thoracic Society: Treatment of tuberculosis and tuberculosis infection in adults and children. Am Rev Respir Dis 1986; 134:335–366.
137. Schatz M, Patterson R, Kloner R, et al: The prevalence of tuberculosis and positive tuberculin skin tests in a steroid-treated asthmatic population. Ann Intern Med 1976; 84:261–265.
138. Dale DC, Fauci AS, Wolff SM: Alternate-day prednisone: Leukocyte kinetics and susceptibility to infection. N Engl J Med 1974; 291:1154–1158.
139. Sherlock P: Adrenal cortical steroids in the patterns of metastasis. JAMA 1962; 181:313–315.
140. Starzl TE, Penn I, Putnam CW, et al: Iatrogenic alterations of immunologic surveillance in man and their influence on malignancy. Transplant Rev 1971; 7:112–145.

141. Scaparro E, Borghi S, Rebora A: Kaposi's sarcoma after immunosuppressive therapy for bullous pemphigoid. Dermatologica 1984; 169:156–159.
142. Leung F, Fam MG, Osoba D: Kaposi's sarcoma complicating corticosteroid therapy for temporal arteritis. Am J Med 1981; 71:320–322.
143. Hoshaw RA, Schwartz RA: Kaposi's sarcoma after immunosuppressive therapy with prednisone. Arch Dermatol 1980; 1280–1282.
144. Blereau RP, Weingarten CM: Diabetic acidosis secondary to steroid therapy. N Engl J Med 1964; 271:836.
145. Boyer MHJ: Hyperosmolar anacidotic coma in association with glucocorticoid therapy. JAMA 1967; 202:95–97.
146. Olefsky J, Kimmerling G: Effects of glucocorticoids on carbohydrate metabolism. Am J Med Sci 1976; 271:202–210.
147. El-Shaboury AH, Hayes TM: Hyperlipidemia in asthmatic patients receiving long-term steroid therapy. Br Med J 1973; 1:85–86.
148. Pennisi AJ, Fiedler J, Lipsey A, et al: Hyperlipidemia in pediatric renal allograft recipients. J Pediatr 1975; 87:249–251.
149. Rebuffé-Scrive M: Steroid hormones and distribution of adipose tissue. Acta Med Scand 1985; (Suppl 723):143–146.
150. Eberlein WR, Bongiovanni AM, Rodriguez CS: The complications of steroid treatment. Pediatrics 1967; 40:279–282.
151. Kaplan JG, Barasch E, Hirschfeld A, et al: Spinal epidural lipomatosis: A serious complication of iatrogenic Cushing's syndrome. Neurology 1989; 39:1031–1034.
152. Rawlings CE, Bullard DE, Caldwell DS: Peripheral nerve entrapment due to steroid-induced lipomatosis of the popliteal fossa. J Neurosurg 1986; 64:666–668.
153. Richards JM, Santiago SM, Klaustermeyer WB: Aseptic necrosis of the femoral head in corticosteroid-treated pulmonary disease. Arch Intern Med 1980; 140:1473–1475.
154. Fisher DE: The role of fat embolism in the etiology of corticosteroid-induced avascular necrosis: Clinical and experimental results. Clin Orthop 1978; 130:68–80.
155. Vakil N, Sparberg M: Steroid-related osteonecrosis in inflammatory bowel disease. Gastroenterology 1989; 96:62–67.
156. Weiner ES, Abeles M: Aseptic necrosis and glucocorticoids in systemic lupus erythematosus: A reevaluation. J Rheumatol 1989; 16:604–608.
157. Fitzsimons R, Grammer LC, Halwig JM, et al: Prevalence of adverse effects in corticosteroid-dependent asthmatics. N Engl Reg Allergy Proc 1988; 8:157–162.
158. Aoki N: Steroid-induced avascular necrosis of bone in neurosurgical patients. Surg Neurol 1986; 25:194–196.
159. Kwong FK, Sue MA, Klaustermeyer WR: Corticosteroid complications in respiratory diseases. Ann Allergy 1987; 58:326–330.
160. Conklin JJ, Alderson PO, Zizic TM, et al: Comparison of bone scan and radiograph sensitivity in the detection of steroid-induced ischemic necrosis of bone. Radiology 1983; 147:221–226.
161. Wang GJ, Daughman SS, Reger SI, et al: The effect of core decompression on femoral head blood flow in steroid-induced avascular necrosis of the femoral head. J Bone Joint Surg [Am] 1985; 67:121–124.
162. Hajiroussou VJ, Webley M: Prolonged low-dose corticosteroid therapy and osteoporosis in rheumatoid arthritis. Ann Rheum Dis 1984; 43:24–27.
163. Baylink OJ: Glucocorticoid-induced osteoporosis. N Engl J Med 1983; 309:306–308.
164. Dykman TR, Gluck OS, Murphy WA, et al: Evaluation of factors associated with glucocorticoid-induced osteopenia in patients with rheumatic diseases. Arthritis Rheum 1985; 28:361–367.
165. Mazanec DJ, Grisanti JM: Drug-induced osteoporosis. Cleve Clin J Med 1989; 56:297–303.
166. Melby J: Systemic corticosteroid therapy: Pharmacology and endocrinologic considerations. Ann Intern Med 1974; 81:505–512.

167. Bowyer SL, LaMothe MP, Hollister JR: Steroid myopathy: Incidence and detection in a population with asthma. J Allergy Clin Immunol 1985; 76:234–242.
168. Ellis EF: Steroid myopathy. J Allergy Clin Immunol 1985; 76:431–432.
169. Horber FF, Scheidegger JR, Grunig BE, et al: Evidence that prednisone-induced myopathy is reversed by physical training. J Clin Endocrinol Metab 1985; 61:83–88.
170. Winter RJ, Kern F, Blizzard RM: Prednisone therapy for alopecia areata. Arch Dermatol 1976; 112:1549–1552.
171. Rooklin A, Lampert S, Jaeger E: Posterior polar cataracts and steroid therapy in children. J Allergy Clin Immunol 1978; 63:383–386.
172. David DS, Berkowitz JS: Ocular effects of topical and systemic corticosteroids. Lancet 1969; 2:149–151.
173. Black RL, Oglesby RB, Von Sallman L, et al: Posterior subcapsular cataracts induced by corticosteroids in patients with rheumatoid arthritis. JAMA 1960; 174:166–171.
174. Castrow FF: Atopic cataracts versus steroid cataracts. J Am Acad Dermatol 1981; 5:64–66.
175. Sevel D, Weinberg EG, Van Niekirk CH: Lenticular complications of long-term steroid therapy in children with asthma and eczema. J Allergy Clin Immunol 1977; 60:215–217.
176. Shiono H, Oonishi M, Yamaguch M, et al: Posterior subcapsular cataracts associated with long-term oral corticosteroid therapy. Clin Pediatr 1977; 16:726–728.
177. Ticho U, Durst A, Licht A, et al: Steroid-induced glaucoma and cataracts in renal transplant recipients. Isr J Med Sci 1977; 13:871–874.
178. Rimsza ME: Complications of corticosteroid therapy. Am J Dis Child 1978; 132:806–810.
179. Weinres RN, Polansky JR, Kramer SG, et al: Acute effects of dexamethasone on intraocular pressure in glaucoma. Invest Ophthalmol Vis Sci 1985; 26:170–175.
180. Dujovne CA, Azarnoff DL: Clinical complications of corticosteroid therapy. Med Clin North Am 1973; 57:1331–1342.
181. Schatz M, Patterson R, Zeitz S, et al: Corticosteroid therapy for the pregnant asthmatic patient. JAMA 1975; 233:804–807.
182. Warrell DW, Taylor R: Outcome for the fetus of mothers receiving prednisolone during pregnancy. Lancet 1968; 1:117–118.
183. Houck W, Melnyk C, Gast MJ: Polymyositis in pregnancy: A case report and literature review. J Reprod Med 1987; 32:208–210.
184. Clee MD, Ferguson J, Browning CK, et al: Glucocorticoid hypersensitivity in an asthmatic patient: Presentation and treatment. Thorax 1985; 40:477–478.
185. Hirschmann JV: Some principles of systemic glucocorticoid therapy. Clin Exp Dermatol 1986; 11:27–33.
186. Saxena AK, Nigam PK: Panniculitis following steroid therapy. Cutis 1988; 42:341–342.
187. Roenigk HH Jr, Haserick JR, Arundell F: Post-steroid panniculitis: Report of a case and review of the literature. Arch Dermatol 1964; 90:387–391.
188. Jasani MK, Boyle JA, Greig WF, et al: Corticosteroid-induced suppression of the hypothalamic-pituitary adrenal axis: Observation on patients given oral corticosteroids for rheumatoid arthritis. Q J Med 1967; 143:261–276.
189. Gordon D, Semple CG, Beastall GH, et al: A study of hypothalamic-pituitary-adrenal suppression following curative surgery for Cushing's syndrome due to adrenal adenoma. Acta Endocrinol [Copenh] 1987; 114:166–170.
190. Graber AL, Ney RL, Nicholson WE, et al: Natural history of pituitary-adrenal recovery following long-term suppression with corticosteroids. J Clin Endocrinol 1965; 5:11–16.
191. Zora JA, Zimmerman D, Carey TL, et al: Hypothalamic-pituitary-adrenal axis suppression after short-term, high-dose glucocorticoid therapy in children with asthma. J Allergy Clin Immunol 1986; 77:9–13.

192. Danowski TS, Bonessi JV, Sabeh C, et al: Probabilities of pituitary-adrenal responsiveness after steroid therapy. Ann Intern Med 1964; 61:11–26.
193. Morris HG, Jorgensen JR: Recovery of endogenous pituitary-adrenal function in corticosteroid-treated children. J Pediatr 1971; 79:480–488.
194. Wilson KS, Gray CE, Lidgard GP, et al: Recovery of hypothalamic-pituitary-adrenal function after intermittent high-dose prednisone and cytotoxic chemotherapy. Postgrad Med J 1977; 53:745–748.
195. Livanov T, Ferriman D, James VHT: Recovery of hypothalamopituitary-adrenal function after corticosteroid therapy. Lancet 1967; 2:856–859.
196. Streck WF, Lockwood DH: Pituitary-adrenal recovery following short-term suppression with corticosteroids. Am J Med 1979; 66:910–914.
197. Spiegel RJ, Vigersky RA, Oliff AI, et al: Adrenal suppression after short-term corticosteroid therapy. Lancet 1979; 1:630–633.
198. Klinefelter HF, Winkenwerder WL, Bledsoe T: Single daily dose prednisone therapy. JAMA 1979; 241:2721–2723.
199. Fuijeda K, Reyes FI, Blankenship J, et al: Pituitary-adrenal function in women treated with low doses of prednisone. Am J Obstet Gynecol 1980; 137:962–965.
200. Shapiro GG: Corticosteroids in the treatment of allergic disease: Principles and practice. Pediatr Clin North Am 1983; 30:955–971.
201. Stern N, Tuck ML: Adrenal insufficiency. In Lavin N (ed): Manual of Endocrinology and Metabolism. Boston: Little, Brown, 1986:113–120.
202. Ackerman GL, Nolan CM: Adrenocortical responsiveness after alternate-day corticosteroid therapy. N Engl J Med 1968; 278:405–409.
203. Fauci AS: Alternate-day corticosteroid therapy. Am J Med 1978; 64:729–731.
204. Avgerinos PC, Schurmeyer TH, Gold PW, et al: Pulsatile administration of human corticotropin-releasing hormone in patients with secondary adrenal insufficiency: Restoration of the normal cortisol secretory pattern. J Clin Endocrinol Metab 1986; 62:816–821.
205. Kehlet H, Binder C: Adrenal-cortical function and clinical course during and after surgery in unsupplemented glucocorticoid-treated patients. Br J Anaesth 1973; 45:1043–1048.
206. Allanby KD: Deaths associated with steroid-hormone therapy. Lancet 1957; 1:1104–1110.
207. Christy N: Clinical significance of pituitary-adrenal suppression by exogenous corticosteroids. J Chronic Dis 1973; 26:261–264.
208. Kahl L, Medsger TA Jr: Severe arthralgias after wide fluctuations in corticosteroid dosage. J Rheumatol 1986; 13:1063–1065.
209. Saltman RJ, Goldberg AC: Adrenal disorders. In Dunagan WC, Ridner ML (eds): Manual of Medical Therapeutics (26th ed). Boston: Little, Brown, 1989, 411–416.

5 | Cytotoxic Agents

Ronald P. Rapini, M.D.
Robert E. Jordon, M.D.
Stephen E. Wolverton, M.D.

The drugs described in this chapter are extremely potent and produce many adverse reactions, especially bone marrow suppression, teratogenicity, and carcinogenicity. Because side effects often make these drugs unsuitable for most benign dermatologic conditions, they are used mainly for malignancies or for immunosuppression. However, they can be extremely valuable, with proper monitoring, in the treatment of certain severe skin diseases.[1, 2] They should be used only by clinicians familiar with their administration and side effects. Several of the drugs are best administered by or after consultation with an oncologist. As with any drug, the potential benefits must be carefully weighed against the risks of adverse effects. The patient must be adequately informed of these risks.[3-6]

Of importance is that myelosuppression is not necessary for a clinical response to occur.[1] Controlled studies have not been done to prove efficacy for the majority of indications listed in this chapter, and experience is largely based on sporadic case reports.

The cytotoxic agents most useful for dermatologic conditions are covered here. Azathioprine, cyclophosphamide, and chlorambucil are covered in the most detail. Mercaptopurine, fluorouracil, melphalan, vinblastine, and hydroxyurea are given less emphasis.

Other drugs used for dermatologic conditions are administered primarily by oncologists and are beyond the scope of this chapter. These include bleomycin (useful intravenously for mycosis fungoides, Kaposi's sarcoma, and squamous cell carcinoma and intralesionally for warts);[3-6] mycophenolic acid (for psoriasis);[7, 8] azaribine (for psoriasis, but removed from the U.S. market);[3, 7] dacarbazine (or DTIC, for metastatic melanoma);[7] actinomycin D (for metastatic melanoma and Kaposi's sarcoma);[3, 7] and procarbazine (for advanced mycosis fungoides).[3]

125

MALIGNANCY RISK FROM CYTOTOXIC AGENTS*

Aside from teratogenicity from the retinoids, there is no more important issue facing dermatologists who administer systemic drugs than the risk of malignancy from cytotoxic agents. Controversy and conflicting data abound. However, careful review of the following studies allows a number of general statements to be made. It is important to avoid broad, sweeping generalizations irrespective of either the clinical setting or the various drugs that are used. There is a great deal of specific information on the risk of malignancy from cytotoxic drugs used for cancer chemotherapy, organ transplantation, rheumatoid arthritis, and to a lesser degree, other benign inflammatory conditions. In addition, there are significant pharmacologic differences that have an impact on the inherent malignancy risk of cyclosporine, alkylating agents such as cyclophosphamide and chlorambucil, and the antimetabolite azathioprine. Cyclosporine is discussed here in addition to the brief review of the drug's malignancy risk in chapter 7.

PATHOGENESIS. There are a number of theories regarding the pathogenesis of malignancies that develop as a result of cytotoxic therapy. The source of foreign antigens that persists within the organ transplantation recipient can overstimulate the recipient's lymphocytes and lead to eventual development of an abnormal clone of malignant lymphoid cells.[9] The theory of malignancy due to altered immunosurveillance suggests that the immune system in normal hosts is frequently faced with small clones of abnormal cells that it can easily eradicate.[9,10] Such small, malignant clones may be allowed to proliferate with therapeutic immunosuppression. Epstein-Barr virus detected in non-Hodgkin's lymphomas (NHLs)[11,12] and human-papillomavirus–induced cutaneous malignancies in renal transplant patients suggest that oncogenic viruses play a significant role.[13] The malignancy may be transferred occultly from the donated organ or may have existed in the recipient at the time of transplantation.[14] Lastly, both chronic renal failure with hemodialysis[15] and rheumatoid arthritis[16,17] are possibly associated with a small increase in risk for malignancy, particularly lymphoreticular malignancies, that is independent of cytotoxic drug therapy.

Thus the most reasonable comparison for the use of cytotoxic drugs in skin disease would be the use of cytotoxic drugs for connective tissue diseases, particularly rheumatoid arthritis.[18–22] There exists a small amount of data on the use of these agents in ocular inflammatory diseases[23] and cutaneous bullous diseases[24] and the consequent risk of malignancy. In these conditions there is no persistent foreign antigen, no prior malignancy, and overall a less debilitated patient population. It is

---

*This section was written by Stephen E. Wolverton.

important to have as similar a comparison population as possible in order to reduce biases that would unfairly constrain the use of these agents in vasculitis, bullous diseases, connective tissue diseases, and neutrophilic dermatoses such as pyoderma gangrenosum.

TRANSPLANTATION CLINICAL STUDIES. The initial report in the transplantation-associated cytotoxic-drug–induced malignancy was in 1969.[25] One decade later, cyclosporine-induced malignancy was reported.[26] A closer look at the transplantation experience, predominantly renal transplantation, is warranted. A large registry of transplantation patients with subsequent malignancy was started in Denver by Penn and Starzl[27] and continued by Penn and Brunson at the University of Cincinnati.[28–30] Although these studies did not establish incidence rates, they are an excellent source of data for patients' risks of various malignancies in comparison with the risks of the population at large. Conventional immunotherapy (azathioprine, prednisone, ± antithymocyte globulin) has an overall risk for malignancy equal to that of cyclosporine. Both of these therapeutic methods in the transplantation patient population have a greater risk of malignancy than that present in the population at large. In general, the malignancy risk is related to the depth of immunosuppression. The higher-dose cytotoxic agent regimens and combination immunosuppression entail a greater risk than do lower-dose regimens and individual drug immunosuppression.

Cyclosporine alone has an increased risk for Kaposi's sarcoma, NHL of predominantly B cell phenotype, and renal carcinoma.[28–30] Conventional immunotherapy exceeds cyclosporine risk for carcinoma in situ of the cervix, carcinoma of the vulva and perineum in women, and cutaneous malignancies. The cyclosporine malignancies tend to occur earlier and are more aggressive. Conventional-immunotherapy–related malignancies tend to develop later and are overall less aggressive than those induced by cyclosporine. The profile of cyclosporine malignancies may resemble that of conventional immunotherapy more closely with longer follow-up.

Increased risks for patients of cytotoxic-drug–induced malignancies, in comparison with those for the general population, are as follows:[28–30] for cutaneous malignancies, 4–21 times; for NHLs, 28–49 times; for carcinoma of the cervix predominately in situ, 11 times; for Kaposi's sarcoma, 400–500 times; and for carcinoma of the vulva and perineum, 100 times.

Even with these troublesome relative risk statistics, the incidence of malignancy overall is 1%–8% in the transplant population.[22, 31] Even with the markedly elevated relative risk figures for NHLs, malignancies are still relatively uncommon in the transplant population. There appears to be no increase of the common, solid tumors such as lung carcinoma, breast carcinoma, colorectal carcinoma, prostate carcinoma, and invasive cervical carcinoma.[32, 33] In several studies, these lymphomas resolved after the immunosuppressive dose was lowered,[34] or they formed more slowly during initial lower-dose immunosuppression.[35]

Specific associations regarding malignancies in the transplantation population are important. Among the B cell lymphomas of the non-Hodgkin's type, a subtype known formerly as reticulum cell sarcoma, and currently as histiocytic lymphoma, predominates.[36–38] These NHLs seldom originate in lymph nodes or gastrointestinal sites, whereas they are present with an unusually high frequency in the central nervous system. The NHLs generally appear within the first year of cyclosporine therapy and present much earlier than with conventional immunotherapy.[30]

Squamous cell carcinoma (SCC) and Kaposi's sarcoma make up the bulk of the cutaneous malignancies associated with immunosuppression in transplantation patients.[39–41] Gupta and colleagues characterized the different pattern of malignancies in these patients.[42] The increased risk of SCCs in renal transplant patients is 18 times that of the general population. In various North American series,[42–44] the rate of occurrence of SCC in these patients is from 0% to 5%, whereas in series from South Africa and Australia, the incidence is 5%–16%.[36, 45, 46] The peak SCC incidence occurs 5–8 years after initiation of therapy. The SCCs are often multiple and are more aggressive; their metastasis rate is 5%–10%. Kaposi's sarcoma tends to be more aggressive than in the non-AIDS (acquired immunodeficiency syndrome), Mediterranean ethnic group type, and it may resolve if the immunosuppressive therapy is decreased or discontinued.[30] There is a smaller increase in basal cell carcinomas.

CONNECTIVE TISSUE DISEASE CLINICAL STUDIES. Patients treated with cytotoxic drugs for connective tissue diseases, particularly rheumatoid arthritis, form a useful population for comparison with dermatology patients.[18–22] Although the issue is controversial, there is probably a small increased risk of lymphoproliferative malignancies in rheumatoid arthritis patients who have never received cytotoxic therapy.[16, 17] The majority of studies of patients treated with cytotoxic drugs demonstrated no increase in malignancies over the expected rate for the rheumatoid arthritis patient population.[47–50] However, a few studies do suggest an increase of NHLs and cutaneous carcinomas, particularly SCC.[18, 51] The risks for common, solid malignancies are not increased.

DRUG COMPARISONS. Critical evaluation of the known clinical pharmacology permits a few general statements. Combination therapy other than with prednisone entails a greater risk than does a single cytotoxic drug alone.[52, 53] Also, a greater risk exists with increasing depth of immunosuppression, regardless of drug choice. In most of the studies of cytotoxic therapy, prednisone is used as an adjunctive therapy. Use of prednisone alone is not associated with any increased risk of malignancy, except in a few studies that suggest a slightly increased risk of Kaposi's sarcoma.[54,55]

The bulk of the evidence for rheumatoid arthritis patients suggests that azathioprine therapy is not associated with any significantly increased risk of malignancy, as seen in the transplantation studies.[47-50] Nevertheless, in a few studies on the use of azathioprine for rheumatoid arthritis, there was only a slightly increased risk of malignancy overall and an increased risk of lymphoma up to eightfold.[18,56]

The alkylating agents cyclophosphamide and chlorambucil have a well-established risk of malignancy, particularly in three areas. Significantly increased is the risk of NHLs of the B cell type, similar to the risk to the overall transplantation population.[20,56,57] Cyclophosphamide therapy increases the risk of transitional cell carcinoma of the bladder about 8–10 times.[20,58,59] The third well-established risk of alkylating agents is for acute nonlymphocytic leukemia; acute myelocytic leukemia predominates in frequency over acute myelomonocytic leukemia.[60,61] Although cyclophosphamide and chlorambucil malignancy risks are probably less than the risks of other alkylating agents, such as nitrogen mustard and melphalan,[62,63] there appears to be a consensus that the risks from cyclophosphamide and chlorambucil for these three categories of malignancy are significantly greater than the risks to the population at large.

Experience with cyclosporine is too limited to permit specific conclusions regarding malignancy in patients with connective tissue diseases.

In general, the more potent immunosuppressive agent cyclosporine and the alkylating agents, cyclophosphamide and chlorambucil, have a greater risk for malignancy induction than does azathioprine. The relative safety of azathioprine is most apparent in the rheumatoid arthritis population studies.[47-50] Still, azathioprine does have a potential risk to those patients that is slightly greater than to the population at large, particularly for NHLs and cutaneous SCCs.

GENERAL PRINCIPLES. Individualized risk/benefit analysis for cytotoxic drug use in dermatology must be undertaken for each individual patient with skin disease. The clinician should appreciate the generally lower inherent disease risk to these patients than to patients with internal malignancies or in organ transplantation. In general, azathioprine would be the drug of choice for cases of severe bullous disorders, vasculitis, and connective tissue diseases when a nonsteroidal immunosuppressive agent is indicated. Such agents are most commonly required when either a steroid-sparing effect is needed or a steroid contraindication exists. All other less toxic, alternative therapies should have been used or considered. The briefest duration with the lowest dose possible is the goal for any immunosuppressive agent. Patients should be instructed in appropriate measures to decrease the malignancy risk. Minimal midday sun exposure and use of sun screens are emphasized for prevention of cutaneous malignancies. Significant intravenous fluids are important for reduction of bladder carcinoma in cyclophosphamide-treated patients. Finally, truly informed consent is necessary.

Although there are no specific guidelines, ongoing surveillance for lymphomas and cutaneous SCCs is important. Regular Pap smears are required for women. With cyclophosphamide therapy, urinalysis, cytology, and cystoscopy for bladder carcinoma are advocated. The routine monitoring of complete blood counts for detection of leukopenia during cytotoxic drug therapy will also allow ongoing surveillance for potential leukemias.

For future dermatologic therapy with these cytotoxic agents, ongoing studies may determine that lower doses of these agents will not be associated with an increase in malignancy risk. Studies performed in vitro, such as sister chromatid exchange, may be useful in following patients at risk from these alkylating agents.[64] Other long-term studies with large numbers of patients, adequate controls, and adequate duration of follow-up are currently under way.

Until the time that more definitive information is available, it is prudent to be very selective in the use of these cytotoxic agents for dermatologic disorders. In general, they should be used only by physicians experienced with all phases of their use. At present, azathioprine appears to have the most optimal risk/benefit ratio for use in many dermatologic conditions.

AZATHIOPRINE (IMURAN)

Azathioprine was developed in the early 1960s as a derivative of 6-mercaptopurine (6-MP). Azathioprine was developed in an attempt to produce a drug with the same activity as 6-MP but with a significantly slower metabolism. Unlike 6-MP, azathioprine is primarily used for immunosuppression, rather than for cancer chemotherapy.

Pharmacology

Structure

Azathioprine is an imidazolyl derivative of 6-MP, to which it is converted in vivo. The drug is therefore classed as a purine analog. More specifically, azathioprine, along with 6-MP and allopurinol, is structurally similar to hypoxanthine, an important precursor in purine metabolism.

Cytotoxic Agents 131

Absorption/Distribution

After oral administration, 50% of azathioprine is absorbed within 2 hours. Also, 30% of circulating azathioprine is bound to serum proteins. Usual doses produce blood levels of less than 1 mcg/ml of both azathioprine and 6-MP. Blood levels are of little value in monitoring therapy because the magnitude and duration of clinical effects correlate with resultant thiopurine nucleotide (thionosinic acid) levels in tissues. The tissue levels are prolonged as a result of the nonenzymatic reaction of azathioprine with various tissue sulfhydryl groups and the subsequent slow release of 6-MP.

Metabolism/Excretion

Azathioprine is converted to 6-MP and subsequently metabolized. Azathioprine is rapidly metabolized (within 8 hours) in erythrocytes and in the liver. Specifically, xanthine oxidase catalyzes the formation of inactive 6-thiouric acid, and metabolism also occurs by methylation of sulfhydryl groups. Proportions of metabolites are significantly different among individual patients, which presumably accounts for the variable magnitude and duration of drug effects. No azathioprine or 6-MP is detected in the urine after 8 hours. Renal clearance (less than 2%) is probably unimportant for most patients, but severely oliguric patients require a reduced dose.

Mechanism of Action

Azathioprine is structurally similar to hypoxanthine. It provides a false precursor and a subsequent impaired adenine and guanine nucleotide formation. Although theoretically effective elsewhere in the cell cycle, azathioprine's greatest inhibition of DNA metabolism occurs in the S phase. Immunosuppressive effects are likely due to impaired DNA synthesis in immunocompetent lymphoid cells. Delayed hypersensitivity and cellular cytotoxicity are suppressed to a greater degree than are antibody responses. The immunosuppression is dose-related. Overall, azathioprine is considered to be a less potent immunosuppressive agent than cyclophosphamide, chlorambucil, or cyclosporine.

Clinical Use (Table 5–1)

Indications

Azathioprine is now the most widely used immunosuppressive drug for dermatologic and autoimmune diseases, although there are only a few controlled studies documenting its efficacy for these indications.[117] Much of the clinical pharmacology of azathioprine is based on its use in renal

Table 5–1. Azathioprine Indications/Contraindications

FDA-Approved Dermatologic Indications

None Specific to Dermatology

    Of interest are official indications for renal transplantation* and rheumatoid arthritis

Other Dermatologic Uses

Vasculitis

    Wegener's granulomatosis[3, 65, 66]
    Allergic granulomatosis (Churg-Strauss)[67]
    Polyarteritis nodosa[68]
    Livedoid vasculitis[69]
    Leukocytoclastic vasculitis[70]

Bullous Dermatoses

    Pemphigoid[24, 71–77]
    Pemphigus[24, 76, 78–80]

Neutrophilic Dermatoses

    Behçet's disease[81–83]
    Pyoderma gangrenosum[84–87]

Connective Tissue Diseases

    Dermatomyositis[88–91]
    Lupus erythematosus
        Systemic[92–98]
        Discoid[99–101]
    Relapsing polychondritis[102]
    Scleroderma[103, 104]

Dermatitis/Papulosquamous

    Severe eczematous dermatitis[105, 106]
    Photodermatitis (photocontact, actinic reticuloid, etc.)[107–110]
    Pityriasis rubra pilaris[111, 112]
    Psoriasis[113]

Miscellaneous

    Sarcoidosis[114]

Contraindications

    Hypersensitivity to azathioprine[115]
    Pregnancy (except when benefit may outweigh risk)[116]
    Prior treatment with alkylating agents (prohibitive risk of neoplasia if subsequently treated with azathioprine)

---

*Azathioprine is generally considered the drug of choice.

transplantation (its use now yielding to use of cyclosporine). Of importance is that the drug is slow-acting. Its full effect may not be realized for 6–8 weeks, and a therapeutic trial should not be considered a failure until after a minimum of 12 weeks. The immunosuppressive effects may persist for several months after the drug is stopped.

DOSAGE GUIDELINES. Azathioprine is given orally at a dose of 1.0 mg/kg/day. It may be increased by 0.5 mg/kg/day after an interval of 6–8 weeks, if there has been no toxicity and no response to the lower dose. Subsequent increases in dosage of 0.5 mg/kg/day may occur every 4 weeks until a maximal dosage of 3.0 mg/kg/day is achieved. A reasonable maximal dose is 2.0 mg/kg/day for dermatologic purposes. Because the drug is supplied as 50-mg scored tablets of Imuran, the starting dosage is 50–100 mg/day (either given in one dose or divided into two daily doses), increasing by increments of 25 mg until the maximal dosage is achieved. Divided dosing may help to prevent gastrointestinal upset. The intravenous form is rarely administered by dermatologists to patients who cannot take the tablets.

LIFE-THREATENING DERMATOSES. In cases of vasculitis, bullous dermatoses, neutrophilic dermatoses, and connective tissue diseases, systemic steroids are often initiated first, and then azathioprine is added later as a steroid-sparing, second-line drug. Some physicians routinely start azathioprine along with prednisone in situations in which azathioprine is certain to be required for steroid-sparing effect. This approach acknowledges the relatively slow onset of immunosuppression from azathioprine and anticipates the drug's full immunosuppresive effects during the tapering phase of prednisone therapy. These physicians often maintain patients' intake of 50–100 mg/day of azathioprine while reducing prednisone to the lowest possible dose. It is uncommon to use azathioprine by itself. Other physicians administer prednisone as monotherapy and add azathioprine only if the patient has a poor response to steroids alone or as a steroid-sparing agent for patients who require chronic therapy. No drugs are consistently useful for the skin changes in systemic scleroderma. Azathioprine merely joins the long list of anecdotal therapies.

OTHER DERMATOSES. For most forms of dermatitis and papulosquamous disorders, topical therapy is usually attempted first. Physicians usually try administering phototherapy, methotrexate, and oral retinoids before resorting to azathioprine. Antimalarials may be worth trying for photodermatitis before azathioprine. Prednisone or antimalarials are usually chosen for severe sarcoidosis before azathioprine. As with all the other potent drugs described in this chapter, azathioprine is generally used only for refractory or severe disease. The potential benefits must be weighed against the possible toxicities.[118, 119]

Adverse Effects

CARCINOGENICITY. Azathioprine entails increased risk of NHLs and cutaneous squamous cell carcinomas; the greatest risk is to transplantation patients. An overview of risk of malignancy from azathioprine, along with cyclophosphamide, chlorambucil, and cyclosporine was presented at the beginning of this chapter.

AZATHIOPRINE MONITORING GUIDELINES[2, 121]

Baseline

- Complete blood count (CBC) with differential and platelet count, serum chemistry profile, urinalysis, tuberculin skin test, complete physical examination

Weeks 1, 2, 3

- CBC with differential and platelet count

Week 4

- CBC with differential and platelet count, serum chemistry profile

Week 6

- CBC with differential and platelet count

Week 8 (then every 1–2 months)

- CBC with differential and platelet count, serum chemistry profile

Periodically (at least every 6 months)

- Lymph node examination, complete physical examination, stool guaiac, chest x-ray, skin cancer examination, Pap smear, amylase level (if indicated)

Note: More frequent surveillance is needed if laboratory values are abnormal or with high-risk patients.

HEMATOLOGIC EFFECTS. The bone marrow suppression effects of azathioprine are dose-related and may occur late in the therapeutic course. The risk appears to be much greater in transplantation patients than in rheumatoid arthritis patients. Most common is leukopenia, which does not correlate with a therapeutic effect. The drug should be discontinued or at least continued with a dose reduction and close laboratory surveillance should the white blood cell count rapidly decrease to below 4,000/cu mm or persist at such a level. Thrombocytopenia and macrocytic anemia occur less commonly.

GASTROINTESTINAL EFFECTS. Nausea and vomiting occur early in therapy in at least 10% of patients. Patients may decrease these symptoms by dividing the dose and taking the tablets after meals. Oral ulcerations may occur but are less frequent than in methotrexate-treated patients. Pancreatitis has also been reported.[120] Hepatotoxicity occurs in less than 1% of nontransplantation patients receiving azathioprine and is generally reversible. Diarrhea and steatorrhea occur uncommonly.

INFECTIONS. Opportunistic infections should always be considered in the treatment of any therapeutically immunosuppressed patient. Overall, these opportunistic fungal, bacterial, viral, and parasitic infections are relatively uncommon in nontransplantation patients.

OTHER ADVERSE EFFECTS. Uncommon (<1%) adverse effects include fever, arthralgia, morbilliform rash, muscle wasting, and alopecia. Chronic high doses of azathioprine may reduce fertility in either sex. Teratogenicity has been reported primarily in patients receiving combined therapy with prednisone and not azathioprine alone. However, usage of azathioprine in pregnancy is contraindicated.

Drug Interactions

Allopurinol inhibits metabolism of azathioprine, necessitating a reduction to 25%–50% of the normal dose of azathioprine. Other concomitant immunosuppressive drugs may accentuate bone marrow depression, infection, or subsequent neoplasia. Viral replication may be uninhibited when live virus vaccines are given along with azathioprine. The neuromuscular blockade of succinylcholine is accentuated by azathioprine. In contrast, neuromuscular blockade induced by D-tubocurarine and pancuronium is antagonized azathioprine.[65]

CYCLOPHOSPHAMIDE (CYTOXAN)

Cyclophosphamide was synthesized in the late 1950s as a derivative of nitrogen mustard. It is classified as an alkylating agent, but this activity is primarily exerted by its many metabolites rather than by cyclophosphamide itself.[122]

Pharmacology

Cyclophosphamide is 2-bis [(2-chloroethyl)amino] tetrahydro-2H-1,3,2-oxazaphosphorine 2-oxide monohydrate. Cyclophosphamide is an example of the chemical class oxazaphosphorines. About 75% of the drug is readily absorbed from the gastrointestinal tract. It is widely distributed through the body, including the brain. Cyclophosphamide itself is not significantly bound to serum albumin. However, the alkylating metabolites are roughly 50% protein-bound.

The drug is predominantly metabolized in the liver. Several metabolites are of particular importance in cyclophosphamide's clinical use and adverse effects. Alkylation is accomplished by phosphoramide mustard and, to a lesser extent, by nornitrogen mustard. The acrolein metabolite is believed to play a central role in bladder toxicity. About 10%–20% of cyclophosphamide is excreted unchanged in urine, whereas more than 50% of the drug's metabolites undergo renal excretion. Plasma half-life ranges from 2 to 10 hours.

Mechanism of Action

Cyclophosphamide primarily depresses B cell function more than it does T cell function. T cell activity may be increased or decreased, depending on whether the drug is given before or after antigen presentation, respectively. T-suppressor cells are affected more than T-helper cells. Some of cyclophosphamide's effects involve inhibition of nuclear DNA replication because of alkylation by cyclophosphamide metabolites. This DNA alkylation is central to the drug's efficacy in neoplasia. It also occurs in normal, rapidly dividing tissues, leading to hematologic, oral, gastrointestinal, and hair-related adverse effects. Cyclophosphamide is a cell-cycle–nonspecific drug.

Clinical Use (Table 5–2)

Indications

Patients should have a white blood cell count greater than 3000/cu mm and a granulocyte count greater than 1000/cu mm before initiating therapy. Also, it is ideal to keep the counts above these levels during maintenance therapy. It must be remembered that leukocyte counts lag behind cyclophosphamide doses by about 8–12 days.

DOSAGE GUIDELINES. Cyclophosphamide is supplied as Cytoxan in 25- and 50-mg tablets. The dosage ranges from 1 to 5 mg/kg/day, typically given as 50–200 mg/day. The ideal maximum is 2 mg/kg/day for nonmalignant dermatologic disease. Patients' tolerance varies greatly. It is best to give the dose in the morning so that patients can drink plenty of fluid

Table 5–2. Cyclophosphamide Indications/Contraindications

FDA-Approved Dermatologic Indications

Mycosis Fungoides (advanced)[2, 123]

Other Dermatologic Uses

Vasculitis
- Wegener's granulomatosis[123–126]*
- Lymphomatoid granulomatosis[127]*
- Polyarteritis nodosa[68, 123]
- Other forms of necrotizing vasculitis[123, 128]
- Cryoglobulinemia[123, 129]
- Rheumatoid vasculitis[123]

Bullous Dermatoses
- Pemphigoid[123, 130]
- Pemphigus[123, 131–133]

Neutrophilic Dermatoses
- Pyoderma gangrenosum[134, 135]
- Behçet's disease[83, 123, 136, 137]

Connective Tissue Diseases
- Dermatomyositis[91, 138–140]
- Lupus erythematosus[97, 98, 123, 141, 142]
- Scleroderma[104, 123]
- Relapsing polychondritis[102]

Malignancies
- Histiocytosis X[3, 143]

Infiltrative Diseases
- Lichen myxedematosus[144]
- Scleromyxedema[145]

Miscellaneous
- Psoriatic arthritis[146]
- Severe eczematous dermatitis[105]

Contraindications

Pregnancy (cyclophosphamide is teratogenic)
Hypersensitivity to cyclophosphamide (may cross-react with chlorambucil)[147, 148]
Severely depressed bone marrow function

*Cyclophosphamide is generally considered the drug of choice.

and can void, preventing cystitis. Some physicians prefer three-times-daily dosing. The dose should be decreased in patients with impaired hepatic or renal function.

Intravenous therapy is rarely used by dermatologists for nonmalignant disease, but monthly intravenous (pulse) treatment has been reported to be an alternative to daily oral treatment. One regimen is to give a monthly bolus of 0.5–1.0 g/sq m body surface area over 60 minutes, followed by vigorous hydration.

CYTOTOXIC DRUG CHOICE. Cyclophosphamide may require more than 6 weeks to bring about a response in the disease. It may be more effective than azathioprine. Still, it is less popular among dermatologists because it has more bone marrow and bladder toxicity and because the risk of malignancy appears to be higher. Some physicians have questioned whether cyclophosphamide should ever be used for benign conditions.

LIFE-THREATENING DERMATOSES. In advanced mycosis fungoides, cyclophosphamide may be used alone or with other drugs, but it is less popular today than are many other modalities. For pemphigus and pemphigoid, cyclophosphamide is usually reserved for combination therapy along with prednisone in those patients for whom prednisone alone or with azathioprine has failed. Cyclophosphamide is generally in third place or lower as a therapeutic choice for most of the diseases listed in Table 5–2, with the exceptions of Wegener's granulomatosis and lymphomatoid granulomatosis, for which it is the drug of choice.

Adverse Effects

CARCINOGENICITY. The increased risk of lymphoma, leukemia, and bladder carcinoma were discussed at the beginning of this chapter. There is a significantly increased risk of cutaneous squamous cell carcinoma.

HEMATOLOGIC TOXICITY. Leukopenia is one of the most common side effects. Thrombocytopenia occurs mainly with higher doses. Anemia is much less common than leukopenia. Complete aplasia may be occasionally encountered, but it is generally reversible.

BLADDER TOXICITY. Hemorrhagic cystitis appears in 5%–40% of patients and is a major problem with this drug. It can be fatal, and it increases the future risk of bladder carcinoma. Excessive fluid intake and frequent voiding should be encouraged.

OTHER ADVERSE EFFECTS. Up to 70% of patients experience anorexia, nausea, vomiting, or stomatitis. These reactions appear to be somewhat dose-dependent. Hemorrhagic colitis rarely occurs. Azoospermia or amenorrhea occurs mainly after prolonged therapy and may be irreversible. Cardiomyopathy is rare, usually occurring with high doses, but it may be fatal. Pneumonitis and pulmonary fibrosis can also occur rarely with higher doses. The dermatologic side effects include alopecia (reversible anagen effluvium in 5%–30% of patients), hyperpigmentation of nails or skin,[149] and rarely urticaria and mucosal ulcers. Other uncommon side effects include fever, anaphylaxis, transient cerebral dysfunction, and water intoxication with the syndrome of inappropriate antidiuretic hormone secretion. As with any immunosuppressive drug, infections may worsen when patients are treated with cyclophosphamide.

CYCLOPHOSPHAMIDE MONITORING GUIDELINES[2]

Baseline

- Complete physical examination, CBC with differential and platelet count, serum chemistry profile, urinalysis

Weekly

- CBC with differential and platelet count, urinalysis (stop treatment if red blood cells appear in urine); frequency of these tests may be reduced to biweekly if results are unremarkable after 3 months of therapy

Monthly

- Serum chemistry profile

Periodically (at least every 6 months)

- Lymph node examination, complete physical examination, stool guaiac, chest x-ray, skin cancer examination, Pap smear

Note: More frequent surveillance is needed if laboratory values are abnormal or with high-risk patients.

Drug Interactions

Allopurinol increases cyclophosphamide toxicity. The effects of agents such as halothane, nitrous oxide, and succinylcholine are enhanced by cyclophosphamide. Chloramphenicol delays cyclophosphamide metabolism, but barbiturates increase the metabolism of cyclophosphamide, which also increase its leukopenic effects. Cyclophosphamide increases the myocardial toxicity of doxorubicin. The decreased immune response seen with cyclophosphamide may reduce the effectiveness of viral vaccines. Other immunosuppressives may have additive immunosuppressive and carcinogenic effects.

CHLORAMBUCIL (LEUKERAN)

Chlorambucil was first synthesized in the 1950s. Chlorambucil, like cyclophosphamide, is a derivative of nitrogen mustard (mechlorethamine) and is classified as a bifunctional alkylating agent.

Pharmacology

The chemical formula for chlorambucil is 4-[bis(chlorethyl) amino]-benzenebutanoic acid. Chlorambucil is rapidly absorbed from the gastrointestinal tract. Peak plasma levels occur at 1 hour after ingestion, and the drug is extensively bound to plasma and tissue proteins. The drug is rapidly metabolized. The plasma half-life is about 1.5 hours. Urinary excretion is extremely low.

Mechanism of Action

A cell-cycle–nonspecific drug, chlorambucil interacts with cellular DNA to produce a cytotoxic cross-linkage. It is the slowest acting and least toxic nitrogen mustard derivative.

Clinical Use (Table 5–3)

Indications

DOSAGE GUIDELINES. Chlorambucil is supplied as sugar-coated 2-mg tablets of Leukeran. The usual oral dosage is 0.05–0.2 mg/kg/day, but dosages for nonmalignant disease should remain at the lower end of this range. Usually, initial dosages are 4–10 mg/day with maintenance dosages of 2–4 mg/day. Chlorambucil can be given in one daily dose because its gastrointestinal side effects are much less frequent than those of most cytotoxic drugs. Overall, chlorambucil is less toxic than cyclophosphamide but is slower acting. Like most of the cytotoxic drugs described in this chapter, it is often given along with prednisone for nonmalignant disease. Short therapeutic courses of 3–6 weeks are believed to be safer than long-term maintenance therapy.

CYTOTOXIC DRUG CHOICE. In today's medicolegal climate, it should be noted that the package insert for Leukeran states that chlorambucil should not be used for treating nonmalignant disease. Clearly, it should be reserved only for well-informed patients experiencing severe morbidity from their benign disorder, if it is used at all. Chlorambucil is not the treatment of choice for any of the diseases listed in Table 5–3. Most referenced articles are anecdotal case reports.

Table 5–3. Chlorambucil Indications/Contraindications

FDA-Approved Dermatologic Indications

None specific to dermatology

Other Dermatologic Uses

Vasculitis

    Cryoglobulinemia[129]
    Wegener's granulomatosis[125]
    Other forms of necrotizing vasculitis[150]

Neutrophilic Dermatoses

    Pyoderma gangrenosum[151]
    Behçet's disease[83,152]

Connective Tissue Diseases

    Dermatomyositis[91]
    Lupus erythematosus[97]
    Relapsing polychondritis[102]
    Scleroderma[3,103]

Malignancies

    Histiocytosis X[143]
    Mycosis fungoides/Sézary's syndrome[3,153]
    Necrobiotic xanthogranuloma with paraproteinemia[154]

Miscellaneous

    Mastocytosis[3,7]
    Sarcoidosis[155]

Contraindications

Hypersensitivity to chlorambucil (may cross-react with cyclophosphamide)[147,148]
Pregnancy

Adverse Effects

Commonly, there is a slowly progressive lymphopenia. Neutropenia may persist for 10 days after the dose is administered. Thrombocytopenia is less common, and irreversible aplasia is infrequently seen. Nausea, vomiting, diarrhea, and oral ulcerations are uncommonly observed. There is a significant incidence of seizures.[156] Azoospermia and amenorrhea may occur and can result in sterility.

    Dermatologic problems are not frequent with this drug. Morbilliform rash, urticaria,[149,157] and alopecia have been reported. Other uncommon side effects include peripheral neuropathy, pulmonary fibrosis, pneumonia, hepatotoxicity, fever, and sterile cystitis. Decreased metabolism of the drug may occur in patients with impaired hepatic function.

> **CHLORAMBUCIL MONITORING GUIDELINES**[2]
>
> **Baseline**
>
> - Complete physical examination, CBC with differential and platelet count, urinalysis
>
> **Weekly**
>
> - CBC with differential and platelet count (see cyclophosphamide monitoring guidelines)
>
> **Monthly**
>
> - Serum chemistry profile, urinalysis
>
> **Periodically (at least every 6 months)**
>
> - Lymph node examination, complete physical examination, stool guaiac, chest x-ray, skin cancer examination, Pap smear
>
> *Note:* More frequent surveillance is needed if laboratory values are abnormal or with high-risk patients.

Drug Interactions

Other immunosuppressives may have additive effect, and a poor immune response may occur when viral vaccines are given.

MERCAPTOPURINE (PURINETHOL)

Mercaptopurine (6-MP) is the active metabolite of azathioprine and is likewise a purine analog. Because of the incomplete and variable absorption of 6-MP, its rapid in vivo degradation, and its more serious side effects, azathioprine has enjoyed much greater popularity among dermatologists. There are currently no approved dermatologic indications for 6-MP. Its primary use in the 1960s and in the early 1970s was for psoriasis at a dosage of 150–250 mg/day.[146, 158, 159] Other dermatologic conditions for which it may be used include histocytosis X,[143, 160] pyoderma gangrenosum,[161] relapsing polychondritis,[102] and polyarteritis nodosa.[68] Because of the general advantages of azathioprine (see earlier discussion) and the far greater efficacy of methotrexate in treating psoriasis, 6-MP is rarely used in dermatology today.

FLUOROURACIL (ADRUCIL)

Fluorouracil (5-FU), a fluorinated pyrimidine analog, was first synthesized in 1957. Its oral absorption is extremely poor, and only the intravenous form is currently available. Intravenous use of 5-FU has been discussed for psoriasis.[162] However, a great deal more work is necessary before its routine use can be recommended. Potential indications would also include metastatic melanoma[7] and scleroderma.[163, 164] Occasional intralesional uses (basal cell carcinoma and keratoacanthoma) and the drug's many topical uses are beyond the scope of this book. 5-FU entails many severe adverse effects, including hematologic and gastrointestinal effects, and an increased risk of malignancy. 5-FU should not be considered for routine dermatologic use, given the narrow risk/benefit ratio and its availability only in the intravenous form.

MELPHALAN (ALKERAN)

Melphalan is a derivative of nitrogen mustard and is classified as an alkylating agent. Although the drug is available orally, absorption by the oral route is highly variable. Again, there are no approved dermatologic indications. However, the drug has an occasional dermatologic use, particularly in the area of scleromyxedema.[145, 165, 166] Melphalan has been used for metastatic melanoma,[149, 167] amyloidosis,[168,169] cryoglobulinemia,[129] necrobiotic xanthogranuloma,[154] pyoderma gangrenosum,[170] and relapsing polychronditis.[102] Frequent adverse effects, such as leukemia,[171] and potentially severe hematologic and gastrointestinal complications, preclude routine use of melphalan in dermatology.

VINBLASTINE (VELBAN, VELSAR)

Vinblastine and closely related vincristine are alkaloids extracted from the periwinkle plant (*Vinca rosea*). Vinblastine is not absorbed from the gastrointestinal tract and must be given intravenously. Approved indications for vinblastine include mycosis fungoides,[3] histiocytosis X,[3] and Kaposi's sarcoma.[172–179] Metastatic melanoma may be another dermatologic indication.[7] Although vinblastine is generally administered by oncologists, dermatologists should be aware of the indications just listed. A low therapeutic index and the availability of only an intravenous route preparation preclude significant use of vinblastine and vincristine in the treatment of skin disease.

HYDROXYUREA (HYDREA)

The chemical structure of hydroxyurea is simply that of urea with an added hydroxyl group. The drug is well absorbed from the gastrointestinal tract. The exact mode of action is uncertain, but most likely its cytotoxic effects involve inhibition of DNA synthesis. The two approved cutaneous indications of interest are metastatic melanoma and squamous carcinoma of the head and neck. Hydroxyurea enjoyed its greatest popularity in the early 1970s as a systemic therapy for psoriasis.[180–183] Given the drug's lesser efficacy and far greater toxicity than currently available systemic agents, hydroxyurea is rarely used for psoriasis today. Other indications have included cryoglobulinemia,[129] hypereosinophilic syndrome presenting as erythema annulare centrifugum,[184] pyoderma gangrenosum,[170] and scleromyxedema.[166]

BIBLIOGRAPHY: Key Reviews/Chapters

Wick MM: Cytotoxic agents in dermatology. In Fitzpatrick TB, Eisen AZ, Wolff R, et al (eds): Dermatology in General Medicine. Philadelphia: Lippincott, 1987, 2577–2582.
Nashel DJ: Mechanisms of action and clinical applications of cytotoxic drugs in rheumatic disorders. Med Clin North Am 1985; 69:817–840.
McDonald CJ: Cytotoxic agents for use in dermatology: I. J Am Acad Dermatol 1985; 12:753–775.
McDonald CJ: Use of cytotoxic drugs in dermatologic diseases: II. J Am Acad Dermatol 1985; 12:965–975.
Ahmed AR, Hombal SM: Cyclophosphamide (Cytoxan): A review on relevant pharmacology and clinical uses. J Am Acad Dermatol 1984; 11:1115–1126.
Ahmed AR, Moy R: Azathioprine. Int J Dermatol 1981; 7:461–467.

REFERENCES

1. McDonald CJ: Cytotoxic agents for use in dermatology. I. J Am Acad Dermatol 1985; 12:753–775.
2. McDonald CJ: Use of cytotoxic drugs in dermatologic diseases. II. J Am Acad Dermatol 1985; 12:965–975.
3. Dantzig PI: Immunosuppressive and cytotoxic drugs in dermatology. Arch Dermatol 1974; 110:393–406.
4. Schwartz RS, Gowans JDC: Guidelines for the use of cytotoxic drugs in rheumatic diseases (letter). Arthritis Rheum 1971; 14:134.
5. Steinberg AD, Plotz PH, Wolff SM, et al: Cytotoxic drugs in the treatment of nonmalignant disease. Ann Intern Med 1972; 76:619–642.
6. Whitehouse JMA: Cytotoxic drugs for non-neoplastic disease. Br Med J 1983; 287:79–80.
7. Moschella SL: Chemotherapy used in dermatology. Cutis 1977; 19:603–612.
8. Gomez EC, Menendez L, Frost P: Efficacy of mycophenolic acid for the treatment of psoriasis. J Am Acad Dermatol 1979; 1:531–537.
9. Penn I: Lymphomas complicating organ transplantation. Transplant Proc 1982; 15:2790–2797.
10. Penn I: The occurrence of cancer in immune deficiencies. Curr Probl Cancer 1982; 6:1–64.
11. Ho M, Miller G, Atchison RW, et al: Epstein-Barr virus infections and DNA hybridi-

zation studies in posttransplantation lymphoma and lymphoproliferative lesions: The role of primary infections. J Infect Dis 1985; 152:876–886.
12. Hanto DW, Sakamoto K, Purtilo DT, et al: The Epstein-Barr virus in the pathogenesis of posttransplant lymphoproliferative disorders. Surgery 1981; 90:204–213.
13. Lutzner MA, Orth G, Dutronquay V: Detection of human papilloma virus type 5 DNA in skin cancers of an immunosuppressed renal allograft recipient. Lancet 1983; 2:422–424.
14. O'Grady JG, Polson RJ, Rolles K, et al: Liver transplantation for malignant disease: Results in 93 consecutive patients. Ann Surg 1988; 207:373–379.
15. Sheil AGR, Flavel S, Disney APS, et al: Cancer development in patients progressing to dialysis and renal transplantation. Transplant Proc 1985; 17:1685–1688.
16. Prior P: Cancer and rheumatoid arthritis: Epidemiologic considerations. Am J Med 1985; 78(Suppl 1A):15–21.
17. Isomaki HA, Hakulinen T, Joutsenlahti V: Excess risk of lymphomas, leukemia and myeloma in patients with rheumatoid arthritis. J Chron Dis 1978; 31:691–696.
18. Silman AJ, Petrie J, Hazleman B, et al: Lymphoproliferative cancer and other malignancies in patients with rheumatoid arthritis treated with azathioprine: A 20-year follow-up study. Ann Rheum Dis 1988; 47:988–992.
19. Tilson JJ, Whisnant J: Pharmaco-epidemiology—drugs, arthritis, and neoplasms: Industry contribution to the data. Am J Med 1985; 78(Suppl 1A):69–76.
20. Baker GL, Kahl LE, Zee BC: Malignancy following treatment of rheumatoid arthritis with cyclophosphamide. Am J Med 1987; 83:1–9.
21. Patapanian H, Graham S, Sambrook PN, et al: The oncogenicity of chlorambucil in rheumatoid arthritis. Br J Rheumatol 1988; 27:44–47.
22. Beveridge T, Krupp P, McKibbin C: Lymphomas and lymphoproliferative lesions developing under cyclosporin therapy. Lancet 1984; 1:788.
23. Palestine AG, Nussenblatt RB, Chan CC: Side effects of systemic cyclosporine in patients not undergoing transplantation. Am J Med 1984; 77:652–656.
24. Burton JL, Greaves MW: Azathioprine for pemphigus and pemphigoid: A 4-year follow-up. Br J Dermatol 1974; 91:103–109.
25. Penn I, Hammond W, Brettschneider L, et al: Malignant lymphomas in transplantation patients. Transplant Proc 1969; 1:106–112.
26. Calne RY, Rolles K, Thiru S, et al: Cyclosporin A initially as the only immunosuppressant in 34 recipients of cadaveric organs. Lancet 1979; 2:1033–1036.
27. Penn I, Starzl TE: A summary of the status of de novo cancer in transplant recipients. Transplant Proc 1972; 4:719–732.
28. Penn I, Brunson ME: Cancers after cyclosporine therapy. Transplant Proc 1988; 20:885–892.
29. Penn I: Cancers after cyclosporine therapy. Transplant Proc 1988; 20:276–279.
30. Penn I: Cyclosporine and oncogenesis. Mt Sinai J Med 1987; 54:460–464.
31. Cockburn I: Assessment of the risks of malignancy and lymphomas developing in patients using Sandimmune. Transplant Proc 1987; 19:1804–1807.
32. Penn I: Cancer in immunosuppressed patients. Transplant Proc 1984; 16:492–494.
33. Hazleman B: Incidence of neoplasms in patients with rheumatoid arthritis exposed to different treatment regimens. Am J Med 1985; 78(Suppl 1A):39–43.
34. Starzl TE, Porter KA, Iwatsuki S, et al: Reversibility of lymphomas and lymphoproliferative lesions developing under cyclosporin-steroid therapy. Lancet 1984; 1:583–587.
35. Brumbaugh J, Baldwin JC, Stinson EB, et al: Quantitative analysis of immunosuppression in cyclosporine-treated heart transplant patients with lymphoma. Heart Transplant 1985; 4:307–311.
36. Sheil AGR: Cancer in renal allograft recipients in Australia and New Zealand. Transplant Proc 1977; 9:1133–1136.

37. Birkeland SA, Kemp E, Hauge M: Renal transplantation and cancer. The Scandia transplant material. Tissue Antigens 1975; 6:28–36.
38. Hoover R, Fraumeni JF Jr: Risk of cancer in renal-transplant recipients. Lancet 1973; 2:55–57.
39. Walder BK, Robertson MR, Jeremy E: Skin cancer and immunosuppression. Lancet 1971; 2:1282–1283.
40. Kinlen LJ, Sheil AGR, Peto J, et al: Collaborative United Kingdom-Australasian study of cancer in patients treated with immunosuppressive drugs. Br Med J 1979; 2:1461–1466.
41. Thompson JF, Allen R, Morris PJ, et al: Skin cancer in renal transplant patients treated with cyclosporin. Lancet 1985; 1:158–159.
42. Gupta AK, Cardella CJ, Haberman HF: Cutaneous malignant neoplasms in patients with renal transplants. Arch Dermatol 1986; 22:1288–1293.
43. Mullen DL, Silverderg SG, Penn I, et al: Squamous cell carcinoma of the skin and lip in renal homograft recipients. Cancer 1976; 37:729–734.
44. Hoxtell EO, Mandell JS, Murray SS, et al: Incidence of skin carcinoma after renal transplantation. Arch Dermatol 1977; 113:436–438.
45. Walder DK, Jeremy D, Charlesworth JA, et al: The skin and immunosuppression. Australas J Dermatol 1976; 17:94–97.
46. Disler PB, MacPhail AP, Meyers AM, et al: Neoplasia after successful renal transplantation. Nephron 1981; 29:119–123.
47. Van Wanghe P, Dequeker J: Compliance and long-term effect of azathioprine in 65 rheumatoid arthritis cases. Ann Rheum Dis 1982; 41(Suppl 1):40–43.
48. Whisnant JK, Pelkey J: Rheumatoid arthritis: Treatment with azathioprine (IMURAN (R)): Clinical side-effects and laboratory abnormalities. Ann Rheum Dis 1982; 41(Suppl 1):44–47.
49. Kirsner AB, Farber SJ, Sheon RP, et al. The incidence of malignant disease in patients receiving cytotoxic therapy for rheumatoid arthritis. Ann Rheum Dis 1982; 41(Suppl 1):32–33.
50. Symington GR, Mackay IR, Lambert RP: Cancer and teratogenesis: Infrequent occurrence after medical use of immunosuppressive drugs. Aust NZ J Med 1977; 7:368–372.
51. Pitt PI, Sultan AH, Malone M, et al: Association between azathioprine therapy and lymphoma in rheumatoid disease. J Roy Soc Med 1987; 80:428–429.
52. Wilkinson AH, Smith JL, Hunsicker LG, et al: Increased frequency of posttransplant lymphomas in patients treated with cyclosporine, azathioprine, and prednisone. Transplantation 1989; 47:293–296.
53. Shah B, First MR, Munda R, et al: Current experience with renal transplantation in older patients. Am J Kidney Dis 1988; 12:516–523.
54. Hoshaw R, Schwartz R: Kaposi's sarcoma after immunosuppressive therapy with prednisone. Arch Dermatol 1980; 116:1280–1282.
55. Leung R, Fam A, Osoba D: Kaposi's sarcoma complicating corticosteroid therapy for temporal arthritis. Am J Med 1982; 71:320–322.
56. Kinlen LJ: Incidence of cancer in rheumatoid arthritis and other disorders after immunosuppressive treatment. Am J Med 1985; 78(Suppl 1A):44–49.
57. Baltus JAM, Boersma JW, Hartman AP, et al: The occurrence of malignancies in patients with rheumatoid arthritis treated with cyclophosphamide: A controlled retrospective follow-up. Ann Rheum Dis 1983; 42:368–370.
58. Pedersen-Bjergaard J, Ersbøll J, Hansen VL, et al: Carcinoma of the urinary bladder after treatment with cyclophosphamide for non-Hodgkin's lymphoma. N Engl J Med 1988; 318:1028–1032.
59. Fairchild WV, Spence CR, Soloman HD, et al: The incidence of bladder cancer after cyclophosphamide therapy. J Urology 1979; 122:163–164.

60. Palmer RG, Denman AM: Malignancies induced by chlorambucil. Cancer Treat Rev 1989; 11:121–129.
61. Berk PP, Goldberg JD, Silverstein MN, et al: Increased incidence of acute leukemia in polycythemia vera associated with chlorambucil therapy. N Engl J Med 1981; 304:441–447.
62. Haas JF, Kittelmann B, Mehnert WH, et al: Risk of leukemia in ovarian tumor and breast cancer patients following treatment by cyclophosphamide. Br J Cancer 1987; 55:213–218.
63. Greene MH, Harris EL, Gershenson DM, et al: Melphalan may be a more potent leukemogen than cyclophosphamide. Ann Intern Med 1986; 105:360–367.
64. Palmer RG, Dore CJ, Denman AM: Cyclophosphamide induces more chromosome damage than chlorambucil in patients with connective tissue diseases. Q J Med 1986; 59:395–400.
65. Ahmed AR, Moy R. Azathioprine: Int J Dermatol 1981; 20:461–467.
66. Fauci AS, Haynes BF, Katz P, et al: Wegener's granulomatosis: Prospective clinical and therapeutic experience with 85 patients for 21 years. Ann Intern Med 1983; 98:76–85.
67. Cooper BJ, Bacal E, Patterson R: Allergic angiitis and granulomatosis. Prolonged remission induced by combined prednisone-azathioprine therapy. Arch Intern Med 1978; 138:367–371.
68. Leib ES, Restivo C, Paulus HE: Immunosuppressive and corticosteroid therapy for polyarteritis nodosa. Am J Med 1979; 67:941–947.
69. Yasue T: Livedoid vasculitis and central nervous system involvement in systemic lupus erythematosus. Arch Dermatol 1986; 122:66–70.
70. Callen JP, af Ekenstam E: Cutaneous leukocytoclastic vasculitis. Clinical experience in 44 patients. South Med J 1987; 80:848–851.
71. Greaves MW, Burton JL, Marks J, et al: Azathioprine in the treatment of bullous pemphigoid. Br Med J 1971; 1:144–145.
72. Dave VK, Vickers CFH: Azathioprine in the treatment of mucocutaneous pemphigoid. Br J Dermatol 1974; 90:183–186.
73. Burton JL, Harman RMM, Peachey RDG, et al: A controlled study of azathioprine in the treatment of pemphigoid. Br J Dermatol 1978; 99(Suppl 16):14.
74. Burton JL, Harman RRM, Peachey RDG, et al: Azathioprine plus prednisone in treatment of pemphigoid. Br Med J 1978; 2:1190–1191.
75. Ahmed AR, Maize JC, Provost TT: Bullous pemphigoid. Clinical and immunologic follow-up after successful therapy. Arch Dermatol 1977; 113:1043–1046.
76. Levene GM: The treatment of pemphigus and pemphigoid. Clin Exp Dermatol 1982; 7:643–652.
77. Mondino BJ, Brown SI: Immunosuppressive therapy in ocular cicatricial pemphigoid. Am J Ophthalmol 1983; 96:453–459.
78. Jablonska S, Chorzelski T: Immunosuppressants in the treatment of pemphigus. Br J Dermatol 1970; 83:315–323.
79. Roenigk HH, Deodhar S: Pemphigus treatment with azathioprine. Clinical and immunologic correlation. Arch Dermatol 1973; 107:353–357.
80. Faber WR, Neumann HA, Flinterman J: Persistent vegetating and keratotic lesions in patients with pemphigus vulgaris during immunosuppressive therapy. Br J Dermatol 1983; 109:459–463.
81. Yazici H, Pazarli H, Barnes CG, et al: A controlled trial of azathioprine in Behçet's syndrome. N Engl J Med 1990; 322:281–285.
82. Nethercott J, Lester RS: Azathioprine therapy in incomplete Behçet's syndrome. Arch Dermatol 1974; 110:432–434.
83. Arbesfeld SJ, Kurban AK: Behçet's disease: New perspectives on an enigmatic syndrome. J Am Acad Dermatol 1988; 19:767–779.

84. Schöpf E, Schulz HJ, Schulz KH: Azathioprin-Behandlung der Dermatitis ulcerosa (Pyoderma gangraenosum). Hautarzt 1969; 20:558–563.
85. Olson K: Pyoderma gangrenosum with systemic L.E. Acta Derm Venereol (Stockh) 1971; 51:233–234.
86. August PG, Wells GC: Pyoderma gangrenosum treated with azathioprine and prednisone. Br J Dermatol 1974; 91(Suppl 10):80–82.
87. Byrne JPH, Hewitt M, Summerly R: Pyoderma gangrenosum associated with active chronic hepatitis. Arch Dermatol 1976; 112:1297–1301.
88. Benson M, Aldo M: Azathioprine therapy in polymyositis. Arch Intern Med 1973; 132:547–551.
89. Niakan E, Pitner SE, Whitaker JN, et al: Immunosuppressive agents in corticosteroid-refractory childhood dermatomyositis. Neurology 1980; 30:286–290.
90. Miller G, Heckmatt JZ, Dubowitz V: Drug treatment of juvenile dermatomyositis. Arch Dis Child 1983; 58:445–450.
91. Ansell BM. Management of polymyositis and dermatomyositis. Clin Rheum Dis 1984; 10:205–213.
92. Corley CC Jr, Lessner HE, Larsen WE: Azathioprine therapy of "autoimmune" diseases. Am J Med 1966; 41:404–412.
93. Sztejnbok M, Stewart A, Diamond H, et al: Azathioprine in the treatment of systemic lupus erythematosus. A controlled study. Arthritis Rheum 1971; 14:639–645.
94. Cade R, Spooner G, Schlein F, et al: Comparison of azathioprine, prednisone, and heparin alone or combined in treating lupus nephritis. Nephron 1973; 10:37–56.
95. Donadio JV, Holley KE, Wagoner RD, et al: Further observations on the treatment of lupus nephritis with prednisone and combined prednisone and azathioprine. Arthritis Rheum 1974; 17:573–581.
96. Hahn BH, Kantor OS, Osterland CK: Azathioprine plus prednisone compared with prednisone alone in the treatment of systemic lupus erythematosus. Ann Intern Med 1975; 83:597–605.
97. Sabbour MS, Osman LM: Comparison of chlorambucil, azathioprine, or cyclophosphamide combined with corticosteroids in the treatment of lupus nephritis. Br J Dermatol 1979; 100:113–125.
98. Dinant HJ, Decker JL, Klippel JH, et al: Alternate modes of cyclophosphamide and azathioprine therapy in lupus nephritis. Ann Intern Med 1982; 96:728–736.
99. Tsokos GC, Caughman SW, Klippel JH: Successful treatment of generalized discoid skin lesions with azathioprine: Its use in a patient with systemic lupus erythematosus. Arch Dermatol 1985; 121:1323–1325.
100. Shehade S: Successful treatment of generalized discoid skin lesions with azathioprine (letter). Arch Dermatol 1986; 122:376–377.
101. Ashinoff R, Werth VP, Franks AG Jr: Resistant discoid lupus erythematosus of palms and soles: Successful treatment with azathioprine. J Am Acad Dermatol 1988; 19:961–965.
102. Cohen PR, Rapini RP: Relapsing polychondritis. Int J Dermatol 1986; 25:280–285.
103. Winkelmann RK, Kierland RR, Perry HO, et al: Management of scleroderma. Mayo Clin Proc 1971; 46:128–134.
104. Steigerwald JC: Progressive systemic sclerosis. Management: III. Immunosuppressive agents. Clin Rheum Dis 1979; 5:284–294.
105. Morrison JGL, Schulz EJ: Treatment of eczema with cyclophosphamide and azathioprine. Br J Dermatol 1978; 98:203–207.
106. Freeman K, Hewitt M, Warin AP: Two cases of distinctive exudative discoid and lichenoid chronic dermatosis of Sulzberger and Garbe responding to azathioprine. Br J Dermatol 1984; 111:215–220.
107. Roed-Peterson J, Thomsen K: Azathioprine in the treatment of airborne contact dermatitis from compositae oleoresins and sensitivity to UVA. Acta Derm Venereol (Stockh) 1980; 60:275–276.

108. Leigh IM, Hawk JL: Treatment of chronic actinic dermatitis with azathioprine. Br J Dermatol 1984; 110:691–695.
109. Haynes HA, Bernhard JD, Gange RW: Actinic reticuloid. Response to combination treatment with azathioprine, hydroxychloroquine, and prednisone. J Am Acad Dermatol 1984; 10:947–952.
110. Toonstra J, Henquet CJM, van Weelden H, et al: Actinic reticuloid. J Am Acad Dermatol 1989; 21:205–214.
111. Hunter GA, Forbes IJ: Treatment of pityriasis rubra pilaris with azathioprine. Br J Dermatol 1972; 87:42–45.
112. Griffiths WAD: Pityriasis rubra pilaris. Clin Exp Dermatol 1980; 5:105–112.
113. Munro DD: Azathioprine in psoriasis. Proc R Soc Med 1973; 66:747–748.
114. Pacheco Y, Marechal C, Marechal F, et al: Azathioprine treatment of chronic pulmonary sarcoidosis. Sarcoidosis 1985; 2:107–113.
115. Saway PA, Heck LW, Bonner JR, et al: Azathioprine hypersensitivity. Case report and review of the literature. Am J Med 1988; 84:960–964.
116. Gebhardt DOE: Azathioprine teratogenicity: Review of the literature and case report (letter). Obstet Gynecol 1983; 61:270.
117. Rosman M, Bertino JR: Azathioprine. Ann Intern Med 1973; 79:694–700.
118. Schein PS, Winokur SH: Immunosuppressive and cytotoxic chemotherapy: Long-term complications. Ann Intern Med 1975; 82:84–95.
119. Speerstra F, Boerbooms AM, van de Putte LB, et al: Side effects of azathioprine treatment in rheumatoid arthritis: Analysis of ten years of experience. Ann Rheum Dis 1982; 41(Suppl 1):37–39.
120. Herskowitz LJ, Olansky S, Lang PG: Acute pancreatitis associated with long-term azathioprine therapy. Arch Dermatol 1979; 115:179.
121. Gendler E: Azathioprine for use in dermatology. J Dermatol Surg Oncol 1984; 10:462–464.
122. Gershwin ME, Goetzl EJ, Steinberg AD: Cyclophosphamide: Use in practice. Ann Intern Med 1974; 80:531–540.
123. Ahmed AR, Hombal SM: Cyclophosphamide (Cytoxan): A review on relevant pharmacology and clinical uses. J Am Acad Dermatol 1984; 11:1115–1126.
124. Novack SN, Pearson CM: Cyclophosphamide therapy in Wegener's granulomatosis. N Engl J Med 1971; 284:938–942.
125. Morton CE, Easton DJ: Cytotoxic therapy for Wegener's granulomatosis (letter). Lancet 1984; 1:1411.
126. DeRemee RA, McDonald TJ, Weiland LH: Wegener's granulomatosis: Observations on treatment with antimicrobial agents. Mayo Clin Proc 1985; 60:27–32.
127. Brodell RT, Miller CW, Eisen AZ: Cutaneous lesions of lymphomatoid granulomatosis. Arch Dermatol 1986; 122:303–306.
128. Fauci AS, Katz P, Haynes BF, et al: Cyclophosphamide therapy of severe systemic necrotizing vasculitis. N Engl J Med 1979; 301:235–238.
129. Ristow SC, Griner PF, Abraham GN, et al: Reversal of systemic manifestations of cryoglobulinemia: Treatment with melphalan and prednisone. Arch Intern Med 1976; 136:467–470.
130. Brody HJ, Pirozzi DJ: Benign mucous membrane pemphigoid. Response to therapy with cyclophosphamide. Arch Dermatol 1977; 113:1598–1599.
131. Ebringer A, Mackay IR: Pemphigus vulgaris successfully treated with cyclophosphamide. Ann Intern Med 1969; 71:125–127.
132. McKelvey EM, Hasegaga J: Cyclophosphamide and pemphigus vulgaris. Arch Dermatol 1971; 103:198–200.
133. Fellner MJ, Katz JM, McCabe JB: Successful use of cyclophosphamide and prednisone for initial treatment of pemphigus vulgaris. Arch Dermatol 1978; 114:889–894.
134. Crawford SE, Sherman R, Farara B: Pyoderma gangrenosum with response to cyclophosphamide therapy. J Pediatr 1967; 71:255–258.

135. Newell LM, Malkinson FD: Pyoderma gangrenosum: Response to cyclophosphamide therapy. Arch Dermatol 1983; 119:495–497.
136. Buckeley CE III, Gillis JR Jr: Cyclophosphamide therapy of Behçet's disease. J Allergy Clin Immunol 1969; 43:273–283.
137. Davatchi F, Baygan F, Chams H, et al: Cyclophosphamide in the treatment of the ocular manifestations of Behçet's disease. J Rheumatol 1984; 11:404–405.
138. El Ghobarch A, Balint GD: Dermatomyositis: Observation on the use of immunosuppressive therapy and review of literature. Postgrad Med 1978; 54:516–527.
139. Yoshioka M, Okuno T, Mikawa H: Prognosis and treatment of polymyositis with particular reference to steroid-resistant patients. Arch Dis Child 1985; 60:236–244.
140. Bombardieri S, Hughes GRV, Neri R, et al: Cyclophosphamide in severe polymyositis (letter). Lancet 1989; 1:1138–1139.
141. Hecht B, Siegel N, Adler M, et al: Prognostic indices in lupus nephritis. Medicine 1976; 55:163–181.
142. McCune WJ, Golbus J, Zeldes W, et al: Clinical and immunological effects of monthly administration of intravenous cyclophosphamide in severe systemic lupus erythematosus. N Engl J Med 1988; 318:1423–1431.
143. Roper SS, Spraker MK: Cutaneous histiocytosis syndromes. Pediatr Dermatol 1985; 3:19–30.
144. Jessen RT, Straight M, Becker LE: Lichen myxedematosus: Treatment with cyclophosphamide. Int J Dermatol 1978; 17:833–839.
145. Gabriel SE, Perry HO, Oleson GB, et al: Scleromyxedema: A scleroderma-like disorder with systemic manifestations. Medicine 1988; 67:58–65.
146. Higgins LC Jr, Thompson JG: Psoriasis with arthritis: Chemotherapy with cyclophosphamide, nitrogen mustard and 6-mercaptopurine. South Med J 1966; 59:1191–1193.
147. Weiss RB, Bruno S: Hypersensitivity reactions to cancer chemotherapy agents. Ann Intern Med 1981; 94:66–72.
148. Kritharides L, Lawrie K, Varigos GA: Cyclophosphamide hypersensitivity and crossreactivity with chlorambucil [letter]. Cancer Treat Rep 1987; 71:1323–1324.
149. Bronner AK, Hood AF: Cutaneous complications of chemotherapeutic agents. J Am Acad Dermatol 1983; 9:645–663.
150. Bradley JD, Brandt KD, Kath BP: Infectious complications of cyclophosphamide treatment for vasculitis. Arthritis Rheum 1989; 32:45–53.
151. Callen JP, Case JD, Sager D: Chlorambucil—An effective corticosteroid-sparing therapy for Pyoderma gangrenosum. J Am Acad Dermatol 1989; 21:515–519.
152. Mamo JG, Azzam SA: Treatment of Behçet's disease with chlorambucil. Arch Ophthalmol 1970; 84:446–450.
153. Hamminga L, Hartgrink-Groenveld CA, van Vloten WA: Sézary's syndrome: A clinical evaluation of eight patients. Br J Dermatol 1979; 100:291–296.
154. Finan MC, Winkelmann RK: Necrobiotic xanthogranuloma with paraproteinemia: A review of 22 cases. Medicine 1986; 65:376–388.
155. Kataria YP: Chlorambucil in sarcoidosis. Chest 1980; 78:36–43.
156. Williams SA, Makker SP, Grupe WE: Seizures: A significant side effect of chlorambucil therapy in children. J Pediatr 1978; 93:516–518.
157. Knisley RE, Settipane GA, Albala MM: Unusual reaction to chlorambucil in a patient with chronic lymphocytic leukemia. Arch Dermatol 1971; 104:77–79.
158. Kravetz RE, Balsam T: Treatment of psoriasis with mercaptopurine. Arch Dermatol 1961; 84:597–600.
159. Baum J, Hurch E, Lewis D, et al: Treatment of psoriatic arthritis with 6-mercaptopurine. Arthritis Rheum 1973; 16:139–147.
160. Hance AJ, Cadranel J, Soler P, et al: Systemic manifestations of pulmonary disease: Pulmonary and extrapulmonary Langerhans' cell granulomatosis (histiocytosis X). Semin Resp Med 1988; 9:349–368.

161. Maldonado N, Torres VM, Mendez-Cashion D, et al: Pyoderma gangrenosum treated with 6-mercaptopurine and followed by acute leukemia. J Pediatr 1968; 72:409–414.
162. Alper JC, Wiemann MC, Rueckl FS, et al: Rationally designed combination chemotherapy for the treatment of patients with recalcitrant psoriasis. J Am Acad Dermatol 1985; 13:567–577.
163. Casas JA, Subauste CP, Alarcón GS: A new promising treatment in systemic sclerosis: 5-fluorouracil. Ann Rheum Dis 1987; 46:763–767.
164. Malaviya AN, Singh RR, Dhar A, et al: Correspondence: 5-fluorouracil in progressive systemic sclerosis: Is it safe? Ann Rheum Dis 1988; 11:964–965.
165. Wright RC, Franco RS, Denton MD, Blaney DJ: Scleromyxedema. Arch Dermatol 1976; 112:63–66.
166. Harris RB, Perry HO, Kyle RA, et al: Treatment of scleromyxedema with melphalan. Arch Dermatol 1979; 115:295–299.
167. Lazarus HM, Herzig RH, Wolff SN, et al: Treatment of metastatic melanoma with intensive melphalan and autologous bone marrow transplantation. Cancer Treat Rep 1985; 69:473–477.
168. Kyle RA, Greipp PR, Garton JP, et al: Primary systemic amyloidosis: Comparison of melphalan/prednisone versus colchicine. Am J Med 1985; 79:708–716.
169. Benson MD: Treatment of AL amyloidosis with melphalan, prednisone, and colchicine. Arthritis Rheum 1986; 29:683–687.
170. Moeller H, Waldenstroem JG, Zettervall O: Pyoderma gangrenosum (dermatitis ulcerosa) and monoclonal (IgA) globulin healed after melphalen treatment. Case report and review of the literature. Acta Med Scand 1978; 203:293–296.
171. Einhorn N: Acute leukemia after chemotherapy (melphalan). Cancer 1978; 41:444–447.
172. Tucker SB, Winkelmann RK: Treatment of Kaposi's sarcoma with vinblastine. Arch Dermatol 1976; 112:958–961.
173. Klein E. Schwartz RA, Laor Y, et al: Treatment of Kaposi's sarcoma with vinblastine. Cancer 1980; 45:427–431.
174. Mintzer DM, Real FX, Jovino L, et al: Treatment of Kaposi's sarcoma and thrombocytopenia with vincristine in patients with the acquired immunodeficiency syndrome. Ann Intern Med 1985; 102:200–202.
175. Volberding PA, Abrams DI, Conant M, et al: Vinblastine therapy for Kaposi's sarcoma in the acquired immunodeficiency syndrome. Ann Intern Med 1985; 103:335–338.
176. Kaplan L, Abrams D, Volberding P: Treatment of Kaposi's sarcoma in acquired immunodeficiency syndrome with an alternating vincristine-vinblastine regimen. Cancer Treat Rep 1986; 70:1121–1122.
177. Volberding PA: The role of chemotherapy for epidemic Kaposi's sarcoma. Semin Oncol 1987; 14:23–26.
178. Gelmann EP, Longo D, Lane HC, et al: Combination chemotherapy of disseminated Kaposi's sarcoma in patients with the acquired immune deficiency syndrome. Am J Med 1987; 82:456–462.
179. Odom RB: Intralesional vincristine "effective" in Kaposi's. Dermatol News 1987; 20:1.
180. Leavell UW, Yarbro JW: Hydroxyurea: A new treatment for psoriasis. Arch Dermatol 1970; 102:144–150.
181. Moschella SL, Greenwald MA. Psoriasis with hydroxyurea: An 18-month study of 60 patients. Arch Dermatol 1973; 107:363–368.
182. Leavell UW, Mersack IP, Smith C: Survey of the treatment of psoriasis with hydroxyurea (letter). Arch Dermatol 1973; 107:467.
183. Smith C, Gelfant S: Effects of methotrexate and hydroxyurea on psoriatic epidermis. Preferential cytotoxic effects on psoriatic epidermis. Arch Dermatol 1974; 110:70–72.
184. Shelley WB, Shelley ED: Erythema annulare centrifugum as the presenting sign of the hypereosinophilic syndrome: Observations on therapy. Cutis 1985; 35:53–55.

6 Methotrexate

Jeffrey P. Callen, M.D., F.A.C.P.
Carol L. Kulp-Shorten, M.D.

In 1951, Gubner and colleagues recognized that the folic acid antagonist aminopterin was effective for the treatment of psoriasis.[1] Shortly after this observation, it was recognized that methotrexate (amethopterin), another folic acid antagonist, was also an excellent therapeutic agent for the control of psoriasis. Despite this discovery, it took nearly 20 years for the U.S. Food and Drug Administration (FDA) to approve methotrexate for use in psoriasis, a nonmalignant condition.[2] Only in the late 1980s was rheumatoid arthritis approved as another indication for the use of methotrexate.[3] Despite large numbers of patients who have been treated with methotrexate, there remain many areas of controversy and confusion regarding the indications for, and the safety of, this chemotherapeutic agent. Included among these controversies are the criteria for selection of the psoriatic patient, the method of laboratory evaluation, and the role of liver biopsies in surveillance. In this chapter we review the existing data on the pharmacology of, the indications for, and the toxicity of methotrexate.

Pharmacology

Structure

Methotrexate (4-amino-N[10]-methyl pteroylglutamic acid) is a potent inhibitor of the enzyme dihydrofolate reductase. It is structurally similar to folic acid, the natural substrate for this enzyme, differing from folic acid in only two areas. The amino group in the 4-carbon position takes the place of a hydroxyl group, and a methyl group at the N[10] position substitutes for the hydrogen atom.

Absorption/Distribution

Methotrexate can be administered orally, intravenously, or intramuscularly. It is rapidly absorbed through the gastrointestinal tract, although peak levels occur more slowly (1 hour after ingestion) through this route than through the other two routes of administration. Although absorption of oral methotrexate may be incomplete and variable with higher doses, this route of administration provides more reliable blood levels than parenteral administration.[4] Concurrent food intake, especially milk-based meals, may decrease bioavailability. However, the drug need not be given when the patient is in a fasting state. Nonabsorbable antibiotics such as neomycin may reduce the absorption of methotrexate significantly. The drug is well distributed throughout the body except in the brain, penetrating the blood–brain barrier poorly.

Metabolism/Excretion

Once absorbed, the level of methotrexate in the plasma has a triphasic reduction. The first phase occurs rapidly (¾ of an hour) and reflects distribution of the drug throughout the body. The second phase of the reduction is represented by renal excretion and occurs over 2–4 hours. Methotrexate is a weak organic acid that is excreted predominantly through the kidney. Such glomeruler filtration and active tubular secretion are susceptible to drug interactions with other weak acids, such as salicylates, probenecid, and sulfonamides. The third phase represents the terminal half-life and varies between 10 and 27 hours. This phase is thought to reflect a slow release of methotrexate, primarily bound to dihydrofolate reductase, from the tissues.

Approximately 50% of methotrexate is bound to plasma proteins, and the active portion of the drug is the free fraction (unbound) in the plasma. Thus any drug that may increase the unbound portion (e.g., sulfonamides, salicylates, tetracycline, chloramphenicol, and phenytoin) may play a role in the tissue effects, as well as in the potential for toxicity. Methotrexate is transported into cells actively, rather than entering by diffusion. It has been felt that methotrexate is not substantially metabolized; however, evidence suggests that the drug is metabolized intracellularly, including within the liver, to polyglutamated forms.[5,6] These metabolites, also potent inhibitors of dihydrofolate reductase, are postulated to play a key role in methotrexate toxicity.

Mechanism of Action

Methotrexate competitively and irreversibly binds to dihydrofolate reductase within 60 minutes with a greater affinity than folic acid. This prevents the conversion of dihydrofolate to tetrahydrofolate. Tetrahydrofolate is a necessary cofactor in the production of 1-carbon units, which are critical for the synthesis of thymidylate and purine nucleotides needed for DNA and RNA synthesis. A less rapid, but partially reversible, competitive inhibition of thymidylate synthetase also occurs within 24 hours after administration of methotrexate.

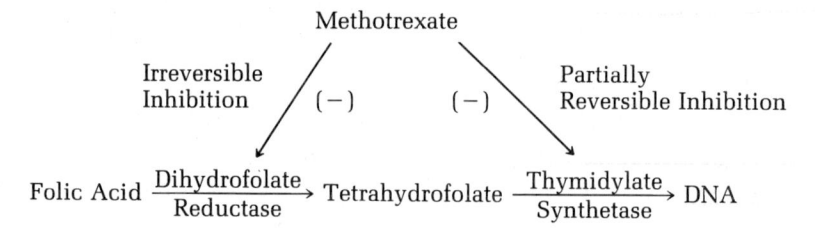

$$\text{Folic Acid} \xrightarrow[\text{Reductase}]{\text{Dihydrofolate}} \text{Tetrahydrofolate} \xrightarrow[\text{Synthetase}]{\text{Thymidylate}} \text{DNA}$$

with Methotrexate causing Irreversible Inhibition (−) of Dihydrofolate Reductase and Partially Reversible Inhibition (−) of Thymidylate Synthetase.

Thus the overall effect of methotrexate is inhibition of cell division, being specific for the S (DNA synthesis) phase of the normal cell cycle. The inhibition of dihydrofolate reductase can be bypassed by leucovorin (N^5-formyl-tetrahydrofolate: folinic acid, citrovorum factor) or thymidine. Leucovorin, a fully reduced, functional folate coenzyme, bypasses the reaction catalyzed by dihydrofolate reductase. Thymidine, coverted to thymidylate by thymidine kinase, bypasses the reaction catalyzed by thymidylate synthetase. Thus acute methotrexate toxicity can be reversed by these agents.

Methotrexate has some activity as an immunosuppressive agent. The effect probably occurs because of inhibition of DNA synthesis in immunologically competent cells. The drug can suppress primary and secondary antibody responses.[7,8] There is no significant effect on cell-mediated immunity. Although methotrexate has potential as a "steroid-sparing" agent, the immunosuppressive effects are relatively weak. Azathioprine and cyclophosphamide are preferred to methotrexate as immunosuppressive agents for dermatologic use.

Clinical Use (Table 6–1)

Indications

Methotrexate is available as a 2.5-mg tablet and is now available in prepackaged weekly doses for low-dose therapy. This prepackaging follows the approval by the FDA of low-dose methotrexate therapy for the treatment of rheumatoid arthritis. Methotrexate is also available in vials of sterile injectable solution, which may be used for intramuscular or intravenous administration (2-ml vials with 2.5 mg/ml and 25 mg/ml available). This agent is approved for use by patients with malignancies, including mycosis fungoides, psoriasis vulgaris, and rheumatoid arthritis. However, it is widely used in dermatology practices for other conditions, including bullous disorders, selected collagen vascular disorders, proliferative conditions such as pityriasis rubra pilaris (PRP) and pityriasis lichenoides et varioliformis acuta (PLEVA), and miscellaneous unrelated diseases.

Table 6-1. Methotrexate Indications/Contraindications

FDA-Approved Dermatologic Indications*

Psoriasis (see text for specifics)[9]
Mycosis Fungoides[10]

   Nondermatologic indication of greatest interest: rheumatoid arthritis

Other Dermatologic Indications*

Proliferative Disorders

   Pityriasis rubra pilaris[11, 12]
   Pityriasis lichenoides et varioliformis acuta[13]
   Reiter's disease[14]

Bullous Dermatoses

   Pemphigus vulgaris[15, 16]
   Bullous pemphigoid[16, 17]

Collagen-Vascular Disorders

   Dermatomyositis/polymyositis[18, 19]
   Lupus erythematosus[20]

Other Dermatoses

   Sarcoidosis[21, 22]
   Keloids[23]
   Lymphomatoid papulosis[24]

Contraindications

Absolute

   Pregnancy or lactation

Relative[9]

   Decreased renal function (dosage must be altered)
   Hepatic disease: abnormal liver function tests, active hepatitis, history of liver disease, cirrhosis
   Severe hematologic abnormalities
   Alcoholism or excessive alcohol intake
   Man or woman contemplating conception (3 months off drug for men, one ovulatory cycle for women)
   Active infectious disease or a history of a potentially serious infection that could be reactivated
   Immunodeficiency syndrome: hereditary or acquired
   Unreliable patient

---

*Methotrexate is not the drug of first choice for any of these conditions.

FDA-Approved Indication

PSORIASIS. The major clinical use of methotrexate in dermatologic practice is in the therapy of psoriasis.[9] The selection of the patient for the initiation of methotrexate therapy should be carefully considered. The benefits and risks of the therapy, as well as available alternative therapies, should be discussed fully before its initiation. In general, the patient who is considered to be a methotrexate candidate should have debilitating disease that either is uncontrolled by conventional methods or is not amenable to more conservative therapies. Physicians should consider each patient on an individual basis, taking into account not only the characteristics of the disease but also the socioeconomic aspects of the individual. For example, it may be impractical for the patient to receive Goeckerman therapy or psoralens plus ultraviolet A (PUVA) therapy because of job-related needs or because the patient may not reside near a phototherapy facility. Similarly, retinoid therapy may be inappropriate because of hyperlipidemia or because the patient may be a woman with childbearing potential. Patients in our practice with recalcitrant psoriasis are presented with the risks and benefits of each of these treatment modalities and participate in the selection of the best therapeutic option for them. Roenigk and colleagues[9] summarized the indications for the use of methotrexate in psoriasis as follows.

INDICATIONS FOR METHOTREXATE THERAPY OF PSORIASIS

- Psoriatic erythroderma
- Psoriatic arthritis: not responsive to conventional therapy
- Pustular psoriasis: generalized or debilitating localized disease
- Psoriasis that adversely affects economics or ability to maintain employment
- Extensive, severe plaque psoriasis: not responsive to conventional therapy

---

The selection of the patient is made after the relative and absolute contraindications to the drug's use are considered. The only true contraindications are pregnancy and lactation. The relative contraindications can be waived when the probable benefits of the therapy outweigh the potential risks. In general, 75%–80% of psoriatics treated with methotrexate will respond, usually within 1–4 weeks. Complete response usually occurs by 2–3 months. Specifics regarding dosing and follow-up of the psoriatic patient are addressed in the Monitoring Guidelines and Therapeutic Guidelines.

Other Dermatologic Uses

OTHER PROLIFERATIVE DISORDERS. Methotrexate has been reported to be useful for several other conditions. Patients with other presumed epidermal proliferative diseases such as PRP,[11, 12] PLEVA,[13] and Reiter's disease[14] have been reported to respond favorably to methotrexate. PRP seems to respond less well to methotrexate than does psoriasis. In general, the doses necessary to control PRP are 1.5–2 times higher than those necessary for control of psoriasis with a similar amount of involved body surface area. Furthermore, anecdotal reports have suggested that for patients with PRP, the drug should be administered on a daily low-dose regimen rather than on a weekly basis.[12] An important disadvantage of this daily-dosage regimen in comparison with the same total weekly dose given over 24 hours is an increased incidence of adverse effects. Methotrexate has only a secondary role in the treatment of this disease with the availability and efficacy of retinoids for PRP.[11] Exquisitely small doses of methotrexate (as little as 2.5–5 mg weekly) often can be used to control the disease process in patients with PLEVA.[13] Reiter's disease can at times be controlled with methotrexate. For this disease, the doses necessary are slightly higher than the doses for psoriasis, and the drug can be beneficial for both the rheumatologic and the cutaneous aspects.[14] Methotrexate therapy can also improve psoriatic arthritis.

IMMUNOLOGIC DISORDERS. Diseases of presumed immunologic origin may also respond to methotrexate. Specifically, bullous diseases such as pemphigus,[15, 16] bullous pemphigoid,[16, 17] and epidermolysis bullosa acquisita may respond. Patients with collagen-vascular diseases such as dermatomyositis,[18, 19] lupus erythematosus,[20] and scleroderma, neutrophilic dermatoses (Sweet's syndrome or pyoderma gangrenosum), and vasculitis may benefit. The drug is most often used for these diseases as a means of sparing the patient from chronic high doses of corticosteroids. Our experience with the use of methotrexate for these disorders (with the exception of dermatomyositis and the neutrophilic dermatoses) has been less rewarding than with the use of other immunosuppressive agents (e.g., azathioprine, cyclophosphamide, or chlorambucil).

In general, methotrexate must be used in weekly doses ranging from 25 to 50 mg to achieve control of these diseases. Methotrexate has been extremely useful to patients with dermatomyositis or polymyositis who either do not respond to corticosteroids or develop steroid-related side effects. It is rarely effective for the control of the skin disease, but it is very effective in the control of the muscle disease. In dermatomyositis the disease may be quantified. Thus one can objectively measure a response by following the muscle strength or the levels of muscle enzymes. The drug is initiated at an empiric weekly dose while the same dose of corticosteroids is maintained. The onset of noticeable improvement is generally within 4–8 weeks. Of the patients treated with methotrexate for dermatomyositis/polymyositis, three fourths will respond, and the dose of systemic corticosteroids can be significantly reduced. Anecdotal reports suggest that methotrexate is beneficial for patients with cutaneous sarcoidosis,[21, 22] keloids,[23] lymphomatoid papulosis,[24] psoriatic arthritis,[25] and mycosis fungoides.[10] Methotrexate is uncommonly used by children for various dermatoses.[26] Great caution should be exercised for use in this age group.

Adverse Effects

HEPATOTOXICITY. Hepatotoxicity resulting from long-term use of methotrexate is the most significant problem that must be considered.[9, 27] Hepatotoxicity differs in the two large populations in which this drug is used on a long-term basis: psoriatics and rheumatoid arthritics. Perhaps there are differences between the populations that may relate to hereditary predisposition to liver disease, the rate of alcoholism, or some other factor as yet unidentified. However, over time it has become evident that among rheumatoid arthritics, methotrexate-related liver damage is possible.[28] Although liver function tests may be abnormal in the presence of liver toxicity, they are frequently normal.[29, 30] Therefore, it is necessary to examine the histologic appearance of the liver during long-term therapy. The data on the risk of methotrexate-induced cirrhosis have varied widely with reported frequencies from 0% to 25%.[9, 27] It appears that the risk of liver damage is low for patients whose cumulative dosage is below 1.5 g.[9] The clinical course of the cirrhosis induced by methotrexate is often nonaggressive. In fact, many of the Scandinavian patients in one study continued therapy without a deterioration of their liver histopathology.[31] The patient who has had an abnormal liver biopsy may with time experience a reversal of the findings while off therapy. Thus it may be possible for that patient to resume therapy.

A noninvasive test to diagnose methotrexate-induced hepatotoxicity would be ideal. Although hepatic ultrasound may be useful according to one study,[32] other studies reported the inability of ultrasound to discriminate fat from fibrosis.[33, 34] Radionuclide scans and the aminopyrine breath test are inadequate to screen for hepatotoxicity that is due to methotrexate.[33, 35] The liver biopsy remains the standard diagnostic test.

PULMONARY TOXICITY. In rare instances, pulmonary toxicity such as acute pneumonitis can occur.[36, 37] This pulmonary toxicity is idiosyncratic, can occur with extremely small doses of methotrexate, and can be life-threatening if the methotrexate is not stopped. In addition, some patients develop a more gradual pulmonary toxicity that is manifest by pulmonary fibrosis on chest x-ray. Chest x-ray studies and pulmonary function testing are not useful in the prediction or the prevention of pulmonary toxicity. The great majority of reports have been about patients with rheumatoid arthritis treated with methotrexate; a prevalence of pulmonary toxicity in up to 5% of these patients has been reported. The frequency is dramatically less among methotrexate-treated psoriatic patients. Methotrexate-induced pneumonitis has infrequently been reported in psoriasis patients.[38–41] Previous guidelines suggested a yearly chest x-ray for methotrexate-treated psoriatic patients.[42] Current guidelines recommend a chest x-ray only if the patient develops symptoms suggesting pneumonitis.[9]

HEMATOLOGIC EFFECTS. Frequent blood counts are important monitors for bone marrow toxicity.[43] Increased susceptibility to infection secondary to leukopenia may develop. Should myelosuppression develop, the patient can be treated with leucovorin, which can bypass the enzyme dihydrofolate reductase and allow normal cell division to resume. This procedure is commonly used for cancer patients treated with much higher doses. Macrocytic indices without anemia are common with dermatologic dosage levels.

GASTROINTESTINAL EFFECTS. Nausea and anorexia are adverse reactions to methotrexate that are commonly encountered. Diarrhea, vomiting, and ulcerative stomatitis are less frequently observed. The presence of ulcerative stomatitis or severe diarrhea requires cessation of the methotrexate therapy. Cautious reinstitution after these problems resolve may be considered.

REPRODUCTIVE EFFECTS. Methotrexate is a potent teratogen and abortifacient, but it has less long-term mutagenic and carcinogenic potential than do the alkylating agents. Women of childbearing years who take methotrexate must use reliable birth control. Previously treated patients do (not) have an increased risk of fetal abnormalities in subsequent pregnancies. Men should be counseled with regard to a possible, reversible oligospermia.

RENAL EFFECTS. High-dose therapy (i.e., 50–250 mg/kg intravenously) may lead to renal toxicity secondary to precipitation of methotrexate in the renal tubules. This toxicity is not likely to be encountered with low-dose therapy for psoriasis.

OTHER ADVERSE EFFECTS. Other reported adverse reactions to methotrexate include mild alopecia, headaches, fatigue, and dizziness. If these reactions occur, the dose can be lowered or stopped. Methotrexate is also felt to be potentially phototoxic.[44] It may cause an unusual reaction in which either a recent sunburn is "recalled" or previously irradiated skin will develop a toxic reaction with the administration of the drug. There is (no) evidence that methotrexate increases the risk of developing a subsequent malignancy.[45, 46]

Monitoring Guidelines

Before the first dose, a thorough evaluation of the patient should be completed. The premethotrexate evaluation begins with a complete history and physical examination. This evaluation will assist the physician in the identification of patients at increased risk for toxicity. The potential for the interaction with other drugs may also be assessed (Table 6–2). The minimal laboratory evaluation should consist of a CBC and a platelet count, tests of renal function, and liver enzyme determinations. For patients at high risk for acquired immunodeficiency syndrome (AIDS), an HIV antibody determination should be part of the screening. The type of renal function testing is a critical issue in elderly patients. Methotrexate is excreted by the kidneys, and even subtle abnormalities in the clearance can result in a markedly prolonged half-life of the drug and eventuate in methotrexate toxicity.[47] Thus in patients over 50 years old, the serum determinations of the blood urea nitrogen and creatinine are (not) sufficient. A creatinine clearance should be determined before the first dose. The drug is contraindicated for patients with creatinine clearance less than 50 ml/minute.

Table 6–2. Some Drugs That May Increase the Potential for Methotrexate Toxicity[9, 49]

Drug	Mechanism of Toxicity
Salicylates	Decreased renal excretion, displacement from plasma proteins
Nonsteroidal anti-inflammatory drugs	Decreased renal excretion, displacement from plasma proteins
Dipyridamole	Intracellular accumulation of methotrexate
Probenecid	Intracellular accumulation, decreased renal tubular function
Retinoids	Hepatotoxicity
Ethanol	Hepatotoxicity
Sulfonamides	Displacement from plasma proteins, decreased renal function
Tetracycline	Displacement from plasma proteins
Chloramphenicol	Displacement from plasma proteins
Phenytoin	Displacement from plasma proteins
Phenothiazines	Displacement from plasma proteins

Adapted from Roenigk HH, Auerbach R, Maibach HI, et al: Methotrexate in psoriasis: Revised guidelines. J Am Acad Dermatol 1988; 19:145–156; Evans WE, Christensen ML: Interactions with methotrexate; J Rheumatol 1985; 12(Suppl 12):15–20.

METHOTREXATE MONITORING GUIDELINES[9]

Baseline

Examination

- Careful history and physical examination
- Identification of patients at increased risk for toxicity
- Recording concomitant medications that may interact with methotrexate

Laboratory

- Complete blood count (CBC) and platelet count
- Liver function tests, liver biopsy (see text)
- Renal function tests: blood urea nitrogen, creatinine, creatinine clearance (see text)
- Human immunodeficiency virus (HIV) testing in high-risk patients

Follow-up

Laboratory

- CBC, platelet count, liver function tests: every week for 4 weeks and 7 days after each dose escalation
- CBC, platelet count, liver function tests: every 3–4 months (long-term after dose stabilization)

Liver Biopsy

- After every 1.5–2.0 g total dose for low-risk patients
- After every 1.0 g total dose for higher risk patients
- Every 6 months for patients with grade IIIA liver biopsy changes (Table 6-3)

Note: More frequent surveillance is needed if laboratory values are abnormal or with high-risk patients.

LIVER BIOPSY. The need for routine liver biopsy before the initiation of therapy has been questioned. In the largest study to date, in which more than 68,000 consecutive liver biopsies were evaluated, 6 deaths occurred.[48] Of importance is that all 6 patients who died had advanced cirrhosis or hepatic malignancies. On the other hand, deaths due to methotrexate-induced cirrhosis in psoriatic patients have occurred. These deaths may be avoidable with proper surveillance.

There are several situations in which pretreatment liver biopsy may not be necessary. Not all patients with psoriasis improve with metho-

Table 6–3. Classification of Liver Biopsy Findings

Grade I	Normal; fatty infiltration, mild; nuclear variability, mild; portal inflammation, mild
Grade II	Fatty infiltration, moderate to severe; nuclear variability, moderate to severe; portal tract inflammation, and necrosis, moderate to severe
Grade III	A: Fibrosis, mild
	B: Fibrosis, moderate to severe
Grade IV	Cirrhosis

Adapted from Roenigk HH, Auerbach R, Maibach HI, et al: Methotrexate in psoriasis: Revised guidelines. J Am Acad Dermatol 1988; 19:145–156.

trexate. Furthermore, some patients cannot tolerate the drug even in small doses. In these instances, performing a pretreatment liver biopsy has placed the patient at risk without any foreseeable benefit. Therefore, many physicians are postponing the initial biopsy until the 3rd–6th month of therapy, when it can be determined that effective, well-tolerated therapy will be continued by an individual patient. In this setting, it is still imperative that a full discussion with the patient take place so that the patient understands that a biopsy will be needed at some time in the near future. One advantage of a premethotrexate liver biopsy is that it impresses on patients the serious nature of the agent with which they are about to be treated.

There are several other instances in which a premethotrexate liver biopsy is necessary. For patients with a personal or familial history of liver disease, a liver biopsy before therapy is helpful. Similarly, for those patients with a history of exposure to known hepatotoxins, including alcohol or intravenous drugs, liver histology is important. Patients with diabetes or obesity are presumed to be at greater risk for liver toxicity, and pretreatment biopsies are deemed necessary. Finally, patients with abnormal baseline liver function tests require a liver biopsy before receiving the first dose of methotrexate.

The need for repeated liver biopsies is based on the total dose taken by the patient. We periodically calculate the cumulative dose and record it in our medical record in order to more effectively deal with the discussion of the need for a liver biopsy. In general, a liver biopsy is repeated after every 1.5–2 g of total dose. The time needed to reach this level of intake varies, depending on the weekly dose. Continuation or discontinuation of methotrexate is based on liver biopsy findings (Table 6–3). The following recommendations have been proposed by Roenigk and colleagues:[9]

1. Patients with grade I or II changes may continue to receive methotrexate therapy.

2. Patients with grade IIIA changes may continue to receive methotrexate therapy but should have another liver biopsy after approximately 6 months of continuous therapy.

3. Patients with grades IIIB and IV should not be given further methotrexate except under exceptional circumstances with careful follow-up of liver biopsies.

The discrimination of grade IIIA versus grade IIIB changes is somewhat subjective, despite the impact on the decision-making process. Equally important is the trend of histologic changes when previous liver biopsies are compared.

LABORATORY MONITORING. The patient should be monitored closely with frequent CBCs and serum multiphasic analyses during the initial phase of therapy, regardless of the disease for which methotrexate is being used. It is our practice to discontinue methotrexate for a white blood count less than 3000/cu mm, a platelet count less than 100,000/cu mm, or a doubling of the upper normal value for liver transaminase levels. The drug may be restarted at a lower dose after a 2- to 3-week rest period if the laboratory abnormality has resolved. After the first month of therapy, monitoring can be conducted less frequently (every 3–4 months). More frequent monitoring is necessary if the dose is being escalated, if there is an intercurrent illness, or if additional systemic therapy with other drugs is begun. Of importance is that published guidelines recommend hematologic laboratory follow-up every month.[9] In practice, it is rare to develop an abnormal white blood cell count or platelet count after the first few months of therapy on a constant or tapering methotrexate dose.

Therapeutic Guidelines

Once the decision has been made to administer methotrexate, the next step is to decide on the dosage and the route of administration. For patients with psoriasis, oral weekly doses are usually effective and reasonably well tolerated. An occasional patient who is poorly compliant may be treated with weekly intramuscular methotrexate, as may the patient who develops nausea from oral, but not parenteral, administration. There are two methods of weekly administration of oral methotrexate: (1) a single weekly dose and (2) three divided doses over a 24-hour period each week. The divided-dose regimen consists of taking the medication on a schedule such as 8 A.M. and 8 P.M. on the first day and 8 A.M. on the second day. With the development of the dose pack, sold under the trade name Rheumatrex (three of the 2.5-mg tablets per dose pack), this schedule may be easier to explain. The rationale behind this schedule relates to the presumed cell cycle kinetics in psoriasis. However, the two methods of administration are equally effective and have similar toxicity.

The initial dose should be fairly conservative in order to prevent myelosuppression. In general, a test dose of 5–10 mg is given, and a CBC and liver function tests are taken 7 days later. The dose is gradually escalated (2.5–5.0 mg/week) to a level that provides reasonable benefit without noticeable toxicity. Patients receiving intramuscular or intravenous methotrexate are able to tolerate higher doses because of more rapid renal clearance. One can measure the response to the drug by quantifying the area of surface involvement or by evaluating the characteristics of an individual lesion such as a scale, erythema, or elevation. On the average, our patients are able to achieve benefits at 10–12.5 mg/week. The total weekly dose rarely exceeds 30 mg. When maximal benefit is reached, the methotrexate may be tapered by 2.5 mg/week in order to determine the lowest possible dosage that provides disease control. For patients treated with intramuscular methotrexate, it may be more convenient to taper by increasing the interval between doses to 2 weeks or more. The dosage and the schedule of administration for other disorders differ from those recommended for psoriasis. These differences have been discussed previously.

BIBLIOGRAPHY: Key Reviews/Chapters

Roenigk HH, Auerbach R, Maibach HI, et al: Methotrexate in psoriasis: Revised guidelines. J Am Acad Dermatol 1988; 19:145–156.
Bickers DR, Hazen PG, Lynch WS: Cytotoxic and immunosuppressive agents. In Clinical Pharmacology of Skin Disease. New York: Churchill Livingstone, 1984, 91–129.
Paller AS: Dermatologic use of methotrexate in children. Pediatr Dermatol 1985; 2:238–243.
Lester RS: Methotrexate. Clin Dermatol 1989; 7(3):128–135.

REFERENCES

1. Gubner R, August S, Ginsberg V: Therapeutic suppression of tissue reactivity: Effect of aminopterin in rheumatoid arthritis and psoriasis. Am J Med Sci 1951; 221:176–182.
2. Weinstein GD: Methotrexate. Ann Intern Med 1977; 86:799–204.
3. Healy LA: The current status of methotrexate use in rheumatoid disease. Bull Rheum Dis 1986; 36(4):1–10.
4. Balis FM, Savitch JL, Bleyer WA: Pharmacokinetics of oral methotrexate in children. Cancer Res 1983; 43:2242–2245.
5. Galivan J, Pupons A, Rhee M: Hepatic parenchymal cell glutamylation of methotrexate studied in monolayer culture. Cancer Res 1986; 46:670–675.
6. Kamen BA, Nylen PA, Camitta DM, et al: Methotrexate accumulation in cells as a possible mechanism of chronic toxicity to the drug. Br J Haematol 1981; 49:355–360.
7. Hersh EM, Carbone PP, Wong VG, et al: Inhibition of primary immune response in man by antimetabolites. Cancer Res 1965; 25:1997–2001.
8. Mitchells MS, Wade ME, DeCenti RC, et al: Immune suppressive effects of cytosine arabinoside and methotrexate in man. Ann Intern Med 1969; 70:535–547.
9. Roenigk HH, Auerbach R, Maibach HI, et al: Methotrexate in psoriasis: Revised guidelines. J Am Acad Dermatol 1988; 19:145–156.

10. McDonald CJ: Cytotoxic agents for use in dermatology: I. J Am Acad Dermatol 1986; 12:753–775.
11. Borrie P: Pityriasis rubra pilaris treated with methotrexate. Arch Dermatol 1967; 79:115–116.
12. Knowles WR, Chernosky ME: Pityriasis rubra pilaris: Prolonged treatment with methotrexate. Arch Dermatol 1970; 102:603–612.
13. Cornelison RL, Knox JM, Everett MA: Methotrexate for the treatment of Mucha-Habermann disease. Arch Dermatol 1972; 106:507–508.
14. Lally EV, Ho G Jr: A review of methotrexate therapy in Reiter syndrome. Semin Arthritis Rheum 1985; 15:139–145.
15. Lever WF, Schaumburg-Lever G: Immunosuppressants and prednisone in pemphigus vulgaris. Arch Dermatol 1977; 13:1236–1241.
16. Levene GM: The treatment of pemphigus and pemphigoid. Clin Exp Dermatol 1982; 7:643–652.
17. Gruber GG, Owen LG, Callen JP: Vesicular pemphigoid. J Am Acad Dermatol 1980; 3:619–622.
18. Metzger AL, Bohan A, Goldberg LS, et al: Polymyositis and dermatomyositis: Combined methotrexate and corticosteroid therapy. Ann Intern Med 1974; 81:182–189.
19. Giannini M, Callen JP: Treatment of dermatomyositis with methotrexate and prednisone. Arch Dermatol 1979; 115:1251–1252.
20. Rothenberg FJ, Graziano FM, Grandone JT, et al: The use of methotrexate in steroid-resistant systemic lupus erythematosus. Arthritis Rheum 1988; 31:612–615.
21. Laeher MJ: Spontaneous remission or response to methotrexate in sarcoidosis. Ann Intern Med 1968; 69:1247–1248.
22. Veien NK, Brodthagen H: Cutaneous sarcoidosis treated with methotrexate. Br J Dermatol 1977; 97:213–216.
23. Onwukwe MF: Treating keloids by surgery and methotrexate. Arch Dermatol 1980; 116:158.
24. Wantzin GL, Thomsen K: Methotrexate in lymphomatoid papulosis. Br J Dermatol 1984; 111:93–95.
25. Kragballe K, Zachariae E, Zachariae H: Methotrexate in psoriatic arthritis: A retrospective study. Acta Derm Venereol 1983; 63:165–167.
26. Paller AS: Dermatologic use of methotrexate in children. Pediatr Dermatol 1985; 2:238–243.
27. Fitzpatrick TB (ed): Methotrexate therapy for psoriasis II: A liver biopsy is indicated in patients who have received more than 2000 mg of methotrexate. Dermatol Capsule & Comment 1980; 2:1–3.
28. Weinblatt ML, Raimer JM: Methotrexate in rheumatoid arthritis. J Am Acad Dermatol 1988; 19:126–128.
29. Newman M, Auerbach R, Feiner H, et al: The role of liver biopsies in psoriatic patients receiving long-term methotrexate. Arch Dermatol 1989; 125:1218–1224.
30. O'Connor GT, Olmstead EM, Zug K, et al: Detection of hepatotoxicity associated with methotrexate therapy for psoriasis. Arch Dermatol 1989; 125:1209–1217.
31. Zachariae H, Sogaard H: Methotrexate-induced liver cirrhosis. Dermatologica 1987; 175:178–182.
32. Miller JA, Dodd H, Rustin MHA, et al: Ultrasound as a screening procedure for methotrexate-induced hepatic damage in severe psoriasis. Br J Dermatol 1985; 113:699–705.
33. Mitchell D, Johnson RD, Testa HJ, et al: Ultrasound and radionuclide scans—Poor indicators of liver damage in patients treated with methotrexate. Clin Exp Dermatol 1987; 12:243–245.
34. Coulson HH, McKenzie J, Neild VS, et al: A comparison of liver ultrasound with liver biopsy histology in psoriatics receiving long-term methotrexate therapy. Br J Dermatol 1987; 116:491–495.

35. Williams CN, McNauley D, Malatjalian DA, et al: The aminopyrine breath test, an inadequate early indicator of methotrexate-induced liver disease in patients with psoriasis. Clin Invest Med 1987; 10:54–58.
36. Sostman HD, Matthay RA, Putman CE, et al: Methotrexate-induced pneumonitis. Medicine 1976; 55:371–388.
37. Searles G, McKendry RJR: Methotrexate pneumonitis in rheumatoid arthritis: Potential risk factors. Four case reports and a review of the literature. J Rheumatol 1987; 14:1164–1171.
38. Phillips TJ, Jones DH, Baker H: Pulmonary complications following methotrexate therapy. J Am Acad Dermatol 1987; 16:373–375.
39. Turck M: Successful psoriasis treatment, then sudden "cytotoxicity." Hosp Prac 1984; 19(8):175–176.
40. Verdich J, Christensen AL: Pulmonary disease complicating intermittent methotrexate therapy of psoriasis. Acta Derm Venereol (Stockh) 1979; 59:471–473.
41. Kaplan RL, Waite DH: Progressive interstitial lung disease from prolonged methotrexate therapy. Arch Dermatol 1978; 114:1800–1802.
42. Roenigk HH, Auerbach R, Maibach HI, et al: Methotrexate guidelines—Revised. J Am Acad Dermatol 1982; 6:145–155.
43. Shupack JL, Webster GF: Pancytopenia following low-dose oral methotrexate therapy for psoriasis. JAMA 1988; 259:3594–3596.
44. Armstrong RB, Poh-Fitzpatrick MB: Methotrexate and ultraviolet radiation. Arch Dermatol 1982; 118:177–178.
45. Bailin TL, Tindall JP, Roenigk HH, et al: Is methotrexate therapy for psoriasis carcinogenic? A modified retrospective—Prospective analysis. JAMA 1975; 232:359–362.
46. Nyfors A, Jensen H: Frequency of malignant neoplasms in 248 long-term methotrexate-treated psoriatics: A preliminary study. Dermatologica 1983; 167:260–261.
47. Ostergard K, Weismann K, Huttes L: Renal function and the rate of disappearance of methotrexate from serum. Eur J Clin Pharmacol 1975; 8:439–444.
48. Piccinino F, Sagnelli E, Pasquale G, et al: Complications following percutaneous liver biopsy: A multicenter retrospective study on 68,276 biopsies. J Hepatol 1986; 2:165–173.
49. Evans WE, Christensen ML: Interactions with methotrexate. J Rheumatol 1985; 12(Suppl 12):15–20.

7 Cyclosporine

Lyn Guenther, M.D., F.R.C.P.C.

CYCLOSPORINE (SANDIMMUNE)

Cyclosporine, also known as cyclosporin A, is a potent immunosuppressive agent that selectively affects helper T cells without suppressing the bone marrow. The clinical use of cyclosporine has primarily been in organ transplantation, in which it has been shown in humans to prolong the survival of kidney, liver, pancreas, heart, heart-lung, and bone marrow allogeneic transplants. It has been in clinical use since 1978. Although its toxicity may limit its use, cyclosporine may prove to be of considerable therapeutic benefit in the treatment of certain dermatologic diseases. In addition, it may help to elucidate their pathogenesis. It is highly efficacious in psoriasis and may be of some benefit in treating lichen planus, pemphigus, bullous pemphigoid, epidermolysis bullosa acquisita, collagen vascular disorders, Behçet's disease, pyoderma gangrenosum, dermatitis, and alopecia areata.

In 1970, Borel at the Sandoz laboratories in Basel, Switzerland, discovered and isolated cyclosporine from the soil fungi *Tolypocladium inflatum gams* and *Cyclindrocarpon lucidum* during a search for antifungal agents.[1,2] Although the drug was found to have only weak antibiotic activity, limited to combating a few fungi and yeasts, it was found to have immunosuppressive properties that were not associated with generalized cytostatic activity.

Pharmacology

Structure

Cyclosporine is a neutral cyclic peptide composed of 11 amino acids, with a total molecular weight of 1202 daltons.[3] The drug Sandimmune is available as an oral solution, in capsules, and as an intravenous preparation. The oral solution contains 100 mg/ml in an olive oil and ethanol base and should be diluted with milk, chocolate drink, or fruit juice in a ratio of 1:10 immediately before it is administered. The soft gelatin capsules have been commercially available since 1988 and are much more convenient. They are available as small, 25-mg pink capsules and as larger, 100-mg dusty rose capsules. The total daily amount should be given in two divided doses.

Absorption/Distribution

Absorption of cyclosporine from the gastrointestinal tract is incomplete and quite variable, with an approximate mean value of 30% of the oral dose. Peak blood levels occur 2–4 hours after it is ingested.[2] There are no significant bioavailability differences between the two oral preparations.[4] For patients unable to take cyclosporine orally, an intravenous preparation can be given with doses reduced to approximately one third of the oral dose. The intravenous concentrate, 50 mg/ml in polyoxyethylated castor oil and ethanol, is diluted with normal saline solution or 5% glucose solution in a 1:20–1:100 ratio immediately before use and administered by slow intravenous infusion over a period of 2–6 hours.

Because cyclosporine is lipophilic, fat has the highest tissue concentration of the drug, approximately 10 times that in plasma.[2] High concentrations are also found in liver, kidney, pancreas, adrenal, and lymphoid tissue, whereas very low levels occur in brain tissue.[2] The distribution in blood is dependent on concentration of the drug, hematocrit, temperature, and lipoprotein concentration.[5] Highest levels are found in erythrocytes and plasma. Approximately 80% of the drug in plasma is bound to proteins, primarily lipoproteins.

Metabolism/Excretion

Irrespective of dose or route of administration, the half-life of cyclosporine is approximately 18 hours. The half-life is prolonged with liver disease and elevated serum bilirubin, but it is not affected by renal disease.[2] Cyclosporine is metabolized in the liver by the cytochrome P-450 microsomal enzymes and undergoes hydroxylation or demethylation.[6] Enterohepatic recirculation occurs, and most of the drug is excreted by way of the bile through feces. Only 6% is excreted in the urine, and of this amount, 0.1% is excreted unchanged.[7]

Mechanism of Action

Cyclosporine influences the early phase of the immune response by affecting the interaction among antigen, antigen-presenting macrophages and dendritic cells, and T cells. Lymphokines such as macrophage-migration inhibition factor are inhibited, which results in decreased recruitment of macrophages. The synthesis and release of interleukin 1

(IL-1) by macrophages and interleukin 2 (IL-2) generation are also inhibited. IL-2 stimulates the secretion of gamma interferon, and it is also critical for helper T cell proliferation. Cyclosporine therefore inhibits gamma interferon production and both primary helper T cell activation and helper T cell–induced maturation of cytotoxic T cells. The activity of cytotoxic T cells is unaffected once they have been produced.

Because helper T cells are inhibited, production of antibodies to T cell–dependent antigens is inhibited. T cell–independent antibodies are unaffected. Suppressor T cells are not inhibited by cyclosporine, and expansion of antigen-specific suppressor T cells may be favored, which allows for graft acceptance.

The primary subcellular action of cyclosporine is likely the inhibition of calcium-dependent signaling events that occur after calcium influx.[8] Cyclosporine binds to and inhibits both calmodulin and cyclophilin, thereby inhibiting the ability of calmodulin to activate cyclic nucleotides, protein kinases, and phospholipase A_2, which initiate the synthesis of protein, messenger RNA, DNA, and prostaglandins.[9] Cyclophilin appears to be the same enzyme as peptidyl-prolyl cis-trans isomerase, an enzyme that unfolds several proteins.[10,11]

Clinical Use (Table 7–1)

Indications

PSORIASIS. A number of open and controlled, blinded studies showed that cyclosporine significantly clears psoriasis;[15–31] these studies include Mueller and Hermann's initial report in 1979.[32] Most of the psoriasis patients studied had severe disease that was refractory to conventional systemic therapy. The drug appears to be at least as good as psoralens plus ultraviolet A (PUVA), ultraviolet B, methotrexate, or retinoid therapy in the treatment of chronic severe plaque psoriasis. Pustular psoriasis appears to be less responsive, and higher doses of cyclosporine may be required. Psoriatic arthritis and psoriatic nail disease also respond well. The response in psoriasis is dose-related. The response is faster and more complete with high doses. Transplantation dosages (15 mg/kg/day) do not appear to be required to treat psoriasis. Lower, putatively safer doses, namely 2.5–5 mg/kg/day, lead to a good response usually within 4–8 weeks. There is no correlation between the clinical response and blood cyclosporine levels. The side effects of nephrotoxicity, immunosuppression, and lymphomas (which will be reviewed later) are putatively minimized with lower doses. In an effort to avoid these complications, cyclosporine might be used to treat acute episodes of psoriasis or to induce remissions. Then other less toxic treatments can be used. Once the psoriasis is controlled with cyclosporine, PUVA therapy can sometimes be used as the sole treatment modality.[21] The combined carcino-

Table 7–1. Cyclosporine Indications/Contraindications

FDA-Approved Dermatologic Indications

None Specific to Dermatology

Nondermatologic Indications
  Prophylaxis of rejection and management of rejection of kidney, liver, and heart transplants*

Canadian-Approved Dermatologic Indications

None Specific to Dermatology

Nondermatologic Indications
  Prophylaxis of graft rejection after solid organ transplantation and bone marrow transplants*
  Treatment of patients with solid organ transplants who are refractory to conventional immunosuppressive therapy*
  Prophylaxis and treatment of graft-versus-host disease[12–14]*

Other Dermatologic Uses

Papulosquamous
  Psoriasis[15–39]
  Lichen planus[40–42]

Bullous Dermatoses
  Pemphigus[43–47]
  Pemphigoid[43, 44, 48, 49]
  Epidermolysis bullosa acquisita[50–52]

Connective Tissue Diseases
  Dermatomyositis/polymyositis[53–58]
  Lupus erythematosus[59–64]
  Sjögren's syndrome[65, 66]
  Scleroderma[67–70]

Neutrophilic Dermatoses
  Behçet's disease[71–75]
  Pyoderma gangrenosum[76–78]

Neoplastic
  Sézary's syndrome[79–81]
  Mycosis fungoides[82–84]

Dermatitis
  Atopic dermatitis[85–88]
  Allergic contact dermatitis[89–92]

Alopecia
  Alopecia areata[93–97]
  Male pattern alopecia[98, 99]

Other Dermatoses
  Allografts/xenografts[100–104]
  Ichthyosis[105, 106]
  Persistent light reaction[107]
  Erhythema nodosum leprosum[108]

Contraindications

Hypersensitivity to cyclosporine
For intravenous form, hypersensitivity to polyethoxylated castor oil

*Cyclosporine is generally considered the drug of choice.

---

genic effects of PUVA and cyclosporine on the skin are unknown. Combined ultraviolet B therapy shows no cyclosporine-sparing effects, and the combined carcinogenic risk is likewise unknown. Combined etretinate therapy shows a modest cyclosporine-sparing effect.[27] Addition of topical clobetasol propionate to cyclosporine results in faster clearing than does cyclosporine alone, but there is no significant difference in relapse rate.[33]

An initial dose of 3–5 mg/kg/day is proposed, and subsequent dosage is adjusted according to the patient's response and adverse effects. Relapse occurs 1–10 weeks after withdrawal, but the high relapse rates may be in part a function of the resistant and persistent cases that have been treated. The psoriasis is usually not worse than before treatment with cyclosporine;[34] however, severe relapse may occur.[35]

Topical cyclosporine is ineffective in treating psoriasis,[36] perhaps because it is inadequately absorbed into the skin. Intradermal cyclosporine, administered in the intravenous concentrate diluted with two parts normal saline solution, results in significant improvement.[37,38]

LICHEN PLANUS. Two patients with recalcitrant generalized lichen planus of 1 and 25 years' duration had complete clearing after 8 weeks of 6 mg/kg/day of cyclosporine. Their disease remained in remission at 10- and 3-month follow-ups.[40] Lichen planus may also improve with topical cyclosporine.[41–42]

PEMPHIGUS AND BULLOUS PEMPHIGOID. Dosages of 5–10 mg/kg/day of cyclosporine have been successfully used as a single agent or in combination with oral corticosteroids in the treatment of several patients with pemphigus and bullous pemphigoid.[43–49] Combination therapy is usually required, and most patients respond. Cyclosporine appears to have a significant steroid-sparing effect.

EPIDERMOLYSIS BULLOSA ACQUISITA. A woman with epidermolysis bullosa acquisita who was responsive only to 80–120 mg/day of prednisone, and unresponsive to azathioprine and sulfapyridine, showed a good response to 9 mg/kg/day of cyclosporine.[50] Three patients with epidermolysis bullosa acquisita who were unresponsive to conventional therapy, including corticosteroids, azathioprine, dapsone, sulfapyridine, methotrexate, phenytoin, vitamin E, gold, isotretinoin, and plasmapheresis, showed an excellent response to cyclosporine in dosages of 6–9 mg/kg/day.[50–52] In the 2 patients in whom anti–basement membrane antibodies were monitored, there was a significant decrease in antibody titers during cyclosporine therapy.[50,52] Two patients discontinued the drug because of side effects, but both patients remained in partial remission.[50,51]

DERMATOMYOSITIS/POLYMYOSITIS. Oral 5- to 10-mg/kg/day dosages of cyclosporine and intravenous 3-mg/kg/day dosages of cyclosporine have been successfully used in the treatment of severe and recalcitrant dermatomyositis and polymyositis.[53–58] Clinical response usually occurs in the first couple of weeks and is associated with decreased muscle enzymes. Clinical and biochemical relapse occurs quickly when the drug is discontinued.

LUPUS ERYTHEMATOSUS. Severe arthralgia in 2 patients with systemic lupus erythematosus (SLE) responded to cyclosporine, but unfortunately drug levels were not monitored, and severe side effects, including renal toxicity, vomiting, and angioedema, occurred.[59] However, in a dosage of 5 mg/kg/day, the drug has been beneficial in a number of steroid-resistant or steroid-dependent SLE patients, and cyclosporine has allowed a significant reduction in the steroid dosage.[60-62] Severe reversible nephrotoxicity may occur in SLE patients with pre-existing renal disease, and one must be cautious when treating such patients with cyclosporine.[63]

One patient with severe, mutilating, progressive discoid lupus erythematosus was unresponsive to hydroxychloroquine, to prednisone in dosages less than 40 mg/day, and to azathioprine; that patient failed to respond to 5.3 mg/kg/day of cyclosporine in combination with 32.5 mg/day of prednisone.[64]

SJÖGREN'S SYNDROME. Double-blind studies have shown that 5 mg/kg/day of cyclosporine improves subjective xerostomia and may improve or arrest the histopathologic changes of the minor labial salivary glands.[65, 66] Xerophthalmia, recurrent parotid gland enlargement, Schirmer's test, and stimulated parotid flow rate do not appear to be affected.

SCLERODERMA. Cyclosporine is also beneficial to patients severely affected with progressive systemic sclerosis. Cyclosporine promotes softening of the sclerotic skin, less frequent occurrence of Raynaud's phenomenon,[67, 68] normalization of respiratory function and esophageal motility, and disappearance of pericardial effusion.[69, 70]

BEHÇET'S DISEASE. Cyclosporine treatment results in a rapid decrease in ocular inflammation, improved visual acuity, and a reduction in ocular attacks in patients with Behçet's disease.[71-75] Nonocular complications, including arthritis, oral and vaginal ulcers, and skin lesions, also improve. Relapse occurs promptly upon discontinuation of the drug. In early studies, researchers employed initial dosages of 10 mg/kg/day. Subsequently, in an effort to minimize nephrotoxicity from cyclosporine, initial dosages of 5 mg/kg/day were suggested. The cyclosporine is increased to a maximal dosage of 7 mg/kg/day if necessary, or 0.2–0.4 mg/kg/day of prednisone is used in conjunction with the lower dosages of cyclosporine.[75]

PYODERMA GANGRENOSUM. Studies have shown that cyclosporine in doses of 6–10 mg/kg/day is highly effective in the treatment of severe idiopathic pyoderma gangrenosum,[76] pyoderma gangrenosum associated with sclerosing cholangitis and ulcerative colitis,[77] and paraproteinemia.[78] Two patients were given maintenance dosages of 3–7.5 mg/kg/day, and their ulcers remained healed.[76] The patient with sclerosing cholangitis and ulcerative colitis also had remission of the cholangitis and inflammatory bowel disease.[77] Relapse did not occur during a 14-month follow-up after discontinuation of cyclosporine.

MYCOSIS FUNGOIDES/SÉZARY'S SYNDROME. Cyclosporine inhibits helper T cell proliferation and has been shown, in vitro, to have cytostatic and cytolytic effects on leukemic T cells but not on B cells.[109] Hence one would expect cyclosporine to be beneficial in the treatment of mycosis fungoides and Sézary's syndrome, diseases characterized by monoclonal proliferation of malignant helper T cells.

Unfortunately, experience to date[79-84] suggests that although cyclosporine may produce short-term clinical improvement and reduction in both the Sézary cell count and the lymphocytic infiltrate on biopsy, long-term remissions have not occurred. Relapses were often associated with an aggressive course. With the exception of 1 patient, cyclosporine has been used only by patients with advanced disease refractory to conventional therapy.

The drug does, however, seem to give rapid relief for the intolerable pruritus that may be seen in these conditions. Suppression of gamma interferon release from Sézary cells has been postulated as the responsible mechanism.

ATOPIC DERMATITIS. Severe atopic dermatitis unresponsive to other treatments, including systemic therapy, has shown prompt and dramatic improvement with cyclosporine treatment.[85-87] Of 10 patients, 9 showed good clinical improvement with dosages of 2-6 mg/kg/day, and dramatic skin improvement was noticed within 3 days in 1 patient.[86] Pruritus also responds quickly.[88] Eczema relapses when treatment is discontinued, and maintenance therapy appears necessary for continued control. The mechanism of action by cyclosporine is unknown, but studies of mice have shown suppression by cyclosporine of spontaneous IgE formation through a T cell-dependent mechanism.[86] Atopic dermatitis patients treated with cyclosporine had suppression of epidermal activation of autoreactive T cells.[87]

ALLERGIC CONTACT DERMATITIS. Subcutaneous and topical cyclosporine inhibit contact dermatitis in mice[89] and guinea pigs,[90] respectively, if they are given either during the early sensitization phase or at the time of antigenic challenge to fully sensitized mice. The effect is shortlived and reversible. Skin patch tests were inhibited in a small percentage of patients treated with topical cyclosporine.[91, 92]

ALOPECIA AREATA. Gebhart and coauthors[93] reported on 1 patient who had had alopecia universalis for more than 30 years; considerable regrowth of eyebrows and scalp hair occurred while the patient was receiving cyclosporine as a renal allograft recipient. Gupta and colleagues[97] treated 6 patients for 12 weeks with 6 mg/kg/day of cyclosporine. Two patients with patchy scalp alopecia areata and 1 with alopecia totalis had cosmetically acceptable results, and the other 3 with alopecia universalis had more than 60% regrowth of terminal scalp hair.[97] Within 3 months of cyclosporine discontinuation, marked hair loss occurred in all patients. A few studies have shown only modest improvement in some patients treated with topical cyclosporine.[94-96]

The mechanism of action of cyclosporine in alopecia areata is unclear. The drug has no significant influence on specific sex hormone actions. Testosterone, cortisol, androstenedione, sex-hormone–binding globulin, dehydroepiandrosterone sulfate, 17-hydroxyprogesterone, and prolactin levels are not affected.[93] This disease is characterized by a peribulbar accumulation of T lymphocytes, and remissions and hair regrowth can be initiated by a local increase in suppressor T cells. Cyclosporine decreases the helper-to-suppressor T cell ratio profoundly by diminishing the helper T cell fraction in the infiltrate. The drug's prevalent mode of action in inducing hair growth, however, appears to be at the cellular level in the hair follicle proper. Extensive general body hair growth has been reported in athymic nude mice after local cyclosporine treatment. It appears that cyclosporine transforms lanugo-hair–producing follicles into vellus or even terminal hair follicles. Cyclosporine may stimulate dormant follicles by shifting them from a resting phase to an active one.

MALE PATTERN ALOPECIA. Preliminary studies suggest that both systemic and topical cyclosporine may be beneficial in treating male pattern alopecia.[98, 99] In one series, 3 of 6 patients treated with systemic cyclosporine for psoriasis developed new scalp hair, and 1 patient's bald spot disappeared after only 6 weeks of treatment. An additional 2 patients felt that their scalp hair was thicker than before. Within 3 months after the cyclosporine treatment was discontinued, the hair reverted back to the precyclosporine status.

SKIN ALLOGRAFTS AND XENOGRAFTS. Cyclosporine can prolong the viability of rat allografts[100, 101] and human skin xenografts[102] in rats. An 11-year-old boy with 85% surface burns and inhalation injury was treated both with skin allografts from several unmatched donors and with cyclosporine in a dose of 8 mg/kg/day for 120 days.[103] No graft rejection was seen either during treatment or in the 2 years after cyclosporine withdrawal.

A 65-year-old man was also successfully treated with allograft skin from 19 donors and a 3-week course of cyclosporine.[104] However, 12 days after cyclosporine was withdrawn, the allografts started to be rejected, but by this time the patient's own donor sites had healed sufficiently to allow a reharvest and complete replacement of the allografted areas by autograft.

Cyclosporine may have potential use in allowing allografts to provide rapid skin cover of burned areas during the period of maximal risk. If immunotolerance is not achieved, the allograft can be replaced whenever donor sites on the patient become available. The cyclosporine is discontinued when the patient is fully autografted.

OTHER DERMATOLOGIC CONDITIONS. One patient receiving cyclosporine and prednisone after a renal transplant had marked incidental improvement of severe ichthyosis vulgaris.[105] This effect was unexpected, given that T lymphocytes play no known role in the pathogenesis of ichthyosis vulgaris. Ho and colleagues found a 4-week course of 6 mg/kg/day of cyclosporine to be ineffective for 5 patients with lamellar ichthyosis.[106]

A 53-year-old man with persistent light reaction, unable to tolerate PUVA and systemic corticosteroids, showed good improvement and an increased UVA threshold from 0.5 to 16 J/sq cm after 4 weeks of 6 mg/kg/day of cyclosporine.[107] There was a gradual deterioration in the cutaneous process and a decrease in the UVA threshold when the cyclosporine was discontinued.

Oral dosages of 6–10 mg/kg/day of cyclosporine were given to 3 patients with chronic steroid-dependent erythema nodosum leprosum; 2 patients achieved excellent results, and the 3rd showed a partial response.[108]

NONDERMATOLOGIC CONDITIONS. Clinical efficacy with cyclosporine has been reported in treatement of diabetes mellitus,[110, 111] Crohn's disease,[112, 113] ulcerative colitis,[114] primary biliary cirrhosis,[67, 115] pulmonary sarcoidosis,[116] aplastic anemia,[117] Graves' ophthalmopathy,[118] and rheumatoid arthritis.[119, 120]

Adverse Effects

Cyclosporine administration carries many risks,[121] the most serious being nephrotoxicity and malignancy. The incidence of adverse effects has greatly decreased with lower cyclosporine doses and close monitoring of cyclosporine levels. The safe therapeutic range for 12-hour trough cyclosporine levels in whole blood is 100–400 ng/ml, as measured by the radioimmunoassay (RIA) method with specific monoclonal antibody. At these levels, side effects are minimized. Levels in plasma and serum levels have been measured, but whole blood levels are recommended. The distribution of cyclosporine in blood can vary and is dependent on the concentration of the drug, hematocrit, temperature, and lipoprotein concentration.[5] The cyclosporine concentration in plasma separated at 37°C will be substantially greater than in plasma separated at room temperature. High-performance liquid chromatography has also been used to assay cyclosporine, but it is being replaced by the RIA method, which is simpler, faster, and more cost efficient.[122]

NEPHROTOXICITY. Nephrotoxicity occurs in approximately one fourth of nontransplant patients treated with cyclosporine and is characterized by a rise in both serum creatinine and blood urea nitrogen, by a decrease in glomerular filtration rate, by sodium retention and hyperkalemia with mild tubular acidosis, or by hypertension. It is frequently associated with high trough levels and is usually reversible when the dose is lowered.[123] However, permanent interstitial fibrosis, tubular atrophy, and glomerular sclerosis may occur even in patients who had normal renal function at the time of biopsy.[124, 125] There appears to be a correlation between the extent of the renal histologic changes and the cumulative cyclosporine. Just as liver biopsies are necessary to monitor methotrexate therapy even with normal liver function tests, renal biopsies may prove necessary to monitor the degree of nephrotoxicity in patients receiving long-term cyclosporine therapy.

MALIGNANCY. Lymphomas have occurred in association with cyclosporine therapy, but the incidence of malignancy seems to be no greater than with other immunosuppressive agents.[126, 127] The incidence of lymphomas in patients treated with cyclosporine alone or with cyclosporine in combination with corticosteroids is approximately 0.2%.[128] Approximately half of the lymphomas are nodal, and half are extranodal. Small bowel involvement occurs in about one fourth of the lymphomas.[127] When lymphoproliferative malignancy occurs, it is often associated with Epstein-Barr virus infection.[129] When the drug dosage is lowered or the drug is discontinued, regression of the lymphomas frequently results. One psoriatic patient treated with cyclosporine developed a benign lymphocytic infiltrate after only 10 days of therapy.[130] The lesions cleared 3 weeks after the cyclosporine was discontinued. Kaposi's sarcoma and squamous cell carcinomas of the skin may also occur.[126, 131, 132] One patient with psoriasis developed a carcinoma of the anal margin after taking cyclosporine for 6 months. The cancer was successfully excised, and the cyclosporine therapy has been continued.[23] (A complete discussion of malignancy risk in which cyclosporine is compared with cytotoxic drugs appears in Chapter 5.)

HYPERTENSION. Hypertension develops in approximately 25% of nontransplant patients. It is usually mild with low-dose cyclosporine therapy and often responds to dose reduction; however, the hypertension may persist after dose reduction or cessation of therapy. It is more common in patients with pre-existing hypertension or renal disease.

HEPATOTOXICITY/GASTROINTESTINAL EFFECTS. A clinically insignificant, dose-dependent elevation of liver enzymes or bilirubin is commonly seen and is reversible when the dose is lowered. Other gastrointestinal side effects include nausea, vomiting, bloating, diarrhea, decreased appetite,[129] and upper gastrointestinal bleeding.[128]

MUCOCUTANEOUS EFFECTS. Gingival hyperplasia occurs in about 30% of renal transplant patients taking cyclosporine.[133, 134] Changes are seen in less than 1 month, progress rapidly, and are most severe in patients with poor oral hygiene. The changes are similar to the gingival hyperplasia induced by phenytoin, except that the latter occurs more slowly, is clinically much firmer, and histologically shows more mature collagen.

Reversible hypertrichosis occurs in approximately half of patients.[23, 135, 136] The condition is determined to be hypertrichosis and not hirsutism, inasmuch as it is not limited to androgen-dependent areas. The face and upper trunk are commonly affected. It usually resolves within 1–2 months after cyclosporine is discontinued.

Other cutaneous side effects include acne, folliculitis, epidermal cysts, keratosis pilaris, sebaceous hyperplasia,[136] Raynaud's phenomenon,[137] and skin cancers (see the Malignancy section).

NEUROLOGIC EFFECTS. Neurologic side effects include paresthesias, hyperesthesias, headache, mild tremor, and (rarely) seizures.[22, 129] Seizures may be associated with hypomagnesemia.

OTHER ADVERSE EFFECTS. Fatigue is quite common. Depression, muscle cramps,[22] benign breast fibroadenomas, breast tenderness, hyperuricemia, normochromic normocytic anemia,[138] myalgias, arthralgias, visual disturbances, hearing loss, sinusitis, and weight loss have also been reported.[128]

An increased incidence of thromboembolic complications was found in 13 patients in a retrospective study of 90 renal transplant patients treated with cyclosporine (10 with pulmonary emboli, 1 with renal vein thrombosis, 3 with deep vein thromboses, and 3 with hemorrhoidal thromboses), in comparison with 1 of 90 treated with standard immunosuppression drugs.[131]

Finally, anaphylaxis with the intravenous preparation of cyclosporine has been reported, presumably because of the cremaphor surfactant in this preparation. Oral cyclosporine has been subsequently given to a patient with intravenous-cyclosporine–associated anaphylaxis, with no ill effects.[140]

Bone marrow toxicity does not occur with cyclosporine, and the incidence and severity of infections appear less than with standard immunosuppression with azathioprine.[141]

CYCLOSPORINE MONITORING GUIDELINES[39]

Baseline

Examination

- Complete history and physical examination
- Recording blood pressure, weight

Laboratory

- Renal function tests: creatinine, blood urea nitrogen, creatinine clearance
- Urinalysis
- Liver function tests: aspartate aminotransferase (serum glutamate oxaloacetate transaminase), alanine aminotransferase (serum glutamate pyruvate transaminase), bilirubin, alkaline phosphatase (gamma glutamyl transferase: optional)
- Complete blood count (CBC) with differential and platelets
- Immunoelectrophoresis
- Miscellaneous chemistries: potassium, uric acid, magnesium

Follow-up

Examination

- Blood pressure every week for 4 weeks, then every 2–4 weeks
- Thorough physical examination every 2–3 months

Laboratory
Every week for 4 weeks, then every 2–4 weeks:
- Creatinine, blood urea nitrogen
- Cyclosporine level

Every 2–4 weeks:
- Urinalysis
- Liver function tests
- CBC with differential and platelets
- Potassium, uric acid, magnesium

Every 2–3 months:
- Creatinine clearance
- Immunoelectrophoresis

Note: More frequent surveillance is needed if laboratory values are abnormal or with high-risk patients.

DRUG INTERACTIONS[142, 143]

Drugs that may decrease cyclosporine levels (cytochrome P–450 induction):
- Anticonvulsants (phenytoin, phenobarbital, carbamazepine, valproate)
- Antibiotics (isoniazid, rifampin, intravenous sulfadimidine-trimethoprim*)

Drugs that may increase cyclosporine levels (cytochrome P–450 inhibition):
- Antibiotics (erythromycin, ketoconazole, amphotericin B, cephalosporins, doxycycline, acyclovir)
- Hormones (corticosteroids, sex hormones)
- Diuretics (thiazides, furosemide)
- Other (warfarin, calcium channel blockers, H_2 antihistamines)

Drugs that may increase nephrotoxicity:
- Antibiotics (aminoglycosides, amphotericin B, trimethoprim-sulfamethoxazole)
- Nonsteroidal anti-inflammatory drugs
- Other (melphalan)

Interaction with the alcohol content of cyclosporine liquid preparation:
- Disulfiram
- Chlorpropamide
- Metronidazole

*Intravenous sulfadimidine-trimethoprim decreases cyclosporine levels by unknown mechanisms (in U.S., sulfadimidine is known as sulfamethazine).

Patients receiving cyclosporine must be monitored closely so that adverse effects can be minimized. A detailed history should include previous treatment that may increase the risk of cutaneous malignancy, such as PUVA, ultraviolet B, and arsenic; a personal or family history of kidney disease, hypertension, or malignancy; and current medications. Patients with renal dysfunction, with uncontrolled hypertension, with past or present malignancy, with a history of epilepsy, with acute infections, who are pregnant or lactating, or who are taking concomitant nephrotoxins should not be treated.[39] Patients should be questioned during each visit about adverse effects and concomitant medication. Drug interactions do occur, and the drugs are listed in the following section.

Dose adjustments should be made if the serum creatinine rises more than 30% above baseline, if the serum potassium rises above the upper limit of normal, if the creatinine clearance decreases by more than 10%–

15%, if the liver enzymes increase by 100% over baseline or above twice the upper limit of normal, or if the diastolic blood pressure rises to above 95 mmHg. The dose is usually reduced by 25%, and the patient is seen a week later. If the abnormality is not corrected during that visit, the drug is usually reduced by another 25%. If the abnormality is not corrected by the next weekly visit, the drug is usually withdrawn. Antihypertensive therapy may be instituted to correct hypertension without discontinuing cyclosporine for patients for whom cyclosporine is potentially life saving.

Summary

In summary, cyclosporine leads to an excellent response in several dermatologic conditions, including psoriasis, Behçet's disease, pyoderma gangrenosum, atopic dermatitis, and alopecia areata. Patients with severe disabling diseases refractory to conventional therapy have dramatically improved with cyclosporine treatment. Despite its profound therapeutic effects, the serious side effects and substantial cost of the drug limit its use. It is likely that systemic cyclosporine treatment will continue to be reserved for patients with severe disabling disease that is unresponsive to conventional therapy, including other systemic therapy. These patients must be willing to accept the possible side effects, and they must be reliable and available for close monitoring. The lowest effective dose of cyclosporine should be sought, and the drug should be used only by physicians who are thoroughly familiar with surveillance for the potential adverse reactions associated with cyclosporine. This surveillance includes repeated, well-directed history and physical examinations, in addition to appropriate laboratory tests.

Although cyclosporine has remarkable efficacy in a number of dermatologic conditions, routine clinical use awaits clarification of several issues. Clinicians must await clear evidence that lower dose cyclosporine regimens reduce malignancy risk, hypertension, and nephrotoxicity to an acceptable range while remaining efficacious. Until that time, cyclosporine should primarily be used in research and tertiary care clinical settings for severe and refractory dermatoses.

BIBLIOGRAPHY: Key Reviews/Chapters

Page EH, Wexler DM, Guenther LC: Cyclosporin A. J Am Acad Dermatol 1986; 14:785–791.
Shuster S: Cyclosporine in dermatology. Transplant Proc 1988; 20(Suppl 4):19–22.
Bos JD, Van Joost TH, Powles AV, et al: Use of cyclosporin in psoriasis. Lancet 1989; 2:1500–1502.
Kahan BD: Drug therapy: Cyclosporine. N Engl J Med 1989; 321:1725–1738.
Gupta AK, Brown MD, Ellis CN, et al: Cyclosporine in dermatology. J Am Acad Dermatol 1989, 21:1245–1256.

REFERENCES

1. Cohen DJ, Loertscher R, Rubin MF, et al: Cyclosporine: A new immunosuppressive agent for organ transplantation. Ann Intern Med 1984; 101:667–682.
2. Nussenblatt RB, Palestine AG: Cyclosporine: Immunology, pharmacology and therapeutic uses. Surv Opthalmol 1986; 31(3):159–169.
3. Wenger R: Chemistry of cyclosporine. In White DJG (ed): Cyclosporin A: Proceedings of the International Symposium, Cambridge, U.K. Amsterdam: Elsevier Biomedical Press, 1982, 19–34.
4. Zehnder C, Beveridge T, Nuesch E, et al: Cyclosporine A capsules: Bioavailability and clinical acceptance study in renal transplant patients. Transplant Proc 1988; 20(Suppl 2):641–643.
5. Lemaire A, Maurer G, Wood AJ: Pharmacokinetics and metabolism. Prog Allergy 1986; 38:93–107.
6. Beveridge T: Pharmacokinetics and metabolism of cyclosporin A. In White DJG (ed): Cyclosporin A: Proceedings of the International Symposium. Cambridge, U.K.: Elsevier Biomedical Press, 1982, 35–44.
7. Britton S, Palacios R: Cyclosporin A: Usefulness, risks and mechanisms of action. Immunol Rev 1982; 65:5–22.
8. Hess AD, Esa AH, Colombani PM: Mechanisms of action of cyclosporine: Effect on cells of the immune system and on subcellular events in T cell activation. Transplant Proc 1988; 20(Suppl 2):29–40.
9. Colombani PM, Robb A, Hess AD: Cyclosporin A binding to calmodulin: A possible site of action on T lymphocytes. Science 1985; 228:337–339.
10. Takahashi N, Hayano T, Suzuki M: Peptidyl-prolyl cis-trans isomerase is the cyclosporin A–binding protein cyclophilin. Nature 1989; 337:473–475.
11. Fischer G, Wittman-Leibold B, Lang K, et al: Cyclophilin and peptidyl-prolyl cis-trans isomerase are probably identical proteins. Nature 1989; 337:476–478.
12. Harper JI, Kendra JR, Desai S, et al: Dermatological aspects of the use of Cyclosporin A for prophylaxis of graft-versus-host disease. Br J Dermatol 1984; 110:469–474.
13. Powles RL, Clink HM, Spence E, et al: Cyclosporin A to prevent graft-versus-host disease in man after allogeneic bone-marrow transplantation. Lancet 1980; 1:327–329.
14. Vogersang GB, Hess AD, Santos GW: Acute graft-versus-host disease: Clinical characteristics in the cyclosporine era. Medicine 1988; 67:163–174.
15. Harper JI, Keat AC, Staughton RC: Cyclosporin for psoriasis [letter]. Lancet 1984; 2:981–982.
16. Van Joost T, Huele F, Stolz E, et al: Short-term use of cyclosporin A in severe psoriasis. Br J Dermatol 1986; 114:615–620.
17. Griffiths CEM, Powles AV, Leonard JN, et al: Clearance of psoriasis with low dose cyclosporin. Br Med J 1986; 293:731–732.
18. Brooks DB: Clearance of psoriasis with low dose cyclosporin. Br Med J 1986; 293:1098–1099.
19. Marks JM: Psoriasis. Br Med J 1986; 293:509.
20. Ellis CN, Gorsulowsky DC, Hamilton TA, et al: Cyclosporine improves psoriasis in a double-blind study. JAMA 1986; 256:3110–3116.
21. Picascia DD, Garden JM, Freinkel RK, et al: Treatment of resistant severe psoriasis with systemic cyclosporine. J Am Acad Dermatol 1987; 17:163–165.
22. Wentzell JM, Baughman RD, O'Connor GT, et al: Cyclosporine in the treatment of psoriasis. Arch Dermatol 1987; 123:163–165.
23. Fry L, Griffiths CEM, Powles AV, et al: Long-term cyclosporine in the management of psoriasis. Transplant Proc 1988; 20(Suppl 4):23–25.

24. Brown MD, Gupta AK, Ellis CN, et al: Cyclosporine for the treatment of psoriasis. Transplant Proc 1988; 20(Suppl 4):26–31.
25. Picascia DD, Garden JM, Freinkel RK, et al: Resistant severe psoriasis controlled with systemic cyclosporine therapy. Transplant Proc 1988; 20(Suppl 4):58–62.
26. Harper JI, Zemelman V, Keat ACS, et al: Cyclosporine for psoriasis: Beneficial effect in refractory skin and joint disease. Transplant Proc 1988; 20(Suppl 4):63–67.
27. Meinardi MMHM, Bos JD: Cyclosporine maintenance therapy in psoriasis. Transplant Proc 1988; 20(Suppl 4):42–49.
28. Huele F, Meinardi MMHM, Van Joost T, et al: Low-dose cyclosporine effective in severe psoriasis: A double-blind study. Transplant Proc 1988; 20(Suppl 4):32–41.
29. Van Joost T, Bos JD, Huele F, et al: Low-dose cyclosporin A in severe psoriasis: A double-blind study. Br J Dermatol 1988; 118:183–190.
30. Marks J: Low-dose cyclosporine A in severe psoriasis. Transplant Proc 1988; 20(Suppl 4):68–71.
31. Finzi AF, Mozzanica N, Cattaneo A, et al: Effectiveness of cyclosporine treatment in severe psoriasis: A clinical and immunologic study. J Am Acad Dermatol 1989; 21:91–97.
32. Mueller W, Hermann B: Cyclosporin A for psoriasis [letter]. N Engl J Med 1979; 301:555.
33. Griffiths CEM, Powles AV, Baker BS, et al: Combination of cyclosporine A and topical corticosteroid in the treatment of psoriasis. Transplant Proc 1988; 20(Suppl 4):50–52.
34. Higgins E, Munro C, Friedmann PS, et al: Risk of relapse upon withdrawal of cyclosporin therapy for psoriasis [letter]. Lancet 1988; 2:802–803.
35. Cacoub P, Artru L, Canesi M, et al: Life-threatening psoriasis relapse on withdrawal of cyclosporin [letter]. Lancet 1988; 2:219–220.
36. Gilhar A, Winterstein G, Golan DT: Topical cyclosporine in psoriasis. J Am Acad Dermatol 1988; 18:378–379.
37. Powles AV, Baker BS, McFadden J, et al: Intralesional injection of cyclosporin in psoriasis. Lancet 1989; 1:537.
38. Ho VC, Griffiths CEM, Ellis CN, et al: Intralesional cyclosporine in the treatment of psoriasis. J Am Acad Dermatol 1989; 22:94–100.
39. Bos JD, Van Joost TH, Powles AV, et al: Use of cyclosporin in psoriasis. Lancet 1989; 2:1500–1502.
40. Ho VC, Gupta AK, Ellis CN, et al: Treatment of severe lichen planus with cyclosporine. J Am Acad Dermatol 1990; 22:64–68.
41. Francès C, Boisnic S, Etienne S, et al: Effect of the local application of ciclosporine A on chronic erosive lichen planus of the oral cavity [letter]. Dermatologica 1988; 177:194–195.
42. Balato N, De Rosa S, Bordone F, et al: Dermatological application of cyclosporine. Arch Dermatol 1989; 125;1430–1431.
43. Thivolet J, Barthélémy H, Rigot-Muller G, et al: Effects of cyclosporin on bullous pemphigoid and pemphigus. Lancet 1985; 1:334–335.
44. Barthélémy H, Biron F, Caludy A, et al: Cyclosporine: New immunosuppressive agent in bullous pemphigoid and pemphigus. Transplant Proc 1986; 18:913–914.
45. Balda BR, Rosenzweig D: Cyclosporin A in der Behandlung von Pemphigus foliaceous und Pemphigus erythematosus. Hautarzt 1986; 37:454–457.
46. Cunliffe WJ: Pemphigus foliaceous and response to cyclosporin. Br J Dermatol 1987; 117:114–116.
47. Barthélémy H, Frappaz A, Cambazard F, et al: Treatment of nine cases of pemphigus vulgaris with cyclosporine. J Am Acad Dermatol 1988; 18:1262–1266.
48. Barthélémy H, Thivolet J, Cambazard F, et al: La ciclosporine dans le traitement de la pemphigöide bulleuse: Étude préliminaire. Ann Dermatol Venereol 1986; 113:309–313.

49. Cunliffe WJ: Bullous pemphigoid and response to cyclosporin. Br J Dermatol 1987; 117:113–114.
50. Connolly SM, Sander HM: Treatment of epidermolysis bullosa acquisita with cyclosporine. J Am Acad Dermatol 1987; 16:890.
51. Zachariae H: Cyclosporine A in epidermolysis bullosa acquisita. J Am Acad Dermatol 1987; 6:1058–1059.
52. Crow LL, Finkle JP, Gammon WR, et al: Clearing of epidermolysis bullosa acquisita with cyclosporine. J Am Acad Dermatol 1988; 5:937–942.
53. Zabel P, Leimenstoll G, Gross WL: Cyclosporin for acute dermatomyositis. Lancet 1984; 1:343.
54. Ejstrup L: Severe dermatomyositis treated with cyclosporin A. Ann Rheum Dis 1986; 45:612–613.
55. Bendtzen K, Tvede N, Andersen V, et al: Cyclosporin for polymyositis. Lancet 1984; 1:792–793.
56. Van der Meer S, Imhof JW, Borleffs JCC: Cyclosporin for polymyositis. Ann Rheum Dis 1986; 45:612.
57. Girardin E, Dayer JM, Paunier L: Cyclosporine for juvenile dermatomyositis. J Pediatr 1988; 112:165–166.
58. Jones DW, Snaith ML, Isenberg DA: Cyclosporine treatment for intractable polymyositis [letter]. Arthritis Rheum 1987; 30:959–960.
59. Isenberg DA, Snaith ML, Al-Khader AA, et al: Cyclosporin relieves arthralgia, causes angioedema. N Engl J Med 1980; 303:754.
60. Feutren G, Querin S, Tron F, et al: The effects of cyclosporine in patients with systemic lupus. Transplant Proc 1986; 18:643–644.
61. Miescher PA, Favre H, Chatelanat F, et al: Combined steroid-cyclosporin treatment of chronic autoimmune diseases. Klin Wochenschr 1987; 65:727–736.
62. Miescher PA, Favre H, Mihatsch MJ, et al: The place of cyclosporine A in the treatment of connective tissue diseases. Transplant Proc 1988; 20(Suppl 4):224–237.
63. Ter Borg EJ, Tegzess AM, Kallenberg CGM: Unexpected severe reversible cyclosporine A–induced nephrotoxicity in a patient with systemic lupus erythematosus and tubulointerstitial renal disease. Clin Nephrol 1988; 29:93–95.
64. Huele F, Van Joost T, Beukers R: Cyclosporine in the treatment of lupus erythematosus. Arch Dermatol 1986; 122:973.
65. Drosos AA, Skopouli FN, Costopoulos JS, et al: Cyclosporin A (CyA) in primary Sjögren's syndrome: A double blind study. Ann Rheum Dis 1986; 45:732–735.
66. Dalavanga YA, Detrick B, Hooks JJ, et al: Effect of cyclosporin A (CyA) on the immunopathological lesion of the labial minor salivary glands from patients with Sjögren's syndrome. Ann Rheum Dis 1987; 46:89–92.
67. Schmitz-Schumann M: Interim report of clinical studies presented at the international symposium on cyclosporin in auto-immune disease, Basel, March 18–20, 1985. Prog Allergy 1986, 38:443–446.
68. Francès C, Branchet MC, Bletry O, et al: Skin collagen from scleroderma patients before and after cyclosporin A treatment. Clin Exp Dermatol 1988; 13:1–3.
69. Appelboom T, Itzkowitch D: Cyclosporine in successful control of rapidly progressive scleroderma [letter]. Am J Med 1987; 82:866–867.
70. Zachariae H, Zachariae E: Cyclosporin A in systemic sclerosis. Br J Dermatol 1987; 116:741–742.
71. Nussenblatt RB, Palestine AG, Rook AH, et al: Treatment of intraocular inflammatory disease with cyclosporin A. Lancet 1983; 2:235–238.
72. Nussenblatt RB, Palestine AG, Chan CC, et al: Effectiveness of cyclosporin therapy for Behçet's disease. Arthritis Rheum 1985; 28:671–679.
73. French-Constant C, Wolman R, Geraint James D: Cyclosporin in Behçet's disease [letter]. Lancet 1983; 2:454–455.

74. Wechsler B, Mertani EB, Le Hoang P, et al: Cyclosporin is effective, but not safe, in the management of Behçet's disease [letter]. Arthritis Rheum 1986; 29:574–575.
75. Nussenblatt RB: The use of cyclosporine in ocular inflammatory disorders. Transplant Proc 1988; 20(Suppl 4):114–121.
76. Magid ML, Gold MH: Treatment of recalcitrant pyoderma gangrenosum with cyclosporine. J Am Acad Dermatol 1989; 20:293–294.
77. Shelley ED, Shelley WB: Cyclosporine therapy for pyoderma gangrenosum associated with sclerosing cholangitis and ulcerative colitis. J Am Acad Dermatol 1988; 18:1084–1088.
78. Penmetcha M, Navaratnam AE: Pyoderma gangrenosum: Response to cyclosporin A. Int J Dermatol 1988; 27:253.
79. Catterall MD, Addis BJ, Smith JL, Coode PE: Sézary syndrome: Transformation to a high grade T-cell lymphoma after treatment with Cyclosporin A. Clin Exp Dermatol 1983; 8:159–169.
80. Puttick L, Pollock A, Fairburn E: Treatment of Sézary syndrome with cyclosporin A. J R Soc Med 1983; 76:1063–1065.
81. Tötterman TH, Scheynius A, Killander A, et al: Treatment of therapy-resistant Sézary syndrome with cyclosporin-A: Suppression of pruritus, leukaemic T cell activation markers and tumour mass. Scand J Haematol 1985; 34:196–203.
82. Maddox AM, Kahan BD, Tucker S, et al: Remission in skin infiltrate of a patient with mycosis fungoides treated with cyclosporine. J Am Acad Dermatol 1985; 12:952–956.
83. Moreland AA, Robertson DB, Heffner LT: Treatment of cutaneous T cell lymphoma with cyclosporin A. J Am Acad Dermatol 1985; 12:886–887.
84. Jansen JR, Thestrup-Pedersen K, Zachariae H, et al: Cyclosporin A therapy for mycosis fungoides. Arch Dermatol 1987; 123:160–163.
85. Van Joost T, Stolz E, Heule F: Efficacy of low-dose cyclosporine in severe atopic skin disease. Arch Dermatol 1987; 166–167.
86. Logan RA, Camp RDR: Severe atopic eczema: Response to oral cyclosporin A. J R Soc Med 1988; 81:417–418.
87. Taylor RS, Baadsgaard O, Headington JT, et al: Epidermal activation of autoreactive T cells in atopic dermatitis: Response to cyclosporine A. Clin Res 1988; 36:699A.
88. Shuster S: Cyclosporine in dermatology. Transplant Proc 1988; 20(Suppl 4):19–22.
89. Rullan PP, Barr RJ, Cole GW: Cyclosporine and murine allergic contact dermatitis. Arch Dermatol 1984; 120:1179–1183.
90. Kakagawa S, Oka D, Jinno Y, et al: Topical application of cyclosporine on guinea pig allergic contact dermatitis. Arch Dermatol 1988; 124:907–910.
91. Lembo G, Balato N, Patrun C, et al: Influence of topical cyclosporin A on patch test reactions. Contact Dermatitis 1989; 20:155–156.
92. Cole GW, Shimomaye S, Goodman M: The effect of topical cyclosporin A on the elicitation phase of allergic contact dermatitis. Contact Dermatitis 1988; 19:129–132.
93. Gebhart W, Schmidt JB, Schemper M, et al: Cyclosporin A–induced hair growth in human renal allograft recipients and alopecia areata. Arch Dermatol Res 1986; 278:238–240.
94. De Prost Y, Teillac D, Paquez F, et al: Placebo-controlled trial of topical cyclosporin in severe alopecia areata. Lancet 1986; 2:803–804.
95. Thomson AW, Aldridge RD, Sewell HF: Topical cyclosporin in alopecia areata and nickel contact dermatitis. Lancet 1986; 2:971–972.
96. Parodi A, Rebora A: Topical cyclosporine in alopecia areata. Arch Dermatol 1987; 123:165–166.
97. Gupta AK, Ellis CN, Cooper KD, et al: Oral cyclosporine for the treatment of alopecia areata. J Am Acad Dermatol 1990; 22:242–250.
98. Picascia DD, Roenigk HH Jr: Effects of oral and topical cyclosporine in male pattern alopecia. Transplant Proc 1988; 20(Suppl 4):109–111.

99. Gilhar A, Pillar T, Etzioni A: Topical cyclosporine in male pattern alopecia. J Am Acad Dermatol 1990; 22:251–253.
100. Towpik E, Kupiec-Weglinski JW, Schneider TM, et al: Cyclosporine and experimental skin allografts. Transplantation 1985; 40:714–718.
101. Gilhar A, Wojciechowski ZJ, Piepkorn MW, et al: Description of and treatment to inhibit the rejection of human split-thickness skin grafts by congenitally athymic (nude) rats. Exp Cell Biol 1986; 54:263–274.
102. Biren CA, Barr RJ, McCullough JL, et al: Prolonged viability of human skin xenografts in rats by cyclosporine. J Invest Dermatol 1986; 86:611–614.
103. Achauer BM, Hewitt CW, Black KS, et al: Long-term skin allograft survival after short-term cyclosporin treatment in a patient with massive burns. Lancet 1986; 1:14–15.
104. Frame JD: Short-term cyclosporin and meshed allograft in burns. Lancet 1987; 1:154–155.
105. Velthius PJ, Jesserun RFM: Improvement of ichthyosis by cyclosporin. Lancet 1985; 1:335.
106. Ho VC, Gupta AK, Ellis CN, et al: Cyclosporine in lamellar ichthyosis. Arch Dermatol 1989;125:511–514.
107. Duschet P, Schwarz T, Oppolzer G, et al: Persistent light reaction. Acta Derm Venereol (Stockh) 1988; 68:176–178.
108. Miller RA, Shen JY, Rea TH, et al: Treatment of chronic erythema nodosum leprosum with cyclosporine A produces clinical and immunohistologic remission. Int J Lepr 1987; 55:441–449.
109. Tötterman TH, Danersund A, Nilsson K, et al: Cyclosporin-A is selectively cytotoxic to human leukemic T cells in vitro. Blood 1982; 59:1103–1107.
110. Stiller CR, Dupre J, Gent M, et al: Effects of cyclosporine immunosuppression in insulin-dependent diabetes mellitus of recent onset. Science 1984; 223:1362–1367.
111. Feutren G, Papoz L, Assan R, et al: Cyclosporin increases the rate and length of remissions in insulin-dependent diabetes of recent onset: Results of a multicentre double-blind trial. Lancet 1986; 2:119–124.
112. Allison MC, Pounder RE: Cyclosporin for Crohn's disease. Lancet 1984; 1:902–903.
113. Bianchi PA, Mondelli M, Quarto di Palo F, et al: Cyclosporin for Crohn's disease. Lancet 1984; 2:1242.
114. Gupta S, Keshavarzian A, Hodgson HJF: Cyclosporin in ulcerative colitis. Lancet 1984; 2:1277–1278.
115. Adams D, Clements D, Elias E: The treatment of primary biliary cirrhosis. J Clin Hosp Pharm 1986; 11(2):65–73.
116. Rebuck AS, Stiller CR, Braude AC, et al: Cyclosporin for pulmonary sarcoidosis. Lancet 1984; 1:1174.
117. Wisloff F, Godal HC: Cyclosporin in refractory severe aplastic anemia. N Engl J Med 1985; 321:1193.
118. McGregor AM, Beck L, Hall R: Cyclosporin A in management of Graves' disease. J R Soc Med 1985; 78:511–512.
119. Amor B, Douglas M: Cyclosporine: Therapeutic effects in rheumatic diseases. Transplant Proc 1988; 20(Suppl 4):218–223.
120. Yocum DE, Klippel JH, Wilder RL, et al: Cyclosporin A in severe, treatment-refractory rheumatoid arthritis: A randomized study. Ann Intern Med 1988; 109:863–869.
121. Kahan BD: Drug therapy: Cyclosporine. N Engl J Med 1989; 321:1725–1738.
122. Keown PA: Optimizing cyclosporine therapy: Dose, levels, and monitoring. Transplant Proc 1988; 20(Suppl 2):382–389.
123. Palestine AG, Nussenblatt RB, Chan CC: Side effects of systemic cyclosporine in patients not undergoing transplantation. Am J Med 1984; 77:652–656.
124. Palestine AG, Austin HA III, Balow JE, et al: Renal histopathologic alterations in patients treated with cyclosporine for uveitis. N Engl J Med 1986; 314:1293–1298.
125. Svenson K, Bohman SO, Hallgren R: Renal interstitial fibrosis and vascular changes.

Occurrence in patients with autoimmune diseases treated with cyclosporine. Arch Intern Med 1986; 146:2007–2010.
126. Penn I, First MR: Development and incidence of cancer following cyclosporine therapy. Transplant Proc 1986; 18(Suppl 1):210–213.
127. Penn I: Cancers after cyclosporine therapy. Transplant Proc 1988; 20(Suppl 1):276–279.
128. Sandimmune. In Kragh CM (ed): Compendium of Pharmaceuticals & Specialties 1989 (24th ed). Ottawa: Canadian Pharmaceutical Association, 1989, 930–934.
129. Bennett WM, Norman DJ: Action and toxicity of cyclosporine. Ann Rev Med 1986; 37:215–224.
130. Brown MD, Ellis CN, Billings J, et al: Rapid occurrence of nodular cutaneous T-lymphocyte infiltrates with cyclosporine therapy. Arch Dermatol 1988; 124:1097–1100.
131. Thompson JF, Allen R, Morris PJ, et al: Skin cancer in renal transplant patients treated with cyclosporin. Lancet 1985; 1:158–160.
132. Bos JD, Meinardi MMHM: Two distinct squamous cell carcinomas in a psoriasis patient receiving low-dose cyclosporine maintenance treatment. J Am Acad Dermatol 1989; 21:1305–1306.
133. Tyldesley WR, Rotter E: Gingival hyperplasia induced by cyclosporin A. Br Dent J 1984; 157:305–309.
134. Adams D, Davies G: Gingival hyperplasia associated with cyclosporin A. A report of two cases. Br Dent J 1984; 157:89–90.
135. Mortimer PS, Thompson JF, Dawber RPR, et al: Hypertrichosis and multiple cutaneous squamous cell carcinomas in association with cyclosporin A therapy. J R Soc Med 1983; 76:786–787.
136. Bencini PL, Montagnino G, Sala F, et al: Cutaneous lesions in 67 cyclosporin-treated renal transplant recipients. Dermatologica 1986; 172:24–30.
137. Deray G, Le Hoang P, Achour L, et al: Cyclosporin and Raynaud phenomenon [letter]. Lancet 1986; 2:1092–1093.
138. Palestine AG, Nussenblatt RB, Chan CC: Side effects of systemic cyclosporine in patients not undergoing transplantation. Am J Med 1984; 77:652–656.
139. Vanrenterghem Y, Roels L, Lerut T, et al: Thromboembolic complications and heamostatic changes in cyclosporin-treated cadaveric kidney allograft recipients. Lancet 1985; 1:999–1002.
140. Chapuis B, Helg C, Jeannet M, et al: Anaphylactic reaction to intravenous cyclosporine. N Engl J Med 1985; 312:1259.
141. Hofflin JM, Potasman I, Baldwin JC, et al: Infectious complications in heart transplant recipients receiving cyclosporine and corticosteroids. Ann Intern Med 1987; 106:209–216.
142. Baciewicz AM, Baciewicz FA: Cyclosporine pharmacokinetic drug interactions. Am J Surg 1989; 157:264–271.
143. Cockburn I: Cyclosporine A: A clinical evaluation of drug interactions. Transplant Proc 1986; 18(Suppl 5):50–55.

8 | Retinoids

Stephen E. Wolverton, M.D.

The term "retinoids" includes all synthetic and natural compounds that have activity like that of vitamin A. The initial understanding of these compounds began in the early 1900s when Antarctic explorers experienced hypervitaminosis A shortly after consuming polar bear liver.[1] In 1931, vitamin A in the form of retinoic acid was purified from liver oil. Four years later, the role of retinal in the visual cycle was identified. In 1946, retinoic acid was synthesized, and its role in growth was determined. The first therapeutic use of vitamin A was in 1941 by Straumfjord for acne vulgaris.[1]

In the early 1960s, Bollag began testing various retinoid compounds in vitro, trying to find those that had a suitable therapeutic index, as determined by the rodent papilloma model.[2] Because of an unsafe therapeutic index for oral tretinoin, only the topical form was subsequently used. In 1969, Kligman and colleagues first used topical tretinoin for acne vulgaris.[3] Isotretinoin, first synthesized in 1955, was initially used in the 1970s for disorders of keratinization.[4] In the late 1970s, isotretinoin was found to be effective for acne vulgaris.[5] It was not until 1972 that etretinate was synthesized. After more than a decade of research, the drug was released in the U.S. in 1986 for use in psoriasis.

More than 1500 retinoids have been developed and tested.[2] Current and future research is being geared toward developing new retinoids with a therapeutic index safer than that of the currently existing retinoids.

Pharmacology

Vitamin A Physiology

In order to completely understand the mechanism of action of the retinoids, it is first useful to understand the physiologic effects of vitamin A in its different forms. The details of vitamin A physiology can be found in several complete reviews.[1,6] Vitamin A exists in three main forms: alcohol (retinol), aldehyde (retinal), and acid (retinoic acid).

Retinyl esters derived from meat and animal products, such as eggs and milk, are the primary dietary form of vitamin A. In the intestines, the retinyl esters are hydrolyzed to retinol. The retinol is absorbed and initially stored in the ester form, particularly as retinal palmitate in the liver. Retinol can also be converted interchangeably to retinal and irreversibly metabolized to retinoic acid.

Beta-carotene, primarily derived from green leafy vegetables and yellow vegetables, is another source of vitamin A. In the intestines, every molecule of beta-carotene is converted into two molecules of retinal; the retinal is then absorbed. There is interchangeable conversion of retinal to retinol and irreversible metabolism to retinoic acid.

These forms of vitamin A are important for vision, reproduction, epithelial differentiation, and normal growth. Retinal is the form important for visual function, whereas retinol is essential to reproduction. Both retinal and retinoic acid play an essential role in epithelial differentiation and normal growth.

A complex of retinol-binding protein (RBP) and transthyretin (formerly known as prealbumin) provides transport in the serum for retinol. Upon hydrolysis of the ester form, retinol is released from the liver. There is a 1:1:1 ratio of retinol, retinol-binding protein, and transthyretin. At the cellular level, retinol is bound to a surface receptor and translocated to the nucleus by cytosolic RBP. There is evidence of a related carrier protein known as nuclear RBP. The function of this nuclear receptor is similar to that of the nuclear receptors for thyroxine, vitamin D_3, and glucocorticosteriods. Synthesis of at least 40 proteins is influenced by retinol and related retinoids.

Physiologically, retinoic acid is predominantly in the all-*trans* form. A small fraction is transported as *cis*-retinoic acid. Serum transport is by albumin. There is a separate cytosolic binding protein known as cytosolic RABP (retinoic acid–binding protein). Subsequent cellular events are similar to those for retinol.

Concentrations of these various binding proteins are central to the physiologic and pharmacologic effects of vitamin A and related synthetic retinoids. The epidermis has a much greater concentration of RBPs than does dermal tissue. Sites devoid of RBP and RABP include serum, cardiac muscle, and skeletal muscle.

Structure

All three forms of vitamin A, as well as all three generations of synthetic retinoids to be discussed, come under the heading of retinoids. Beta-carotene, which serves as a precursor for retinal, is not considered a retinoid.

The first-generation (nonaromatic) retinoids include isotretinoin and tretinoin.[6] Because of unacceptable systemic toxicity from tretinoin, this drug is not discussed further. First-generation retinoids are formed by manipulation of the polar end and the polyene side chain. The second generation (monoaromatic) consists of etretinate and acitretin (etretin). These drugs were formed through replacement of the cyclic end with various substituted and nonsubstituted ring systems. The third generation (polyaromatic) are known as the arotinoids. The arotinoids are formed through cyclization of the polyene side chain. Drugs currently being investigated include arotinoid ethylester, the carboxylic acid derivative of arotinoid ethylester (arotinoid acid), and arotinoid ethyl sulfone.

In the following discussion, the focus is primarily on isotretinoin and the two monoaromatic retinoids, etretinate and acitretin. The arotinoids have a thousandfold increase in potency, in spite of maintaining the same therapeutic index as the second-generation retinoids. The arotinoids are discussed only briefly later in the chapter.[7,8]

Absorption/Distribution

Isotretinoin has 25% oral bioavailability that can be improved slightly with meals. The effect of meals, particularly with lipid content, is greater with the second generation of retinoids. Both etretinate (40% bioavailability with food) and acitretin (60% bioavailability with food) have a significant increase in bioavailability when taken with food.[9-11] Although the lipophilic nature of etretinate would make this increase reasonable, a twofold elevation in the bioavailability of acitretin occurs in spite of its hydrophilic nature.

All three drugs demonstrate peak levels that behave in a linear pharmacokinetic fashion with dose plotted against plasma level. Isotretinoin levels peak about 3 hours after ingestion, and etretinate (4 hours) and acitretin (4 hours) peak somewhat later.[9]

As discussed earlier, retinol and naturally occurring retinoic acid are transported by RBP/transthyretin and by albumin, respectively.[1,6,12] Isotretinoin, being the cis-isomer of all-trans retinoic acid, is 99.9% bound to plasma albumin. The second-generation retinoids are bound both by lipoproteins and by albumin. Etretinate is 99% protein-bound, predominantly to plasma lipoproteins. The hydrophilic compound acitretin binds predominantly to albumin, and a lesser amount binds to lipoproteins.

As with vitamin A, there is significant concentration of all the synthetic retinoids in the liver.[1,6] They have a lesser affinity than vitamin A for storage in hepatocytes and in Ito stellate fibroblasts. When retinoid absorption exceeds liver storage capacity, symptoms of hypervitaminosis A result. Because isotretinoin and acitretin are water-soluble, there is very little lipid deposition.[9] The unique feature of etretinate is its extensive and prolonged storage in fat because of its lipid solubility.[1,6] Implications of this storage are discussed subsequently with regard to the prolonged half-life and resultant prolonged risk of teratogenicity with etretinate.

Metabolism/Excretion

The major metabolite of isotretinoin is produced by oxidation, which forms 4-oxo-isotretinoin. Lesser amounts of tretinoin and 4-oxo-tretinoin are produced. With etretinate there is significant first-pass metabolism by hydrolysis to the active metabolite acitretin. Glucuronidation conjugates are subsequently formed from acitretin.

There are important differences in the terminal elimination half-lives of the three synthetic retinoids.[9] Isotretinoin has a half-life of 10–20 hours. Etretinate has a prolonged half-life of 80–160 days. After etretinate therapy is discontinued, the serum levels quickly drop to very low levels. However, these levels may persist for up to 2.9 years.[13] Acitretin is more like isotretinoin, with a half-life of 50 hours and subsequent complete elimination by 3 weeks. Both isotretinoin and acitretin are completely cleared from the body within a month after the drug is stopped. This gives both drugs a definite advantage over etretinate for use by women of childbearing age.

All three drugs are equally excreted in the urine and feces.[9] Conjugated metabolites appear in the bile with subsequent excretion in the feces. Isotretinoin demonstrates limited enterohepatic recirculation.

Mechanism of Action

There are numerous pharmacologic effects of the synthetic retinoids.[1] However, several of these effects to be detailed are believed to be most central to the therapeutic benefits obtained from the retinoids.

IMMUNOLOGIC/ANTI-INFLAMMATORY EFFECTS. Psoriasis is a useful model of retinoid pharmacodynamics. Both arachidonic acid metabolism and polyamine synthesis are altered in psoriasis.[1] Retinoid reduction of leukotriene and hydroxyeicosatetraenoic acid (HETE) products decreases the neutrophil chemotactic effects of these compounds. The retinoids directly inhibit ornithine decarboxylase and lessen the inflammatory proliferative state that results from an activation of this enzyme.[1]

Other retinoid effects include decreased immunoglobulin production from B cells and decreased mitogen stimulation of peripheral lymphocytes.[1] There is no effect on antibody-dependent cellular cytotoxicity.

SEBUM EFFECTS. When isotretinoin is administered at a dosage of 40 mg twice a day, there is an initial reduction of sebaceous gland size accompanied by decreased differentiation to mature sebocytes. The result is a 70%–90% decrease in sebum production and an altered sebum composition with less wax ester and squalene production.[14, 15] Within 1 month after cessation of therapy, the sebum composition returns to normal, whereas the amount produced remains decreased an average of 40% from baseline.[14, 15] Although complete explanation of this sebaceous gland inhibition is lacking, there is no evidence of suppressed androgen synthesis. Levels of peripheral androgens and gonadotropins remain unchanged.[15] Second- and third-generation retinoids produce little or no reduction in or altered composition of sebaceous gland lipids.[16, 17]

Acne pathogenesis includes altered follicular keratinization, which leads to microcomedo formation and subsequent inflammatory lesions. Retinoid-induced normalization of this abnormal keratinization leads to decreased follicular occlusion.[18-20] With the reduced sebum production, the growth of *Propionobacterium acnes* and subsequent conversion of triglycerides to free fatty acids are decreased.[14, 15] Inhibition of neutrophil chemotaxis is believed to be important for the beneficial effects in acne vulgaris.[21] In addition, neutrophil chemotaxis inhibition by retinoids may be important in psoriasis therapy.[22]

ANTITUMOR/ANTIPROLIFERATIVE EFFECTS. Perhaps the most exciting potential benefit from synthetic retinoids is the inhibition of tumor promotion in certain malignant and premalignant conditions. It has long been known that various epithelial structures undergo squamous metaplasia during vitamin A deficiency.[6, 23] The subsequent replacement of vitamin A normalizes this altered keratinization. Lippman and colleagues recently reviewed retinoid effects on polyamine synthesis.[23] Phorbol ester (e.g., phorbol myristate acetate and triphorbol acetate) and diacyl glycerol activation of protein kinase-C leads to activation of ornithine decarboxylase.[23, 24] Ornithine decarboxylase is the rate-limiting enzyme in production of the polyamines spermine, spermidine, and putrescine. This polyamine pathway has been associated with the initiation and promotion of rodent papillomas, which are a useful model of human actinic keratoses.[23, 24] Retinoids inhibit both ornithine decarboxylase activation and the proliferation associated with increased polyamine synthesis.

Activation of oncogenes may be central to virus-induced, radiation-induced, and chemical-induced carcinogenesis.[23, 24] Retinoid inhibition of expression of these oncogenes may likewise decrease the possibility of malignant conversion of various premalignant lesions.

In animal models and human trials, various epithelial premalignant conditions are prevented from undergoing malignant conversion as long as the retinoid therapy is sustained. Benefits have been noted for oral, pharyngeal, pulmonary, bladder, uterine-cervical, and breast epithelial malignancies.[25, 26] The primary retinoid benefit may be mediated by an antipromotion effect that lessens the probability of the malignant conversion stage of carcinogenesis. For a more complete discussion on this subject, see articles by a number of investigators.[23-30]

MISCELLANEOUS EFFECTS. Retinoids are known to inhibit collagenase activity, which suggests possible efficacy in recessive dystrophic epidermolysis bullosa.[1] Altered cell-to-cell interactions are important effects. Altered glycosaminoglycan and glycoprotein composition may be important as well.

SUMMARY. Although vitamin A has an important role in vision, reproduction, epithelial differentiation, and growth, the effects of synthetic retinoids used in dermatology are mostly epithelial. Through normalization of epithelial growth and differentiation, benign inflammatory proliferative diseases, such as psoriasis, and premalignant and malignant conditions may respond to retinoids. The improvement in disorders of keratinization is also primarily the result of these epithelial effects. By normalizing keratinization, retinoids play a central role in therapy of pilosebaceous disorders such as acne vulgaris. There is no doubt that other anti-inflammatory, immunologic, and cell-to-cell interaction effects play a major role in the therapeutic benefits of these compounds.

Clinical Use (Table 8–1)

Indications

The five categories listed in Table 8–1 are psoriasis, acne and related disorders, disorders of keratinization, neoplastic disorders, and miscellaneous inflammatory conditions. For each disease, it is important to focus on which synthetic retinoid is most efficacious, whether the patient needs short-term versus long-term therapy, the likelihood of sustained remission, alternative modes of therapy, and the risk-benefit ratio.

PSORIASIS. The single indication approved by the U.S. Food and Drug Administration (FDA) for etretinate is severe recalcitrant psoriasis. The forms most responsive to etretinate or acitretin as monotherapy include the generalized pustular[33-37] and erythrodermic forms.[44, 45, 48, 49] Localized pustular psoriasis may benefit as well with retinoids used as monotherapy.[38-41] Etretinate use in severe plaque-type psoriasis generally leads to partial improvement and often is more effective when combined with other treatment modalities. Potential combinations include retinoids with psoralens plus ultraviolet A (Re-PUVA), in which retinoids are given 10–14 days before PUVA is initiated. Retinoid therapy is then subsequently tapered once remission has occurred. Later PUVA doses are likewise reduced.[52-61] Etretinate or acitretin, in combination with ultraviolet B,[62, 63] topical steroids,[64, 65] anthralin,[66] and methotrexate,[67, 68] has been beneficial in selected patients. The possibility of synergistic liver toxicity with methotrexate limits this particular combination.[149]

Table 8–1. Retinoid Indications/Contraindications

FDA-Approved Dermatologic Indications

Acne Vulgaris (isotretinoin)
    Recalcitrant nodulocystic

Psoriasis (etretinate)
    Pustular
    Erythrodermic
    Severe plaque type

Dermatologic Uses

Psoriasis
  OVERVIEWS[30–32]
  MONOTHERAPY
    Pustular[33–41]
    Severe plaque type[42–49]
    Erythrodermic[37, 44, 45, 48, 49]
    Nail changes[50]
    Psoriatic arthritis[51]
  COMBINATION THERAPY
    Retinoid/PUVA—RePUVA[52–61]
    Retinoid/ultraviolet B[62, 63]
    Retinoid/topical steroid[64, 65]
    Retinoid/anthralin[66]
    Retinoid/methotrexate[67, 68]

Acne Vulgaris/Related Disorders
  Acne vulgaris
    Overviews[14, 69, 70]
    Clinical studies[5, 71–77]
  Rosacea[78–80]
  Gram-negative folliculitis[80]
  Hidradenitis suppurativa[81, 82]

Disorders of Keratinization
  Overviews[83–87]
  Darier's disease[88–90] (*for severe cases)
  Pityriasis rubra pilaris[91–93]*
  Ichthyosis[4, 94–99] (*for lamellar ichthyosis)
  Keratodermas[100–108]
  Epidermal nevi[83]

Premalignant/Malignant Conditions
  Overviews[23–27]
  Premalignant lesions[26, 109–116]
  Syndromes with increased risk of
    cutaneous malignancies[26]
      Xeroderma pigmentosum[117]
      Basal cell nevus syndrome[118]
      Epidermodysplasia verucciformis[119]
  Cutaneous malignancies[26]
    Multiple basal cell carcinomas[120, 121]
    Mycosis fungoides[122–124]
    Melanoma[26]

Miscellaneous Inflammatory Conditions
  Lupus erythematosus[125–128]
  Lichen planus[129–132]
  Lichen sclerosus et atrophicus[133–135]
  Sarcoidosis[136]
  Other dermatoses[137–142]

Arotinoid Use
  Overviews[7, 8]
  Psoriasis[143, 144]
  Psoriatic arthritis[145]
  Mycosis fungoides/other neoplasms[146–148]

Contraindications

Absolute
  Pregnancy or patient's likelihood of becoming pregnant
  Sensitivity to parabens (isotretinoin: present in gel capsule)

Relative
  Severe hypertriglyceridemia or hypercholesterolemia, particularly if other coronary artery disease risk factors are present
  Significant hepatic dysfunction

*Retinoids are generally considered the drugs of choice.

Etretinate and acitretin therapy is usually begun at 0.75–1 mg/kg/day in divided dosages. A maximal dosage of 1.5 mg/kg/day is recommended, with a maintenance dosage of 0.5–0.75 mg/kg. This maintenance dosage can generally be used after 8–16 weeks of therapy. Erythrodermic patients may respond initially at 0.25 mg/kg/day but may require gradual increases of 0.25 mg/kg/day.

Although the recommended drug holidays are theoretically sound, most patients actually suffer relapse within 2 months after discontinuing etretinate. In my experience, a reasonable alternative is to reduce dosages to as low as 25 mg every day or even 25 mg every other day for long-term maintenance therapy.

Although methotrexate may be a better treatment option for psoriatic arthritis, etretinate improves psoriatic arthritis in 60% of patients.[51]

The *Physicians' Desk Reference* recommends using etretinate only for patients who have been treated with methotrexate and systemic steroids. Given the general contraindication for systemic steroids in psoriasis, this step is unnecessary. With the inherent risks of methotrexate, retinoid therapy is often indicated before methotrexate for psoriasis. Acitretin has been studied alone[42–44] and in direct comparison with etretinate.[48, 49] These studies suggest similar efficacy and side effect profiles for these two drugs. Acitretin has a better pharmacokinetic profile than etretinate because it is completely eliminated from the body by 1 month. Women of childbearing age in particular will be at less risk with this more rapid elimination than with etretinate.

ACNE. After multiple successful clinical studies[5, 71–73] isotretinoin was released in September 1982. The sole indication was severe recalcitrant nodulocystic acne vulgaris. Although the same indication holds today, there is a greater need for more careful patient selection, particularly with women of childbearing potential.[150, 151] Appropriate patients have severe nodulocystic acne with a tendency for scarring that has been refractory to maximal management, including several systemic antibiotics. Typically, 0.5–1 mg/kg/day is given in divided doses. An initial response is seen by 8 weeks, and improvement continues through the end of 20 weeks' administration.[14, 69, 70] Comparisons of 0.1, 0.5, and 1.0 mg/kg/day suggest similar initial efficacy at all dosages; however, the two lower dosage options allow more frequent relapses.[74–76] More significant and frequent adverse effects at 1.0 mg/kg/day may make 0.5 mg/kg/day more suitable for less severe cases. Should another isotretinoin course be necessary, the recommendation is to wait 8 weeks after completion of the first course. There may be continued improvement even during the 2 months after cessation of therapy. For trunk involvement and unusually recalcitrant cases, dosages up to 2 mg/kg/day may be required.[14, 69, 70] An early flare-up of disease activity is generally due to cessation of previous systemic antibiotics in addition to the altered cutaneous barrier function that leads to increased granulation tissue and *Staphylococcus aureus* superinfection.[14] Second-generation (aromatic) retinoids do not have the sebostatic effect of isotretinoin and have no role in acne therapy.[16, 17, 77]

With proper selection of patients, the use of isotretinoin for severe acne can be exceedingly gratifying because of the potential for long-term sustained improvement. In my experience, however, only a minority of patients experience complete clearing, whereas the majority of patients demonstrate marked improvement that is maintained by less aggressive acne therapy after the discontinuation of isotretinoin.

ROSACEA. Only a small number of studies have addressed the use of isotretinoin in rosacea.[78–80] Therapeutic response has been greatest in treatment of the papulopustular variety and minimal in treatment of the vascular form of rosacea. At least two thirds of patients have a good response. The majority of rosacea patients have sustained improvement for more than a year after isotretinoin discontinuation. The dosage range, the rate of response, and the total duration of therapy are similar to those of isotretinoin use in acne vulgaris. Granulomatous rosacea appears to respond. However, the relatively small number of patients treated to date do not provide sufficient experience for definitive guidelines.[78–80]

HIDRADENITIS SUPPURATIVA. Only a few reports describe the use of retinoids in hidradenitis suppurativa.[81, 82, 138] The response to isotretinoin is less than in acne vulgaris or rosacea. Also, dosages in the range of 1–2 mg/kg/day are required. One half of the patients cleared or improved significantly with 0.7–1.2 mg/kg/day of isotretinoin in a study by Dicken and colleagues.[81] Acitretin produced significant improvement in a single case report.[82]

DARIER'S DISEASE. Since the initial report detailing retinoid use in lamellar ichthyosis, Darier's disease, and pityriasis rubra pilaris, first- and second-generation retinoids have been the mainstay of treatment in most disorders of keratinization.[4] Disorders of keratinization typically respond better to etretinate/acitretin than to isotretinoin.[83–85] A possible exception to this generalization would be isotretinoin for Darier's disease.[88] However, etretinate and acitretin may be useful in Darier's disease.[86, 89, 90] Episodic drug use, particularly in the months when the disease is expected to flare up (warm seasons of the year), is prudent. Four- to six-month courses during these months allow maintenance therapy by topical measures the remainder of the year. Although dosages of 0.5–1 mg/kg/day of all three drugs are generally recommended, Happle and colleagues recommended starting at 0.2–0.3 mg/kg/day to prevent the initial flare-up commonly seen in many patients treated with retinoids.[83]

Retinoids are most effective in patients with widespread hyperkeratotic forms of Darier's disease.[83, 84] Patients with moist intertriginous presentation tend to respond less optimally, and their disease may flare up significantly with retinoid treatment.

PITYRIASIS RUBRA PILARIS. Studies of retinoid use in pityriasis rubra pilaris were reviewed by Cohen and Prystowsky in 1989.[91] A dosage range of 1–1.5 mg/kg/day for isotretinoin and generally 1 mg/kg/day for etretinate induced significant improvement in approximately 70% of the patients. A small but significant percentage of the patients achieved a sustained remission with therapy. Most studies focused on only a few cases. Goldsmith and colleagues' evaluation of 45 patients with pityriasis rubra pilaris treated with isotretinoin is a notable exception.[92]

ICHTHYOSIS. In ichthyosis management, etretinate and acitretin have distinctive advantages over isotretinoin.[83–85] The most frequent indication is lamellar ichthyosis. In this form of ichthyosis, the response to retinoid therapy and acceptance of the side effect profile are superior to those of other forms of ichthyosis.[4, 83, 85, 94, 95] In ichthyosis vulgaris and x-linked recessive ichthyosis, the limited severity of the disease generally does not require retinoid use, even though these are retinoid-responsive conditions.[83, 96] Retinoid therapy for epidermolytic hyperkeratosis (bullous congenital ichthyosiform erythroderma) may lead to an initial increase in bullae. The bullae formation is less likely when the initial dosage of etretinate is 0.25 mg/kg/day and is increased gradually.[83] Lamellar ichthyosis associated with Sjögren-Larssen syndrome typically responds well.[85, 97] Ichthyosis variants such as ichthyosis linearis circumflexa, erythrokeratoderma variabilis, and systemic progressive erythrokeratoderma likewise may respond well.[84, 95, 98] There is a single case report of sustained improvement with Harlequin fetus.[99]

In comparison with the isotretinoin dosage needed to improve ichthyosis (2 mg/kg/day or more), etretinate or acitretin therapy leads to good responses in the range of 0.5–1.0 mg/kg/day.[83, 84] A significant response typically occurs in the first 2 months of therapy. After that time the maintenance dose can generally be reduced to 25 mg/day. As with Darier's disease, most patients with the severe forms of ichthyosis are willing to tolerate the significant side effects of the retinoids, given the lack of efficacious alternatives.

Because most cases of ichthyosis present in childhood, careful risk-benefit analysis needs to be addressed. The lower maintenance dose required of the second-generation (aromatic) retinoids may decrease the risk of premature epiphyseal closure and DISH- (diffuse idiopathic skeletal hyperostosis-) like complications.[83, 84]

KERATODERMAS/EPIDERMAL NEVI. The response rate and the dosage range for second-generation (aromatic) retinoids for various forms of keratodermas are quite similar to those of ichthyosis.[87, 100–102] Keratoderma subtypes responding well included the Unna-Thost and punctate forms with or without epidermolytic hyperkeratosis. The recessive forms with transgrediens, such as Papillon-Lefèvre syndrome and mal de Meleda, likewise respond well.[83, 103–105] In Vohwinkel's syndrome (keratoderma hereditaria mutilans), both the keratoderma and the pseudoainhium respond.[83, 106, 107] In addition, the pachyonychia congenita–associated palmar and plantar keratoderma have been successfully treated.[108] Caution should be exercised in patients with associated epidermolytic hyperkeratosis. These patients should be treated starting at low doses and gradually increasing the dose to avoid a flare-up in the number of erosions or bullae.[83]

Systematized verrucous epidermal nevi improve somewhat, particularly if they have a prominent verrucous component. Papillomatous and organoid varieties and inflammatory linear verrucous epidermal nevus (ILVEN) respond minimally.[83]

PREMALIGNANT CUTANEOUS DISEASES. Patients with actinic keratoses, arsenical keratoses, and Bowen's disease all benefit from retinoid therapy.[23, 26, 109–112] Keratoacanthomas and bowenoid papulosis are also retinoid-responsive.[113–116] Only patients with widespread conditions that are unresponsive to other basic modes of therapy should be treated with retinoids. Of importance is that therapy needs to be sustained indefinitely to maintain clinical improvement.[23, 26]

SYNDROMES WITH INCREASED RISK OF CUTANEOUS MALIGNANCY. Successful retinoid therapy has been reported in patients with basal cell nevus syndrome, xeroderma pigmentosum, widespread epidermal dysplasia, and epidermodysplasia verruciformis.[117–119] In long-term therapy for chemoprevention of basal cell nevus syndrome and xeroderma pigmentosum, researchers have administered high-dosage isotretinoin therapy, at least 2 mg/kg/day.[26] At this level therapeutic benefits are significantly countered by significant adverse reactions. Lower dosages of isotretinoin and etretinate at 1 mg/kg/day or below hopefully will prove to be equally effective. In neoplastic conditions, the retinoid dose needs to be sustained indefinitely to avoid relapse.[23, 26]

MALIGNANT CUTANEOUS DISEASES. Peck and colleagues demonstrated a marked reduction in formation of new basal cell carcinomas with isotretinoin at an average maintenance dosage of 1.5 mg/kg/day. The patients had previously formed numerous basal cell carcinomas as a result of actinic damage and did not have basal cell nevus syndrome.[120, 121]

There have been multiple studies on the use of systemic retinoids in mycosis fungoides primarily in combination with either PUVA or systemic chemotherapy. The best response is noted in patch and early plaque-stage disease.[122–124] In spite of several problems in study design,

Zachariae and colleagues demonstrated a marked improvement in mycosis fungoides with advanced disease. Etretinate plus traditional chemotherapy was far more effective than traditional chemotherapy alone.[123]

A less impressive response has been noted in metastatic melanoma patients.[26] Retinoid therapy currently has no significant role in management of melanoma.

Although there are no good long-term data, prevention of numerous actinic keratoses and squamous cell carcinomas that commonly form in renal transplantation patients would be a most useful area of retinoid therapy in malignancies. Although cutaneous malignancies are common in other organ transplantation settings, this problem seems to be the greatest for the renal transplant patient. In addition, premalignant lesions of the oral mucosa, the larynx, the trachea, the bladder, and the cervix have all responded to systemic retinoid therapy.[25, 26] An important area of research would be to maximize the therapeutic benefit through proper drug and dose selection with hopes of minimizing the significant adverse effect profile that limits long-term therapy of these conditions.

LUPUS ERYTHEMATOSUS. Both isotretinoin and etretinate have been used successfully by patients with various cutaneous forms of lupus erythematosus.[125–127] A good response occurs in the hyperkeratotic variety of discoid lupus erythematosus.[128] Patients with generalized discoid lupus (without hyperkeratosis) and subacute lupus erythematosus have also responded.[125–127] Both isotretinoin and etretinate have been beneficial in the range of 1 mg/kg/day with response by 4 weeks in the majority of patients. This response is typically not sustained after discontinuation of the drug. Overall, retinoid efficacy in treating cutaneous lupus erythematosus is roughly equal to that of the antimalarials. Many of the patients treated have not responded to systemic steroids and antimalarials.

LICHEN PLANUS. Both isotretinoin and etretinate used in the range of 1 mg/kg/day give equally mediocre results.[129–132] Although many patients respond by 4 weeks, the majority have insufficient improvement to warrant long-term retinoid therapy, in view of the significant adverse effects that these drugs create. The important retinoid use would be for erosive oral lichen planus, for which retinoids alone or in combination with low-dose steroids may be beneficial.

MISCELLANEOUS CONDITIONS. Retinoids may present an alternative to topical testosterone for some patients with vulvar lichen sclerosus et atrophicus.[133–135] Significant response to isotretinoin has been reported in several patients with sarcoidosis.[136] Reviews by Ellis and Voorhees and by Dicken are useful sources for uncommon, anecdotal retinoid uses.[137, 138] Retinoid use in these conditions should be considered experimental.

AROTINOIDS. The arotinoids represent the third generation of retinoids. Arotinoid ethyl ester, its metabolite arotinoid acid, and arotinoid ethyl sulfone are currently being evaluated in a variety of dermatoses.[7, 8] The arotinoids are distinguished by a thousandfold increase in potency over that of first- and second-generation retinoids, with a dosage range of 20–150 mcg/day. In spite of this dosage range, the in vitro therapeutic index is similar to those of other synthetic retinoids. The low dosage in the microgram range produces serum levels that are difficult to measure. Nevertheless, the pharmacokinetics of arotinoid ethyl ester are believed to be similar to those of etretinate (an ethyl ester), and the metabolite arotinoid acid is analogous to acitretin (both are carboxylic acid derivatives). The arotinoids have a reduced effect on serum lipids, in comparison with those of first- and second-generation retinoids. Hyperostoses have been reported.[8]

Several successful therapeutic trials with the arotinoids have been reported for psoriasis.[7, 8, 143, 144] Psoriatic arthritis has responded favorably as well.[145] Mycosis fungoides and other neoplasms show promising results in several reports.[146-148] Finally, lichen planus, lamellar ichthyosis, prurigo nodularis, and several other cutaneous disorders have been treated with the arotinoids.[7, 8]

Adverse Effects

An imposing list of potential adverse effects should be considered when the synthetic retinoids are prescribed. An individualized, careful assessment of risk-benefit ratio followed by diligent surveillance for adverse effects is of paramount importance. The following discussion of potential adverse effects emphasizes overall frequency, relative frequency between first- and second-generation retinoids, and which patients are at high risk for a specific adverse effect. Measures to minimize the risk of adverse effects, monitoring guidelines, and management of the adverse effects are also discussed.

TERATOGENICITY. Teratogenicity is the most important adverse effect of the retinoids. The most common retinoid-induced malformations include those of the central nervous system (hydrocephaly, cranial nerve abnormalities), craniofacial anomalies (anotia, microtia, absent external auditory canal), cardiac anomalies (septal defects, aortic arch abnormalities), and thymus anomalies (aplasia, hypoplasia).[152-154] These abnormalities occur in almost 50% of full-term pregnancies in which there was first-trimester exposure to isotretinoin.[154] Etretinate-induced teratogenicity occurs less frequently, perhaps because the patient population receiving etretinate is older and the drug was released for commercial use later than isotretinoin.[155] Spontaneous abortions occur in one third of exposed pregnancies, and there is an increased number of stillbirths.[154] Etretinate has not been associated with cardiac abnormalities to date. However, numerous acral skeletal abnormalities are known to occur with exposure to the drug during pregnancy.[156]

The putative mechanism involves effects on cephalic neural crest development, particularly with exposure between 3 and 6 weeks of gestation.[155] Patients at greatest risk are young patients and those patients who cannot comply with contraceptive measures. Of all isotretinoin-associated pregnancy reports in which contraceptive history was available, no contraceptive was used in 50% of patients.[151]

An American Academy of Dermatology task force has offered guidelines for the use of isotretinoin. Women of childbearing age should be on adequate contraception for at least 1 month before starting the drug, have a negative pregnancy test within 2 weeks of starting the drug, and begin the drug on the 2nd or 3rd day of a normal menstrual period.[150] Because etretinate may persist in detectable amounts in the blood circulation for up to 2 years and 11 months after the last dose, it is not known how soon after etretinate use that conception would be safe.[13] Particular care regarding patient selection, patient education, and truly informed consent are of major importance. Effective contraceptive measures were reviewed by Grimes.[157]

OCULAR EFFECTS. Retinoid adverse effects can involve the eyelids, the conjunctiva, the cornea, the lens, the retina, and the optic nerve.[158–160] In addition, a variety of congenital abnormalities may occur. The initial report of ocular adverse effects was in 1979, describing isotretinoin-induced blepharoconjunctivitis.[161] Conjunctivitis occurs in 20%–50% of patients. With isotretinoin, S. aureus superinfection is a common event. Corneal erosions leading to corneal opacities may occur. These opacities will slowly resolve after discontinuation of the drug. In rare instances, cataracts have been reported. Abnormalities of retinal function with abnormal night vision can occur. Pseudotumor cerebri, manifested by abnormal vision with nausea and vomiting, headache, and papilledema, has been reported primarily with isotretinoin (see also the Central Nervous System Effects section).[158] Congenital abnormalities not mentioned in the Teratogenicity section include microphthalmia, cortical blindness, and optic nerve atrophy.[158, 159]

The mechanism responsible for the corneal and conjunctival adverse effects is believed to be decreased tear formation, as well as decreased lipid content in the tears.[158] Abnormalities of night vision are most likely due to interference of the retinoids with steps in the visual pigment (rhodopsin) cycle.

There are no specific ocular monitoring guidelines. However, any abnormality of vision that is not corrected with the use of artificial tears should be evaluated. Patients with visual abnormalities accompanied by headache, nausea, and vomiting should be examined for papilledema. If these findings are present, prompt referral to a neurologist is essential. Ophthalmologic evaluation for altered night vision includes dark-adaptation testing and possibly an electroretinogram or electro-oculogram.[159]

It is important to be aware of the potentially irreversible adverse effects. There have been rare cases of persistent dry eyes and persistent abnormal night vision.[158] Cataracts, although rare, are irreversible. The congenital defects are likewise irreversible. Serious but reversible and rare problems include optic neuritis and pseudotumor cerebri.[158]

In general, management of symptoms from dry eyes is the most frequent patient intervention. Artificial tears used regularly may alleviate symptoms of blepharoconjunctivitis. Particularly with isotretinoin, topical antistaphylococcal antibiotics may be useful.

BONE EFFECTS. Adverse effects associated with the synthetic retinoids closely resemble the bone findings of hypervitaminosis A.[6] The findings include decalcification, primarily of the long bones; cortical hyperostosis; periosteal thickening; and epiphyseal closure. The possibility of premature epiphyseal closure in growing children should be carefully considered, particularly with high-dose, long-term retinoid therapy. Three cases of premature epiphyseal closure have been reported, involving both isotretinoin and etretinate therapy.[162-165] The epiphyseal closure is generally partial, associated with a very high dose and with prolonged retinoid therapy, and accompanied by other confounding factors such as concomitant or prior vitamin A use. The initial report of retinoid-induced skeletal toxicity was by Pittsley and Yoder in 1983.[166] Findings resembling DISH are detected in up to 30% of etretinate patients. Specific findings include osteophytes, with or without bridging, in the absence of disk space narrowing, along with anterior spinal ligament calcification and extraspinal calcification of other tendons and ligaments.[167-169] This condition should be considered in the treatment of patients with disorders of keratinization because long-term therapy is generally required. Of importance is that spinal cord compression with neurologic deficit after long-term etretinate therapy has been reported.[170]

Although the pattern of abnormalities closely resembles the findings in hypervitaminosis A, the pathogenesis of retinoid bone adverse effects is not known. The risk of retinoid-induced hyperostoses and of DISH-syndrome–like findings in psoriasis, in disorders of keratinization, and in acne therapy has been studied by many investigators, with conflicting results.[168, 169, 171-177] In addition, patients are frequently asymptomatic at sites where there is calcification.[178] High-risk patients are those taking any retinoid at high doses for long durations. Older patients and those with previous arthritis are probably at increased risk. Numerous axial skeletal changes may exist in psoriatic patients in the absence of prior retinoid therapy, which complicates the assessment of skeletal adverse effects.[179] One should carefully consider the risk to children of premature epiphyseal closure and other effects on the developing skeleton.

Surveillance for DISH-like findings is optimal when directed at the ankle; the knee and pelvis are less frequently involved.[137, 168, 169] For axial skeleton involvement, a lateral thoracic spine x-ray, possibly including cervical spine films, would be the best way to screen for retinoid-induced hyperostosis.[166, 172] Radiographs of significantly symptomatic sites are considered useful. There are no official guidelines for monitoring for bone-related adverse effects. Yearly screening x-rays of high-risk sites should be considered optional. Bone scans may be more sensitive in detecting premature epiphyseal closure.[163]

In addition, musculoskeletal complaints in the absence of radiographic changes are very common, occurring in up to 20% of retinoid-treated patients.[138] In general, musculoskeletal complaints are managed with conservative anti-inflammatory drugs and rest. The retinoid dose can be reduced if the symptoms persist.

LIPID EFFECTS. The most frequently detected laboratory abnormalities involve abnormal blood lipids. In multiple studies, researchers have evaluated the risk of hyperlipidemia due to retinoid therapy.[180-182] Isotretinoin, etretinate, and acitretin elevate triglycerides in 50% of patients and cholesterol in 30% of patients.[155, 178] Decreased high-density lipoprotein cholesterol occurs less frequently. Although the concern regarding hyperlipidemia and atherosclerosis is greater with long-term etretinate therapy, the lipid elevations are generally higher with isotretinoin.

The mechanism responsible for hyperlipidemia is not known. Elevated lipoproteins, particularly apolipoprotein B, have been noted.[183] Decreased lipoprotein catabolism and lipoprotein lipase activity have been demonstated. Patients at high risk for retinoid-associated hyperlipidemia include those with diabetes mellitus, obese patients, those with significant alcohol intake, and patients consuming a high-saturated-fat, high-cholesterol diet.[155, 183] Although pretreatment lipid levels reportedly do not predict subsequent lipid abnormalities, the highest lipid elevations are, in my experience, generally seen in patients with previous hyperlipidemia.

The most important unanswered question is the long-term effect of etretinate on the coronary arteries. Patients with a family history of coronary artery disease or significant risk factors, such as cigarette smoking and hypertension, probably should not receive long-term etretinate. Proper patient selection and dietary management of these problems are essential. Omega-3 fatty acids (such as those found in fish oil) have been reported to decrease triglycerides and increase high-density lipoprotein cholesterol in psoriatic patients treated with etretinate or acitretin. Low-density lipoprotein cholesterol levels are not altered significantly.[184]

The package insert recommendation for both isotretinoin and etretinate is to monitor lipids every 1–2 weeks until they are stable, which generally occurs in 4–8 weeks.[137] Initial lipid determinations every month are probably adequate for patients without risk factors for retinoid-induced hyperlipidemia who have normal baseline lipids. The lipids are subsequently drawn with other laboratory tests, initially every month and then every 3 months. Patients who develop triglyceride levels over 600 or cholesterol levels over 300–350 should have the retinoid withdrawn until the laboratory abnormalities are corrected. Although the risk for coronary artery disease from hypertriglyceridemia is unknown, triglyceride levels over 800 give significant risk for pancreatitis and eruptive xanthomas.[185]

LIVER EFFECTS. Transient transaminase (aspartate aminotransferase [serum glutamate oxaloacetate transaminase], or AST [SGOT], and alanine aminotransferase [serum glutamate pyruvate transaminase], or ALT [SGPT]) abnormalities are noted in 20%–30% of the etretinate-treated patients and at a lower frequency with isotretinoin.[155, 178] Elevations of alkaline phosphatase, lactate dehydrogenase, and bilirubin occur much less frequently. These changes usually occur between 2 and 8 weeks after treatment is begun. Severe or persistent alterations in liver enzymes are rare, occurring in about 1% of etretinate-treated patients.[137] There have been four etretinate-associated deaths from liver failure.[155]

Although the mechanism of hepatotoxicity is unknown, synthetic retinoids are stored in the liver at a concentration far greater than serum concentration. Patients at high risk for liver toxicity include those with diabetes mellitus, obesity, prior or concurrent methotrexate use, alcohol abuse, and patients with abnormal results of pretreatment liver function tests. As with lipid abnormalities, proper patient selection is very important for instituting etretrinate therapy, ideally avoiding therapy in the high-risk groups just listed.

Guidelines for both isotretinoin and etretinate include liver function tests every 2 weeks for the first month of treatment, monthly tests until 6 months of therapy have elapsed, and tests every 3 months thereafter.[137] Transaminase elevations greater than twice the upper normal range should lead to retinoid discontinuation. Once the laboratory findings return to normal, therapy can be resumed with more frequent monitoring. With smaller enzyme elevations, the levels generally return to baseline while the patient is still receiving therapy without sequelae.[155, 186] Long-term retinoid therapy is uncommonly associated with abnormal liver biopsies.[186–190] Liver biopsies do not reveal hepatotoxicity that has not been suspected on routine liver function tests. At this time there is no official recommendation concerning liver biopsy of retinoid-treated patients.

CENTRAL NERVOUS SYSTEM EFFECTS. Changes of pseudotumor cerebri, although infrequent, are the most important central nervous system adverse effects. Transient headaches are relatively common early in therapy. However, accompanying nausea, vomiting, and visual changes should prompt further evaluation to exclude pseudotumor cerebri.[160, 191, 192] In an early report on pseudotumor cerebri associated with isotretinoin use, half the patients were taking tetracycline or minocycline concomitantly.[70] Combined therapy with isotretinoin and tetracycline or minocycline should be avoided. Uncommon adverse effects include depression, peripheral sensory changes, and vertigo.[193]

The mechanism for these neurologic changes is unknown. Patients' awareness of key neurologic symptoms to report is the most important aspect of surveillance for neurologic adverse effects. These neurologic adverse effects appear to be reversible upon discontinuation of the retinoid therapy.

MUCOCUTANEOUS EFFECTS. The most common adverse effect is cheilitis; 90% of patients experience this problem. Dry skin with increased fragility occurs in 80% of patients. Etretinate, in particular, leads to palm, sole, and fingertip desquamation and increased skin fragility.[137, 194] The dermatitic changes associated with this dryness, which is known as retinoid dermatitis, can mimic a number of other conditions, including pityriasis rosea,[195] rosacea,[196] mycosis fungoides,[197] and eczema craquelé.[198] An erythrodermic eruption may represent the most severe form of retinoid dermatitis.[199] Many patients taking etretinate complain of a sticky sensation of their skin, which is probably due to increased mucus deposition.[200] Dryness of the mouth occurs in 30% of patients. Nosebleeds due to nasal mucosa dryness are seen in 15% of patients. Contact lens intolerance is associated with the ocular changes mentioned previously.

In isotretinoin-treated acne patients, several specific problems may occur. First, S. aureus colonization due to decreased sebum production may lead to blepharoconjunctivitis, nasal colonization, and impetiginization in sites of abnormal skin.[201] Second, pyogenic-granuloma–like proliferations of granulation tissue occur early in therapy.[202, 203] Finally, photosensitivity is noted particularly with isotretinoin and is probably due to reduction of thickness of the stratum corneum.[204]

Abnormal sebum production, reduced stratum corneum thickness, and areas of altered skin barrier function are all central to the mucocutaneous adverse effects. No particular groups are at high risk for these effects. Cheilitis, nasal dryness, and cutaneous fragility are most common and most troublesome in the seasons with low humidity. Liberal use of emollients, preceded by skin hydration, and periodic use of topical steroids are the mainstays of management. Oral antibiotics may be necessary for the staphylococcal infections. Intralesional steroids, topical steroids, or even bursts of systemic steroids can be useful for the areas of excessive proliferation of granulation tissue.[202, 203]

MUSCLE EFFECTS. Myalgias are noted in roughly 15% of isotretinoin-treated patients. An increased frequency and severity of these myalgias can be seen in patients undergoing physical training programs involving heavy exertion, particularly when new programs are being initiated. These symptoms have been accompanied by markedly elevated creatine phosphokinase levels but have not been accompanied by rhabdomyolysis.[205, 206] Several researchers have reported abnormalities on electromyogram and muscle biopsy testing in these patients.[207, 208] These muscle effects are associated mostly with isotretinoin therapy. Generalized increase of muscle tone due to etretinate has been reported.[209]

The mechanism involved in muscle adverse effects is not known. High-risk patients would be those whose professions or hobbies include heavy exertion. Attempts should be made to moderate these activities or avoid retinoid therapy during prolonged periods of heavy exertion. There are no official guidelines for laboratory monitoring. However, patients with severe myalgias should have at least a creatine phosphokinase determination. One should keep in mind that in the absence of retinoids, creatine phosphokinase elevations up to 20 times baseline levels can be seen in healthy runners 24 hours after a marathon race.[210]

HAIR/NAIL EFFECTS. The risk of telogen effluvium due to the retinoids has been reported to vary over a range of 10%–75%.[137, 155] The risk is greater for etretinate and acitretin and much less with isotretinoin. Hair loss is a dose-related effect and is reversible starting 2 months after either discontinuation of therapy or a significant dose reduction. Changes in the hair shaft have been noted only infrequently.[211] Fragile nails, nail dystrophy, and onycholysis occur infrequently.[212]

The mechanism of hair loss is unknown. However, it resembles the changes seen with hypervitaminosis A. Women seem to have a more noticeable hair loss, particularly if there is already a mild androgenic alopecia. Persistent hair loss has been associated with retinoid therapy. In general, reassurance about the reversibility of the hair loss is sufficient to alleviate patients' concerns. Dose reduction or even cessation of therapy may be necessary in more severe cases.

OTHER SYSTEMIC EFFECTS. Proteinuria and cellular casts on urinalysis are transient effects noted in 10% of patients.[213] Infrequent hematologic changes include anemia, leukopenia, and both elevated and depressed platelet counts.[155] Elevated erythrocyte sedimentation rates occur in up to 40% of patients. In rare instances, patients with diabetes may have more difficult glucose control while taking retinoids. Finally, development of inflammatory bowel disease during retinoid therapy has been reported.[214, 215]

Hypersensitivity reactions are distinctly uncommon. Both erythema multiforme and erythema nodosum have been associated with isotretinoin use.[214] The Adverse Drug Reaction Reporting System for dermatology has reported an effect like that of Antabuse (disulfiram) after ethanol consumption.[214]

SUMMARY. Surveillance for unsuspected pregnancy, for ocular findings, and for bone, lipid, and liver effects is of tremendous importance. Given that pregnancy prevention has been adequately enforced, possible irreversible adverse effects include ocular (dry eyes, decreased night vision, cataracts) and bone abnormalities (osteophytes, DISH, premature epiphyseal closure). The uncertainties regarding the potentially increased risk for coronary artery disease also should be presented to patients who are considering retinoid therapy. In addition, the remote possibility of etretrinate-induced chronic hepatitis and liver failure needs to be discussed, and laboratory values must be followed carefully. Patients' and physicians' awareness of these risks, careful surveillance, and prompt discontinuation of the drug when any serious or potentially irreversible adverse effect develops are most important clinical strategies for the retinoids.

Drug Interactions

There are four main types of drug interactions involving the retinoids. First, there is an additive toxicity if the patient is taking significant doses of vitamin A in addition to synthetic retinoids. Doses above the minimal daily requirement of 5000 units/day of vitamin A entail the risk of significant additive toxicity when synthetic retinoids are taken. Concomitant administration of methotrexate probably increases the risk of hepatotoxicity.[149] Of importance is that combined use of either tetracycline or minocycline with isotretinoin has been associated with half of the initial cases of retinoid-associated pseudotumor cerebri.[70] Finally, concomitant use of the topical acne products that dry the skin will increase the dryness that occurs with the administration of isotretinoin.

Also of importance is that current evidence suggests no adverse interaction between retinoids and oral contraceptives. Estrogen and gonadotropin levels are not changed by the retinoids.[216]

Therapeutic Guidelines

Two key issues influence the decision-making process regarding the retinoids. First, retinoids are the single most effective category of drugs

RETINOID MONITORING GUIDELINES[70, 137]

Baseline

- Pregnancy test: serum (in women of childbearing potential)
- Complete blood count (CBC) with platelets
- Liver function tests: AST (SGOT), ALT (SGPT), alkaline phosphatase, bilirubin
- Lipid profile during fasting* (triglycerides, cholesterol, high-density lipoprotein cholesterol)
- Renal function tests (blood urea nitrogen, creatinine)
- Urinalysis
- Other routine chemistries

Follow-up

- Clinical evaluation monthly for first 4–6 months, then every 3 months

At 2 weeks:

- Liver function tests
- Triglyceride and cholesterol levels during fasting*

Monthly for first 4–6 months, then every 3 months:†

- CBC with platelets
- Liver function tests
- Triglyceride and cholesterol levels during fasting*
- Renal function tests, urinalysis‡

Periodically as indicated by symptoms:

- Pregnancy test: serum
- X-ray of significantly symptomatic joints with long-term therapy
- Yearly x-ray of ankle or thoracic spine (optional)

Note: More frequent surveillance is needed if laboratory values are abnormal or with high-risk patients.

*Lipids should be drawn after a 12-hour fast and a 36-hour abstinence from ethanol.

†When isotretinoin is used for a 20-week acne course, it is reasonable to discontinue laboratory monitoring after 8–12 weeks if laboratory results remain normal.

‡Renal function tests and urinalyses are infrequently altered by retinoids; consider performing them every other time a laboratory evaluation is done.

available for acne vulgaris and the disorders of keratinization. Second, major systemic side effects such as teratogenicity and ocular, bone, lipid, and liver adverse effects make careful patient selection and ongoing laboratory surveillance critical. Issues regarding the unknown long-term risk for coronary artery disease and bone toxicity need further resolution.

One can best perform individualized risk-benefit analysis by addressing the following issues:

1. Patients' age and sex: Particular caution should be used in retinoid therapy for children and for women of childbearing age.

2. Disease responsiveness: The most effective retinoid drug choice, dose, and duration and the possibility of remissions for the disease to be treated need to be considered.

3. Disease severity: In general, indications for retinoids are conditions that are significantly disabling, on either a physical or an emotional basis.

4. Alternative treatments available: Are there other therapeutic options, and have they been adequately tried?

The following issues should be addressed to make the retinoid use as safe as possible:

1. Dose/duration: A patient should take the lowest possible dose for the briefest possible period of time, either tapering completely or reducing to the lowest effective dose for chronic therapy.

2. Combination treatment: Topical and systemic adjunctive therapy should be strongly considered in all cases.

3. Laboratory surveillance: This should be done as outlined in the Monitoring Guidelines section.

4. Patient education: This should, in particular, include ocular, bone, central nervous system, and muscle adverse effects, as these areas have no routine examination or laboratory monitoring guidelines except when indicated by important symptoms.

5. Treatment of side effects: Maximized patient compliance and satisfactory therapy require patient education regarding methods to minimize mucocutaneous side effects and awareness of expected hair and nail effects.

Finally, female patients must avoid pregnancy at all costs while using retinoids. Although there are specific guidelines from Roche Dermatologics, the following are general guidelines that I have found useful:

1. Patient selection: A female patient's capability of understanding the teratogenicity risk and reliability in avoiding pregnancy are essential.

2. Patient education: Optimal education involves both the physician's explanation and information handouts that address the important issues regarding teratogenicity. After the patient has heard and read these instructions, she should have an adequate opportunity to ask any ques-

tions that she may have. Current packaging of isotretinoin provides a reminder of the pregnancy risk.

3. Informed consent (see Chapter 17): Whether the documentation occurs in the progress notes or on a signed specific form, well-documented informed consent is essential.

4. Contraception: With isotretinoin and acitretin, adequate contraception 1 month before therapy through 1 month after therapy is essential for women. The indefinite persistence at detectable serum levels of etretinate prohibits use by women of childbearing potential. Acceptable contraception methods for isotretinoin include oral contraceptives, hormonal injections, intrauterine devices, and sterilization (see Grimes' review[157]).

5. Exclusion of pregnancy: Pregnancy tests should be obtained within 2 weeks before a woman starts taking the drug, and the retinoids should be started on the 2nd or 3rd day of a normal menstrual period.

6. The female patient must consider available options if pregnancy occurs *before* retinoid therapy is commenced. It is helpful to document her thoughts on this subject in the medical record.

Only through addressing all these issues can an optimal risk-benefit ratio be achieved. Even then, there are still significant potential risks with synthetic retinoid therapy. Only physicians thoroughly familiar with these risks, with monitoring guidelines, and with elements of patient education should prescribe the retinoids. Some of the most gratifying clinical results can be obtained through the appropriate use of synthetic retinoids.

BIBLIOGRAPHY: Key Reviews/Chapters

Ellis CN, Voorhees JJ: Etretinate therapy. J Am Acad Dermatol 1987; 16:267–291.
Dicken CH: Retinoids: A review. J Am Acad Dermatol 1984; 11:541–552.
David M: Adverse effects of retinoids. Med Toxicol 1988; 3:273–288.
Peck GL, DiGiovanna JJ: Retinoids. In Fitzpatrick TB, Eisen AZ, Wolff K, et al (eds): Dermatology in General Medicine. Philadelphia: JB Lippincott, 1987, 2582–2609.
Lowe NJ, David M: New retinoids for dermatologic diseases. Dermatol Clin 1988; 6:539–552.
Boyd AS: An overview of the retinoids. Am J Med 1989; 86:568–574.
Silverman AK, Ellis CN, Voorhees JJ: Hypervitaminosis A: Paradigm of retinoid side effects. J Am Acad Dermatol 1987; 16:1027–1039.

REFERENCES

1. Peck GL, DiGiovanna JJ: Retinoids. In Fitzpatrick TB, Eisen AZ, Wolff K, et al (eds): Dermatology in General Medicine. Philadelphia: JB Lippincott, 1987, 2582–2609.
2. Bollag W: The development of retinoids in experimental and clinical oncology and dermatology. J Am Acad Dermatol 1983; 9:797–805.

3. Kligman AM, Fulton JE Jr, Plewig G: Topical vitamin A acid in acne vulgaris. Arch Dermatol 1969; 99:469–476.
4. Peck GL, Yoder FW: Treatment of lamellar ichthyosis and other keratinizing dermatoses with a synthetic retinoid. Lancet 1976; 2:1172–1174.
5. Peck GL, Olsen TG, Yoder FW, et al: Prolonged remissions of cystic and conglobate acne with 13-cis retinoic acid. N Engl J Med 1979; 300:329–333.
6. Silverman AK, Ellis CN, Voorhees JJ: Hypervitaminosis A: Paradigm of retinoid side effects. J Am Acad Dermatol 1987; 16:1027–1039.
7. Saurat JH, Mérot Y, Borsky M, et al: Arotinoid acid (Ro 13–7410): A pilot study in dermatology. Dermatologica 1988; 176:191–199.
8. Mérot Y, Caminzind M, Geiger JM, et al: Arotinoid ethyl ester (RO 13–6298): A long-term pilot study in various dermatoses. Acta Derm Venereol (Stockh) 1987; 67:237–242.
9. Vahlquist A, Rollman O: Clinical pharmacology of 3 generations of retinoids. Dermatologica 1987; 175(Suppl 1):20–27.
10. DiGiovanna JJ, Gross EG, McClean SW, et al: Etretinate: Effect of milk intake on absorption. J Invest Dermatol 1984; 82:636–640.
11. McNamara PJ, Jewell RC, Jensen BK, et al: Food increases the bioavailability of acitretin. J Clin Pharmacol 1988; 28:1051–1055.
12. Siegenthaler G, Saurat JH, Salomon D, et al: Skin cellular retinoid–binding proteins and retinoid responsive dermatoses. Dermatologica 1986; 173:163–173.
13. DiGiovanna JJ, Zeck LA, Ruddel ME, et al: Etretinate: Persistent levels of a potent teratogen [abstract]. J Invest Dermatol 1984; 82:434.
14. Jones DH: The role and mechanism of action of 13-cis-retinoic acid in the treatment of severe (nodulocystic) acne. Pharmacol Ther 1989; 40:91–106.
15. Strauss JS, Stewart ME, Downing DT: The effect of 13-cis-retinoic acid on sebaceous glands. Arch Dermatol 1987; 123:1538a–1541.
16. Harms M, Philippe I, Radeff B, et al: Arotinoid Ro 13–6298 and etretin: Two new retinoids inferior to isotretinoin in sebum suppression and acne treatment. Acta Derm Venereol (Stockh) 1986; 66:149–154.
17. Goldstein JA, Solha-Szott A, Thomsen RJ, et al: Comparative effect of isotretinoin and etretinate on acne and sebaceous gland secretion. J Am Acad Dermatol 1982; 6:760–765.
18. Vahlquist A, Torma H: Retinoids and keratinization. Current concepts. Int J Dermatol 1988; 27:81–95.
19. Elias PM: Retinoid effects on the epidermis. Dermatologica 1987; 175(Suppl 1):28–36.
20. Leyden JJ, McGinley KJ, Foglia AN: Qualitative and quantitative changes in cutaneous bacteria associated with systemic isotretinoin therapy for acne conglobata. J Invest Dermatol 1986; 86:390–393.
21. Norris DA, Osborn R, Robinson W, et al: Isotretinoin produces significant inhibition of monocyte and neutrophil chemotaxis in vivo in patients with cystic acne. J Invest Dermatol 1987; 89:38–43.
22. Ellis CN, Kang NA, Grekin RC, et al: Etretinate reduces polymorphonuclear leukocyte chemotaxis–enhancing properties of psoriatic serum. J Am Acad Dermatol 1985; 13:437–443.
23. Lippman SM, Kessler JF, Meyskens FL Jr: Retinoids as preventive and therapeutic anticancer agents (Part I). Cancer Treat Rep 1987; 71:391–405.
24. Krinsky NI: Theoretical basis for anticarcinogenic effects of retinoids. J Cut Aging Cosm Dermatol 1988; 1:55–59.
25. Peck GL: Retinoids and cancer. J Invest Dermatol 1985; 85:87–88.
26. Lippman SM, Kessler JF, Meyskens FL Jr: Retinoids as preventive and therapeutic anticancer agents (Part II). Cancer Treat Rep 1987; 21:493–515.
27. Editorial: Retinoids and control of cutaneous malignancy. Lancet 1988; 2:545–546.

28. Boutwell RK, Verma AK, Takigawa M, et al: Retinoids as inhibitors of tumor promotion. In Saurat JH (ed): Retinoids: New Trends in Research and Therapy. Basel, Switzerland: Karger, 1985, 83–96.
29. Yuspa JH, Lichti U: Retinoids and skin carcinogenesis: A mechanism of anticarcinogenesis by the modulation of epidermal differentiation. In Saurat JH (ed): Retinoids: New Trends in Research and Therapy. Basel, Switzerland: Karger, 1985, 56–65.
30. Matt L, Lazarus N, Lowe NJ: Newer retinoids for psoriasis—Early clinical studies. Pharmacol Ther 1989; 40:157–169.
31. Lowe NJ, Lazarus V, Mall L: Systemic retinoid therapy for psoriasis. J Am Acad Dermatol 1988; 19:186–191.
32. Goldfarb MT, Ellis CN, Voorhees JJ: Short-term and long-term considerations in the management of psoriasis with retinoids. Dermatologica 1987; 175(Suppl 1):100–106.
33. Shelnitz LS, Esterly NB, Honig DJ: Etretinate therapy for generalized pustular psoriasis in children. Arch Dermatol 1987; 123:230–233.
34. Wolska H, Jablonska S, Langner A, et al: Etretinate therapy in generalized pustular psoriasis (Zumbusch type): Immediate and long-term results. Dermatologica 1985; 171:297–304.
35. Lorand T, Pierard-Franchimont C, de la Brassinne M: Treatment of generalized pustular psoriasis with Ro-10–9359. Dermatologica 1983; 167:159–160.
36. Moy RL, Kingston TP, Lowe NJ: Isotretinoin vs. etretinate therapy in generalized pustular and chronic psoriasis. Arch Dermatol 1985; 121:1297–1301.
37. Wolska H, Jablonska S, Bounameaux Y: Etretinate in severe psoriasis: Results of double-blind study and maintenance therapy in pustular psoriasis. J Am Acad Dermatol 1983; 9:883–889.
38. White SI, Marks JM, Shuster S: Etretinate in pustular psoriasis of palms and soles. Br J Dermatol 1985; 113:581–585.
39. Foged E, Holm P, Larsen PO: A randomized trial of etretinate (Tigason) in palmoplantar pustulosis. Dermatologica 1983; 166:120–123.
40. van de Kerkhof PCM, Chang A, van Dooren-Greebe R, et al: Intraepidermal accumulation of polymorphonuclear leukocytes in persistent palmoplantar pustulosis during treatment with acitretin. Acta Derm Venereol (Stockh) 1988; 68:499–503.
41. Lassus A, Geiger JM: Acitretin and etretinate in the treatment of palmoplantar pustulosis: A double-blind comparative trial. Br J Dermatol 1988; 119:755–759.
42. Goldfarb MT, Ellis CN, Gupta AK, et al: Acitretin improves psoriasis in a dose-dependent fashion. J Am Acad Dermatol 1988; 18:655–662.
43. Berbis P, Geiger JM, Vaisse C, et al: Benefit of progressively increasing doses during the initial treatment with acitretin in psoriasis. Dermatologica 1989; 178:88–92.
44. Lassus A, Nyblom M, Virranliski T, et al: Treatment of severe psoriasis with etretin (Ro 10–1670). Br J Dermatol 1987; 117:333–341.
45. Ellis CN, Hermann RC, Gorsulowsky DC, et al: Etretinate reduces inpatient treatment of psoriasis. J Am Acad Dermatol 1988; 19:191–196.
46. Dubertret L, Chastang C, Beylot C, et al: Maintenance therapy of psoriasis by Tigason. Br J Dermatol 1985; 113:323–330.
47. Ehmann CW, Voorhees JJ: International studies of the efficacy of etretinate in the treatment of psoriasis. J Am Acad Dermatol 1982; 6:692–696.
48. Kragballe K, Jansen CT, Geiger JM, et al: A double-blind comparison of acitretin and etretinate in the treatment of severe psoriasis. Acta Derm Venereol (Stockh) 1989; 69:35–40.
49. Gollnick H, Bauer R, Brindley C, et al: Acitretin versus etretinate in psoriasis: Clinical and pharmacokinetic results of a German multicenter study. J Am Acad Dermatol 1988; 19:458–469.
50. Galosi A, Plewig G, Braun-Falco O: The effects of aromatic retinoid Ro 10–9359 (etretinate) on fingernail growth. Arch Dermatol Res 1985; 277:138–140.

51. Chieregato GC, Leon A: Treatment of psoriatic arthropathy with etretinate: A two-year follow-up. Acta Derm Venereol (Stockh) 1986; 66:321–324.
52. Honigsmann H, Wolff K: Results of therapy for psoriasis using retinoid and photochemotherapy (RePUVA). Pharmacol Ther 1989; 40:67–73.
53. Lauharanta J, Juvakoski T, Lassus A: A clinical evaluation of the effects of an aromatic retinoid (Tigason), combination of retinoid and PUVA, and PUVA alone in severe psoriasis. Br J Dermatol 1981; 104:325–332.
54. Grupper C, Berretti B: Treatment of psoriasis by oral PUVA therapy combined with aromatic retinoid (Ro 10–9359; Tigason). Dermatologica 1981; 162:404–413.
55. Roenigk RK, Gibstine C, Roenigk HH Jr: Oral isotretinoin followed by psoralens and ultraviolet A or ultraviolet B for psoriasis. J Am Acad Dermatol 1985; 13:153–155.
56. Honigsmann H, Wolff K: Isotretinoin-PUVA for psoriasis. Lancet 1983; 1:236.
57. Saurat JH, Geiger JM, Amblard D, et al: Randomized double-blind multicenter study comparing acitretin-PUVA, etretinate-PUVA and placebo-PUVA in the treatment of severe psoriasis. Dermatologica 1988; 172:218–224.
58. Lassus A, Lauharanta J, Eskelinen A: The effect of etretinate compared with different regimens of PUVA in the treatment of persistent palmoplantar pustulosis. Br J Dermatol 1985; 112:455–459.
59. Lawrence CM, Marks J, Parker S, et al: A comparison of PUVA–etretinate and PUVA-placebo for palmoplantar pustular psoriasis. Br J Dermatol 1984; 110:221–226.
60. Lauharanta J, Geiger JM. A double-blind comparison of acitretin and etretinate in combination with bath PUVA in treatment of extensive psoriasis. Br J Dermatol 1989; 121:107–112.
61. Vaatainen N, Hollmen A, Fraki JE: Trimethylpsoralen plus ultraviolet A combined with oral retinoid (etretinate) in the treatment of severe psoriasis. J Am Acad Dermatol 1985; 12:52–55.
62. Iest J, Boer J: Combined treatment of psoriasis with acitretin and UVB phototherapy compared with acitretin alone and UVB alone. Br J Dermatol 1989; 120:665–670.
63. Orfanos CE, Stiegleder GK, Pullmann H, et al: Oral retinoid and UVB radiation: A new alternative treatment for psoriasis on an outpatient basis. Acta Derm Venereol (Stockh) 1979; 59:241–244.
64. Poland MK, van der Rhee HJ, van der Schroeff JG: A three-year follow-up study of psoriasis patients treated with low dosages of etretinate orally and corticosteroids topically. Acta Derm Venereol (Stockh) 1982; 62:361–364.
65. van der Rhee HJ, Tijssen JGP, Herrmann WA, et al: Combined treatment of psoriasis with a new aromatic retinoid (Tigason) in low dosage orally and triamcinolone acetonide cream topically: A double-blind trial. Br J Dermatol 1980; 102:203–212.
66. Orfanos CE, Runne U: Systemic use of a new retinoid with and without local dithranol treatment in generalized psoriasis. Br J Dermatol 1976; 98:101–103.
67. Tuyp E, MacKie RM: Combination therapy for psoriasis with methotrexate and etretinate. J Am Acad Dermatol 1986; 14:70–73.
68. Rosenbaum MM, Roenigk HH Jr: Treatment of generalized pustular psoriasis with etretinate (Ro 10–9359) and methotrexate. J Am Acad Dermatol 1984; 10:357–361.
69. Leyden JJ: Retinoids and acne. J Am Acad Dermatol 1988; 19:164–168.
70. Shalita AR, Cunningham WJ, Leyden JJ, et al: Isotretinoin treatment of acne and related disorders: An update. J Am Acad Dermatol 1983; 9:629–638.
71. Hennes R, Mack A, Schell H, et al: 13-cis-retinoid acid in conglobate acne: A follow-up study of 14 trial centers. Arch Dermatol Res 1984; 276:209–215.
72. Peck GL, Olsen TH, Butkus D, et al: Isotretinoin versus placebo in the treatment of cystic acne. J Am Acad Dermatol 1982; 6:735–745.
73. Farrell LN, Strauss JS, Stranieri AM: The treatment of severe cystic acne with 13-cis retinoic acid. J Am Acad Dermatol 1980; 3:602–611.
74. Strauss JS, Rapini RP, Shalita AR, et al: Isotretinoin for acne: Results of a multicenter dose-response study. J Am Acad Dermatol 1984; 10:490–496.

75. van der Meeren HLM, van der Schroeff JG, Stijnen T, et al: Dose-response relationship in isotretinoin for conglobate acne. Dermatologica 1983; 167:299–303.
76. Jones DH, King K, Miller AJ, Cunliffe WJ: A dose-response study of 13-cis-retinoic acid in acne vulgaris. Br J Dermatol 1983; 108:333–343.
77. Menter A, Boyd A: Cystic acne in patients undergoing etretinate therapy. J Am Acad Dermatol 1988; 18:751–752.
78. Hoting E, Paul E, Plewig G: Treatment of rosacea with isotretinoin. Int J Dermatol 1986; 25:660–663.
79. Turjanmaa K, Reunala T.: Isotretinoin treatment of rosacea. Acta Derm Venereol (Stockh) 1986; 66:89–91.
80. Plewig G, Nikolowski J, Wolff HH: Action of isotretinoin in acne rosacea and gram-negative folliculitis. J Am Acad Dermatol 1982; 6:766–785.
81. Dicken CH, Powell ST, Spear KL: Evaluation of isotretinoin treatment of hidradenitis suppurativa. J Am Acad Dermatol 1984; 11:500–502.
82. Hogan DJ: Successful treatment of hidradenitis suppurativa with acitretin. J Am Acad Dermatol 1988; 18:355–356.
83. Happle R, van de Kerkhof PCM, Traupe H: Retinoids in disorders of keratinization: Their use in adults. Dermatologica 1987; 175(Suppl 1):107–124.
84. Ruiz-Maldonado R, Tamayo L: Retinoids in disorders of keratinization in children. Dermatologica 1987; 175(Suppl 1):125–132.
85. Traupe H, Happle R: Etretinate therapy in children with severe keratinization defects. Eur J Pediatr 1985; 143:66–169.
86. Mahrle G, Meyer-Hamme S, Ippen H: Oral treatment of keratinizing disorders of skin and mucous membranes with etretinate: Comparative study of 113 patients. Arch Dermatol 1982; 118:97–100.
87. Viglioglia PA: Therapeutic evaluation of the oral retinoid Ro 10–9359 in several non-psoriatic dermatoses. Br J Dermatol 1980; 103:483–487.
88. Dicken CH, Bauer EA, Hazen PG, et al: Isotretinoin treatment of Darier's disease. J Am Acad Dermatol 1982; 6:721–726.
89. Lauharanta J, Kanerva L, Turjanmaa K, et al: Clinical and ultrastructural effects of acitretin in Darier's disease. Acta Derm Venereol (Stockh) 1988; 68:492–498.
90. Löwhagen GB, Michaëlsson G, Mobacken H, et al: Effects of etretinate (Ro 10–9359) on Darier's disease. Dermatologica 1982; 168:123–130.
91. Cohen PR, Prystowsky JH: Pityriasis rubra pilaris: A review of diagnosis and treatment. J Am Acad Dermatol 1989; 20:801–807.
92. Goldsmith LA, Weinrich AE, Shupack J: Pityriasis rubra pilaris response to 13-cis-retinoic acid (isotretinoin). J Am Acad Dermatol 1982; 6:710–715.
93. Dicken CH: Isotretinoin treatment of pityriasis rubra pilaris. J Am Acad Dermatol 1987; 16:297–301.
94. El-Ramly M, Zachariae H: Long-term oral treatment of two pronounced ichthyotic conditions: Lamellar ichthyosis and epidermolytic hyperkeratosis with the aromatic retinoid Tigason (Ro 10–9359). Acta Derm Venereol (Stockh) 1983: 63:452–456.
95. Tamayo L, Ruiz-Maldonado R: Oral retinoid (Ro 10–9359) in children with lamellar ichthyosis, epidermolytic hyperkeratosis and symmetrical progressive erythrokeratoderma. Dermatologica 1980; 161:305–314.
96. Bruckner-Tuderman L, Sigg C, Geiger JM, et al: Acitretin in the symptomatic therapy for severe recessive x-linked ichthyosis. Arch Dermatol 1988; 124:529–532.
97. Jagell S, Liden S: Treatment of the ichthyosis of Sjögren-Larson syndrome with etretinate (Tigason). Acta Derm Venereol (Stockh) 1983; 63:89–91.
98. Fixler ZC: Treatment of erythrokeratoderma variabilis with oral synthetic retinoids. Cutis 1980; 25:300–304.
99. Lawlor F, Pieris S: Harlequin fetus successfully treated with etretinate. Br J Dermatol 1985; 112:585–590.

100. Sybert VP, Dale BA, Holbrook KA: Palmar-plantar keratoderma: A clinical, ultrastructural, and biochemical study. J Am Acad Dermatol 1988; 18:75–86.
101. Christiansen JV: Keratoderma punctata hereditaria treated with etretinate (Tigason). Acta Derm Venereol (Stockh) 1983; 63:181.
102. Deschamps P, Leroy D, Pedailles S, et al: Keratoderma climacterum (Haxthausen's disease): Clinical signs, laboratory findings, and etretinate treatment in 10 patients. Dermatologica 1986; 172:258–262.
103. Kellum RE: Papillon-Lèfevre syndrome in four siblings treated with etretinate: A nine-year evaluation. Int J Dermatol 1989; 9:605–608.
104. Nazzaro V, Blanchet-Bardon C, Mimoz C, et al: Papillon-Lèfevre syndrome: Ultrastructural study and successful treatment with acitretin. Arch Dermatol 1988; 124:533–539.
105. Brambilla L, Pigatto PD, Boneschi V, et al: Unusual cases of meleda keratoderma treated with aromatic retinoid etretinate. Dermatologica 1984; 168:283–286.
106. Rivers JK, Duke EE, Justus DW: Etretinate: Management of keratoderma hereditaria mutilans in four family members. J Am Acad Dermatol 1985; 13:43–49.
107. Camisa C, Rossana C: Variant of keratoderma hereditaria mutilans (Vohwinkel's syndrome): Treatment with orally administered isotretinoin. Arch Dermatol 1982; 120:1323–1328.
108. Thomas DR, Jorizzo JL, Brysk MM, et al: Pachyonychia congenita: Electron microscopic and epidermal glycoprotein assessment before and during treatment. Arch Dermatol 1984; 120:1475–1479.
109. Shuttleworth D, Salaman JR, Marks R: Etretinate treatment of severe cutaneous dysplasia in renal transplant recipients. Br J Dermatol 1987; 117(Suppl 32):24.
110. Moriarty M, Dunn J, Darragh A, et al: Etretinate in treatment of actinic keratosis: A double-blind crossover study. Lancet 1982; 1:364–365.
111. Coburn PR, Cream JJ, Glaser M: Arsenical keratoses—Response to etretinate and electron beam therapy. Br J Dermatol 1983; 109(Suppl 24):72.
112. Sharma SC, Simpson NB: Treatment of arsenical keratosis with etretinate. Acta Derm Venereol (Stockh) 1983; 63:449–452.
113. Blanchet-Bardon C, Puissant A, Lutzner M: Etretinate in bowenoid papulosis. Lancet 1981; 2:1348–1349.
114. De Mari F, Rampen FH, van Everdingen JJ: Etretinate in bowenoid papulosis [letter]. Lancet 1981; 2:936–937.
115. Cristofolini M, Piscioli F, Zumiani G, et al: The role of etretinate in management of keratoacanthoma. J Am Acad Dermatol 1985; 12:633–638.
116. Benoldi D, Alinovi A: Multiple persistent keratoacanthomas: Treatment with oral etretinate. J Am Acad Dermatol 1984; 10:1035–1038.
117. Moshell AN: Prevention of skin cancer in xeroderma pigmentosum with oral isotretinoin. Cutis 1989; 43:485–490.
118. Cristofolini M, Zumiani G, Scappini P, et al: Aromatic retinoid in the chemoprevention of the progression of nevoid basal cell carcinoma syndrome. J Dermatol Surg Oncol 1984; 10:778–781.
119. Lutzner MA, Blanchet-Bardon C: Oral retinoid treatment of human papillomavirus type 5–induced epidermodysplasia verruciformis. N Engl J Med 1980; 302:1091.
120. Peck GL, Gross EG, Butkus D: Chemoprevention of basal cell carcinoma with isotretinoin. J Am Acad Dermatol 1982; 6:815–823.
121. Peck GL, DiGiovanna JJ, Sarnoff DS, et al: Treatment and prevention of basal cell carcinoma with oral isotretinoin. J Am Acad Dermatol 1988; 19:176–185.
122. Claudy AL, Rouchouse B, Bucheron S, et al: Treatment of cutaneous lymphoma with etretinate. Br J Dermatol 1983; 109:49–56.
123. Zachariae H, Grunnet E, Thestrup-Pedersen K, et al: Oral retinoid in combination with bleomycin, cyclophosphamide, prednisone and transfer factor in mycosis fungoides. Acta Derm Venereol (Stockh) 1982; 62:162–164.

124. Molin L, Thomsen K, Volden G, et al: 13-cis-retinoic acid–mycosis fungoides. In Saurat JH (ed): Retinoids: New Trends in Research and Therapy. Basel, Switzerland: Karger, 1985, 371–374.
125. Ruzicka T, Meurer M, Bieder T: Efficiency of acitretin in treatment of cutaneous lupus erythematosus. Arch Dermatol 1988; 124:897–902.
126. Newton RC, Jorizzo JL, Solomon AR, et al: Mechanism-oriented assessment of isotretinoin in chronic or subacute cutaneous lupus erythematosus. Arch Dermatol 1986; 122:170–176.
127. Ruzicka T, Meurer M, Braun-Falco O: Treatment of cutaneous lupus erythematosus with etretinate. Acta Derm Venereol (Stockh) 1985; 65:324–329.
128. Green SG, Piette W: Successful treatment of hypertrophic lupus erythematosus with isotretinoin. J Am Acad Dermatol 1987; 17:364–368.
129. Camisa C, Allen CM: Treatment of oral erosive lichen planus with systemic isotretinoin. Oral Surg Oral Med Oral Pathol 1986; 62:393–396.
130. Ferguson MM, Simpson NB, Hammersley N: The treatment of erosive lichen planus with a retinoid—Etretinate. Oral Surg Oral Med Oral Pathol 1984; 58:283–287.
131. Sloberg K, Hersle K, Mobacken H, et al: Severe oral lichen planus: Remission and maintenance with vitamin A analogues. J Oral Pathol 1983; 12:473–477.
132. Hersle K, Mobacken H, Sloberg K, et al: Severe oral lichen planus: Treatment with an aromatic retinoid (etretinate). Br J Dermatol 1982; 106:77–80.
133. Romppanen U, Rantala I, Lauslahti K, et al: Light- and electron-microscopic findings in lichen sclerosus of the vulva during etretinate treatment. Dermatologica 1987; 175:33–40.
134. Mørk NJ, Jensen P, Hoel PS: Vulvar lichen sclerosus et atrophicus treated with etretinate (Tigason). Acta Derm Venereol (Stockh) 1986; 66:363–365.
135. Neuhofer J, Fritsch P: Treatment of localized scleroderma and lichen sclerosus with etretinate. Acta Derm Venereol (Stockh) 1984; 64:171–174.
136. Waldinger TP, Ellis CN, Quint K, et al: Treatment of cutaneous sarcoidosis with isotretinoin. Arch Dermatol 1983; 119:1003–1005.
137. Ellis CN, Voorhees JJ: Etretinate therapy. J Am Acad Dermatol 1987; 16:267–291.
138. Dicken CH: Retinoids: A review. J Am Acad Dermatol 1984; 11:541–552.
139. Lassus A, Eskelinen A, Saila K, et al: Treatment of Reiter's disease with etretinate. In Saurat JH (ed): Retinoids: New Trends in Research and Therapy. Basel, Switzerland: Karger, 1985, 391–396.
140. Norris JF, Cunliffe WJ: Phenytoin-induced gum hypertrophy improved by isotretinoin. Int J Dermatol 1987; 26:602–603.
141. Hong WK, Endicott J, Itri L, et al: 13-cis-retinoic acid in the treatment of oral leukoplakia. N Engl J Med 1989; 315:1501–1505.
142. Fritsch P, Klein G, Aubock J, et al: Retinoid therapy of recessive dystrophic epidermolysis bullosa. J Am Acad Dermatol 1983; 9:766–767.
143. Tsambaos D, Orfanos CE: Antipsoriatic activity of a new synthetic retinoid: The arotinoid Ro 13–6298. Arch Dermatol 1983; 119:746–751.
144. Ott F, Geiger JM. Therapeutic effect of arotinoid Ro 13–6298 in psoriasis. Arch Dermatol Res 1983; 275:257–258.
145. Fritsch P, Rauschmeier W, Zussner C: Arotinoid in psoriatic arthropathy. In Saurat JH (ed): Retinoids: New Trends in Research and Therapy. Basel, Switerland: Karger, 1985, 384–390.
146. Sherman MI, Truitt GA: Prevention and therapy of tumors with arotinoids. Eur J Clin Oncol 1988; 24:359–362.
147. Hoting E, Meissner K: Arotinoid-ethylester: Effectiveness in refractory cutaneous T-cell lymphoma. Cancer 1988; 62:1044–1048.
148. Tousignant J, Raymond GP, Light MJ: Treatment of cutaneous T-cell lymphoma with arotinoid Ro 13–6298. J Am Acad Dermatol 1987; 16:167–171.
149. DiGiovanna JJ, Peck GL: Retinoid toxicity. Prog Dermatol 1987; 21:1–8.

150. Pochi PE, Ceilley RI, Coskey RJ, et al: Guidelines for prescribing isotretinoin (Accutane) in the treatment of female acne patients of childbearing potential. J Am Acad Dermatol 1988; 19:920.
151. Strauss JS, Cunningham WJ, Leyden JJ, et al: Isotretinoin and teratogenicity. J Am Acad Dermatol 1988; 19:353–354.
152. Stern RS: When a uniquely effective drug is teratogenic: The case of isotretinoin. N Engl J Med 1989; 320:1007–1009.
153. Teelmann K: Retinoids: Toxicology and teratogenicity to date. Pharmacol Ther 1989; 40:29–43.
154. Lammer EJ, Chen CT, Hoar RM, et al: Retinoic acid embryopathy. N Engl J Med 1985; 313:837–841.
155. David M: Adverse effects of retinoids. Med Toxicol 1988; 3:273–288.
156. Rosa FW, Wilk AL, Kelsey FO: Teratogen update: Vitamin A congeners. Teratology 1986; 33:355–364.
157. Grimes DA: Reversible contraception for women at high risk of fetal anomalies. J Am Acad Dermatol 1987; 17:148–155.
158. Gold JA, Shupack JL, Nemel MA: Ocular side effects of the retinoids. Int J Dermatol 1989; 28:218–225.
159. Lebowitz MA, Berson DS: Ocular effects of oral retinoids. J Am Acad Dermatol 1988; 19:209–211.
160. Fraunfelder FT, LaBraico JM, Meyer SM: Adverse ocular reactions possibly associated with isotretinoin. Am J Ophthalmol 1985; 100:534–537.
161. Blackman HJ, Peck GL, Olsen TG, et al: Blepharoconjunctivitis: A side effect of 13-cis-retinoic acid therapy for dermatologic diseases. Ophthalmology (Rochester) 1979; 86:753–759.
162. Marini JC, Hill S, Zasloff MA: Dense metaphyseal bands and growth arrest associated with isotretinoin therapy. Am J Dis Child 1988; 142:316–318.
163. Glover MT, Atherton DJ: Etretinate and premature epiphyseal closure. J Am Acad Dermatol 1987; 17:853–854.
164. Prendiville J, Bingham EA, Burrows D: Premature epiphyseal closure—A complication of etretinate therapy in children. J Am Acad Dermatol 1986; 15:1259–1262.
165. Milstone LM, McGuire J, Ablow RC: Premature epiphyseal closure in a child receiving oral 13-cis-retinoic acid. J Am Acad Dermatol 1982; 7:663–666.
166. Pittsley RA, Yoder FW: Skeletal toxicity associated with long-term administration of 13-cis-retinoic acid for refractory ichthyosis. N Engl J Med 1983; 308:1012–1014.
167. White SI, MacKie RM: Bone changes associated with oral retinoid therapy. Pharmacol Ther 1989; 40:137–144.
168. DiGiovanna JJ, Helfgott RK, Gerber LH, et al: Extraspinal tendon and ligament calcification associated with long-term therapy with etretinate. N Engl J Med 1986; 315:1177–1182.
169. DiGiovanna JJ, Helfgott RK, Gerber LH: Extraspinal tendon and ligament calcification after long-term isotretinoin therapy [abstract]. J Invest Dermatol 1987; 88:485.
170. Tfelt-Hansen P, Knudsen B, Petersen E: Spinal cord compression after long-term etretinate. Lancet 1989; 2:325–326.
171. Kilcoyne RF, Cope R, Cunningham W, et al: Minimal spinal hyperostosis with low dose isotretinoin therapy. Invest Radiol 1986; 11:624–627.
172. Pennes DR, Martel W, Ellis CN, et al: Evolution of skeletal hyperostosis caused by 13-cis-retinoic acid therapy. AJR 1988; 151:967–973.
173. Carey BM, Parkin GJS, Cunliffe WJ, et al: Skeletal toxicity with isotretinoin therapy: A clinico-radiologic evaluation. Br J Dermatol 1988; 119:609–614.
174. Ellis CN, Pennes DR, Martel W, et al: Radiographic bone surveys after isotretinoin therapy for cystic acne. Acta Derm Venereol (Stockh) 1985; 65:83–85.
175. Halkier-Sorensen L, Laurberg G, Andresen J: Bone changes in children on long-term treatment with etretinate. J Am Acad Dermatol 1987; 16:999–1006.

176. Glover MT, Peters AM, Atherton DJ: Surveillance for skeletal toxicity of children treated with etretinate. Br J Dermatol 1987; 116:609–614.
177. Gilbert M, Ellis CN, Voorhees JJ: Lack of skeletal radiographic changes during short-term etretinate therapy for psoriasis. Dermatologica 1986; 172:160–163.
178. Lowe NJ, David M: New retinoids for dermatologic diseases. Dermatol Clin 1988; 6:539–552.
179. Dale K, Vinje O: Radiography of the spine and sacro-iliac joints in ankylosing spondylitis and psoriasis. Acta Radiol [Diagn] (Stockh) 1985; 26:145–159.
180. Bershad S, Rubinstein A, Paterniti JR, et al: Changes in plasma lipids and lipoproteins during isotretinoin therapy for acne. N Engl J Med 1985; 313:981–985.
181. Zech LA, Gross EG, Peck GL, et al: Changes in plasma cholesterol and triglyceride levels after treatment with oral isotretinoin. Arch Dermatol 1983; 119:987–993.
182. Vahlquist C, Michaelsson G, Vahlquist A, et al: A sequential comparison of etretinate (Tigason) and isotretinoin (Roaccutane) with special regard to their effects on serum lipoproteins. Br J Dermatol 1985; 112:69–76.
183. Marsden J: Hyperlipidemia due to isotretinoin and etretinate: Possible mechanisms and consequences. Br J Dermatol 1986; 114:401–407.
184. Ashley JM, Lowe NJ, Borok ME, et al: Fish oil supplementation results in decreased hypertriglyceridemia in patients with psoriasis undergoing etretinate or acitretin therapy. J Am Acad Dermatol 1988; 19:76–82.
185. Brunzell JD, Austin MA: Plasma triglycerides and coronary disease. N Engl J Med 1989; 320:1273–1275.
186. Roenigk HH Jr: Liver toxicity of retinoid therapy. J Am Acad Dermatol 1988; 19:199–208.
187. Camuto P, Shupack J, Orbuch P, et al: Long-term effects of etretinate on the liver in psoriasis. Am J Surg Pathol 1987; 11:30–37.
188. Roenigk HH Jr, Cibstine C, Glazer S, et al.: Serial liver biopsies in psoriatic patients receiving long-term etretinate. Br J Dermatol 1985; 112:77–81.
189. Glazer SK, Roenigk HH Jr, Yokoo H, et al: Ultrastructural survey and tissue analysis of human livers after a 6-month course of etretinate. J Am Acad Dermatol 1984; 10:632–638.
190. Zachariae H, Foged E, Bjerring P, et al: Liver biopsy during etretinate (Tigason) treatment. In Saurat JH (ed): Retinoids: New Trends in Research and Therapy. Basel, Switzerland: Karger, 1985, 494–497.
191. Roytman M, Frumkin A, Bohn TG: Pseudotumor cerebri caused by isotretinoin. Cutis 1988; 42:399–400.
192. Viraben R, Mathieu C, Fontan B: Benign intracranial hypertension during etretinate therapy for mycosis fungoides. J Am Acad Dermatol 1985; 13:515–517.
193. Hazen PG, Carney JF, Walker AE, et al: Depression—A side effect of 13-cis-retinoic acid therapy. J Am Acad Dermatol 1983; 9:278–279.
194. Williams ML, Elias PM: Nature of skin fragility in patients receiving retinoids for systemic effect. Arch Dermatol 1981; 117:611–619.
195. Helfman RJ, Brickman M, Fahey J: Isotretinoin dermatitis simulating acute pityriasis rosea. Cutis 1984; 33:297–300.
196. Crivellato E: A rosacea-like eruption induced by Tigason (Ro 10–9359). Acta Derm Venereol (Stockh) 1982; 62:450–451.
197. Molin L, Thomsen K, Volden G, et al: Retinoid dermatitis mimicking progression in mycosis fungoides: A report from the Scandinavian mycosis fungoides group. Acta Derm Venereol (Stockh) 1985; 65:69–71.
198. Taïeb A, Maleville J: Retinoid dermatitis mimicking "eczéma craquelé" [letter]. Acta Derm Venereol (Stockh) 1985; 65:570.
199. Levin J, Almeyda J: Erythroderma probably due to etretinate. Br J Dermatol 1985; 112:373–374.
200. Ellis CN, Gold RC, Grekin RC, et al: Etretinate therapy stimulates deposition of mucus-

like material in epidermis of patients with psoriasis. J Am Acad Dermatol 1982; 6:699–704.
201. Graham ML, Corey R, Califf R, et al: Isotretinoin and *Staphylococcus aureus* infection. Arch Dermatol 1986; 122:815–817.
202. Puig L, Moreno A, Llistosella E, et al: Granulation tissue proliferation during isotretinoin treatment. Int J Dermatol 1986; 25:191–193.
203. Hodak E, David M, Feverman EJ: Excess granulation tissue during etretinate therapy. J Am Acad Dermatol 1984; 11:1166–1167.
204. Ferguson J, Johnson BE: Retinoid associated phototoxicity and photosensitivity. Pharmacol Ther 1989; 40:123–135.
205. Jacyk WK: Elevated creatine phosphokinase levels associated with the use of etretinate. J Am Acad Dermatol 1986; 15:710.
206. Lipinski JT, Schwimmer B: Elevated CPK and isotretinoin [letter]. J Am Acad Dermatol 1985; 12:581–585. [Replies by McBurney EI and Rosen DA, Chen D, and Rofsky HE.]
207. David M, Hodak E, Sandbank M, et al: Electromyographic abnormalities in patients undergoing long-term therapy with etretinate. J Am Acad Dermatol 1988; 19:273–275.
208. Hodak E, David M, Gadoth N, et al: Etretinate-induced skeletal muscle damage. Br J Dermatol 1987; 116:623–626.
209. Ellis CN, Gilbert M, Cohen KA, et al: Increased muscle tone during etretinate therapy. J Am Acad Dermatol 1986; 14:907–909.
210. Dressendorfer RH, Wade CE: The muscular overuse syndrome in long-distance runners. Phys Sports Med 1983; 11:116–130.
211. Hays SB, Camisa C: Acquired pili torti in two patients treated with synthetic retinoids. Cutis 1985; 35:466–468.
212. Ferguson MM, Simpson NB, Hammersly N: Severe nail dystrophy associated with retinoid therapy. Lancet 1983; 2:974.
213. Ginsberg H, Rubenstein A, Brown WV: Medical complications of isotretinoin. Clin Dermatol 1986; 4(1):183–189.
214. Bigby M, Stern RS: Adverse drug reactions to isotretinoin. A report from the Adverse Drug Reaction Reporting System. J Am Acad Dermatol 1988; 18:543–552.
215. Schleicher SM: Oral isotretinoin and inflammatory bowel disease. J Am Acad Dermatol 1985; 13:834–835.
216. Torok L, Kasa M: Spermatologic and endocrinologic examinations. *In* Saurat J-H (ed): Retinoids: New Trends in Research and Therapy. Basel, Switzerland: Karger, 1985, 407–410.

9 Psoralens

Robert B. Skinner, Jr., M.D.

Psoralens belong to the furocoumarin class of compounds. They are unusual in that when taken alone they have no clinical effect. However, when combined with long-wave ultraviolet (UVA) light (320–400 nm) irradiation of the skin, they become biologically active and are used to treat psoriasis, vitiligo, and a number of other dermatoses. The two psoralens that are currently available in the United States are 8-methoxypsoralen (methoxsalen, 8-MOP) and 4,5′,8-trimethylpsoralen (trioxsalen, TMP). Another psoralen, 5-methoxypsoralen (bergapten, 5-MOP), is available in Europe.

Psoralens have been used therapeutically for thousands of years. Sufferers of vitiligo ("white leprosy"), a socially devastating, depigmenting condition, have been treated since about 1400 B.C. in Egypt and about 1550 B.C. in India with naturally occurring psoralens and sunlight. Psoralens are found in parsley, celery, parsnips, and citrus fruits, and they function in the plants' defense against insects (phytoalexins).[1] *Psoralea corylifolea* Linnaeus seed was a source of psoralen in India. The Egyptian plant *Ammi majus L.* contains 8-MOP and 5-MOP.[2] Extracts of these plants were either applied topically or taken orally, and the patient was then exposed to sunlight. Kuske in 1938 first linked photosensitization of skin caused by plants containing psoralens and isolated 5-MOP from oil of bergamot.[3]

In 1947, Fahmy and Abu-Shady reported isolation of ammoidin (8-MOP) from *Ammi majus L.*[4] They successfully repigmented vitiligo lesions by using this 8-MOP preparation and sunlight. El Mofty developed the use of oral crystalline or topical 8-MOP plus sunlight in the treatment of vitiligo.[5] Fitzpatrick and associates demonstrated that oral psoralen plus sunlight was phototoxic and increased melanin pigmentation.[6] They also established that the maximal phototoxic effect occurred 1.5–2.0 hours after ingestion of psoralen. The first controlled trial in the treatment of psoriasis with oral 8-MOP and exposure to a high-intensity, artificial source of UVA radiation (320–400 nm) was conducted at Harvard University in 1974. Parrish and co-workers demonstrated in a paired comparison that photochemotherapy, or PUVA (psoralen plus UVA), was an effective treatment of psoriasis.[7] Since 1974, thousands of psoriasis patients have been successfully treated with PUVA in multicenter clinical trials in the U.S. and in Europe.[8,9] In addition, thousands of vitiligo patients have been treated with PUVA since the 1950s.[10]

In the U.S., 8-MOP has been available since 1951, and TMP since 1964. Currently, 5-MOP is being evaluated in the U.S. through clinical trials. The Bureau of Radiological Health of the Food and Drug Administration (FDA) published specifications for UVA irradiation in the May 20, 1982, *Federal Register* and approved PUVA for the treatment of psoriasis.

Pharmacology

Structure

Psoralens are furocoumarin tricyclic hydrocarbon compounds. They are formed by the linear fusion of a furan ring with a benzpyrene, coumarin. The furan ring is attached at its 3'2' bond to the 6'7' bond of the coumarin molecule. Methoxyl groups located on the 8 or 5 positions produce 8-MOP or 5-MOP, whereas methyl groups added at the 4, 5', and 8 positions produce TMP. Psoralens are photoactive reagents capable of being intercalated into double-stranded nucleic acids and forming covalent bonds at either the furan or the coumarin end of a molecule.[11] The psoralen can therefore bind to both sides of a double-stranded nucleic acid helix (bifunctional adducts), producing a covalent crosslink. This reaction occurs only with concomitant ultraviolet radiation in the 320–400 nm (UVA) range.

Absorption/Distribution

The oral form of 8-MOP is the main psoralen in dermatologic use at the present time. There is significant interindividual variation in absorption that depends in part on the formulation of psoralen. The drug is poorly soluble in water and poorly absorbed. As a consequence, the gastric emptying time and bowel transit time play an important role in psoralen pharmacology. The maximal serum concentration occurs 1–4 hours after ingestion of psoralen. Results have been variable with regard to the effect of food on psoralen absorption. Ehrsson and co-workers found an increased maximal serum concentration of psoralen taken with food.[12] However, most authors have found that food intake delays but does not alter the psoralen absorption. Herfst and de Wolff looked at 8-MOP plasma levels in 20 psoriatic patients treated with PUVA under fasting and nonfasting conditions.[13] They found that 8-MOP was more quickly absorbed without food in the stomach, but the mean peak serum concentration was not affected by whether the patient had eaten. Levins and colleagues studied Oxsoralen, a crystalline preparation, and Oxsoralen Ultra, a liquid preparation (ICN Pharmaceuticals).[14] The liquid formulation produced earlier phototoxicity than did the crystalline formulation and produced earlier phototoxicity when given with a low-fat diet than with a high-fat diet. Roelandts and colleagues found no difference in the absorption of 8-MOP with a low-fat diet and with fasting, but a high-fat diet caused a significant decrease in 8-MOP levels.[15] The bioavailability of 8-MOP was greater after a low-fat meal than on an empty stomach.[12] Therefore, the data suggest that maximal absorption is obtained when 8-MOP is taken with a low-fat meal. The drug 5-MOP is absorbed in a similar manner as 8-MOP, and plasma levels are similar when the drugs are given in an aqueous solution.[16]

Many studies have been done on various preparations of oral psoralens. Several studies have shown considerable blood level variation in crystalline preparations of 8-MOP.[17-19] Stolk and associates were the first to demonstrate that the serum concentration could be increased by the administration of 8-MOP as an aqueous solution, in comparison with a powder in a gelatin capsule.[20] Hönigsmann and co-workers found that a liquid preparation of 8-MOP yielded a peak serum concentration in 1 hour, in comparison with 2 hours after a crystalline preparation.[21] The liquid preparation produced threefold greater serum levels. The amount of liquid 8-MOP needed to clear psoriasis was only 40% of the necessary dose of the crystalline 8-MOP. The liquid preparation was eliminated more rapidly, and the degree of photosensitization was more reproducible because of more consistent absorption. When taken in a solution in soft gelatin capsules, 8-MOP produced higher serum levels than it did in micronized powder in hard gelatin capsules.[21-24] Currently, 8-MOP in a solution in soft gelatin capsules (Oxsoralen Ultra) seems to be the best-absorbed formulation. The older formulation, Oxsoralen, is no longer available in the U.S.

In various studies, researchers have found that psoralens are widely distributed in body tissues.[25, 26] Muni and colleagues found the highest levels of 8-MOP in the gastrointestinal tract, the blood, the liver, and the skin.[26] The drug is 84% bound to serum albumin. Tolbutamide can increase the free fraction (and resultant photosensitivity) of 8-MOP by displacing the drug from binding sites.[27]

Metabolism/Excretion

Schmid and co-workers demonstrated a profound saturable first-pass effect after 8-MOP absorption.[28] This first-pass effect results in a loss of active drug that reaches the circulation that is due to liver metabolism. Of low doses of 8-MOP, little reaches the circulation, whereas higher doses of 8-MOP saturate liver enzymes and serum levels are markedly increased. Andrew and colleagues reported a twenty-fivefold increase in 8-MOP plasma levels after the dosage of 8-MOP is increased from 10 mg to 40 mg.[29] After oral administration of 5-MOP as a solution, its absorption and plasma levels are similar to those of 8-MOP.[16]

TMP is less water-soluble than 8-MOP or 5-MOP, and the tablet formulation of TMP is therefore absorbed more slowly than 8-MOP or 5-MOP tablets. Both Schmid and co-workers[16] and Kligman and Goldstein[30] demonstrated that an enhanced first-pass effect with hepatic metabolism produced very low TMP levels in the blood. The solution formulation of TMP produced more rapid absorption and enhanced photosensitivity with low plasma levels.

Psoralens are metabolized in the liver. After oral administration of 8-MOP, 5%–10% of radiolabeled psoralen is found in the feces.[31] About 90% of the psoralen is found in the urine in the form of 8-hydroxypsoralen, 4'5' dihydrodiol 8-MOP, 3,4 dihydrodiol 8-MOP, furocoumaric acid, and unmetabolized 8-MOP.[32] The metabolites originate in the degradation of the furan moiety.[33] The major pathways for the metabolism of 8-MOP are hydroxylation, glucuronide formation, epoxidation, and hydrolysis.[34] Both 8-MOP and 5-MOP seem to induce the production of hepatic microsomal drug-metabolizing enzymes and cytochrome P-450, whereas TMP does not induce these enzymes, and 5-MOP shows similar metabolic pathways as 8-MOP.

The metabolites of 8-MOP are quickly eliminated; they have a serum half-life of approximately 1 hour.[35] This rapid elimination is important in order to avoid prolonged risk of photosensitivity that is due to incidental UVA exposure.

TMP is metabolized more rapidly than 8-MOP, and the main metabolite of TMP is 4,8-dimethyl-5'-carboxypsoralen.[32] The metabolic attack is on the methyl groups that produce alcohols and carbonic acids.

Mechanism of Action

Psoralens have no effect unless combined with long-wave ultraviolet radiation (320–400 nm). The maximal absorption of psoralens is considered to occur with 210–330 nm of ultraviolet radiation, whereas the action spectrum for PUVA is 320–335 nm.[36,37] Without exposure to UVA, psoralens are intercalated between base pairs of nucleic acids.[38] With UVA absorption, the first step is the oxygen-independent formation of cyclobutane adducts that are monofunctional (i.e., that interact with a single DNA strand) and are not photosensitizing. The result is covalent bonding of the 3,4 double bond of the coumarin ring, or the 4,5 double bond of the furan ring of psoralens, with the 5,6 double bond of thymidine.[39] This is followed by formation of bifunctional adducts that cross-link between the pyrimidine bases of two strands of DNA.[40] This effect of PUVA is well documented, but the definitive role of these bifunctional pyrimidine adducts in psoriasis therapy is uncertain.[41, 42] Psoralens that produce bifunctional adducts cause photosensitization.[41] It is thought that the therapeutic effect seen in psoriasis is due to a decreased DNA synthesis,[43] mitosis, and epidermal proliferation[44] from the psoralen-DNA effects.[45, 46] PUVA-induced immunologic alterations may also play a role in improving psoriasis.[47, 48]

PUVA can damage DNA by production of reactive oxygen species that may cause DNA strand breaks. Pathak and Joshi demonstrated that 8-MOP plus UVA induced production of singlet oxygen and superoxide radicals,[49] and 5-MOP and TMP have been shown to induce singlet oxygen production.[50] Psoralens have also been shown to damage mitochondria[51] and to interact with RNA and proteins.[52]

In normal skin, PUVA exposure produce inflammation and melanogenesis. Inflammation from PUVA peaks 48–72 hours after treatment and lasts longer than inflammation from ultraviolet B (UVB; 280–320 nm), which peaks 24 hours after treatment. Both PUVA and UVB evoke a prostaglandin-mediated erythema. Epidermal changes are similar in PUVA- and UVB-induced erythema.[53, 54] PUVA and UVB produce pigmentation in a similar manner, and PUVA-induced pigmentation can be predicted by the ability to tan with UVB exposure. PUVA increases the number of melanocytes and the number and transfer of melanosomes to keratinocytes. The combination 8-MOP plus UVA does not affect the size or distribution of melanosomes,[55] unlike topical TMP plus UVA.[56] The repigmentation of vitiligo is thought to be due to PUVA-induced inflammation and subsequent melanogenesis. Proliferation and migration of viable melanocytes from hair follicles into adjacent depigmented skin may also be responsible for vitiligo repigmentation. TMP is less phototoxic than 8-MOP and is used mainly for treatment of vitiligo.

Clinical Use (Table 9–1)

Approved Indications

PSORIASIS. PUVA has been shown in many clinical trials to be an effective treatment for psoriasis.[7-9, 57-65] The first clinical trials were half-body paired comparisons of oral 8-MOP followed by exposure to high-intensity, long-wave ultraviolet light (UVA) versus conventional ultraviolet light (UV) therapy. Parrish and co-workers initially reported in 1974 that they found complete clearing of generalized psoriasis in 21 patients.[7] In paired-comparison studies, PUVA was found to be more effective than conventional UV (275–380 nm). Wolff and colleagues found complete clearing of the PUVA-treated side in 90% of the psoriatic patients, and 85% remained in remission with maintenance treatments for up to 400 days.[60] PUVA was found to be superior to conventional UV (250–400 nm) in all cases.

Table 9–1. PUVA Indications/Contraindications

FDA-Approved Dermatologic Indications

Psoriasis Vulgaris[7-9, 57-66]
Vitiligo*[6, 10, 67-74]
Increasing Tolerance to Sunlight/Enhancing Pigmentation†[75]

Other Dermatologic Uses

Neoplastic
  Mycosis fungoides/Sézary's syndrome[57, 76-86]
  Histiocytosis X[87]

Dermatitis/Papulosquamous
  Atopic eczema[88, 89]
  Chronic hand eczema[90, 91]
  Nickel contact dermatitis[92]
  Pustulosis palmoplantaris[93]
  Parapsoriasis[76]
  Lichen planus[94, 95]
  Pityriasis lichenoides/lymphomatoid papulosis[96, 97]

Photosensitivity Dermatoses
  Polymorphous light eruption[98, 99]
  Solar urticaria[100]
  Actinic reticuloid[101]
  Chronic actinic dermatitis/prurigo[102, 103]
  Erythropoietic protoporphyria[104]

Other Pruritic Dermatoses
  Pruritus with HIV infection[105]
  Dermographism[106]
  Urticaria pigmentosa[107, 108]
  Prurigo nodularis[109]

Granulomatous Dermatoses
  Generalized granuloma annulare[110, 111]
  Sarcoidosis[112]

Other Immunologic Dermatoses
  Alopecia areata[113-116]
  Pemphigus vulgaris[117]
  Graft-versus-host disease[118-120]

Miscellaneous Dermatoses
  Transient acantholytic dermatosis[121]
  Progressive pigmented purpuric dermatoses[122]
  Icthyosis linearis circumflexia[123]
  Scleromyxedema[124]

Contraindications

History of idiosyncratic reactions to psoralen compounds
A specific history of light-sensitive disease such as lupus erythematosus, porphyria cutanea tarda, erythropoietic protoporphyria, variegate porphyria, xeroderma pigmentosum, and albinism
Prior ionizing radiation, inorganic arsenic exposure, or topical nitrogen mustard: increases the risk of skin cancer
Melanoma or history of melanoma
History of invasive cutaneous squamous cell carcinoma
Aphakia: increased risk of retinal damage with absence of lens
Pregnancy or lactation
Severe cardiac disease: difficulty with prolonged standing, heat intolerance (relative contraindication)
Severe liver disease: altered psoralen metabolism (relative contraindication)
Patient under 12 years of age (relative contraindication)
Concomitant use of other photosensitive agents (relative contraindication)

*PUVA is generally considered the treatment of choice.
†Trioxsalen is approved only for this indication.

In the PUVA follow-up study in 1976 (U.S. Cooperative Clinical Trial), Melski and colleagues reviewed the treatment of 1380 psoriatic patients at 16 centers.[8] They found 88% clearing of the patients; guttate psoriasis cleared most rapidly, and erythrodermic psoriasis cleared most slowly. It was demonstrated that maintenance therapy with PUVA was needed to prevent recurrence and that long-term therapy was associated with side effects. A multicenter European study revealed a clearing rate of 89% in 3174 patients treated with PUVA.[9] Failure rates and recurrences were more frequent with erythrodermic psoriasis and with more severe disease in general. Generalized pustular psoriasis may respond to PUVA, although it is typically less responsive than plaque-type psoriasis.[61, 62] Of interest is that psoriatic arthritis frequently responds to PUVA.[66] Boer and associates compared PUVA and UVB treatment for 183 psoriasis patients.[63] PUVA resulted in a higher therapeutic score (95%–100% clearance), particularly if more than 50% of skin surface was involved. Also, PUVA-treated patients needed less maintenance therapy. Stern and coauthors reported in a 7.2-year study of 1380 patients that PUVA was an effective outpatient therapy for severe psoriasis.[64] Outpatient PUVA was more cost-effective than daycare centers or inpatient hospitalization. Stern and Melsk identified four factors that are likely to make patients with less than 70% skin involvement discontinue therapy: age of more than 70 years, fair or poor general health, multiple previous hospitalizations for psoriasis, and unusual reactions to sunlight.[65] In practical terms, the distance that a patient has to travel to receive PUVA and the patient's intolerance to psoralens are more common limiting factors.[61]

In general, PUVA should be used by patients with severe, recalcitrant, disabling psoriasis that is not responsive to other forms of topical therapy and UVB phototherapy. Patients should be informed of possible long-term side effects such as skin cancer and cataracts, as well as the need for maintenance therapy.

VITILIGO. Psoralens (topical or oral) plus UVA (artificial or natural sunlight) have been reported to produce repigmentation of vitiligo lesions.[6, 67–74] Morison reported that approximately 70% of vitiligo patients have some repigmentation of lesions after up to 200 PUVA treatments over 1–2 years.[67] Bleehen treated 32 vitiligo patients with oral TMP and various sources of UVA, including natural sunlight.[68] Patients were treated once or twice a week over 4–28 months. Six patients showed considerable repigmentation, and 9 others had significant cosmetic improvement. Vitiligo of the face, the neck, and the trunk were more responsive than that of the arms and the legs. In this study, natural sunlight worked better than artificial UVA. Parrish and colleagues found that 73% of patients improved with oral 8-MOP or oral TMP and UVA.[69] However, no patients had complete repigmentation in all areas. Parrish and colleagues found no correlation between improvement and extent of involvement, duration of vitiligo, or age of patient. Side effects were mild. Singh and coauthors reported nearly complete repigmentation in 18 of 20 vitiligo patients who used daily oral TMP and sunshine.[70]

Other Dermatologic Uses

PUVA therapy can be used for a variety of conditions with diverse pathogenesis. Mycosis fungoides is the most widely accepted indication for PUVA that is not FDA-approved. Several other dermatoses are briefly discussed in this section as well. The reader is encouraged to review the cited references before PUVA is used for these indications. Aside from the brief course of therapy for polymorphous light eruption, the protocols for using PUVA therapy for the conditions to be described are quite similar to protocols used in psoriasis therapy (see the Therapeutic Guidelines section).

MYCOSIS FUNGOIDES. Gilchrist and coauthors in 1976 first reported the effectiveness of PUVA in the treatment of mycosis fungoides.[76] Nine patients with stage II or more advanced disease were treated successfully for up to 28 months. Since then, numerous reports have confirmed these results.[77-86]

Gupta and Anderson reviewed the existing studies on PUVA for mycosis fungoides.[61] More than 80% of patients with stage I or II disease demonstrated complete clearing with PUVA therapy. Stage III disease (tumors or ulcerative lesions) completely cleared in less than 40% of cases. Patients with stage IV (lymph node involvement) and stage V (visceral involvement) disease generally experienced worsening of disease activity with PUVA therapy. Topical nitrogen mustard may be used adjunctively for body sites shielded from UVA exposure. Sézary's syndrome and, to a lesser degree, mycosis fungoides are responsive to extracorporeal photopheresis.[77, 78] With this modality, leukocyte-rich plasmapheresed blood plus a psoralen is exposed to a UVA source before it is returned to the patient. Further details of extracorporeal photopheresis are beyond the scope of this chapter.

ATOPIC DERMATITIS. PUVA therapy has in several studies been beneficial to atopic dermatitis patients.[88, 89] These patients are typically less responsive to PUVA and relapse more rapidly after stopping PUVA than psoriasis patients.

LICHEN PLANUS. Patients with generalized lichen planus that is unresponsive to topical or systemic glucocorticosteroids are good candidates for PUVA therapy. In one study, remission was achieved by 6 of 7 patients who required a total of 17–48 treatments.[95]

POLYMORPHOUS LIGHT ERUPTION (PMLE). Prophylactic treatment of PMLE involves a 4-week course of PUVA administered three times per week in the spring.[98, 99] The therapeutic benefit is due to increased stratum corneum thickness (hardening), increased melanization, and perhaps immunologic mechanisms. Initial and subsequent UVA doses are similar to those used in psoriasis therapy (Table 9–2).

ALOPECIA AREATA. Mitchell and Krull comprehensively reviewed alopecia areata, including the use of PUVA by the patients.[113] Good to excellent results were obtained by 60%–70% of patients studied. Although topical or oral 8-MOP plus localized UVA irradiation of the scalp may be used,[114] there is evidence that total body UVA irradiation and oral 8-MOP give superior results.[115]

Acute Adverse Effects

The most frequent acute adverse effect of PUVA treatment is erythema.[7] The PUVA-induced erythema occurs after 24–36 hours and usually peaks after 48–72 hours. This condition can last up to 1 week and can vary from mild redness to severe blister formation and skin necrosis. If significant local pain and erythema occur during treatment, the affected site can be shielded with a drape or with sunscreens during subsequent UVA exposure until these findings resolve. Widespread PUVA-induced erythema and pain necessitate temporary cessation of therapy until these findings have resolved. A small UVA dosage reduction and more gradual increments are then appropriate.

Other acute adverse effects are pruritus, transient nausea (less with TMP than with 8-MOP), headache, and Koebner's phenomenon (appearance of psoriasis in areas of significant photosensitivity).[9] Pruritus induced by PUVA treatments can usually be controlled with emollients alone or with topical steroids. Localized pruritic sites may benefit from sunscreens applied before UVA exposure. Widespread, recalcitrant pruritus that is unresponsive to oral antipruritic medication or to UVA dosage reduction generally requires discontinuation of PUVA. Nausea

Table 9–2. Skin Types and Appropriate UVA Exposure[61]

Skin Type	History/Physical Examination	Initial Dose Joules/sq cm	Increments Joules/sq cm
I*	Always burn, never tan	0.5–1.0	0.25–0.5
II	Always burn, but sometimes tan	1.0–2.0	0.5
III	Sometimes burn, but always tan	1.5–3.0	0.5–1.0
IV	Never burn, always tan	2.0–4.0	1.0
V	Moderately pigmented	2.5–5.0	1.0
VI	Blacks	3.0–6.0	1.0–1.5

*Vitiligo patients and erythrodermic psoriatic patients should be classified as having type I skin.

due to psoralens is common. Splitting the psoralen into two doses, administered half an hour apart, is generally beneficial. For patients with refractory nausea, a psoralen dosage reduction and a corresponding increase in UVA exposure may allow tolerance of the psoralen medication.

Tanning beds (UVA) and psoralens, used in combination, are strictly forbidden. Severe photosensitivity may result from this combination because of the lack of medical supervision and reliable dosimetry. A fatality that was due to psoralen intake and subsequent excessive UVA exposure from a commercial tanning bed underscores this point (*Chicago Sun-Times*, May 22, 1989).

Chronic Adverse Effects

OPHTHALMOLOGIC EFFECTS. Animal studies have shown variable results in the effect of PUVA on the eye. Cloud and co-workers found anterior cortical cataracts in albino mice and guinea pigs treated with high doses of 8-MOP and UVA.[125] Parrish and colleagues found no cataracts in PUVA-treated Dutch-belted rabbits,[126] and Freeman and Troll found no cataracts in guinea pigs treated with PUVA.[127]

Back and associates found no ocular pathology in 13 patients treated with methoxsalen for vitiligo.[128] However, bilateral cataracts were reported in a patient treated with PUVA for 2½ years for vitiligo.[129] Woo and coauthors reported cataracts associated with psoralen photoproducts in a PUVA-treated psoriasis patient.[130] Boukes and Bruynzeel evaluated 408 patients for up to 6 years after the initial PUVA exposure.[131] In 3 patients, all under 40 years of age, cataracts developed without alternative explanation within the 1st year. The role of noncompliance with UVA-blocking glasses was not addressed. Lafond and associates followed 78 PUVA patients for a mean of 10.8 months.[132] Two younger patients developed cataracts; noncompliance with instructions to wear protective glasses played a major role in the cataract development. Both anterior and posterior cortical cataracts were noted in these studies. PUVA-induced photokeratoconjunctivitis[133] and transient visual defects[134] have also been reported.

Stern and co-workers, in a 5-year prospective study of 1299 psoriatic patients treated with PUVA, found no significant increase in cataracts overall.[135] However, in patients who received more than 100 PUVA treatments, there was a small increase in nuclear sclerosis (a relative risk of 2.3) and posterior subcapsular opacities (a relative risk of 3.0). The patients with these findings had no alteration in visual acuity that was due to the opacities. Patients wore UVA-blocking eyeglasses for 12 hours after ingestion of 8-MOP and when exposed to sunlight. Similar results have been reported in other long-term follow-up studies of PUVA patients.[136–138] Abdullah and Keczkes reported no cataracts, lens opacities, or decreased visual acuity in 198 patients treated with PUVA over a 10-year period.[137]

Ultraviolet radiation in the range of 300–400 nm passes through the cornea and is absorbed by the lens.[139] Normally, 8-MOP diffuses out of the lens 12–24 hours after ingestion, but with exposure to UVA, 8-MOP can photobind to lens proteins[135] and form photoadducts.[140] With repeated ingestion of 8-MOP and exposures to UVA, psoralen-protein complexes can potentially build up in the lens and lead to cataracts. In order to prevent the possibility of cataract development, it is recommended that patients wear UVA-blocking wraparound glasses from the time of psoralen ingestion until 24 hours later.[141] One study also suggested wearing eye protection on the day after drug ingestion and in rooms with windows.[142] Ophthalmologic examinations should be performed before treatment, every 6 months for 1 year, and at yearly intervals thereafter.[141]

In summary, the risk of cataracts from PUVA is neglible in patients who comply with wearing UVA-blocking wraparound glasses for 12–24 hours after ingesting psoralen. An additional 24 hours of wearing these glasses is probably unnecessary. The majority of cataracts just described developed in the first few years after initiation of PUVA therapy. The long-term risk of PUVA-induced cataracts is unknown, and so yearly ophthalmologic examinations are indicated indefinitely.

CUTANEOUS CARCINOMA INDUCTION. Stern and co-workers, in a prospective study of 1367 psoriasis patients, found the same risk of cutaneous cancer as in the general population,[143] and Halprin and associates found an increased incidence of skin cancer in non–PUVA-treated psoriatics, in comparison with matched diabetic patients.[144]

In a prospective study of 1373 PUVA-treated psoriasis patients, Stern and co-workers found a risk of cutaneous carcinoma to be 2.6 times that of the general population and found a higher ratio (1.5:1) of squamous cell carcinoma (SCC) to basal cell carcinomas (BCC) than expected (0.3:1).[145] The PUVA-induced SCC occurred more frequently in non–sun-exposed areas than expected. Two subsequent evaluations of the same cohort of PUVA-treated psoriasis patients have been published.[146, 147] In the 1988 study, there was an elevenfold increase in cutaneous SCC in patients who received more than 260 PUVA treatments, in comparison with patients who received fewer than 160 treatments.[147] The biologic behavior of these malignancies was similar to that of cutaneous SCC from other etiologies. Only when patients were followed for at least 10 years after initiation of PUVA was a modest dose-related increase in BCC detected.[147] In all three studies, an adjustment for prior exposure to ionizing radiation and tar was made.[145–147] Forman and colleagues followed 551 patients for up to 10 years in another U.S. study group, the PUVA-48 cooperative study.[148] BCC occurred in 2.4%, and SCC in 1.6%, of the patients studied.

In contrast, multiple European studies have revealed no increase in cutaneous carcinoma in PUVA-treated patients.[149-153] Hönigsmann and coauthors reported that previous arsenic exposure was the main risk factor for PUVA-induced skin cancer, although exposure to ionizing radiation or methotrexate also were factors.[149] Lindskov found skin cancer risk factors to be exposure to ionizing radiation, to methotrexate, to arsenic, or to topical nitrogen mustard and a history of cutaneous malignancy.[150] Reshad and colleagues found, in a 7-year follow-up of 216 PUVA-treated psoriatics, an SCC:BCC ratio of 2.5:1. Half of the carcinomas occurred on non–sun-exposed skin, and many patients had multiple cutaneous malignancies.[151]

Abdullah and Keczkes reviewed 198 of 292 patients treated with long-term PUVA chemotherapy for various skin diseases over a 10-year period.[137] They found 1 patient who developed an SCC and 1 patient who had a lentigo maligna. Of importance is that multiple studies have failed to demonstrate an increased cutaneous melanoma risk in PUVA-treated patients.[154]

A report by Stern and Members of the Photochemotherapy Follow-Up Study disclosed an almost 300-fold increased risk of invasive SCC of the genitalia in male patients receiving prolonged, high-dose PUVA.[155] A small increase (a 4.6 relative risk) in male genital SCC due to high levels of UVB radiation was noted as well. Overall, 1.6% of 892 men studied developed genital neoplasms (including in situ SCC and keratoacanthomas). These data clearly mandate adequate protection of the male genitalia during PUVA and UVB therapy.

In summary, there is an increased risk of cutaneous SCC to patients with high exposure levels to PUVA in cohorts studied in the U.S. European studies consistently fail to demonstrate a similar increased risk. Possible explanations for this discrepancy include different therapeutic approaches used and a different incidence of cutaneous malignancies in the respective countries. The risk of metastasis from PUVA-induced SCC appears to be no greater than the risk of metastasis from SCC that occurs in the absence of PUVA therapy. Patients should be informed about the SCC risk and advised regarding cutaneous self-examination and physician monitoring for skin cancer detection. It is hoped that new combination treatments, such as etretinate and PUVA, will limit the amount of long-term exposure to PUVA. Avoidance of PUVA by patients with skin type I (and perhaps type II), prior arsenic exposure, prior ionizing radiation, or a history of skin cancer should also decrease the risk of subsequent SCC.

PIGMENTED MACULES. Chronic PUVA therapy can induce hyperpigmented macules on light-exposed areas of skin. Kanerva and Lauharanta reported a 41% incidence of PUVA-induced freckling.[156] Sun-reactive skin types I,[157] II,[157] and III[158] are more prone to develop these lesions.

The higher the cumulative number of PUVA treatments[159] and the total amount of UVA radiation,[160] the greater the chance of developing these pigmented macules. Histologically, the pigmented lesions show a lentiginous proliferation of functionally active melanocytes, some of which appear atypical.[161] Other names for pigmented macules include freckles,[162] lentigines,[163] persistent ashen-gray macules,[164] stellate hyperpigmented freckling,[165] and nevus spilus–like spots.[166] It is not known whether the pigmented macules induced by PUVA will progress to melanocytic dysplasia and eventually melanoma. Thus far, the number of melanomas reported in patients treated with PUVA is no greater than would be expected in the general population.[154, 167]

IMMUNOLOGIC EFFECTS. Circulating white blood cells are exposed to 5% of the skin surface UVA radiation during PUVA therapy.[168] PUVA treatment has been shown to suppress the number and function of blood lymphocytes,[169] polymorphonuclear leukocytes,[170] monocytes,[170] and macrophages.[171] In addition, PUVA may decrease total T cells, T cell surface markers, suppressor T cells,[172] helper T cells,[173] natural killer cell activity, and mitogen response.[174]

PUVA causes decreased delayed hypersensitivity with resultant decreased response to contact allergens.[175] Dinitrochlorobenzene contact hypersensitivity has been shown to be decreased by PUVA treatment. This suppression occurs in both the induction and the elicitation phases of delayed hypersensitivity by systemic and local actions of PUVA.[176] There is a decrease in the number of Langerhans cells after PUVA therapy, which may contribute to the decreased contact hypersensitivity. The long-term effect of this immunosuppression produced by PUVA therapy is not known. The risk of immunosuppression-related opportunistic infections or lymphomas does not appear to be increased.[177]

BULLOUS PEMPHIGOID INDUCTION. Bullous pemphigoid has been reported to occur in patients during PUVA therapy.[178–181] PUVA apparently can cause pre-existing bullous pemphigoid to flare up and can induce or unmask latent bullous pemphigoid. This adverse effect is quite uncommon.

LUPUS ERYTHEMATOSUS INDUCTION. Lupus erythematosus has been reported to develop during PUVA therapy.[182–184] However, there are reports of both increased incidence of antinuclear antibodies (ANA) with PUVA[185, 186] and no increase in ANA.[187, 188] ANA-positive patients have been safely treated with PUVA for up to 28 months.[189] Dowdy and coauthors reported PUVA-induced skin lesions typical of subacute cutaneous lupus erythematous associated with pancytopenia, antibodies to double-stranded DNA, and hypocomplementemia, all of which improved or resolved with discontinuation of PUVA.[190]

PUVA MONITORING GUIDELINES[75, 142]

Baseline

Ocular

- Gross examination
- Slit-lamp examination of lens and cornea
- Funduscopic examination of retina
- Assessment of visual acuity

Cutaneous

- Skin examination for skin cancer, premalignant lesions, freckling, and actinic damage
- Skin biopsy of suspicious lesions for histologic diagnosis

Laboratory

- Complete blood count (CBC)
- Liver function tests: aspartate aminotransferase (serum glutamate oxaloacetate transaminase), alanine aminotransferase (serum glutamate pyruvate transaminase), alkaline phosphatase, bilirubin, lactate dehydrogenase
- Renal function tests: blood urea nitrogen, serum creatinine
- ANA: perhaps optional after 1 year
- Urinalysis

Follow-Up

Ocular

- Repeat examination after 6 months, after 1 year, and yearly

Cutaneous

- Periodic complete skin examination at least every 6–12 months by physician; ideally, monthly self-examination by patient

Laboratory

- Repeat after 1 month, after 6 months, after 1 year, and yearly*

Note: More frequent surveillance is needed if laboratory values are abnormal or with high-risk patients.

*Published guidelines do not suggest laboratory testing after 1 month, although this timing is optimal for detection of idiosyncratic adverse effects.

MISCELLANEOUS CUTANEOUS ADVERSE EFFECTS. PUVA-induced cutaneous lesions include acne,[191] seborrheic dermatitis,[192] pruritus,[193] painful skin,[194,195] vitiligo,[196] hypertrichosis,[197] disseminated superficial actinic porokeratosis,[198] onycholysis,[199] nail pigmentation,[200] Bowen's disease, keratoacanthoma,[201] and xeroderma pigmentosum–like changes.[202] A poikilodermatous appearance is common in patients who have received long-term PUVA (usually more than 100 treatments).

MISCELLANEOUS SYSTEMIC ADVERSE EFFECTS. Reported systemic reactions to chronic PUVA treatment include hepatotoxicity,[203-205] preleukemia,[206] acute myeloid leukemia,[207] nephrotic syndrome,[208] exacerbation of gouty arthritis,[209] and bronchonconstriction.[210,211]

Drug Interactions

Tolbutamide can displace psoralens from protein-binding sites and therefore increase their photosensitizing potential.[27] Concomitant use of drugs with known photosensitizing potential such as sulfonamides, tetracyclines, griseofulvin, phenothiazines, and thiazide diuretics should be prescribed with appropriate caution (see Oxsoralen Ultra package insert).

Therapeutic Guidelines

PSORIASIS MANAGEMENT. PUVA is administered as oral 8-MOP followed by exposure to a controlled dosage of artificial, high-intensity UVA radiation. The dosage of oral 8-MOP and the interval between treatments are fixed during the induction phase of therapy, whereas the amount of UVA exposure varies according to the clinical response of the patient. Resolution of lesion scale, thickness, and erythema are used to gauge the therapeutic response.

Traditionally, 0.6 mg/kg of crystalline 8-MOP (Oxsoralen) was administered approximately 2 hours before UVA exposure. The newer liquid 8-MOP formulation (Oxsoralen Ultra) is given in a dosage of 0.3–0.4 mg/kg approximately 1½ hours before UVA exposure. Both the 0.6 and the 0.3–0.4 mg/kg dosages are based on lean body weight. The starting dosage of UVA is determined by sun-reactive skin type, which is based on sunburn and tanning history (see Table 9–2). Alternatively, the starting UVA dosage can be determined by measurement of the minimal phototoxic dose (MPD, or minimal amount of UVA administered with 8-MOP necessary to produce faint erythema 48 hours after UVA exposure). The MPD test range should consist of 0.5–1.0 J/sq cm increments in the predicted initial dose range (Table 9–2) to at least 1–2 J/sq cm above this range. The starting dosage as determined by MPD testing (typically ½–¾ of the MPD) is frequently higher than the dosage suggested by sun-reactive skin type. Increments of UVA are usually 0.5–

1.0 J each treatment, depending on skin type, until psoriasis clearing or significant erythema or pruritus occurs. The clinician should keep in mind during this phase that Koebner's phenomenon is a risk of excessively rapid UVA increments. UVA dose is precisely controlled and monitored with photometers. Total cumulative dose measured in J/sq cm is recorded for each patient. Treatments are usually given two or three times per week and are avoided on consecutive days. Typically, 18–30 PUVA treatments are required to induce a remission.

After clearing, a maintenance regimen is usually begun to prevent relapse.[58, 60, 64, 65, 212] The UVA dose that induced clearing is continued during the maintenance phase, and the interval between treatments is gradually increased. A reasonable maintenance protocol is as follows: two to four weekly PUVA treatments; two to four PUVA treatments with 2-week intervals between treatments; two to four PUVA treatments with 3-week intervals between treatments; then PUVA treatments with 4-week intervals between treatments.[61] This maintenance treatment program can be continued indefinitely. However, one can periodically attempt to discontinue PUVA during any of these treatment intervals. In one large series, an average of 30 treatments per year were required during the maintenance phase of PUVA therapy.[212] Should a disease flare-up occur during the maintenance phase, the frequency of treatments should increase to the last effective interval.

Patients should wear UVA opaque goggles in the irradiation chamber, during the 1st day of PUVA treatment (absolute requirement), and perhaps during the 2nd day after PUVA treatment (relative requirement).[141] Patients should avoid exposure to sunlight for 8 hours after the PUVA treatment by using protective clothing, hats, and sunscreens.[141] Patients should use adjunctive topical therapy for psoriatic lesions of scalp, intertriginous sites, and the plantar surfaces of the feet.

BATH PUVA FOR PSORIASIS. Patients may be exposed to psoralens added to bath water, instead of orally ingesting them, to prevent systemic side effects of nausea and headache.[213] The risk of cataracts is neglible because of minimal systemic psoralen absorption. TMP seems to be more effective than 8-MOP,[213] and TMP baths followed by exposure to UVA have been shown to be a safe and effective treatment of psoriasis.[214] Turjanmaa and colleagues compared bath PUVA (50-mg TMP in 150 liters of water) with oral PUVA and found 75% and 77% clearing of chronic plaque psoriasis with relapses of 61% and 58%, respectively, after 1 year.[215] The cumulative UVA dose was significantly lower with bath PUVA. Both bath PUVA and oral PUVA often produced significant erythema, although this led to discontinuation of therapy more frequently by bath-PUVA patients.

COMBINATION THERAPY FOR PSORIASIS. The combination of PUVA and other modalities is used to reduce adverse effects of treatment, increase

PUVA efficacy, and reduce the cost of treatment.[61] PUVA has been combined with corticosteroids,[216] anthralin,[217] UVB,[218, 219] methotrexate,[220] and retinoids[221-223] in the treatment of psoriasis. Resistant lesions or involved sites not accessible to PUVA are appropriate situations for using adjunctive topical corticosteroids.[216] In one study, anthralin and PUVA in combination produced clearing of psoriasis more quickly than did PUVA alone.[217] Several studies have demonstrated more rapid clearing of psoriasis and reduced cumulative UVA doses by a combination of UVB and PUVA therapy.[219, 220] Three weekly courses of methotrexate before PUVA therapy is initiated followed by concomitant methotrexate and PUVA, can decrease the number of UVA exposures, decrease the cumulative UVA exposure, and improve the overall efficacy of PUVA.[221] The possible synergistic carcinogenicity of these two modalities makes this combination therapy a questionable option.[150-151] Re-PUVA (retinoid and PUVA) is a useful combination therapy.[221-223] Typically, etretinate is started 10-14 days before PUVA therapy is begun. After the psoriasis clears, the etretinate is tapered down and the patient switches to the PUVA maintenance protocol. The advantages of this combination include reduced cumulative UVA dose, reduced retinoid dose, and possibly reduced risk of cutaneous malignancy due to the anti-tumor-promotion effect of retinoids.

VITILIGO MANAGEMENT. Vitiligo lesions can be repigmented by ingestion of oral 8-MOP or TMP, followed by exposure to natural sunlight or UVA radiation from an artificial UVA light source. Patients who are well motivated are optimal candidates because of the prolonged course of PUVA that is necessary to induce repigmentation. Although children may repigment more readily than adults, PUVA therapy in children under age 12 is not generally recommended.[61]

According to Hönigsmann and coauthors, the usual method of treating vitiligo is to use a combination of oral TMP and artificial UVA or natural sunlight.[75] UVA doses are based on the involved depigmented skin's being similar to type I skin (see Table 9-2). Gradual increments are used to maintain just perceptible erythema without pain. The treatments are generally given twice a week. TMP is recommended because it is less phototoxic than 8-MOP. Patients start treatment with 0.6 mg/kg of TMP and proceed to 0.9 mg/kg if there is no response after 25 treatments. If there is still no response after another 25 treatments, 0.3 mg/kg of 8-MOP is used instead of TMP. If there is no response after another 25 treatments, the 8-MOP dose is increased to 0.6 mg/kg. A combination of 0.3 mg/kg of 8-MOP and 0.6 mg/kg of TMP may be considered in selected cases. If there is no repigmentation after these steps, the disease should be considered unresponsive.

An alternative, more practical regimen, is to use TMP and natural sunlight. A TMP dose of 10-15 mg is administered 2 hours before midday sunlight exposure (as per the Trisoralen package insert). The initial exposure of 15 minutes is gradually increased to the point of producing just perceptible erythema without pain, which occurs 48 hours after the exposure. The exposure should remain at this level. PUVA in which natural sunlight is used should be performed at most two or three times per week on alternate days. This method of PUVA administration is probably less successful than PUVA with artificial UVA and should be prescribed only for very reliable patients.

A positive result is the appearance of perifollicular macular repigmentation. Reversal of an initial response can result from Koebner's phenomenon. If this occurs, treatment should be stopped for 4 weeks and then resumed with sub-MPD UVA exposure.

Body sites that respond poorly to PUVA include mucosal surfaces (lips), distal dorsal hands, tips of fingers, bony prominences, palms, soles, and nipples. These areas should be shielded with sunscreens.

Repigmentation may reverse if therapy is discontinued before complete repigmentation has taken place. Development of new vitiligo lesions while a patient is receiving PUVA therapy indicates suboptimal treatment or Koebner's phenomenon. Usually 150–200 PUVA treatments are necessary for repigmentation, but only a few patients totally repigment, and 30% do not respond at all.[75] Sunscreens are important to use at all times, both to protect the depigmented sites and to minimize the pigment contrast of uninvolved skin.

BIBLIOGRAPHY: Key Reviews/Chapters

Gupta AK, Anderson TF: Psoralen photochemotherapy. J Am Acad Dermatol 1987; 17:703–734.
Bickers DR: Position paper—PUVA therapy. J Am Acad Dermatol 1983; 8:265–270.
Hönigsmann H, Wolff K, Fitzpatrick TB, et al: Oral photochemotherapy with psoralens and UVA (PUVA): Principles and practice. In Fitzpatrick TB, Eisen AZ, Wolff K, et al (eds): Dermatology in General Medicine (3rd ed). New York: McGraw-Hill, 1987, 1533–1558.
de Wolff FA, Thomas TV: Clinical pharmacokinetics of methoxsalen and other psoralens. Clin Pharmacokinet 1986; 11:62–75.
McEvoy MT, Stern RS: Psoralens and related compounds in the treatment of psoriasis. Pharmacol Ther 1987; 34:75–97.
Stern RS: PUVA and the induction of skin cancer. In Conti CJ, Slaga TJ, Klein-Szanto AJ (eds): Skin Tumors: Experimental and Clinical Aspects. New York: Raven Press, 1989, 85–101.

REFERENCES

1. Berenbaum M, Feeny P: Toxicity of angular furanocoumarins to swallowtail butterflies: Escalation in a coevolutionary arms race? Science 1981; 212:927–929.
2. Stolk LML, Siddiqui AH: Biopharmaceutics, pharmacokinetics and pharmacology of psoralens. Gen Pharmacol 1981; 19:649–653.

3. Kuske H: Experimentelle Untersuchungen zur Photosensibilisierung der Haut durch pflanzliche Wirkstoffe: Lichtsensibilisierung durch Furocoumarine als Ursache verschiedener phytogener Dermatosen. Arch Dermatol Syph 1938; 178:112–123.
4. Fahmy IR, Abu-Shady H: Ammi majus Linn: Pharmacognostical study and isolation of crystalline constituent, ammoidin. Quart J Pharm Pharmacol 1947; 20:281–291.
5. El Mofty AM: A preliminary clinical report on the treatment of leukoderma with Ammi majus Linn. Egypt Med Assoc 1948; 31:651–656.
6. Fitzpatrick TB, Hopkins CE, Blickenstaff DD, et al: Augmented pigmentation and other responses of normal human skin to solar radiation following oral administration of 8-methoxypsoralen. J Invest Dermatol 1955; 25:187–190.
7. Parrish JA, Fitzpatrick TB, Tanenbaum L, et al: Photochemotherapy of psoriasis with oral methoxsalen and longwave ultraviolet light. N Engl J Med 1974; 291:1207–1211.
8. Melski JW, Tanenbaum L, Parrish JA, et al: Oral methoxsalen photochemotherapy for the treatment of psoriasis: A cooperative clinical trial. J Invest Dermatol 1977; 68:328–335.
9. Henseler T, Wolff K, Hönigsmann H, et al: Oral 8-methoxy-psoralen photochemotherapy for psoriasis. The European PUVA study: A cooperative study among 18 European centres. Lancet 1981; 1:853–857.
10. Parrish JA, Stern RS, Fitzpatrick TB: Evaluation of PUVA—1980: Its basic nature and toxicity. In Moschella SL (ed): Dermatology Update-Reviews for Physicians. New York: Elsevier, 1980, 313–337.
11. Kanne D, Straub K, Rapoport H, et al: Psoralen-deoxyribonucleic acid photoreaction: Characterization of the monoaddition products from 8-methoxypsoralen and 4,5'8 trimethylpsoralen. Biochemistry 1982; 21:861–871.
12. Ehrsson H, Nilssow SO, Ehrnebo M, et al: Effect of food on kinetics of 8-methoxypsoralen. Clin Pharmacol Ther 1979; 25:167–171.
13. Herfst MJ, de Wolff FA: Influence of food on the kinetics of 8-methoxypsoralen in serum and suction blister fluid in psoriatic patients. Eur J Clin Pharmacol 1983; 23:75–80.
14. Levins PC, Gange RW, Momtaz-T K, et al: Bioactivity of a new liquid formulation of 8-methoxypsoralen (8-MOP): Time course and effect of diet. J Invest Dermatol 1983; 80:305–306.
15. Roelandts R, VanBoven M, Adriaens P: Methoxsalen serum level variations in psoralen and ultraviolet-A (PUVA) therapy [letter]. Arch Dermatol 1981; 117:758.
16. Schmid J, Brickl R, Busch U, et al: Comparison of pharmacokinetics, pharmacodynamics and metabolism of 8-MOP, 5-MOP and TMP. In Proceedings International Psoralens Symposium, 1984, 109–116.
17. Ljunggren B, Carter DM, Albert J, et al: Plasma levels of 8-methoxypsoralen determined by high-pressure liquid chromatography in psoriatic patients ingesting drug from two manufacturers. J Invest Dermatol 1980; 74:59–62.
18. Anderson KE, Menne T, Gammeltoft M, et al: Pharmacokinetics and clinic comparison of two 8-methoxypsoralen brands. Arch Dermatol Res 1980; 268:23–29.
19. Menne T, Anderson KE, Larsen E, et al: Pharmacokinetic comparison of seven 8-methoxypsoralen brands. Acta Derm Venereol (Stockh) 1981; 61:137–140.
20. Stolk LM, Kammeijer A, Cormane RH, et al: Serum levels of 8-methoxypsoralen: Differences between two oral methods of administration. Br J Dermatol 1980; 103:417–420.
21. Hönigsmann H, Jaschke E, Nitsche V, et al: Serum levels of 8-methoxypsoralen in two different drug preparations: Correlation with photosensitivity and dose requirements for photochemotherapy. J Invest Dermatol 1982; 79:233–236.
22. Langner A, Wolska H: New galenical form of 8-methoxypsoralen in photochemotherapy of psoriasis. Arch Dermatol Res 1981; 271:461–462.
23. Monbaliu JG, Bogaert MG, DeBersaques J, et al: Problems with commercial formulations of 8-methoxypsoralen. Dermatologica 1981; 163:468–473.

24. Nitsche V, Raff M, Bardach H: 8-Methoxypsoralen (8-MOP) in neuer galenischer Zubereitung und seine Beziehung zum 8-MOP serumspiegel. Arch Dermatol Res 1981; 271:11–17.
25. Wulf HC, Hart J: Distribution of tritium-labelled 8-methoxypsoralen in the rat, studied by whole body autoradiography. Acta Derm Venereol (Stockh) 1979; 59:97–103.
26. Muni IA, Schneider H, Olsson TA, et al: Absorption, distribution, and excretion of 8-methoxypsoralen in HRA/SKH mice. Natl Cancer Inst Monogr 1984; 66:85–90.
27. de Wolff FA, Thomas TV: Clinical pharmacokinetics of methoxsalen and other psoralens. Clin Pharmacokinet 1986; 11:62–75.
28. Schmid J, Prox A, Zipp H, et al: The use of stable isotopes to prove the saturable first-pass effect of methoxsalen. Biomed Mass Spectrom 1980; 7:560–564.
29. Andrew E, Nilsen A, Thune P, et al: Photochemotherapy in psoriasis—Clinical response and 8-MOP plasma concentrations at two dose levels. Clin Exp Dermatol 1981; 6:591–600.
30. Kligman AM, Goldstein FP: Ineffectiveness of trioxalen as an oral photosensitizer. Arch Dermatol 1973; 107:413–414.
31. Pathak MA, Fitzpatrick TB, Parrish JA: Pharmacologic and molecular aspects of psoralen photochemotherapy. In Farber EM, Cox AJ (eds): Psoriasis: Proceedings of the Second International Symposium. New York: Yorke Medical Books, 1977, 262–271.
32. Bickers DR, Pathak MA: Psoralen pharmacology: Studies on metabolism and enzyme induction. Natl Canc Inst Monogr 1984; 66:77–84.
33. Schmid J, Prox A, Reuter A, et al: The metabolism of 8-methoxypsoralen in man. Eur J Drug Metab Pharmacokinet 1980a; 5:81–92.
34. McEvoy MT, Stern RS: Psoralens and related compounds in the treatment of psoriasis. Pharmacol Ther 1987; 34:75–97.
35. Herfst MJ, de Wolff FA: Intraindividual and interindividual variability in 8-methoxypsoralen kinetics and effect in psoriatic patients. Clin Pharmacol Ther 1983; 34:117–124.
36. Harber LC, Bickers DR: Photosensitivity Diseases (1st ed). Philadelphia: WB Saunders 1981, 45–55.
37. Fleming MG, Brody N: Biologic effectiveness of black light fluorescent lamps for PUVA [letter]. J Am Acad Dermatol 1985; 12:894–895.
38. Cole RS: Psoralen monoadducts and interstrand cross-links in DNA. Biochim Biophys Acta 1971; 254:30–39.
39. Song PS, Tapley KI: Photochemistry and photobiology of psoralens. Photochem Photobiol 1979; 29:1177–1197.
40. Johnston BH, Johnson MA, Moore CB, et al: Psoralen-DNA photoreaction: Controlled reaction of mono and diadducts with nanosecond ultraviolet laser pulses. Science 1977; 197:906–908.
41. Cech T, Pathak MA, Biswas RK: An electron microscopic study of the photochemical cross-linking of DNA in guinea pig epidermis by psoralen derivatives. Biochim Biophys Acta 1979; 562:342–360.
42. Lerche A, Sondergaard J, Wadskov S, et al: DNA interstrand crosslinks visualized by electron microscopy in PUVA-treated psoriasis. Acta Derm Venereol (Stockh) 1979; 59:15–20.
43. Walter JF, Voorhees JJ, Kelsey WH, et al: Psoralen plus black light inhibits epidermal DNA synthesis. Arch Dermatol 1973; 107:861–865.
44. Fritsch PO, Gschnait F, Kaaserer G, et al: PUVA suppresses the proliferative stimulus produced by stripping on hairless mice. J Invest Dermatol 1979; 73:188–190.
45. Pathak MA: Mechanisms of psoralen photosensitization reactions. Natl Cancer Inst Monogr 1984; 66:41–46.
46. Pohl J, Christophers E: Photo inactivation of skin fibroblasts by fractionated treatment with 8-methoxypsoralen and UVA. J Invest Dermatol 1979; 73:176–179.

47. Cormane RH, Hamerlinck F, Siddiqui AH: Immunologic implications of PUVA therapy in psoriasis vulgaris. Arch Dermatol Res 1979; 265:245–267.
48. Okamoto H, Takigawa M, Horio T: Alteration of lymphocyte functions by 8-methoxypsoralen and longwave ultraviolet radiation: I. Suppressive effects of PUVA on T-lymphocyte migration in vitro. J Invest Dermatol 1985; 84:203–205.
49. Pathak MA, Joshi PC: Production of active oxygen species ($^1O_2$ and O_2^-) by psoralens and ultraviolet radiation (320–400 nm). Biochim Biophys Acta 1984; 798:115–126.
50. Vedaldi D, Dall'Acqua F, Gennaro A: Photosensitized effects of furocoumarins: The possible role of singlet oxygen. Z Naturforsch [C] 1983; 38:866–869.
51. Fisher T: Topical psoralen ultraviolet radiation. In Roenigk HH, Maibach HI (eds): Psoriasis (1st ed). New York: Dekker, 1985:493–504.
52. Rodighiero G, Dall'Acqua F: In vitro photoreactions of selected psoralens and methylangelicins with DNA, RNA, and proteins. Natl Cancer Inst Monogr 1984; 66:31–40.
53. Hönigsmann H, Wolff K, Konrad K: Epidermal lysosomes and ultraviolet light. J Invest Dermatol 1974; 63:337–342.
54. Rosario R, Mark GJ, Parrish JA, et al: Histological changes produced in skin by equally erythemogenic doses of UVA, UVB, UVC and UVA with psoralens. Br J Dermatol 1979; 101:299–308.
55. Zaynoun S, Konrad K, Gschnait F, et al: The pigmentary response to photochemotherapy. Acta Derm Venereol (Stockh) 1977; 57:431–440.
56. Toda K, Pathak MA, Parrish JA, et al: Alteration of racial differences in melanosome distribution in human epidermis after exposure to ultraviolet light. Nature [New Biol] 1972; 236:143–145.
57. Parrish JA, LeVine MA, Fitzpatrick TB: Oral methoxsalen photochemotherapy of psoriasis and mycosis fungoides. Int J Dermatol 1980; 19:379–386.
58. Wolff K, Hönigsmann H: Clinical aspects of photochemotherapy. Pharmacol Ther 1981; 12:381–418.
59. Roenigk HH, Farber EM, Stons F, et al: Photochemotherapy for psoriasis. Arch Dermatol 1979; 115:576–579.
60. Wolff K, Fitzpatrick TB, Parrish JA, et al: Photochemotherapy for psoriasis with orally administered methoxsalen. Arch Dermatol 1976; 112:945–950.
61. Gupta AK, Anderson TF: Psoralen photochemotherapy. J Am Acad Dermatol 1987; 17:703–734.
62. Hönigsmann H, Gschnait F, Konrad K, et al: Photochemotherapy for pustular psoriasis (von Zumbusch). Br J Dermatol 1977; 97:119–126.
63. Boer J, Hermans J, Schothorst AA, et al: A comparison of phototherapy (UVB) and photochemotherapy (PUVA) for clearing and maintenance therapy of psoriasis. Arch Dermatol 1989; 120:52–57.
64. Stern RS: Long-term use of psoralens and ultraviolet A for psoriasis: Evidence for efficacy and cost savings. J Am Acad Dermatol 1986; 14:520–526.
65. Stern RS, Melsk JW: Long-term continuation of psoralen and ultraviolet-A treatment of psoriasis. Arch Dermatol 1982; 118:400–403.
66. Perlman SG, Gerber LH, Roberts M, et al: Photochemotherapy and psoriatic arthritis. Ann Intern Med 1979; 91:717–722.
67. Morison WL: Phototherapy and Photochemotherapy of Skin Disease. New York: Praeger, 1983, 75–79.
68. Bleehen SS: Treatment of vitiligo with oral 4,5′,8-trimethylpsoralen (Trisoralen). Br J Dermatol 1972; 86:54–60.
69. Parrish JA, Fitzpatrick TB, Shea C, et al: Photochemotherapy of vitiligo. Use of orally administered psoralens and a high-intensity long-wave ultraviolet light system. Arch Dermatol 1976; 112:1531–1534.
70. Singh M, Kanwar AJ, Bharija SC, et al: Daily psoralen therapy in vitiligo [letter]. Arch Dermatol 1987; 123:1279–1280.
71. Ortel B, Tanew A, Hönigsmann H: Vitiligo treatment. In Hönigsmann H, Stingl G

(eds): Current Problems in Dermatology (vol 15). Basel, Switzerland: Karger, 1986, 265–271.
72. Grimes PE, Minus HR, Chakrabarti SG, et al: Determination of optimal topical photochemotherapy for vitiligo. J Am Acad Dermatol 1982; 7:771–778.
73. Fulton JE Jr, Leyden J, Papa C: Treatment of vitiligo with topical methoxsalen and blacklite. Arch Dermatol 1969; 100:224–229.
74. Elliot JA: Methoxsalen in the treatment of vitiligo. Arch Dermatol 1959; 77:237–243.
75. Hönigsmann H, Wolff K, Fitzpatrick TB, et al: Oral photochemotherapy with psoralens and UVA (PUVA): Principles and practice. In Fitzpatrick TB, Eisen AZ, Wolff K, et al (eds): Dermatology in General Medicine (3rd ed). New York: McGraw-Hill, 1987, 1533–1558.
76. Gilchrist BA, Parrish JA, Tanenbaum L, et al: Oral methoxsalen photochemotherapy of mycosis fungoides. Cancer 1976; 38:683–689.
77. Heald PW, Edelson RL: Photopheresis therapy of cutaneous T cell lymphoma. Keio J Med 1988; 37(2):155–167.
78. Edelson R, Berger C, Gasparro F, et al: Treatment of cutaneous T cell lymphoma by extracorporeal photochemotherapy: Preliminary results. N Engl J Med 1987; 316:297–303.
79. Thomsen K, Hammar H, Molin L, et al: Retinoids plus PUVA (RePUVA) and PUVA in mycosis fungoides, plaque stage: A report from the Scandinavian Mycosis Fungoides Group. Acta Derm Venereol (Stockh) 1989; 69:536–538.
80. Abel EA, Sendagorta E, Hoppe RT, et al: PUVA treatment of erythrodermic and plaque-type mycosis fungoides. Ten-year follow-up study. Arch Dermatol 1987; 123:897–901.
81. Roenigk HH: Photochemotherapy for mycosis fungoides. Arch Dermatol 1977; 113:1047–1051.
82. Warin AP: Photochemotherapy in the treatment of psoriasis and mycosis fungoides. Clin Exp Dermatol 1981; 6:651–657.
83. Molin L, Thomsen K, Volden G, et al: Photochemotherapy (PUVA) in the tumour stage of mycosis fungoides: A report from the Scandanavian Mycosis Fungoides Study Group. Acta Derm Venereol (Stockh) 1981; 61:52–54.
84. Lowe NJ, Cripps DJ, Dufton PA, et al: Photochemotherapy for mycosis fungoides: A clinical and histological study. Arch Dermatol 1979; 115:50–53.
85. Hönigsmann H, Brenner W, Rauschmeier W, et al: Photochemotherapy for cutaneous T cell lymphoma. J Am Acad Dermatol 1984; 10:238–245.
86. Niema KM: PUVA treatment in mycosis fungoides. Dermatologica 1979; 158:462–467.
87. Neumann C, Kolde G, Bonsmann G: Histiocytosis X in an elderly patient. Ultrastructure and immunochemistry after PUVA photochemotherapy. Br J Dermatol 1988; 119:385–391.
88. Morison WL, Parrish JA, Fitzpatrick TB: Oral psoralen photochemotherapy of atopic eczema. Br J Dermatol 1978; 98:25–30.
89. Atherton DJ, Carabott F, Glover MT, et al: The role of psoralen photochemotherapy (PUVA) in the treatment of severe atopic eczema in adolescents. Br J Dermatol 1988; 118:791–795.
90. Sheehan-Dare RA, Goodfield MJ, Rowell NR: Topical psoralen photochemotherapy (PUVA) and superficial radiotherapy in the treatment of chronic hand eczema. Br J Dermatol 1989; 121:65–69.
91. Rosén K, Jontell M, Mobacken H, et al: Epidermal Langerhans' cells in chronic eczematous dermatitis of the palms treated with PUVA and UVB. Acta Derm Venereol (Stockh) 1989; 69:200–205.
92. Kalimo K, Lammintausta K, Viander M, et al: PUVA treatment of nickel contact dermatitis: Effect on dermatitis, patch test sensitivity, and lymphocyte transformation reactivity. Photodermatol 1989; 6:16–19.
93. Rosén K: Pustulosis palmoplantaris and chronic eczematous hand dermatitis. Treat-

ment, epidermal Langerhans' cells and association with thyroid disease. Acta Derm Venereol (Stockh) 1988; 137(Suppl):1–52.
94. Lehtinen R, Happonen RP, Kuusilehto A, et al: A clinical trial of PUVA treatment in oral lichen planus. Proc Finn Dent Soc 1989; 85:29–33.
95. Ortonne JD, Thivolet J, Sannwald C: Oral photochemotherapy in the treatment of lichen planus: Clinical results, histological and ultrastructural observations. Br J Dermatol 1978; 99:77–88.
96. Boelen RE, Faber WR, Lambers JCCA, et al: Long-term follow-up of photochemotherapy in pityriasis lichenoides. Acta Derm Venereol (Stockh) 1982; 62:442–444.
97. Wantzin GL, Thomsen K: PUVA-treatment in lymphomatoid papulosis. Br J Dermatol 1982; 107:687–690.
98. Gschnait F, Hönigsmann H, Brenner W, et al: Induction of UV light tolerance by PUVA in patients with polymorphous light eruption. Br J Dermatol 1978; 99:293–296.
99. Morison WL: Phototherapy and photochemotherapy of skin disease. New York: Praeger, 1983, 80–81.
100. Parrish JA, Jaenicke KF, Morison WL, et al: Solar urticaria: Treatment with PUVA and mediator inhibitors. Br J Dermatol 1982; 106:575–580.
101. Ashinoff R, Buchness MR, Lim HW: Lymphoma in a black patient with actinic reticuloid treated with PUVA: Possible etiologic considerations. J Am Acad Dermatol 1989; 21:1134–1137.
102. Sinclair SW, Hindson C: PUVA therapy of chronic actinic dermatitis. Australas J Dermatol 1988; 29:117–119.
103. Farr PM, Diffey BL: Treatment of actinic prurigo with PUVA: Mechanism of action. Br J Dermatol 1989; 120:411–418.
104. Ross AM: PUVA therapy for erythropoietic protoporphyria. Photodermatol 1988; 5:148–149.
105. Gorin I, Lessana-Leibowitch M, Fortier P, et al: Successful treatment of the pruritus of human immunodeficiency virus infection and acquired immunodeficiency syndrome with psoralens plus ultraviolet A therapy. J Am Acad Dermatol 1989; 20:511–513.
106. Logan RA, O'Brien TJ, Greaves MW: The effect of psoralen photochemotherapy (PUVA) on symptomatic dermographism. Clin Exp Dermatol 1989; 14:25–28.
107. Christophers E, Hönigsmann H, Wolff K, et al: PUVA-treatment of urticaria pigmentosa. Br J Dermatol 1978; 98:701–702.
108. Kolde G, Frosch PJ, Czarnetzki BM: Response of cutaneous mast cells to PUVA in patients with urticaria pigmentosa: Histomorphometric, ultrastructural, and biochemical investigations. J Invest Dermatol 1984; 83:175–178.
109. Vaatainen N, Hannuksela M, Karvonew J: Local photochemotherapy in nodular prurigo. Acta Derm Venereol (Stockh) 1980; 59:544–547.
110. Hindson TC, Spiro JG, Cochrane H: PUVA therapy of diffuse granuloma annulare. Clin Exp Dermatol 1988; 13:26–27.
111. Kerker BJ, Huang CP, Morison WL: Photochemotherapy of generalized granuloma annulare. Arch Dermatol 1990; 126:359–361.
112. Patterson JW, Fitzwater JEW: Treatment of hypopigmented sarcoidosis with 8-methoxypsoralen and long wave ultraviolet light. Int J Dermatol 1984; 120:121–122.
113. Mitchell AJ, Krull EA: Alopecia areata: Pathogenesis and treatment. J Am Acad Dermatol 1984; 11:763–775.
114. Lassus A, Kianto U, Johansson E, et al: PUVA treatment for alopecia areata. Dermatologica 1980; 161:298–304.
115. Claudy AL, Gagnaire D: PUVA treatment of alopecia areata. Arch Dermatol 1983; 119:975–978.
116. Brown AC: Treatment of alopecia areata [letter]. Arch Dermatol 1985; 121:308–309.

117. Rook AH, Jegasothy BV, Heald P, et al: Extracorporeal photochemotherapy for drug-resistant pemphigus vulgaris. Ann Intern Med 1990; 112:303–305.
118. Jaschonek K, Einsele H, Schmidt J, et al: 8-methoxypsoralen and ultraviolet A therapy for cutaneous manifestations of graft-versus-host disease [letter]. Lancet 1988; 1:599.
119. Kapoor N, Wolverton SE, Copelan EA, et al: Psoralen and ultraviolet A radiation (PUVA) in the treatment of resistant chronic graft-versus-host disease (GVHD) [abstract]. Blood 1989; 74(Suppl):51a.
120. Hymes SR, Morison WL, Farmer ER, et al: Methoxsalen and ultraviolet A radiation in treatment of chronic cutaneous graft-versus-host reaction. J Am Acad Dermatol 1985; 12:30–37.
121. Paul BS, Arndt KA: Response of transient acantholytic dermatosis to photochemotherapy. Arch Dermatol 1984; 120:121–122.
122. Nožičková M, Bělobrádek, M: Progressive pigmented purpuric dermatosis: Effect of psoralens and ultraviolet A irradiation. Sb Ved Pr Lek Fak Karlovy Univerzity Hradci Kralove 1989; 32:45–55.
123. Manabe M, Yoshiike T, Negi M, et al: Successful treatment of icthyosis linearis circumflexa with PUVA. J Am Acad Dermatol 1983; 8:905–907.
124. Farr PM, Ive FA: PUVA treatment of scleromyxedema. Br J Dermatol 1984; 110:347–350.
125. Cloud T, Hakim R, Griffin AC: Photosensitization of the eye with methoxsalen: II. Chronic effects. Arch Ophthalmol (Chicago) 1962; 66:689–694.
126. Parrish JA, Chylack L, Woehler M, et al: Dermatological and ocular examinations of rabbits chronically photosensitized with methoxsalen. J Invest Dermatol 1979; 73:256–258.
127. Freeman RG, Troll D: Photosensitization of the eye by 8-methoxypsoralen. J Invest Dermatol 1969; 53:449–453.
128. Back O, Hollstrom E, Liden S, et al: Absence of cataracts 10 years after treatment with 8-methoxypsoralen. Acta Derm Venereol (Stockh) 1980; 60:79–80.
129. Pedvis-Leftick A, Crylin MN, Solomon LM: Cataracts in a patient with vitiligo with received photochemotherapy. Arch Dermatol 1979; 115:1253–1254.
130. Woo TY, Wong RC, Wong JM, et al: Lenticular psoralen photoproducts and cataracts of a PUVA-treated psoriatic patient. Arch Dermatol 1985; 121:1307–1308.
131. Boukes AJ, Bruynzeel DP: Ocular findings in 340 long-term treated PUVA patients. Photodermatol 1985; 2:178–180.
132. Lafond G, Roy PD, Grenier R: Lens opacities appearing during therapy with methoxsalen and long-wave radiation. Can J Ophthalmol 1984; 19:173–175.
133. Backman HA: The effects of PUVA on the eye. Am J Optom Physiol Opt 1982; 59:86–89.
134. Fenton DA, Wilkinson JD: Dose-related visual defects in patients receiving PUVA therapy [letter]. Lancet 1983; 1:1106.
135. Stern RS, Parrish JA, Fitzpatrick TB: Ocular findings in patients treated with PUVA. J Invest Dermatol 1985; 85:269–273.
136. Hammershoy O, Jessen F: A retrospective study of cataract formation in 96 patients treated with PUVA. Acta Derm Venereol (Stockh) 1982; 62:444–446.
137. Abdullah AN, Keczkes K: Cutaneous and ocular side effects of PUVA photochemotherapy: A 10-year follow-up study. Clin Exp Dermatol 1989; 14:421–424.
138. Cox NH, Jones SK, Downey DJ, et al: Cutaneous and ocular side-effects of oral photochemotherapy: Results of an 8-year follow-up study. Br J Dermatol 1987; 116:145–152.
139. Boettner EA, Wolter J: Transmission of the ocular media. Invest Ophthalmol 1962; 1:776–783.
140. Lerman S: Ocular side effects of psoriasis therapy. N Engl J Med 1980; 303:941–942.
141. Farber EM, Epstein JH, Nall L, et al: Current status of oral PUVA therapy for psoriasis. J Am Acad Dermatol 1982; 6:851–855.

142. Morison WL, Strickland PT: Environment UVA radiation and eye protection during PUVA therapy. J Am Acad Dermatol 1983; 9:522–525.
143. Stern R, Zierler S, Parrish JA: Psoriasis and the risk of cancer. J Invest Dermatol 1982; 78:147–149.
144. Halprin KM, Comerford M, Richard-Taylor J: Cancer in patients with psoriasis. J Am Acad Dermatol 1982; 7:633–638.
145. Stern RS, Thibodeau LA, Kleinerman RA, et al: Risk of cutaneous carcinoma in patients treated with oral methoxsalen photochemotherapy for psoriasis. N Engl J Med 1979; 300:809–813.
146. Stern RS, Laird N, Melski J, et al: Cutaneous squamous cell carcinoma in patients treated with PUVA. N Engl J Med 1984; 310:1156–1161.
147. Stern RS, Lange R: Non-melanoma skin cancer occurring in patients treated with PUVA five to ten years after first treatment. J Invest Dermatol 1988; 91:120–124.
148. Forman AB, Roenigk HH Jr, Caro WA, et al: Long-term follow-up of skin cancer in the PUVA-48 cooperative study. Arch Dermatol 1989; 125:515–519.
149. Hönigsmann H, Wolff K, Gschnait F, et al: Keratoses and non-melanoma skin tumors in long-term photochemotherapy (PUVA). J Am Acad Dermatol 1980; 3:406–414.
150. Lindskov R: Skin carcinomas and treatment with photochemotherapy (PUVA). Acta Derm Venereol (Stockh) 1983; 63:223–226.
151. Reshad H, Challoner F, Pollock DJ, et al: Cutaneous carcinoma in psoriatic patients treated with PUVA. Br J Dermatol 1984; 110:299–305.
152. Lassus A, Renaula J, Idanpaa-Heikkila J, et al: PUVA treatment and skin cancer. A follow-up study. Acta Derm Venereol (Stockh) 1981; 61:141–145.
153. Henseler T, Christophers E, Hönigsmann H, et al: Skin tumors in European PUVA study: Eight-year follow-up of 1,643 patients treated with PUVA for psoriasis. J Am Acad Dermatol 1987; 16:108–116.
154. Gupta AK, Stern RS, Swanson NA, et al: Cutaneous melanomas in patients treated with psoralens plus ultraviolet A: A case report and the experience of the PUVA follow-up study. J Am Acad Dermatol 1988; 19:67–76.
155. Stern RS, and Members of the Photochemotherapy Follow-up Study. Genital tumors among men with psoriasis exposed to psoralens and ultraviolet A radiation (PUVA) and ultraviolet B radiation. N Engl J Med 1990; 322:1093–1097.
156. Kanerva L, Lauharanta J: PUVA-lentigo. Photodermatology 1985; 2:49–51.
157. Ros A, Wennersten G, Lagerholm B: Long-term photochemotherapy for psoriasis: A histopathological and clinical follow-up study with special emphasis on tumor incidence and behavior of pigmented lesions. Acta Derm Venereol (Stockh) 1983; 63:215–221.
158. Abel EA, Reid H, Wood C, et al: PUVA-induced melanocytic atypia: Is it confined to PUVA lentigines? J Am Acad Dermatol 1985; 13:761–768.
159. Rhodes AR, Stern RS, Melski JW: The PUVA lentigo: An analysis of predisposing factors. J Invest Dermatol 1983; 81:459–463.
160. Niemi KM, Niemi A, Kanerva L: Morphologic changes in epidermis of PUVA-treated patients with psoriasis with or without a history of arsenic therapy. Arch Dermatol 1983; 119:904–909.
161. Rhodes AR, Harrist TJ, Momtaz-T K: The PUVA-induced pigmented macule: A lentiginous proliferation of large, sometimes cytologically atypical, melanocytes. J Am Acad Dermatol 1983; 9:47–58.
162. Bleehen SS: Freckles induced by PUVA treatment. Br J Dermatol 1978; 99(Suppl): 20–21.
163. Kietzmann H, Goos M, Christophers E: PUVA-lentigines with atypical melanocyte hyperplasia after long-term photochemotherapy [abstract]. In Second International Symposium on the Treatment of Psoriasis, Herzl, Israel, 1981.
164. Kanerva L, Lauharanta L, Niemi KM, et al: Persistent ashen-gray maculae and freckles induced by long-term PUVA treatment. Dermatologica 1983; 166:281–286.

165. Miller RA: Psoralens and UVA-induced stellate hyperpigmented freckling. Arch Dermatol 1982; 118:619–620.
166. Hofmann C, Plewig G, Braun-Falco O: Ungewöhnliche Nebenwirkungen bei oraler Photochomeotherapie (PUVA-therapie) der Psoriasis. Hautarzt 1977; 28:583–588.
167. Marx JL, Auerbach R, Possick P, et al: Malignant melanoma in sites in two patients treated with psoralens and ultraviolet A. J Am Acad Dermatol 1983; 9:904–911.
168. Friedman PS, Rogers S: Photochemotherapy of psoriasis: DNA damage in blood lymphocytes. J Invest Dermatol 1980; 74:440–443.
169. Viander M, Jansen CT, Eskola J: Influence of whole-body PUVA treatments on peripheral blood: NK cell activity. Photodermatol 1984; 1:23–29.
170. Bredberg A, Forsgren A: Effects of in-vitro PUVA on human leukocyte function. Br J Dermatol 1984; 111:159–168.
171. Verhagen AR, Bergers M, deJongh G, et al: Effects of PUVA on human blood monocytes in-vitro. J Invest Dermatol 1983; 81:201–203.
172. Guilhou JJ, Cloth J, Guillot B, et al: Immunological aspects of psoriasis: IV. Presence of circulating immune complexes in patients before and after PUVA therapy: Correlation with T-cell markers. Br J Dermatol 1980; 102:173–178.
173. Moscicki RA, Morison WL, Parrish JA, et al: Reduction of fraction of circulating helper-inducer T-cells identified by monoclonal antibodies in psoriatic patients treated with long-term psoralen/ultraviolet-A radiation (PUVA). J Invest Dermatol 1982; 79:205–208.
174. Scherer R, Kern B, Braun-Falco O: UVA induced inhibition of proliferation of PHA-stimulated lymphocytes from humans treated with 8-methoxypsoralen. Br J Dermatol 1977; 97:519–528.
175. Kalimo K, Koulu L, Jansen CT: Effect of single UVB or PUVA exposure on immediate and delayed skin hypersensitivity reactions in humans. Arch Dermatol Res 1983; 275:374–378.
176. Moss C, Friedman PS, Shuster S: How does PUVA inhibit delayed cutaneous hypersensitivity? Br J Dermatol 1982; 107:511–516.
177. Stern RS, Lange R: Cardiovascular disease, cancer, and cause of death in patients with psoriasis: 10 years prospective experience in a cohort of 1,380 patients. J Invest Dermatol 1988; 91:197–201.
178. Thomsen K, Schmidt H: PUVA-induced bullous pemphigoid. Br J Dermatol 1976; 95:568–569.
179. Robinson JK, Baughman RD, Provost TT: Bullous pemphigoid induced by PUVA therapy. Br J Dermatol 1978; 99:709–713.
180. Albergo RP, Gilgor RS: Delayed onset of bullous pemphigoid after PUVA and sunlight treatment of psoriasis. Cutis 1982; 30:621–624.
181. Abel EA, Bennett A: Bullous pemphigoid: Occurrence in psoriasis treated with psoralens plus long-wave ultraviolet radiation. Arch Dermatol 1979; 115:988–989.
182. Millins JL, McDuffie FC, Muller SA, et al: Development of photosensitivity and an SLE-like syndrome in a patient with psoriasis. Arch Dermatol 1978; 114:1177–1181.
183. Eyanson S, Greist MC, Brandt KS, et al: Systemic lupus erythematosus. Association with psoralen-ultraviolet. A treatment of psoriasis. Arch Dermatol 1979; 115:54–56.
184. Bruze M, Krook G, Ljunggren B: Fatal connective tissue disease with antinuclear antibodies following PUVA therapy. Acta Derm Venereol (Stockh) 1984; 64:157–160.
185. Bjellerup M, Bruze M, Forsgren A, et al: Antinuclear antibodies during PUVA therapy. Acta Derm Venereol (Stockh) 1978; 59:73–75.
186. Bruze M, Ljunggren B: Antinuclear antibodies appearing during PUVA therapy. Acta Derm Venereol (Stockh) 1985; 65:31–36.
187. Stern RS, Morison WL, Thibodeau LA, et al: Antinuclear antibodies and oral methoxsalen photochemotherapy (PUVA) for psoriasis. Arch Dermatol 1979; 115:1320–1324.
188. Levin DL, Roenigk HH Jr, Caro WA, et al: Histologic, immunofluorescent, and

antinuclear antibody findings in PUVA-treated patients. J Am Acad Dermatol 1982; 6:328–333.
189. Kubba R, Steck WD, Clough JD: Antinuclear antibodies and PUVA photochemotherapy. Arch Dermatol 1981; 117:474–477.
190. Dowdy MJ, Nigra TP, Barth WF: Subacute cutaneous lupus erythematosus during PUVA therapy for psoriasis: Case report and review of the literature. Arthritis Rheum 1989; 32:343–346.
191. Jones C, Bleehen SS: Acne induced by PUVA treatment. Br Med J 1977; 2:866.
192. Tegner E: Seborrheic dermatitis of the face induced by PUVA treatment. Acta Derm Venereol (Stockh) 1983; 63:335–339.
193. Rogers S, Marks J, Shuster S: Itch following photochemotherapy for psoriasis. Acta Derm Venereol (Stockh) 1981; 61:178–180.
194. Tegner E: Severe skin pain after PUVA treatment. Acta Derm Venereol (Stockh) 1979; 59:467–470.
195. Miller J, Munro DD: Severe skin pain following PUVA. Acta Derm Venereol (Stockh) 1980; 60:187.
196. Todes-Taylor N, Abel EA, Cox AJ: The occurrence of vitiligo after psoralens and ultraviolet A therapy. J Am Acad Dermatol 1983; 9:526–532.
197. Rampen FHJ: Hypertrichosis in PUVA-treated patients. Br J Dermatol 1983; 109:657–660.
198. Reymond JL, Beani JC, Amblard P: Superficial actinic porokeratosis in a patient undergoing long-term PUVA therapy. Acta Derm Venereol (Stockh) 1980; 60:539–540.
199. Rau RC, Flowers FP, Barnett JL: Photo-onycholysis secondary to psoralen use. Arch Dermatol 1978; 114:448.
200. Nalk RPC, Paramesuara YR: 8-methoxypsoralen-induced nail pigmentation. Int J Dermatol 1982; 21:275–276.
201. Hofman C, Plewig G, Braun-Falco O: Bowenoid lesions, Bowen's disease and keratoacanthomas in long-term PUVA-treated patients. Br J Dermatol 1979; 101:685–692.
202. Lorette G, Jafar R, Grojean MF, et al: Xeroderma pigmentosum–like changes [letter]. Arch Dermatol 1983; 119:873–874.
203. Bjellerup M, Bruze M, Hansson A, et al: Liver injury following administration of 8-methoxypsoralen during PUVA therapy. Acta Derm Venereol (Stockh) 1979; 59:371–372.
204. Pariser DM, Wyles RJ: Toxic hepatitis from oral methoxsalen photochemotherapy (PUVA). J Am Acad Dermatol 1980; 3:248–250.
205. Freeman K, Warin AP: Deterioration of liver function during PUVA therapy. Photodermatol 1984; 1:147–148.
206. Wagner J, Mauthrope R, Philip P, et al: Preleukemia (haemopoietic dysplasia) developing in a patient with psoriasis treated with 8-methoxypsoralen and ultraviolet light (PUVA) treatment. Scand J Haematol 1978; 21:299–304.
207. Hansen NE: Development of acute myeloid leukemia in a patient with psoriasis treated with oral 8-methoxypsoralen and long wave ultraviolet light. Scand J Haematol 1979; 22:57–60.
208. Lam Thuon Mine LTK, Williams RP, Anderson JL, et al: Nephrotic syndrome after treatment with psoralens and ultraviolet-A. Br Med J (Clin Res) 1983; 287:94–95.
209. Burnett JW: Acute gout secondary to psoriasis exacerbated by photochemotherapy. Arch Dermatol 1982; 118:211.
210. Anderson CD, Frodin T: Unusual adverse effects of methoxypsoralen: Bronchial reaction during photochemotherapy. J Am Acad Dermatol 1984; 10:298.
211. Ramsey B, Marks JM: Bronchoconstriction due to 8-methoxypsoralen. J Am Acad Dermatol 1988; 119:83–86.
212. Melski JW, Stern RS: Annual rate of psoralen and ultraviolet-A treatment of psoriasis after initial clearing. Arch Dermatol 1982; 118:404–408.

213. Fisher T, Alsins J: Treatment of psoriasis with trioxsalen baths and dysprosium lamps. Acta Derm Venereol (Stockh) 1976; 56:383–390.
214. Hannuksela M, Karvonen J: Trioxsalen bath plus UVA effective and safe in the treatment of psoriasis. Br J Dermatol 1978; 99:703–707.
215. Turjanmaa K, Salo H, Reunala T: Comparison of trioxsalen bath and oral methoxsalen PUVA in psoriasis. Acta Derm Venereol (Stockh) 1985; 65:86–88.
216. Schmoll M, Henseler T, Christophers E: Evaluation of PUVA, topical corticosteroids, and the combination of both in the treatment of psoriasis. Br J Dermatol 1978; 99:693–702.
217. Cripps DJ, Lowe NJ: Photochemotherapy for psoriasis remission times: Psoralens and UVA and combined photochemotherapy with anthralin. Clin Exp Dermatol 1979; 4:477–483.
218. Momtaz-T K, Parrish JA: Combination UVB and PUVA in the treatment of psoriasis [abstract]. J Invest Dermatol 1981; 76:303.
219. Diette KM, Momtaz-T K, Parrish JA, et al: Psoralens and UV-A and UV-B twice weekly for treatment of psoriasis. Arch Dermatol 1984; 120:1169–1173.
220. Morison WL, Momtaz-T K, Mosher K, et al: Combined methotrexate–PUVA in the treatment of psoriasis. J Am Acad Dermatol 1982; 6:46–51.
221. Fritsch PO, Hönigsmann H, Jaschke E, et al: Augmentation of oral methoxsalen-photochemotherapy with an oral retinoic acid derivative. J Invest Dermatol 1978; 70:178–182.
222. Grupper C, Berretti B: Treatment of psoriasis by oral PUVA therapy combined with aromatic retinoids (Ro 10–9359; Tigason). Dermatologica 1981; 162:404–413.
223. Hönigsmann H, Wolff K: Isotretinoin–PUVA for psoriasis [letter]. Lancet 1983; 1:236.

10 | Dapsone and Sulfapyridine

Kenneth E. Greer, M.D.

Fromm and Wittmann first synthesized dapsone (diaminodiphenylsulfone, or DDS) in 1908; in 1937, the chemically related sulfonamides were shown to possess antibacterial activity in experimental streptococcal infections in mice.[1] The first use of dapsone in humans occurred in 1938, also against streptococcal infections, but the very large dosages that were prescribed (1–2 g/day) resulted in severe hemolytic anemia and methemoglobinemia. Thus the early use of sulfones was limited in humans, especially because the sulfonamides were more effective against common bacterial infections at lower dosages. However, in 1940, sulfones were found to be effective in treating experimental tuberculosis in animals, and shortly thereafter they gained prominence as the first truly effective therapy for leprosy. Dapsone remains the mainstay of therapy of leprosy for more than two million people around the world today. The sulfones were also used for their antimalarial effects in the 1940s, and it was documented in 1960 that there was a low prevalence of malaria in dapsone-treated leprosy patients.[1]

Early in their history, the sulfones were shown to possess antiinflammatory activity for various dermatologic diseases, primarily dermatitis herpetiformis (in the early 1950s) and subcorneal pustular dermatosis (in 1956). More recently, the sulfones have been widely used for a host of dermatologic diseases, quite successfully for some (dermatitis herpetiformis, subcorneal pustular dermatosis, erythema elevatum diutinum, bullous lupus erythemathosus) and with marginal benefit for a number of other diseases (pemphigus, granuloma faciale, bullous pemphigoid, etc.). The antibiotic spectrum of dapsone has been expanded to include *Pneumocystis carinii* infection in patients with acquired immunodeficiency syndrome (AIDS), as well as cutaneous leishmaniasis.

The history of the development of sulfapyridine, which is actually a sulfonamide and not a sulfone, is less well described in the literature, inasmuch as its antibacterial activity was not as strong as that of the other sulfonamides. In addition, the absorption of sulfapyridine after its oral administration is slow and erratic, and it is difficult to predict blood levels, which often limits its usefulness. The drug was, however, shown to be effective against dermatitis herpetiformis (DH), as well as acrodermatitis continua (or Hallopeau's acrodermatitis), before dapsone's effectiveness was established. Sulfapyridine is still used today, albeit less frequently than dapsone, for DH and, rarely, for other dapsone-responsive dermatoses. Salicylazosulfapyridine (sulfasalazine), a compound in common use for ulcerative colitis, is actually broken down in the body to aminosalicylic acid and sulfapyridine, but the absorption of salicylazosulfapyridine is much less than that of sulfapyridine alone and thus has limited usefulness for dermatologic diseases.

Pharmacology

Structure

The chemical structures of the sulfones and sulfapyridine are different. Sulfapyridine has linkage of sulfur to atoms other than oxygen, namely nitrogen. Dapsone is an odorless, white crystalline powder with a slightly bitter taste. It is poorly soluble in water but is freely soluble in alcohol. Dapsone may discolor after exposure to light, although there is no chemical change after discoloration. Diasone (sulfoxone sodium) is a substituted form of dapsone and is more water-soluble than dapsone, but its absorption is irregular, and it must be metabolized to dapsone before it is effective. Diasone has no advantage over dapsone and is no longer used in the U.S., although it is still available in Canada and in Europe.

Sulfapyridine is actually an intermediate-acting antibacterial sulfonamide and occurs in the form of white, odorless crystals or powder and, like dapsone, is more soluble in alcohol than in water. It also darkens when exposed to light.

Absorption/Distribution

Dapsone is absorbed slowly, but almost completely, from the gastrointestinal tract. Because other sulfones must be metabolized to dapsone in the body for effectiveness, dapsone is the major sulfone used in clinical medicine today. Plasma concentrations generally peak within 6 hours after oral administration of the drug, but the serum levels vary remarkably from patient to patient. This variation in serum levels occurs for a number of reasons, including differences in body weight, in absorption, and in degree of acetylation. The steady-state serum level is achieved in 1 week. Interestingly, and without explanation, higher dapsone blood concentrations are found in women than in men.[2] Dapsone is distributed in all tissues, but it concentrates in the skin, the liver, the muscles, and the kidneys. Levels in the skin may be as high as ten times that in the serum. Trace concentrations of dapsone may be present in the tissues up to 3 weeks after discontinuation of the drug. Dapsone is also distributed to sweat, saliva, tears, sputum, bile, and breast milk. Dapsone does cross the placenta. It does not penetrate ocular tissue well, which is of significance in patients with ocular involvement by leprosy. Sulfapyridine is absorbed slowly but incompletely from the gastrointestinal tract, and peak blood concentrations are also reached within 6 hours.

Metabolism/Excretion

Dapsone is approximately 70% protein-bound and is metabolized in the liver and eliminated primarily by the kidneys. There is remarkable interindividual variation in its half-life in plasma, which may range from 10 to 83 hours but averages 20–30 hours. Of a single 100-mg oral dose, 90% is eliminated within 9 days. Metabolism in the liver includes acetylation, but deacetylation occurs simultaneously, and equilibrium between acetylated and nonacetylated dapsone is reached rapidly. The acetylator status (slow/fast) of the patient has no effect on either the clinical efficacy or the associated adverse effects of dapsone.[3] Dapsone and its acetylated derivative are conjugated with glucuronic acid in the liver and are excreted by the kidneys. Approximately 10% of the drug is excreted in the bile.

Sulfapyridine may undergo acetylation (but not deacetylation), hydroxylation, and conjugation with glucuronic acid in the liver. More than 50% of patients are slow acetylators, and they may experience an increased incidence of adverse effects. Sulfapyridine and its metabolites are excreted principally in the urine. The drug is available in 500-mg tablets, and the dosage for the treatment of DH in adults is 1.5–2.0 g/day.

Mechanism of Action

Like antimalarials, sulfones have antimicrobial as well as anti-inflammatory effects, and the mode of action is different in microbial-induced diseases than in the noninfectious dermatologic disorders.

ANTIBACTERIAL ACTIVITY. Sulfones have antimicrobial activity against leprosy and other infectious diseases that is similar to that of other sulfonamides in that they act as antimetabolites against para-aminobenzoic acid in folate synthesis. Dapsone readily penetrates the bacterial cells and is both bactericidal and bacteriostatic against *Mycobacterium leprae*. Dapsone is also somewhat effective against all multiplying stages in the life cycle of plasmodia and appears to retain full activity against plasmodia that have developed resistance to 4-aminoquinoline antimalarials, such as chloroquine.[4] Sulfapyridine has the same mechanism of action as the other antibacterial sulfonamides, but it is not used for infectious diseases because of its toxicity and relative lack of efficacy when compared with currently used sulfonamides.

ANTI-INFLAMMATORY ACTIVITY. The exact mechanism of action of sulfone and sulfapyridine in noninfectious diseases has not been elucidated, but dapsone has been shown to suppress nonspecific inflammation, the Arthus reaction, and adjuvant-induced arthritis in a manner comparable with that of corticosteroids and indomethacin.[3] Many of the cutaneous diseases that are responsive to dapsone are thought to be autoimmune in nature or, in particular, to be diseases in which polymorphonuclear leukocytes (PMLs) have a prominent pathophysiologic role.[4] Activated PMLs generate superoxide radicals through the action of reduced nicotinamide adenine dinucleotide phosphate (NADPH) oxidase on O_2. Superoxide dismutase in turn generates H_2O_2 from superoxide simultaneously with PML myeloperoxidase release. Dapsone is believed to inhibit myeloperoxidase generation of toxic oxygen intermediates derived from H_2O_2.[4] In addition, dapsone interferes with the formation of hypochlorite and other strong oxidants produced from the halide component of the PMLs myeloperoxidase-peroxide-halide system. Dapsone can also inhibit mitogen-stimulated lymphocyte transformation but does not appear to have an effect on complement deposition, at least in DH or in normal skin. There are effects on membrane-associated phospholipid metabolism, lysosomal enzymes, tissue proteinases, neutrophil chemotaxis, and a variety of cells of the host defense system, but the specific mechanism of action of dapsone and how it affects such a wide spectrum of dermatologic diseases are unknown.

The literature contains very little information concerning the mechanism of action of sulfapyridine in noninfectious dermatologic disorders.

Clinical Use (Table 10–1)

Approved Indications

Dapsone is approved for use for infectious and noninfectious diseases, and the *Physicians' Desk Reference* lists two disorders (leprosy and DH) under indications and usage. There are other disorders against which dapsone may be efficacious (see Table 10–1). Sulfapyridine is used almost exclusively for noninfectious diseases and predominantly for DH and closely related disorders, such as chronic bullous dermatosis of childhood. Dapsone is available in 25-mg and 100-mg scored tablets. Sulfapyridine is available only in 500-mg tablets.

DERMATITIS HERPETIFORMIS. Dapsone is the drug of choice in the

Table 10–1. Dapsone/Sulfapyridine Indications/Contraindications

FDA-Approved Dermatologic Indications

Dermatitis Herpetiformis[5–10]*
Leprosy[11,12]*

Other Dermatologic Uses

Bullous Diseases

   Linear IgA bullous dermatosis/chronic bullous dermatosis of childhood[13–17]*
   Bullous systemic lupus erythematosus[18–21]*
   Subcorneal pustular dermatosis[22,23]*
   Vesicular/bullous pemphigoid[24–26]
   Cicatricial pemphigoid[27,28]
   Pemphigus (superficial subtypes)[29–31]
   Hailey-Hailey disease[32,33]

Vasculitis

   Erythema elevatum diutinum[34,35]*
   Granuloma faciale[36,37]
   Vasculitis (leukocytoclastic)[38–40]

Neutrophilic Dermatoses (Neutrophilic Vascular Reactions)

   Pyoderma gangrenosum[41]
   Sweet's syndrome[42,43]
   Behçet's disease/aphthous ulcers[44,45]

Pilosebaceous Diseases

   Acne (nodulocystic)[46,47]
   Granulomatous rosacea[48]

Infectious Diseases

   Actinomycotic mycetoma[49]
   Malaria (chloroquine resistant)[50]
   Cutaneous leishmaniasis[51]
   Pneumocystis carinii pneumonia in AIDS[52]

Other Dermatoses

   Pustular psoriasis[53]
   Brown recluse spider bites[54]*
   Panniculitis[55]
   Relapsing polychondritis[56]
   Granuloma annulare[57]

Contraindications

   Dapsone is contraindicated for patients who are hypersensitive to the drug, and the same can be said for sulfapyridine, although cross-sensitivity between the two drugs is uncommon.

Note: FDA = Food and Drug Administration.
*Dapsone is generally considered the drug of choice.

treatment of DH. The response rate approaches 100%, assuming that the patient can tolerate the drug.[5-8] In fact, before the availability of various diagnostic laboratory tests became widespread, a dapsone trial was frequently used as confirmation of a suspected diagnosis of DH. However, a number of other bullous dermatoses may also respond to dapsone, and a specific diagnosis of DH cannot be made by means of the therapeutic trial alone. Patients with DH who can adhere to a gluten-restricted diet for at least 6–12 months may be able to reduce the required dosage of dapsone for adequate control of their disease, and for some patients the medication may be completely tapered.[9,10] For the majority of DH patients, their disease can be controlled by several weeks of 100 mg or less of dapsone per day. An occasional patient may require as much as 300 mg/day, a level at which significant toxicity is often encountered.

Different regimens have been recommended for initiating therapy with dapsone for DH patients. Toxicity appears to be less if one starts with a low dosage of dapsone (50 mg/day) and increases the dosage slowly (50 mg/week) until disease control is attained. Patients must be monitored carefully, both clinically and with laboratory tests, for the development of adverse effects (see Monitoring Guidelines). Dapsone is more effective than sulfapyridine for DH, but exceptions do occur. Adverse effects are usually less prevalent with sulfapyridine, however; it is generally used by patients who cannot tolerate dapsone. The dosage of sulfapyridine for DH averages 1.5–2.0 g/day. The drug is either ineffective against or rarely used for other dapsone-responsive dermatologic diseases listed in Table 10–1.

LEPROSY. The recommendations for the treatment of leprosy are in a constant state of flux, and they vary from country to country for the various forms of the disease. Many strains of Mycobacterium leprae are now resistant to dapsone.[11] Most experts from the World Health Organization agree that combination therapy is indicated for all cases of multibacillary disease and most cases of paucibacillary leprosy.[12] The agents that are commonly recommended by the World Health Organization are dapsone (1–2 mg/kg of body weight 6 days a week), rifampin (rifampicin), clofazimine, and prothionamide. There is a repository form of dapsone (acedapsone) in an oily vehicle for intramuscular injection that is occasionally used. The 225-mg (1.5 ml) dosage provides a steady plasma level that is above the minimal inhibitory concentration for dapsone-sensitive M. leprae.

Other Dermatologic Uses

For a large number of other dermatologic and infectious disorders against which dapsone has been reported to be effective, experience in treating them is so limited that it is difficult to make definite conclusions concerning whether the drug is truly efficacious. The drug is usually very effective in certain uncommon bullous dermatoses (chronic bullous dermatitis of childhood, bullous lupus erythematosus, etc.) and in erythema elevatum diutinum. Dapsone may be the drug of choice in the early treatment of brown recluse spider bites. There are reports, however, that the drug can be used efficaciously in a wide variety of disorders.

LINEAR IMMUNOGLOBULIN A (IgA) BULLOUS DERMATOSIS/CHRONIC BULLOUS DERMATOSIS OF CHILDHOOD. These subepidermal bullous diseases with linear deposition of IgA at the basement membrane zone respond to dapsone or sulfapyridine but are clinically distinct from DH. They do not respond to a gluten-free diet and often involve the mucous membranes, and patients may require supplemental oral corticosteroids to control the diseases. Also, unlike DH, the diseases (especially in childhood) may remit within a few months. At times the diseases may mimic bullous erythema multiforme clinically but not immunologically.[17]

BULLOUS SYSTEMIC LUPUS ERYTHEMATOSUS. Dapsone is especially beneficial for patients with the relatively uncommon bullous dermatosis associated with systemic lupus erythematosus (SLE), often at a dosage as low as 50 mg/day.[18-21] These patients usually have granular IgA deposits along the basement membrane zone in perilesional and nonlesional skin, a finding that is seen in only 17% of patients with SLE without the bullous component. The disease has been seen in children as well as in adults, and bullae may be the presenting findings of lupus erythematosus. Of importance is that dapsone generally eradicates the cutaneous lesions of bullous SLE without affecting other, noncutaneous components of this systemic disease. Dapsone has also been reported to be effective in the treatment of subacute cutaneous lupus erythematosus.[21]

SUBCORNEAL PUSTULAR DERMATOSIS. This vesicopustular eruption, which affects mainly middle-aged women, was described as a distinct entity in 1956 by Sneddon and Wilkinson. They included in their reports descriptions of patients who responded dramatically to dapsone.[22] Chimenti and Ackerman subsequently proposed that the disease is a form of pustular psoriasis, and a significant number of patients have not responded to dapsone.[23] The exact nosology of this disease has yet to be fully defined.

VESICULAR/BULLOUS PEMPHIGOID. A number of patients with bullous pemphigoid have been reported to respond to dapsone and sulfapyridine, but it is probable that some had IgA bullous dermatoses.[24-26] Some pemphigoid patients with subepidermal linear IgG deposition present predominantly with vesicular lesions. These patients may respond well to dapsone. There have been reports of dapsone's providing a steroid-sparing effect in patients with bullous pemphigoid, and dapsone is certainly worth considering for patients with chronic and recalcitrant forms of the disease.

CICATRICIAL PEMPHIGOID. Rogers and coauthors reported that of 24 patients with cicatricial pemphigoid, 20 had partial or complete control of their disease with dapsone, usually at a dosage of 100–200 mg/day.[27] I have found the drug to be minimally effective for the majority of patients with this chronic disabling disease, which usually responds to cyclophosphamide (75–150 mg/day). I always give dapsone as the initial drug because it has a better toxicity profile than cyclophosphamide. However, I end up using cyclosphosphamide in most cases.

PEMPHIGUS. Dapsone has been used sparingly as sole therapy for the treatment of pemphigus, although there are reports of its efficacy as the initial form of therapy for patients with more superficial forms of the disease (pemphigus foliaceus and erythematosus). Five of 8 patients responded to an initial dosage of 200–300 mg/day.[29] There are a few reports of efficacy of dapsone for other forms of pemphigus, including pemphigus vegetans.[30,31]

HAILEY-HAILEY DISEASE. Chronic benign familial pemphigus was described by Hailey and Hailey in 1939. Numerous therapeutic modalities have been described as being efficacious, at least at certain times, for this notoriously recalcitrant disease,[32] and dapsone is included in this list.[33] The beneficial effects of most forms of therapy for Hailey-Hailey disease are usually short-lived, and physicians often have a whole armamentarium of agents that they use interchangeably for the disease.

ERYTHEMA ELEVATUM DIUTINUM. The majority of patients with the localized form of vasculitis known as erythema elevatum diutinum (EED) will respond to dapsone, but as in DH, the drug is not curative. Dapsone only suppresses disease activity, and the lesions quickly recur when dapsone is discontinued.[34] The etiology of EED is unknown, although many patients show an unusual hypersensitivity to streptococcal infections.[35] It is doubtful, however, that the beneficial effects of dapsone for EED are related to antibacterial activity.

GRANULOMA FACIALE. In the majority of reported cases of granuloma faciale, the disease has followed a long-term course that is notoriously resistant to a host of therapeutic modalities, including topical and intralesional steroids, cryotherapy, radiation, surgical excision, antimalarial agents, dermabrasion, and sulfones.[36] There are isolated reports, however, of dramatic responses to 25–100 mg/day of dapsone.[36–37] Because the disease may remit spontaneously, the percentage of patients whose disease can be effectively managed with dapsone is unknown.

VASCULITIS-LEUKOCYTOCLASTIC. Interest in the use of dapsone in the treatment of leukocytoclastic vasculitis, including hypocomplementemic urticarial vasculitis, has increased.[38] Although not all patients respond, the drug may be especially helpful in the chronic and purely cutaneous forms of the disease, for which prolonged use of systemic steroids should be avoided.[39] According to one report, the drug was effective in the treatment of the vasculitis in Henoch-Schönlein disease.[40]

NEUTROPHILIC VASCULAR REACTIONS. As mentioned earlier, many of the cutaneous diseases that are responsive to dapsone are diseases with a prominent infiltrate of polymorphonuclear leukocytes. Several of these diseases have been grouped under the heading of neutrophilic vascular reactions in which there is often leukocytoclasia but without true vasculitis. Dapsone has been used successfully in the treatment of occasional patients with pyoderma gangrenosum,[41] Sweet's syndrome,[42,43] and Behçet's disease.[44,45] These diseases are usually treated initially with oral corticosteriods, but dapsone may be useful, especially as a steroid-sparing agent.

PILOSEBACEOUS DISEASES. Dapsone has been reported to be effective in the management of nodulocystic acne, but the evidence to support this has been largely anecdotal and based on single-case reports.[46] Dapsone was shown to be clearly inferior to 13-cis retinoic acid in a randomly allocated study.[47] In at least one report, dapsone was helpful in rosacea when tetracycline was not sufficient.[48]

INFECTIOUS DISEASES. Sulfones were first used for actinomycotic mycetoma in 1946, and according to a number of reports, dapsone has been effective therapy for disease caused by both aerobic and anaerobic actinomycetes (predominantly *Nocardia braziliensis*, *Nocardia asteroides*, and *Actinomyces israelii*).[49]

Dapsone has antiprotozoal activity and has been used in the treatment and chemoprophylaxis of malaria, especially for chloroquine-resistant strains of *Plasmodium falciparum*.[50]

Dapsone was first used to treat cutaneous leishmaniasis, as reported in 1986. Of 50 patients with the disease due to *Leishmania tropica*, 40 were cured after 21 days of dapsone, 2 mg/kg of body weight as a single daily dose.[51] This study contrasted sharply with previous studies in which dapsone had been reported ineffective against the diffuse type of cutaneous leishmaniasis, which is usually resistant to most of the prevalent antileishmanial drugs (pentavalent antimonial compounds such as sodium stibogluconate and pentamidine). The 80% cure rate reported in this Indian study has led to further interest in the use of dapsone for cutaneous leishmaniasis, especially because the drug is inexpensive and more easily administered than other therapeutic modalities for this disease.

Also in 1986, dapsone combined with trimethoprim was shown to be effective in the treatment of Pneumocystis carinii pneumonia in patients with AIDS.[52] This regimen has been used because more than 50% of patients treated with either of the approved regimens (trimethoprim-sulfamethoxazole or pentamidine isethionate) develop such severe adverse reactions that the treatment must be discontinued. In addition, pentamidine is given parenterally, and trimethoprim-sulfamethoxazole is poorly tolerated when given orally in the high dosages used for this form of pneumonia. The combination of dapsone (100 mg/day) plus trimethoprim (20 mg/kg/day) was felt to be at least as effective as, and to have a lower frequency of adverse effects than, other treatments for this life-threatening infection in patients with AIDS.

OTHER DERMATOSES. There are reports in the literature of the efficacy of dapsone for a variety of unrelated conditions. In most of these cases, dapsone is not necessarily the drug of choice and may be beneficial in only a small percentage of patients. However, dapsone does provide an alternative therapy when other modalities are either unsuccessful or too toxic. Pustular psoriasis, both the generalized and the palmoplantar types, has been treated effectively with dapsone, although etretinate is probably the drug of choice for the generalized form of the disease.[53] In one study, dapsone was found to be very helpful in preventing both skin necrosis and delayed wound healing in patients with brown recluse spider bites.[54] Dapsone, either alone or in combination with infusions of alpha-1-proteinase inhibitor concentrate, has been beneficial in the treatment of the rare patient with panniculitis associated with a deficiency of alpha-1-antitrypsin.[55] Some, but certainly not all, patients with relapsing polychondritis may be effectively treated with dapsone, although prednisone may well be the drug of choice for severe forms of the disease.[56] Finally, there have been sporadic reports of patients with generalized granuloma annulare who responded favorably to treatment with dapsone.[57]

Adverse Effects

The toxicity of dapsone has been well established. Some of the adverse effects are pharmacologic and predictable, but there are allergic and idiosyncratic reactions as well. Other than patients with a deficiency of glucose-6-phosphate dehydrogenase (G6PD), most people tolerate this drug well, except when very high dosages are used. There are several million patients with leprosy who take dapsone daily with minimal toxicity, but the dosages for leprosy are often lower than those required to treat most dermatologic diseases. The higher the dosage, the more likely the development of intolerable adverse effects. There are conflicting reports concerning cross-sensitivity of dapsone and sulfapyridine, although it appears that one can proceed cautiously with sulfapyridine in dapsone-sensitive patients and vice versa.[3] The most frequent adverse effects of dapsone are hematologic, but dapsone may have an effect on the liver, the kidneys, the skin, and the nervous system. Pretreatment baseline evaluation is listed in the monitoring guidelines and should include a complete blood count (CBC), a chemistry profile, a urinalysis, and an analysis of the G6PD level.

HEMATOLOGIC EFFECTS. Hematologic effects of dapsone and sulfapyridine include hemolysis, methemoglobinemia, leukopenia, and in rare cases, agranulocytosis. Further details regarding the mechanism of dapsone-induced hemolysis and methemoglobinemia can be found in an excellent review by Uetrecht.[58] Dapsone hydroxylamine metabolites are believed to have a central role in the pathogenesis of both processes. Hemolysis and methemoglobinemia are dosage-related, and the former occurs in patients with or without G6PD deficiency, although it is much more severe in patients with a deficiency of this enzyme. Most patients without G6PD deficiency will have a 2-g/dl drop in hemoglobin at standard dapsone doses, with a subsequent re-equilibration at 1-g/dl hemoglobin below pretreatment baseline values. The sulfones are strong oxidizers and accelerate both the aging process of red blood cells and the destruction of the older red blood cells, which lead to hemolysis. Hemolysis and the resulting anemia may be severe in patients treated with 200–300 mg/day of dapsone but rarely produce major problems, except in patients with cardiovascular compromise. Reticulocyte counts are a useful means of assessing the amount of dapsone-induced hemolysis and the body's reserve of nutritional hemoglobin precursors (i.e., iron, vitamin B_{12}, and folate).

Methemoglobinemia may produce obvious cyanosis in some patients, but it is usually clinically significant only in patients with cardiovascular disease. With methemoglobin, iron has been oxidized from the ferrous to the ferric state. This oxidized form of hemoglobin cannot carry oxygen, and it also impedes the release of oxygen from normal hemoglobin; both these characteristics result in tissue hypoxia. Rare patients with a deficiency of methemoglobin reductase are particularly susceptible to methemoglobinemia with dapsone. The rarity of this syndrome precludes routine screening for this enzyme deficiency.

A rare but dreaded complication of dapsone and sulfapyridine is agranulocytosis. The typical syndrome includes fever, sore throat with necrotic white pharyngeal pseudomembranes, pyoderma or cellulitis, and occasionally a morbilliform rash. The white blood cell count is generally less than 2000/cu mm with markedly decreased or absent granulocytes. Death, when it occurs, is due to bacterial sepsis. The last fatal case was reported in 1970.[59, 60] Ognibene reported an unusual series of cases in which 16 soldiers in Vietnam developed agranulocytosis 3–12 weeks after starting low dosages of dapsone used in conjunction with chloroquine for malaria prophylaxis.[60] Eight fatalities due to sepsis occurred in this series. Dapsone-associated agranulocytosis has been reported for dapsone use in acne,[61] granuloma annulare,[62] and leprosy.[63] Associated conditions have included a reversible monoclonal IgD gammopathy,[64] pseudoleukemia,[65] and reversible aplastic anemia.[63] Agranulocytosis due to sulfapyridine has been reported as well.[66]

Although in the 1980s reports of agranulocytosis were very rare and no fatalities were reported, the possibility of agranulocytosis should always be considered by the clinician who prescribes dapsone and sulfapyridine. The patient should be strongly advised to discontinue dapsone and see a physician if there is a significant fever, particularly if this is accompanied by pharyngitis or other signs of infection. The risk appears to be greatest between the 4th and the 12th weeks of therapy, and the monitoring for leukopenia and agranulocytosis should be at least every 2 weeks during this interval. The occurrence of agranulocytosis after 3 months is extremely uncommon.

DAPSONE HYPERSENSITIVITY SYNDROME. Cutaneous hypersensitivity reactions are uncommon and have been reported with sulfapyridine more frequently than with dapsone. Although theoretical cross-reaction between these two drugs is possible, the general consensus is that simple hypersensitivity manifested only by a morbilliform eruption to one drug does not preclude use of the other. Additional reactions include erythema multiforme, erythema nodosum, and toxic epidermal necrolysis.[58] An unusual but potentially fatal infectious-mononucleosis–like syndrome is known as the *dapsone hypersensitivity syndrome* (sulfone syndrome). The syndrome was reviewed by Smith, who detailed 27 cases that occurred in the 1980s.[67] The syndrome is characterized by fever, malaise, and lymphadenopathy. A maculopapular (morbilliform) eruption initially presents after 5–6 weeks of dapsone treatment and frequently progresses to an exfoliative erythroderma. Hepatomegaly with jaundice accompanies the rash. Laboratory findings include abnormal liver function tests either on a hepatocellular or on a cholestatic basis. Eosinophilia and an increased number of atypical lymphocytes are generally noted. Partial manifestation of the syndrome with prominent liver involvement has been reported.[68] At least 5 fatal cases of dapsone hypersensitivity syndrome have been reported since 1950.[69–73] In these cases, the cause of death when known was severe hepatitis with liver failure.

The mononucleosis-like syndrome just described is generally recognized clinically; however, periodic liver function tests are important for surveillance. The patient should be taught the key symptoms of this dapsone hypersensitivity syndrome and should be instructed to discontinue the drug and notify the physician if they occur.

HEPATOTOXICITY AND NEPHROTOXICITY. Toxic hepatitis and cholestatic jaundice may occur with dapsone. The former often occurs as part of the dapsone hypersensitivity syndrome. The cholestasis is generally rapidly reversible upon discontinuation of the drug. Very rare instances of renal papillary necrosis and the nephrotic syndrome have been reported with dapsone.[74] Sulfapyridine may cause crystalluria, which results from the accumulation of the poorly water-soluble acetylated metabolite in the kidneys. One can minimize this problem by increasing fluid intake while taking sulfapyridine. Periodic urinalysis is thus important in the follow-up of patients taking sulfapyridine.

NERVOUS SYSTEM EFFECTS. Dapsone may cause axon damage, which results in a peripheral neuropathy that affects motor nerves much more frequently than sensory nerves.[75-77] This adverse effect on the peripheral nerves generally occurs in patients who are taking large daily dosages of dapsone and may occur after prolonged therapy with the drug. Patients should be monitored for the development of weakness, loss of sensation, and paresthesias. Even after the drug is discontinued, recovery may take years. Psychosis may also occur in patients taking dapsone, especially in patients with a prior or current history of mental disturbance.

OTHER ADVERSE EFFECTS. A number of bothersome, but rarely serious, side effects occur in patients taking dapsone and sulfapyridine. They include nausea, vomiting, headache, weakness, fatigue, dizziness, and shortness of breath.

Warnings

Extreme caution must be used in treating patients with leukopenia, severe anemia, G6PD or methemoglobin-reductase deficiency, liver disease, and renal disease. Dapsone has been used safely during pregnancy by many patients with leprosy, but use of the drug by pregnant women has not been studied adequately for clinicians to assume that it is completely safe for the fetus. Dapsone is distributed into breast milk and should be avoided by nursing women whenever possible.

Drug Interactions

Probenecid should be avoided by patients who are taking dapsone because it may reduce renal excretion of dapsone. However, adequate studies supporting this potential interaction have not been done.

> **DAPSONE/SULFAPYRIDINE* MONITORING GUIDELINES**[3]
>
> **Baseline**
>
> - CBC with differential white blood cell count
> - Reticulocyte count
> - Chemistry profile (including tests for renal and hepatic function)
> - Urinalysis
> - Glucose-6-phosphate dehydrogenase level†
>
> **Follow-up**
>
> - CBC and reticulocyte count at least every 2 weeks for first 3 months, then every 3 months‡
> - Periodic evaluation of renal function and liver function, including urinalysis (suggested monthly for the first 3–6 months, then every 3–6 months)
> - Methemoglobin levels (only as clinically indicated, such as in patients with cardiopulmonary disease or methemoglobin-reductase deficiency)
> - Periodic screening evaluation of neurologic function (especially at higher dosage levels), done by dermatologist (e.g., having patients walk on their toes)
>
> Note: More frequent surveillance is needed if laboratory values are abnormal or with high-risk patients.
>
> *There are no specific guidelines for sulfapyridine, and the only laboratory tests followed routinely are the CBC and the urinalysis.[58]
>
> †Although G6PD deficiency is most common in blacks and patients of Mediterranean descent, screening is best done before therapy is instituted for all dapsone-treated patients.
>
> ‡The Food and Drug Administration guidelines suggest a weekly CBC during the 1st month of dapsone therapy, monthly for the next 6 months, then periodically thereafter. In reality, the risk for agranulocytosis is greatest between the 4th and the 12th weeks of treatment. Given the patient's awareness of key symptoms to report, the CBC guidelines in this table are most reasonable.

Rifampin decreases the half-life of dapsone by inducing liver enzymes that are responsible for inactivation of the drug, although a dosage change is not generally required during concomitant therapy for patients with leprosy. Serum dapsone levels may be lower in patients taking rifampin concomitantly, but it is not known whether this affects the clinical results.

Caution should be used by patients taking drugs that can also cause adverse hematologic effects, such as anemia or leukopenia. There is some evidence that dapsone may interfere with the anti-inflammatory effects of clofazimine, although clofazimine does not affect the pharmacokinetics of dapsone.

BIBLIOGRAPHY: Key Reviews/Chapters

Uetrecht J: Dapsone and sulfapyrindine. Clin Dermatol 1989; 7:111–120.
Wozel G: The story of sulfones in tropical medicine and dermatology. Int J Dermatol 1989; 28:17–21.
Katz SI: Dapsone. In Fitzpatrick TB, Eisen AZ, Wolff K, et al (eds): Dermatology in General Medicine (3rd ed). New York: McGraw-Hill, 1987, 2570–2574.
Lang PG Jr: Sulfones and sulfonamides in dermatology today. J Am Acad Dermatol 1979; 1:479–492.

REFERENCES

1. Wozel G: The story of sulfones in tropical medicine and dermatology. Int J Dermatol 1989; 28:17–21.
2. Pieters FAJM, Zuidema J: The pharmacokinetics of dapsone after oral administration to healthy volunteers. Br J Clin Pharmacol 1986; 22:491–494.
3. Lang PG Jr: Sulfones and sulfonamides in dermatology today. J Am Acad Dermatol 1979, 1:479–492.
4. Wozel G, Barth J: Current aspects of modes of action of dapsone. Int J Dermatol 1988; 27:547–552.
5. Fry L: The treatment of dermatitis herpetiformis. Clin Exp Dermatol 1982; 7:633–642.
6. Katz SI: Commentary: Sulfoxone (diazone) in the treatment of dermatitis herpetiformis. Arch Dermatol 1982; 118:809–812.
7. Morgan JK, Marsden CW, Coburn JG, et al: Dapsone in dermatitis herpetiformis. Lancet 1955; 1:1197–1200.
8. Alexander J O'D: Dapsone in the treatment of dermatitis herpetiformis. Lancet 1955; 1:1201–1202.
9. Mobacken H, Anderssohn H, Dahlberg E, et al: Relationship of dietary gluten intake to dapsone dose in dermatitis herpetiformis. Acta Derm Venereol (Stockh) 1987; 67:267–270.
10. Reunala T, Blomquist K, Tarpila S, et al: Gluten-free diet in dermatitis herpetiformis. Br J Dermatol 1977; 97:473–480.
11. Pearson JMH, Rees RJW, Waters MFR: Sulphone resistance in leprosy: A review of one hundred proven cases. Lancet 1975; 2:69–72.
12. Shaw J, Brooks PM, McNeil JJ, et al: The management of leprosy. Med J Austral 1987; 146:593–598.
13. Wojnarowska F, Marsden RA, Bhogal B, et al: Chronic bullous dermatosis of childhood, childhood cicatricial pemphigoid, and linear IgA disease of adults: A comparative study demonstrating clinical and immunopathologic overlap. J Am Acad Dermatol 1988; 19:792–805.
14. Easterly NB, Furey NL, Kirschner BS, et al: Chronic bullous dermatosis of childhood. Arch Dermatol 1977; 113:42–46.
15. Marsden RA: The treatment of benign chronic bullous dermatosis of childhood, and dermatitis herpetiformis and bullous pemphigoid beginning in childhood. Clin Exp Dermatol 1982; 7:653–663.
16. Ratnam KV: IgA dermatosis in an adult Chinese population: A 10-year study of linear IgA and dermatitis herpetiformis in Singapore. Int J Dermatol 1988; 27:21–24.
17. Argenyi ZB, Bergfeld WF, Valenzuela R, et al: Linear IgA bullous dermatitis mimicking erythema multiforme in adults. Int J Dermatol 1987; 26:513–517.

18. Camisa C: Vesiculobullous systemic lupus erythematosus: A report of four cases. J Am Acad Dermatol 1988; 18:93–100.
19. Rock B, Patel HP: Bullous eruption in a patient with lupus erythematosus. Arch Dermatol 1987; 123:938–939.
20. Kettler AH, Bean SF, Duffy JO, et al: Systemic lupus erythematosus presenting as a bullous eruption in a child. Arch Dermatol 1988; 124:1083–1087.
21. Fenton DA, Black MM: Low-dose dapsone in the treatment of subacute cutaneous lupus erythematosus. Clin Exp Dermatol 1986; 11:102–103.
22. Sneddon LB, Wilkinson DB: Subcorneal pustular dermatosis. Br J Dermatol 1956; 68:385–394.
23. Chimenti S, Ackerman AB: Is subcorneal pustular dermatosis of Sneddon and Wilkinson an entity sui generis? Am J Dermatopathol 1981; 3:363–376.
24. Joblanska S, Chorzelski T: When and how to use sulfones in bullous dermatoses. Int J Dermatol 1981; 20:103–105.
25. Rogers RS: Dapsone and sulfapyridine therapy of pemphigoid diseases. Australas J Dermatol 1986; 27:58–63.
26. Pierson JR: Bullous pemphigoid responding to sulfapyridine and the sulfones. Arch Dermatol 1977; 113:610–615.
27. Rogers, RS, Seehafer JR, Perry HO: Treatment of cicatricial (benign mucous membrane) pemphigoid with dapsone. J Am Acad Dermatol 1982; 6:215–223.
28. Bean SF: Diagnosis and management of chronic oral mucosal bullous dermatoses. Dermatol Clin 1987; 5:751–760.
29. Bassett N, Guillot B, Michel B: Dapsone as initial treatment in superficial pemphigus. Arch Dermatol 1987; 123:783–785.
30. Rodan KP, Hu C, Nickoloff BJ: Malodorous intertriginous pustules and plaques. Arch Dermatol 1987; 123:396–397.
31. Piamphongsant T: Pemphigus controlled by dapsone. Br J Dermatol 1976; 94:681–686.
32. Michel B: Commentary: Hailey-Hailey disease. Arch Dermatol 1982; 118:781–783.
33. Sire DJ, Johnson BL: Benign familial chronic pemphigus treated with dapsone. Arch Dermatol 1971; 103:262–265.
34. Katz SI, Gallin JI, Hertz KC, et al: Erythema elevatum diutinum: Skin and systemic manifestations, immunologic studies, and successful treatment with dapsone. Medicine 1977; 56:443–455.
35. Fort SL, Rodman OG: Erythema elevatum diutinum response to dapsone. Arch Dermatol 1977; 113:819–822.
36. Anderson CR: Dapsone in granuloma faciale. Lancet 1975; 1:642.
37. Guill MA, Aton JK: Facial granuloma responsive to dapsone therapy. Arch Dermatol 1982; 118:332–335.
38. Fortson JS, Zone JJ, Hammond ME, et al: Hypocomplementemic urticarial vasculitis syndrome responsive to dapsone. J Am Acad Dermatol 1986; 15:1137–1142.
39. Fredenberg MF, Malkinson FD: Sulfone therapy in the treatment of leukocytoclastic vasculitis. Report of three cases. J Am Acad Dermatol 1987; 16:772–778.
40. Ledermann JA, Hoffbrand BI: Dapsone in allergic vasculitis: Its use in Henoch-Schönlein disease following vaccination. J R Soc Med 1983; 76:613–614.
41. Wernikoff S, Merritt C, Briggaman RA, et al: Malignant pyoderma or pyoderma gangrenosum of the head and neck. Arch Dermatol 1987; 123:371–375.
42. Aram H: Acute febrile neutrophilic dermatosis (Sweet's syndrome). Response to dapsone. Arch Dermatol 1984; 120:245–247.
43. Greer KE, Cooper PH: Sweet's syndrome (acute febrile neutrophilic dermatosis). Clin Rheum Dis 1982; 8:427–441.

44. Convit J, Goihman-Yahr M, Rondon-Lugo AJ: Effectiveness of dapsone in Behçet's disease. Br J Dermatol 1984; 111:629–630.
45. Sharquie KE: Suppression of Behçet's disease with dapsone. Br J Dermatol 1984: 110:493–494.
46. Lorincz AL, Pearson RW: Sulfapyridine and sulfone type drugs in dermatology. Arch Dermatol 1962; 85:42–56.
47. Prendiville JS, Logan RA, Russell-Jones R: A comparison of dapsone with 13-cis retinoic acid in the treatment of nodular cystic acne. Clin Exp Dermatol 1988; 13:67–71.
48. Wilkin JK: Rosacea. Int J Dermatol 1983; 22:393–400.
49. Rogers RS 3rd, Muller SA: Treatment of actinomycetoma with dapsone. A report of infection with Nocardia asteroides. Arch Dermatol 1974; 109:529–534.
50. Chiodini PL: The chemoprophylaxis of malaria. J Antimicrob Chemother 1987; 20:297–302.
51. Dogra J, Lal BB, Misra SN: Dapsone in the treatment of cutaneous leishmaniasis. Int J Dermatol 1986; 25:398–400.
52. Leoung GS, Mills J, Hopewell PC, et al: Dapsone-trimethoprim for Pneumocystis carinii pneumonia in the acquired immunodeficiency syndrome. Ann Intern Med 1986; 105:45–48.
53. Macmillan AL, Champion RH: Generalized pustular psoriasis treated with dapsone. Br J Dermatol 1973; 88:183–185.
54. Rees RS, Altenbern DP, Lynch JB, et al: Brown recluse spider bites: A comparison of early surgical excision versus dapsone and delayed surgical excision. Ann Surg 1985; 202:659–663.
55. Smith KC, Pittelkow MR, Su WP: Panniculitis associated with severe α 1-antitrypsin deficiency: Treatment and review of the literature. Arch Dermatol 1987; 123:1655–1661.
56. Barranco VP, Minor DB, Solomon H: Treatment of relapsing polychondritis with dapsone. Arch Dermatol 1976; 112:1286–1288.
57. Saied N, Schwartz RA, Estes SA: Treatment of generalized granuloma annulare with dapsone. Arch Dermatol 1980; 116:1345–1346.
58. Uetrecht J: Dapsone and sulfapyridine. Clin Dermatol 1989; 7:111–120.
59. Ten-Broeke JE, Cunningham LD: Agranulocytosis following dapsone administration. Dermatologica 1973; 146:21–24.
60. Ognibene AJ: Agranulocytosis due to dapsone. Ann Intern Med 1970; 72:521–524.
61. Firkin FC, Mariani AF: Agranulocytosis due to dapsone. Med J Aust 1977; 2:247–251.
62. Potter MN, Yates P, Slade R, et al: Agranulocytosis caused by dapsone therapy for granuloma annulare. J Am Acad Dermatol 1977; 20:87–88.
63. Foucald J, Uphouse W, Berenberg J: Dapsone and aplastic anemia. Ann Intern Med 1985; 102:139.
64. Lahuerta-Palacios JJ, Gomez-Pedraja JF, Montalban MA, et al: Proliferation of IgD kappa plasma cells after agranulocytosis induced by dapsone. Br Med J [Clin Res] 1985; 290:282–283.
65. Levine PH, Weintraub LR: Pseudoleukemia during recovery from dapsone-induced agranulocytosis. Ann Intern Med 1968; 68:1060–1065.
66. Rosenthal N, Vogel P: Granulocytopenia caused by sulfapyridine in children. JAMA 1939; 113:584–587.
67. Smith WC: Are hypersensitivity reactions to dapsone becoming more frequent? Lepr Rev 1988; 59:53–58.
68. Johnson DA, Cattau EL Jr, Kuritsky JN, et al: Liver involvement in the sulfone syndrome. Arch Intern Med 1986; 146:875–877.

69. Smith WC: Hypersensitivity reactions to dapsone. Lepr Rev 1986; 57:179–180.
70. Frey HM, Gershon AA, Borkowisky W, et al: Fatal reactions to dapsone during treatment of leprosy. Ann Intern Med 1981; 94:777–779.
71. Jamrozik K: Dapsone syndrome occurring in two brothers. Lepr Rev 1986; 57:57–62.
72. Leiker DL: The mononucleosis syndrome in leprosy patients treated with sulfones. Int J Lepr 1956; 24:402–405.
73. Allday EJ, Barnes J: Toxic effects of diaminodiphenylsulphone in treatment of leprosy. Lancet 1951; 2:205–206.
74. Hoffbrand BI: Dapsone and renal papillary necrosis. Br Med J 1978; 1:78.
75. Helander I, Partanen J: Dapsone-induced distal axonal degeneration of the motor neurons. Dermatologica 1978; 156:321–324.
76. Gutmann L, Martin JD, Welton W: Dapsone motor neuropathy—An axonal disease. Neurology 1976; 26:514–516.
77. Ahrens ED, Meckler RJ, Callen JP: Dapsone-induced peripheral neuropathy. Int J Dermatol 1986; 25:314–316.

11 Antimalarials

Charles Camisa, M.D.

The antimalarial drugs used for dermatologic diseases are quinacrine, chloroquine, and hydroxycholoroquine. They were developed in that order as alternatives to quinine in the prophylaxis and suppressive treatment of *Plasmodium* malaria.

The popular use of antimalarials in the treatment of skin diseases began after Page's 1951 report of improvement of discoid lupus erythematosus with quinacrine.[1] The mechanism or mechanisms of action of the drugs in malaria, or any skin disease (except perhaps for porphyria cutanea tarda), are not precisely known, and some dermatologists object to the use of the term *antimalarials*. Although these compounds may also have anti-inflammatory and immunomodulatory effects, their rich history as antimalarials since the 1930s defies a change in classification at this point. Therefore, for the purpose of familiarity, this chapter will refer to quinacrine and the 4-aminoquinolines as the antimalarials.

An extensive research effort began in Germany during World War I to synthesize antimalarials when normal supplies of quinine decreased.[2] Quinacrine was the first, introduced in 1930. Despite rapid professional acceptance, its structure remained obscure as a result of inadequate patent disclosure until its degradation and synthesis by Russian scientists in 1934. When quinine became unavailable to the Allies in World War II, large-scale production and distribution of quinacrine to servicemen in endemic areas began. Although quinacrine was three times more potent than quinine, its toxicity and inability to cure malaria or act as a true causal prophylactic led to the search for more effective drugs in the U.S.

Chloroquine is one of thousands of compounds synthesized and tested for activity against malaria in ducks and for toxicity in mammals. Of 10 compounds studied in human volunteers with experimentally induced malaria, chloroquine was most promising. It was released for field trial in 1944 and introduced into clinical medicine in 1947. The introduction of a hydroxyl group into one of the N-ethyl groups of chloroquine resulted in the synthesis of hydroxychloroquine in 1946. In the same bioassays, its antimalarial activity was similar to chloroquine, but it was only about 40% as toxic.

Another ironic twist in the development of antimalarials deserves mention. After World War II, it was discovered that chloroquine, under the name of Resochin, had been synthesized in 1934 and submitted to the U.S. Patent Office on December 14, 1939, by Andersag.[3]

Pharmacology

Structure (Table 11–1)

Most antimalarials are substituted 4-aminoquinolines. Quinacrine has an extra benzene ring and is considered an acridine compound.

Absorption/Distribution

Antimalarials are bitter, water-soluble, crystalline powders that are absorbed rapidly and completely from the gastrointestinal tract. Quinacrine is bright yellow; chloroquine and hydroxychloroquine are white. Maximal plasma levels of quinacrine are achieved in 1–3 hours after ingestion. However, the drug binds avidly to tissue protein; its concentrations are highest in liver, spleen, and kidney tissues, mainly in nuclei and mitochondria. It takes 4–6 weeks to attain equilibrium between daily intake and excretion.

Various single and repeated dosage regimens for chloroquine and hydroxychloroquine yield nearly identical plasma level curves with peaks at 5 and 4 hours, respectively.[4] Distributions of the two drugs in

Table 11–1. Antimalarials Used in Dermatology

Generic Name	Trade Name	Chemical Structure	Tablet Form	Equivalent Dose	Cost to Pharmacist
Chloroquine	Aralen		Chloroquine phosphate 250 mg (150-mg base) or 500-mg base (300-mg base)	250 mg	$0.03
Hydroxy-chloroquine	Plaquenil		Hydroxychloroquine sulfate 200 mg (155-mg base)	400 mg	$0.90
Quinacrine	Atabrine		Quinacrine hydrochloride 100 mg	100 mg	$0.21

tissue are qualitatively similar: they are least in bone, skin, fat, and brain tissues and greater in (in ascending order) muscle, eye, heart, kidney, liver, lung, spleen, and adrenal gland tissues. The absolute amounts are 2.5 times higher for chloroquine. It is possible for some tissue to accumulate concentrations of these 4-aminoquinolines several hundred times those in plasma.

Metabolism/Excretion

The major pathway of biotransformation is not known, but alteration must be extensive. About 11% of a daily dose is excreted in the urine, and smaller amounts are detected in feces, sweat, breast milk, saliva, and bile.[4]

The terminal half-lives of chloroquine and hydroxychloroquine are similar: 40–50 days.[5] The long half-lives are attributed to extensive tissue uptake. The attainment of steady-state concentrations in 3–4 months may account for the slow appearance of therapeutic benefit. Hydroxychloroquine can be detected in whole blood 5 months after a single dose.

Their metabolism differs in one respect: chloroquine breaks down into one first-stage metabolite (desethylchloroquine) and hydroxychloroquine breaks down into two (desethylhydroxychloroquine and desethylchloroquine). The first-stage desethyl compounds break down in turn to the primary amine.[4]

There is also a difference in the relative amounts of drug excreted in urine and feces. After a single dose, approximately three times more chloroquine than hydroxychloroquine can be accounted for in urine, and three times more hydroxychloroquine than chloroquine can be accounted for in feces. The data suggest that hydroxychloroquine forms an ether glucuronide that is excreted in bile. The low proportion of unchanged hydroxychloroquine eliminated by the kidneys indicates that no dosage adjustment is necessary for patients with mild to moderate renal function impairment.

Mechanism of Action

ANTIMALARIAL EFFECTS. Since the introduction of quinacrine and the 4-aminoquinolines in 1939, their mechanism of action in malaria and other diseases has remained enigmatic. The drugs are suppressive; that is, they do not prevent infection. Instead, they inhibit the erythrocytic stage of development of the malaria parasites, so that the infected person is kept free of the clinical manifestations of disease.[6]

The antimalarial effect of these drugs may be due to their intercalation in DNA, which stabilizes the double helix form and prevents separation of complementary strands. Replication of DNA and transcription of RNA are thus inhibited. The stoichiometry is one chloroquine molecule bound to 4.5 bases and is in agreement with the statistic estimate of maximally one intercalant with 4.2 bases.[3] Pharmacologic concentrations can be achieved in plasmodium-erythrocyte systems. Thus the chemotherapeutic effect of the antimalarials as blood schizontocides may be due to inhibition of DNA-primed nucleic acid polymerase reactions.

OVERVIEW OF DERMATOLOGIC EFFECTS. Many pharmacologic effects of antimalarials have been reported for concentrations that are much greater than that achieved in plasma at recommended daily dosages (1×10^{-6} M). This concentration multiplied by 1000 may be found in melanin-containing tissues, particularly the choroid and ciliary body of the eye (1×10^{-3} M).[7] The concentration of the drugs is 5–15 times higher in the epidermis than in the dermis.[8] Potential mechanisms of action of antimalarials in the treatment of skin and rheumatic diseases include the following: sunscreen effects, DNA interactions, anti-inflammatory activity, and immunosuppressive effects. The mechanism of action in porphyria cutanea tarda is considered separately.

SUNSCREEN EFFECTS. It seems only logical to begin with this possible mechanism because antimalarials are used to treat many skin diseases that are either induced or aggravated by light. Moreover, quinacrine and chloroquine exhibit three peaks of absorption in aqueous solution: 280, 424, 444 nm and 222, 328, 343 nm, respectively.[2,9]

In his landmark article, Page suggested that oral administration of quinacrine reduced the minimal erythema dose after only 10 days of treatment.[1] Sams and Carroll applied aqueous solutions of chloroquine in concentrations varying from 0.001% to 5%.[10] After exposure to an artificial ultraviolet (UV) light source, diminished erythema was seen only with chloroquine concentrations above 0.5%. These experiments and others, all performed in the 1950s and 1960s, suggested that antimalarials have weak UV-screening effects and can alter abnormal reactions to UV when given topically or intradermally.[11] These effects are probably not secondary to their high affinity for melanin. Defining a role for the antimalarials and their metabolites in light filtration can now be accomplished through the exploitation of monochromatic light and through sophisticated methods of analyzing drug-melanin complexes in tissue. However, any such effect on light filtration could not explain the action of antimalarials on the visceral manifestations of lupus erythematosus, rheumatoid arthritis, and sarcoidosis.

DNA INTERACTIONS. If intercalation into DNA and action as "DNA template poisons" were the major mechanism of action,[3–6] then one would expect to see more toxicity in those host tissues that concentrate the drug. Chloroquine and hydroxychloroquine inhibited the reaction of denatured calf thymus DNA with sera from patients with lupus erythematosus, as measured by quantitative complement fixation. This suggested that the drugs were inhibiting this reaction by binding to the DNA rather than to the antibodies.[13] In another experiment,[14] incubation of chloroquine with sera containing antinuclear factor was more likely to inhibit reaction with calf thyroid nuclei than was prior treatment of the tissue sections. These results suggested a preferential, direct effect on the antibody, rather than on the nuclear antigen.

ANTI-INFLAMMATORY EFFECTS. Chloroquine accumulates in lysosomes, and it stabilizes the lysosomal membrane against such labilizers as vitamin A and UV light.[8] The activity of hydrolytic enzymes might be reduced by an increased pH in the lysosome, their release into the external milieu prevented or delayed, or their activity directly inhibited by chloroquine. The combination of all these effects may reduce local tissue damage.

In modified Boyden chamber assays, chloroquine inhibits chemotaxis of polymorphonuclear leukocytes (PMLs)[15] and eosinophils.[16] Phagocytosis of zymosan particles by PMLs could be inhibited by greater concentrations of chloroquine than those necessary to inhibit chemotaxis. In an experimental immunologic vasculitis model (reversed passive Arthus reaction in guinea pigs), edema and erythema could be inhibited by treatment with chloroquine. The antigen or complement was found fixed to vessel walls, but few PMLs were seen in this location.[15] This suggests that chloroquine did not prevent either immune complex formation or complement fixation, but it did inhibit migration of PMLs to the area and the subsequent release or activity of mediators of inflammation.

IMMUNOSUPPRESSIVE EFFECTS. Early work showed that rabbit antibody response to sheep red blood cells, diphtheria toxoid, and typhoid antigens was (not) diminished by chloroquine.[17] There was no effect on delayed hypersensitivity to tuberculin in animals known to be tuberculin-positive. Chloroquine in high concentrations demonstrated marked inhibition of complement-mediated hemolysis (CH_{50} assay) in a dose-response fashion. Neblett and coauthors suggested that depression of complement activity was an important mechanism of action of chloroquine in connective tissue diseases.[18]

Long-term treatment of patients with rheumatoid arthritis produces a decrease in acute phase reactants and rheumatoid factor titer.[19] Panayi and co-workers showed that peripheral blood lymphocytes of rheumatoid arthritis patients treated with 250 mg/day of chloroquine exhibited reduced responsiveness to phytohemagglutinin (PHA) in comparison with cells of patients treated with aspirin.[20] This was the first indication of a suppressive effect of chloroquine on cell-mediated immunity. Unfortunately, patients were not used as their own controls. Therefore, it is possible that decreased PHA responsiveness is secondary to the improvement of inflammatory arthritis by chloroquine. Mackenzie believed that the effectiveness of the 4-aminoquinolines in rheumatoid arthritis is related to interference with intracellular vesicle fusion processes.[21] Large quantities of cellular membrane, including receptors such as those that recognize PHA, are sequestered within the cell in the increased number of lysosomal vesicles. This depletion of cell surface receptors may decrease the rate or efficiency with which a cell responds to its environment.

Salmeron and Lipsky studied the effect of chloroquine on PHA and concanavalin A–induced lymphocyte proliferation.[22] Chloroquine, at a concentration of 12 mcg/ml, produced significant inhibition of tritiated thymidine incorporation with either mitogen. When fresh autologous mitomycin C–treated monocytes were added back to the cultures of cells preincubated with chloroquine, their mitogen responsiveness was restored. These data suggest that chloroquine selectively depresses a "helper" function of monocytes.

Chloroquine, at a very low concentration (0.8 mcg/ml), markedly suppressed the generation of immunoglobulin-secreting cells from peripheral blood mononuclear cells incubated for 7 days with *Staphylococcus aureus*.[22] Chloroquine may thus block an early step in the sequence of events that result in the generation of antibody-synthesizing cells. Salmeron and Lipsky showed that this effect was the result of chloroquine's interference with the secretion of interleukin-1 by monocytes.

MECHANISM OF ACTION IN PORPHYRIA CUTANEA TARDA (PCT). Felsher and Redeker and many others clearly demonstrated that chloroquine and hydroxychloroquine caused a marked increase in urinary uroporphyrin excretion with accompanying elevations in serum transaminases when administered to patients with PCT.[23] In each case, complete clinical and nearly complete biochemical remission appeared within weeks and persisted during an extended period of observation. In 2 patients, the hepatic uroporphyrin concentration was reduced to half the pretreatment value. Felsher and Redeker suggested that a complex between chloroquine and uroporphyrin formed in liver cells and was released and excreted in urine and feces.

Scholnick and colleagues confirmed in a PCT rat model that chloroquine induced massive urinary excretion associated with a marked decrease in hepatic porphyrin content without changing the activity of the rate-controlling enzyme of porphyrin biosynthesis, delta-aminolevulinic acid synthetase.[24] They further showed that chloroquine induced a shift in the absorption maximum of coproporphyrin I or uroporphyrin III, which indicated that a physical interaction occurred. Chloroquine acted in a concentration-dependent manner in effecting the release of coproporphyrin from a liver homogenate. The results suggested that chloroquine and porphyrin formed a water-soluble complex or that chloroquine competed with porphyrin for specific binding sites. Taljaard and associates noted that urinary iron excretion increased simultaneously with porphyrinuria during chloroquine administration.[25] They reasoned that if liver cell necrosis is not an essential part of the process, an alternative explanation for the lengthy remissions following chloroquine use must be sought. Hepatic iron overload seems to be pertinent to the pathogenesis of PCT, and the beneficial effect of phlebotomy has been attributed to reduction in iron stores. Taljaard and associates suggested that chloroquine depletes a fraction of the liver iron stores that is responsible for continued overproduction and storage in the liver of higher carboxylated porphyrins.

Clinical Use (Table 11-2)

Approved Indications

Except for lupus erythematosus, all other approved indications for antimalarials are nondermatologic. Quinacrine became obsolete for malaria and tapeworm infections as equally effective and less toxic alternatives were introduced.[12] The major indication for quinacrine is currently in the treatment of giardiasis at a dosage of 100 mg three times a day for 5 days. Microorganisms disappear from stools, and symptoms clear rapidly.

Hydroxychloroquine is used as a disease-modifying agent in rheumatoid arthritis. Improvement is seen overall in about 63% of patients, but about 12% achieve complete remission.[32]

LUPUS ERYTHEMATOSUS. After Page's report,[1] numerous studies confirmed the efficacy of quinacrine and other antimalarials in the treatment of discoid skin lesions. Until Kraak and coauthors reported the first double-blind, placebo-controlled trial of hydroxychloroquine,[26] the improvement of discoid lupus erythematosus (DLE) during antimalarial therapy was dismissed as spontaneous remission, placebo-effect, or "publication artifact." Their data showed that hydroxychloroquine was significantly more effective than placebo after 3 months and 1 year of treatment and that hydroxychloroquine given for 3 months after a year of placebo treatment was more effective than the reverse.

There have been no extensive double-blind studies of effects of antimalarials in systemic lupus erythematosus (SLE), but Dubois believed that up to 95% of patients with DLE and SLE skin lesions would show moderate to marked improvement.[27] In their textbook, Wallace and Dubois stated that antimalarials improved polyarthralgia, pleuritis, low-grade pericarditis, malaise, and lethargy. They may have a steroid-sparing effect but are not considered effective for acutely ill patients with fever or central nervous system, hematologic, or renal involvement.

Antimalarials

Table 11–2. Antimalarial Indications/Contraindications

FDA-Approved Dermatologic Indication

Lupus erythematosus[1, 26–30] (*in selected cases)†
Nondermatologic indications of interest include rheumatoid arthritis (hydroxychloroquine),[31–33] malaria* (all three malarials).[6, 12]

Other Dermatologic Uses

Photosensitivity Dermatoses

Polymorphous light eruption (PMLE)[34, 35]†
Porphyria cutanea tarda[36–41]†
Dermatomyositis (cutaneous features)[42]†
Solar urticaria[43, 44]

Granulomatous Dermatoses

Sarcoidosis[45]†
Granuloma annulare (generalized)[46]

Lymphocytic Infiltrates

Lymphocytoma cutis[47]
Lymphocytic infiltrate of Jessner[48]

Other Conditions

Reticular erythematous mucinosis syndrome[49, 50]
Atopic dermatitis[51]
Urticarial vasculitis[52]
Localized scleroderma[53]
Panniculitis (idiopathic)[54]

Contraindications

The main contraindications to the use of antimalarials are pregnancy and lactation, because the drugs can cross the placenta and are secreted in breast milk. They are also contraindicated in patients who have myasthenia gravis. In several other situations, antimalarials may be used with caution and proper monitoring: for children, for patients with G6PD deficiency, and for psychotic patients.

Note: FDA = Food and Drug Administration.
*Antimalarials are generally considered the drug of choice.
†Antimalarials are definitely effective.

Antimalarials should be reserved for those patients with localized cutaneous disease who have not responded to reasonable efforts at sun avoidance, liberal use of broad-spectrum sunscreens, and potent topical or intralesional corticosteroids. Significant scalp involvement with alopecia and disseminated discoid, annular, or papulosquamous skin lesions also warrant antimalarials. Systemic corticosteroids are generally not effective for DLE and probably should not be used for this purpose.

The recommended dosages (see Table 11–1) and usage of the three antimalarials are closely tied to their toxicity and clinical efficacy and will be discussed in the Therapeutic Guidelines section.

Other Dermatologic Uses

PHOTOSENSITIVITY DERMATOSES. The photodermatoses, including polymorphous light eruption (PMLE), dermatomyositis, and solar urticaria, may be ameliorated by treatment with antimalarials. Reticular erythematous mucinosis syndrome can be photoaggravated and may benefit from antimalarial therapy.[49, 50] In a double-blind trial of hydroxychloroquine completed during the summer months, 28 patients with PMLE showed moderate improvement in both symptoms and skin rash.[35] Murphy and coauthors and others agree that antimalarials should be reserved for the months in which risk for the eruption is highest in those patients who fail to respond to sunscreens or prophylactic "hardening of the skin" with UVB phototherapy or psoralens plus ultraviolet A (PUVA).[43] Some cases of a similar but distinct entity, lymphocytic infiltration of the skin (Jessner), may respond to antimalarials.[48]

The skin manifestations of dermatomyositis are notoriously difficult to treat. They are often resistant to systemic and topical corticosteroid treatment. However, if the patient has active myositis and is being treated aggressively with corticosteroids and methotrexate or immunosuppressives, the skin may improve. Callen showed that hydroxychloroquine improved skin lesions in 10 of 11 patients.[42] The drug did not affect the myopathy, but it did allow tapering of steroids that were being used to treat the skin.

GRANULOMATOUS DERMATOSES. In placebo-controlled trials, antimalarials, particularly chloroquine, have been shown to suppress pulmonary and cutaneous granulomas of sarcoidosis. For localized skin lesions, superpotent topical corticosteroids may be all that is necessary. Destructive acral or lupus pernio lesions may require intralesional corticosteroids. Systemic corticosteroids are usually reserved for symptomatic pulmonary disease but may be used for disseminated skin lesions, ulcerations, or cicatricial alopecia due to sarcoidosis. Alternatively, antimalarials may be used alone or combined with alternate-day dosage regimens of oral corticosteroids. Relapse of skin lesions may occur after withdrawal of antimalarial therapy.[45] Disseminated granuloma annulare also may respond to antimalarials.[46]

OTHER INDICATIONS. Quinacrine has several other interesting uses in medicine that deserve mention.[6] Because of its avid binding to nucleoprotein, quinacrine has been used as a probe for nucleolar function, as well as for analysis of specific regions of human chromosomes (Q-banding). Quinacrine is used in the palliative treatment of malignant pleural effusions and ascites. Instillation into these body cavities causes reabsorption of fluid; subsequent thickening and adhesion of serosal surfaces prevent fluid reaccumulation.

Adverse Effects

An impressive list of possible side effects has been published,[30,55] and almost any organ system can be affected. All the adverse reactions can occur with any of the three antimalarials, with two notable exceptions. First, quinacrine therapy produces a yellowish stain of the skin and the sclera in about a third of patients after months of therapy, whereas the other drugs do not. The stain is most marked on the dorsal surface of hands, feet, and arms, and in skin folds. The yellow pigment disappears gradually after therapy is stopped, and it is harmless. The cosmetic appearance can be troublesome to fair-skinned patients. Second, quinacrine is not toxic to the retina, whereas chloroquine and hydroxychloroquine potentially are.

MISCELLANEOUS SYSTEMIC ADVERSE EFFECTS. Gastrointestinal side effects, nausea, vomiting, and diarrhea are the most common reasons for early decreases in dosage or discontinuation of treatment. Approximately 10% of patients are unable to tolerate chloroquine. Infrequent central nervous system effects that may be seen in susceptible patients or with higher-than-recommended dosages include restlessness, excitement, confusion, headache, seizures, myasthenia, and toxic psychosis.[56] Rare but potentially fatal bone marrow toxicity has been reported, including aplastic anemia (quinacrine) and agranulocytosis (chloroquine). Chloroquine has been associated with hemolysis in glucose-6-phosphate dehydrogenase (G6PD) deficiency, although this is considered more of a problem with the 8-aminoquinoline primaquine.

CUTANEOUS ADVERSE EFFECTS. A bluish-gray to black hyperpigmentation may occur in 10%–30% of patients treated for 4 months or longer with any of the drugs.[57] The pigmentation typically affects the shins (resembling ecchymoses), the face, the palate (with a sharp line demarcating the hard and soft palates), and the nail beds (as tranverse bands).[58] Biopsies show both hemosiderin around capillaries and dermal melanin. The pigmentation may take many months to fade after discontinuation of therapy. Progressive bleaching of the hair roots of the scalp, the face, and the body is another unusual pigmentary disturbance that may appear in as many as 10% of patients taking chloroquine.[59,60] This phenomenon is also reversible.

The incidence of pruritus and "dermatitis" associated with antimalarial use has been reported to be 10%–20%.[61] The rashes included urticaria, morbilliform, eczematous, lichenoid, exfoliative dermatitis, and erythema annulare centrifugum patterns.[62] Bauer estimated the incidence of rashes in servicemen during World War II at 1 of 2000 and 1 of 500 for 100 and 200 mg/day of quinacrine, respectively.[63] He also reported that 3 of the most severely affected servicemen with lichen planus–like histology developed the late sequela of palmar squamous cell carcinoma, two with metastases to the axilla. However, all 3 had received low-dosage radiation therapy.

The controversial issue of whether antimalarials exacerbate pre-existing psoriasis has received attention in the dermatologic and rheumatologic literature. Interestingly, these drugs are used in the treatment of psoriatic arthropathy. The incidence of flare-up actually varies from 0% to 100%![64] Kuflik studied the effect of malaria prophylaxis (200 mg/week of chloroquine and 15 mg/week of primaquine) on 48 patients with psoriasis.[65] Psoriasis worsened in 42% of patients, but only 6% were resistant to topical treatment. For this reason, Kuflik concluded that prophylactic antimalarial treatment was not contraindicated for psoriasis patients traveling to endemic areas. Slagel and James reviewed the literature and reported an overall incidence of 31% for acute generalized eruptions (including both flare-ups of psoriasis and other drug-related eruptions).[66] Quinacrine was responsible for the greatest frequency of exfoliative erythroderma, whereas chloroquine was most commonly responsible for significant psoriasis flare-ups. A markedly lower incidence for both types of reactions was noted for hydroxychloroquine than for the other antimalarials. Psoriatic flare-ups and recalcitrance to conventional therapy are probably very low risks inasmuch as hydroxychloroquine is now used almost exclusively for arthritis. A prospective study of large numbers of patients with psoriatic arthritis who are treated with either antimalarial or other drugs and are followed for at least 6 months is required to help define the risk.

ACUTE POISONING. Fatal reactions have been reported after accidental or intentional overdosage with chloroquine. The particular sensitivity of very young children (aged 1–3 years) to only 1 g has been emphasized.[67, 68] Irreversible cardiac arrest occurred in some patients within 1–2 hours of drug ingestion. Intubation, gastric lavage, and acidification of urine to increase excretion may be lifesaving measures. Rasmussen pointed out that adults show the same sensitivity to chloroquine on a milligram per kilogram basis.[69]

Although special precautions should be taken to prevent poisoning (as with any medication), antimalarials are not contraindicated for children. Malaria prophylaxis should be given according to guidelines in the Aralen and Plaquenil package inserts. Hydroxychloroquine, although not approved by the FDA for this purpose, is used in the treatment of juvenile rheumatoid arthritis.

OCULAR TOXICITY. The antimalarials can cause several ocular adverse effects, but it is the inherent retinal toxicity of chloroquine and hydroxychloroquine, first reported in 1959[70] and later confirmed,[71, 72] that forms the basis for current treatment and ocular safety monitoring guidelines. Several reviews on this topic are available.[73, 74]

As mentioned earlier, chloroquine has an affinity for melanin-containing tissues and accumulates in the eye (iris, choroid, pigmented epithelium of the retina). Here it persists for years after cessation of therapy. It has been suggested that this abnormal concentration of drug blocks the normal protective light-absorbing action of melanin. Mackenzie speculated that 4-aminoquinolines might interfere with phagolysosome function of retinal pigmented epithelial cells, which leads to inefficient elimination of photoreceptor cell debris and retinal dystrophy.[31]

CORNEA. Antimalarials are deposited in the basal epithelium as early as the first few weeks of therapy. Although usually asymptomatic, patients may complain of halos around lights as a result of these deposits. Visual acuity is not reduced.

Easterbrook reported a striking difference in the prevalence and appearance of the corneal changes of patients treated with chloroquine (95%) and hydroxychloroquine (<20%).[75] In the latter, the deposits were "very mild and difficult to visualize" when the pupils were dilated and the corneas were retroilluminated with the slit lamp. The finding of corneal deposits is not considered a contraindication to continued treatment, unless the patient has troublesome visual symptoms. The deposits disappear completely 6–8 weeks after antimalarial drugs are discontinued, and there is no residual corneal damage.

CILIARY BODY. A reduction in the accommodative power of the eye and a change in extraocular muscle balance may occur soon after the initiation of chloroquine therapy. If the symptoms bother the patient, the dosage should be reduced. No loss of accommodation has been reported in patients receiving hydroxychloroquine.

RETINA. The incidence of true retinopathy is low; only about 300 cases have been described in the world's literature. The classic picture of chloroquine retinopathy consists of granular or stippled hyperpigmentation of the macula, surrounded first by a clear zone of depigmentation and then by another ring of pigmentation. This "bull's-eye" lesion represents an advanced stage of retinopathy with a more serious visual field deficit (absolute scotomas) and possible progression of the scotoma and loss in visual acuity even after the drug is discontinued. The onset of retinopathy may be delayed up to 7 years after cessation of chloroquine therapy.[76, 77]

It is clearly the duty of dermatologic therapists to use these drugs at a dosage that minimizes the risk of developing retinopathy and to monitor patients in such a way that a reversible preretinopathy (premaculopathy) state can be detected. The clinical findings that represent these reversible states have been defined by various authors.[78, 79]

Previous authors have suggested that it was either the lifetime accumulated dose of antimalarial drugs (100–300 g) or the duration of treatment (in years) that was associated with the risk of retinopathy. Mackenzie, however, showed, and Easterbrook confirmed, in 900 and 1500 patients, respectively, that long-term daily dosages of 3.5 mg/kg of chloroquine or 6.5 mg/kg of hydroxychloroquine lie below the threshold at which retinal toxicity was found to develop.[31, 75]

Easterbrook and Bernstein carefully studied and analyzed the frequency and types of ophthalmologic examinations available.[75, 78] Their recommendations for the detection of patients with relative paracentral

---

ANTIMALARIAL MONITORING GUIDELINES[75, 78, 80, 81]

Baseline

Ocular
- Baseline slit-lamp and funduscopic examination, assessment of visual acuity
- Visual field testing by both static and kinetic techniques with a 3-mm red test object
- Asking patients to test themselves with the Amsler grid (Fig. 11–1) every 2 weeks; patients test each eye separately by occluding the opposite eye with reading glasses on and looking for "faded" squares

Laboratory
- Complete blood count (CBC)
- G6PD screening
- Automated chemistry profile (emphasis on liver function tests)
- Random or 24-hour urinary porphyrin screening

Follow-up

Ocular
- Reviewing subjective visual complaints, slit-lamp and funduscopic test results, and visual acuity (every 6 months)
- Repeating visual field testing if patients complain of difficulty in reading ("missing" words and letters) and demonstrate reproducible bilateral "fading" of Amsler grid squares
- Discontinuing chloroquine or hydroxychloroquine treatment if bilateral field defects are confirmed

Laboratory
- CBC (monthly for 3 months, then every 4–6 months)
- Automated chemistry profile (after 1 month, after 3 months, and then every 4–6 months)

Note: More frequent surveillance is needed if laboratory values are abnormal or with high-risk patients.

278   *Antimalarials*

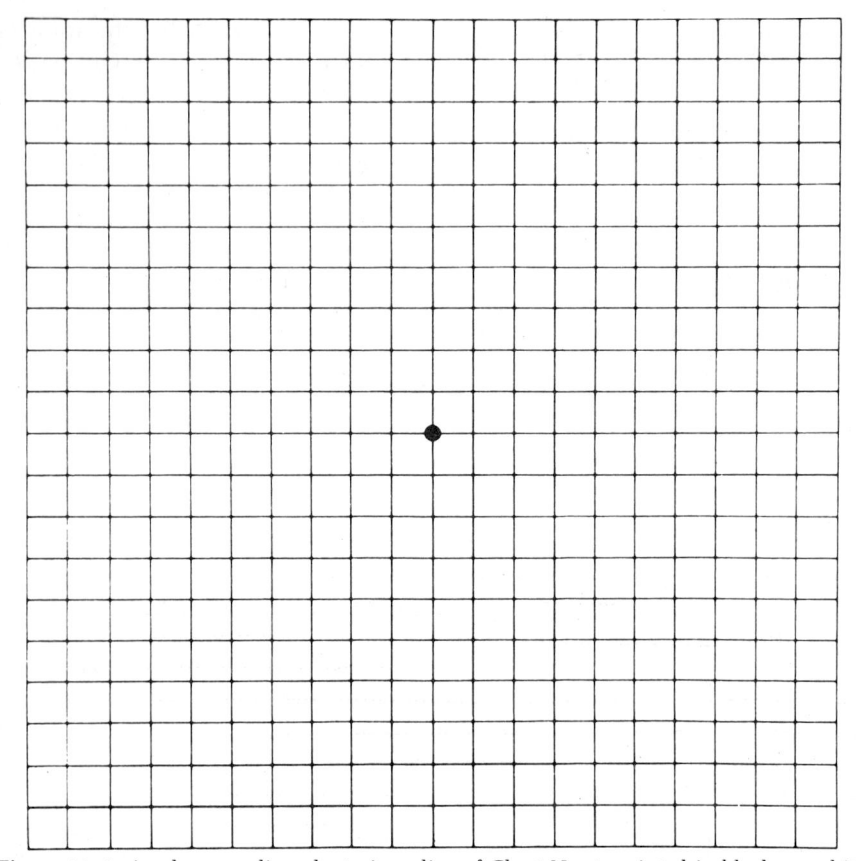

Figure 11–1. Amsler recording chart. A replica of Chart No. 1, printed in black on white for convenience of recording.

scotomas, which usually disappear within 3 months after cessation of antimalarial therapy, are included in the Monitoring Guidelines.

In general, time-consuming specialized tests, including fluorescein angiography, electro-oculograms, and electroretinograms, are positive only in late stages of retinopathy. They are therefore not useful for screening for reversible toxicity. Fluorescein angiography may be useful in some elderly patients with pre-existing senile macular degeneration or in whom visual field testing may not be reliable.

Drug Interactions

The only significant drug interactions of concern are those between antimalarials. Chloroquine and hydroxychloroquine should not be administered concurrently because of the additive retinotoxic potential. The combination of chloroquine and primaquine used for malaria prophylaxis is more likely to induce hemolysis in the G6PD-deficient patient. Although the combinations are not formally approved, rheumatologists routinely use hydroxychloroquine together with methotrexate, prednisone, and nonsteroidal anti-inflammatory drugs in the treatment of SLE, rheumatoid arthritis, and psoriatic arthritis without significant drug interaction.[33] Digoxin levels may be elevated by antimalarials.

Therapeutic Guidelines

The following dosage recommendations apply to treatment of all the dermatologic indications except PCT (see the following section). Travelers to endemic areas should contact the Centers for Disease Control for the latest recommendations for malaria prophylaxis that have been influenced by the emergence and dissemination of chloroquine-resistant strains of Plasmodium falciparum.

The treatment of DLE was reviewed in 1989.[30] The antimalarial of first choice is hydroxychloroquine at a daily dosage of 6.5 mg/kg calculated from the patient's ideal (lean) body weight, or 400 mg, whichever is less. (For sarcoidosis, it may be preferable to start with chloroquine 3.5–4.0 mg/kg/day or 250 mg, whichever is less.[45]) It may take up to 4–8 weeks of therapy before a clinical response is seen and several more months for maximal benefit. Theoretically, priming a patient with an antimalarial may decrease the time necessary to reach equilibrium between plasma and tissues. An initial priming dosage of an antimalarial is used in the treatment of the acute attack of vivax or falciparum malaria. For chloroquine, this consists of 1 g followed by an additional 500 mg after 6–8 hours and 500 mg daily for the next 2 days, a total dosage of 2.5 g over 3 days.[82] In general, priming is not necessary for the chronic and non–life-threatening conditions. Higher dosages may increase the risk of gastrointestinal irritation and retinal toxicity. If nausea, vomiting, or diarrhea becomes problematic, stopping the drug and restarting at a lower dosage may circumvent the problem. Patients who develop a drug-related eruption must discontinue the antimalarial. However, patients who are intolerant of or "allergic" to hydroxychloroquine may tolerate chloroquine, and vice versa.

In patients who do not obtain maximal benefit for their skin disease after 3 months, 100 mg/day of quinacrine may be added to the regimen without increasing the risk of retinotoxicity. Quinacrine may be a better choice as the initial antimalarial for darkly pigmented races because the expected pigmentary alteration may be less detectable. It is also possible that a given patient may respond better to equivalent dosages of either chloroquine or hydroxychloroquine. Suggested safety monitoring tests adapted from package inserts and reviews[75, 78, 80, 81] are shown in the Monitoring Guidelines.

For patients who have developed retinopathy or rashes from either or both 4-aminoquinolines, or who are unreliable in keeping regular follow-up appointments, quinacrine may be used alone at a dosage of 100–200 mg/day.

After maximal improvement is achieved, the dosage of antimalarial should be decreased gradually by about 25% every 3–6 months. Relapse occurs frequently at low dosages. It therefore may be necessary to maintain some patients on one or two tablets per week in order to suppress severe or extensive skin lesions. Some patients with seasonal, light-aggravated disease can be treated only during the problematic months; the pre-seasonal treatment time needed for equilibration should then be taken into account.

TREATMENT OF PCT. For patients with PCT, ingestion of all exogenous hepatotoxins (alcohol, estrogens, and iron supplements) should first be discontinued. Phlebotomy is still considered the treatment of first choice for PCT. Units of whole blood are removed gradually or rapidly in order to achieve a hemoglobin level of 10–11 g/dl.[39] Numerous publications have shown that antimalarial treatment achieves results equivalent to phlebotomy.[36-38] Therefore, these drugs are reserved for either patients who are already anemic or patients in whom phlebotomy is impractical or technically not feasible.

A test dose of 200 mg of hydroxychloroquine or 125 mg of chloroquine is administered, and liver function tests are performed 1 week later. This dose is then repeated twice a week for 6–12 months. Higher dosages may lead to hepatotoxicity as a result of rapid mobilization of hepatic porphyrin stores. Clinical remission and a nearly normal biochemical profile of porphyrin excretion occurs in all patients so treated. Harber and Bickers recommended continued treatment until the total urinary porphyrin level is less than 300 mcg/day.[39] Relapse generally occurs within 1–2 years, but some patients have remained in remission for more than 4 years.[38] The combination of phlebotomy and low dosages of chloroquine has been tried, but a convincing advantage over either treatment alone has not been shown.[40,41]

BIBLIOGRAPHY: Key Reviews/Chapters

Willoughby JS, Shear NH: Antimalarials. Clin Dermatol 1989; 7(3):60–68.
Portnoy JZ, Callen JP: Ophthalmologic aspects of chloroquine and hydroxychloroquine therapy. Int J Dermatol 1983; 22:273–278.
Isaacson D, Elgart M, Turner ML: Antimalarials in dermatology. Int J Dermatol 1982; 21:379–395.
Lo JS, Berg RE, Tomecki KJ: Treatment of discoid lupus erythematosus. Int J Dermatol 1989; 28:497–507.
Titus ED: Recent developments in the understanding of the pharmacokinetics and mechanisms of action of chloroquine. Ther Drug Monit 1989; 11:369–379.
Wallace DJ, Dubois EL (eds): Dubois' Lupus Erythematosus. Philadelphia: Lea & Febiger, 1987, 512–526.

REFERENCES

1. Page F: Treatment of lupus erythematosus with mepacrine. Lancet 1951; 2:755–758.
2. Wolfe AD: Quinacrine and other acridines. In Corcoran JW, Hahn FE (eds): Mechanisms of Action of Antimicrobial and Antitumor Agents: Vol. 3. Antibiotics. New York: Springer-Verlag, 1975, 203–233.
3. Hahn FE: Chloroquine (Resochin). In Corcoran JW, Hahn FE (eds): Mechanisms of Action of Antimicrobial and Antitumor Agents: Vol. 3. Antibiotics. New York: Springer-Verlag, 1975, 58–78.
4. McChesney EW: Animal toxicity and pharmacokinetics of hydroxychloroquine sulfate. Am J Med 1983; 75(1A):11–18.
5. Tett SE, Cutler DJ, Day RO, et al: A dose-ranging study of the pharmacokinetics of hydroxychloroquine following intravenous administration to healthy volunteers. Br J Clin Pharmacol 1988; 26:303–313.
6. DiPalma JR: Chemotherapy of protozoan infections I: Malaria. In DiPalma JR (ed): Drill's Pharmacology in Medicine. New York: McGraw-Hill, 1971, 1770–1792.
7. Tanenbaum L, Tuffanelli DL: Animalarial agents: Chloroquine, hydroxychloroquine, and quinacrine. Arch Dermatol 1980; 116:587–591.
8. Sams WM: Chloroquine: Mechanisms of action. Mayo Clin Proc 1967; 42:300–309.
9. Hong DD: Chloroquine phosphate. In Florey K (ed): Analytical Profiles of Drug Substances: Vol. 1. New York: Academic Press, 1972, 61–85.
10. Sams WM, Carroll NV. The "spectral shift" phenomenon of chloroquine. Arch Dermatol 1966; 93:123–128.
11. Lester RS, Burnham TK, Fine G, et al: Immunologic concepts of light reactions in lupus erythematosus and polymorphous light eruptions: I. The mechanism of action of hydroxychloroquine. Arch Dermatol 1967; 96:1–10.
12. Rollo IM: Miscellaneous drugs used in the treatment of protozoal infections. In Gilman AG, Goodman LS, Gilman A (eds): Goodman and Gilman's The Pharmacological Basis of Therapeutics (6th ed). New York: Macmillan, 1980, 1070–1079.
13. Stollar D, Levine L: Antibodies to denatured DNA in lupus erythematosus serum: V. Mechanism of DNA–anti-DNA inhibition by chloroquine. Arch Biochem Biophys 1963; 101:335–341.
14. Bencze G, Johnson GD: Inhibition of antinuclear factor reaction by chloroquine. Immunol 1965; 9:201–202.
15. Ward PA: The chemosuppression of chemotaxis. J Exp Med 1966; 124:209–226.
16. Gauderer CA, Gleich GJ: Inhibition of eosinophilotaxis by chloroquine and corticosteroids. Proc Soc Exp Biol Med 1978; 157:129–133.
17. Kalmanson GM, Guze LB: Studies of the effects of hydroxychloroquine on immune responses. J Lab Clin Med 1965; 65:484–489.
18. Neblett TR, Burnham TK, Kay W: Chloroquine: Its mechanism of action upon immune phenomena. Arch Dermatol 1965; 92:720–725.
19. Sheon RP: Results of two year study of the effect of chloroquine phosphate on rheumatoid factor titre and rheumatoid arthritis [abstract]. Arthritis Rheum 1968; 11:840–841.
20. Panayi GS, Neill WA, Duthie JJR, et al: Action of chloroquine phosphate in rheumatoid arthritis: I. Immunosuppressive effect. Ann Rheum Dis 1973; 32:316–318.
21. Mackenzie AH: Pharmacologic actions of 4-aminoquinoline compounds. Am J Med 1983; 75(1A):5–10.
22. Salmeron G, Lipsky PE: Immunosuppressive potential of antimalarials. Am J Med 1983; 75(1A):19–24.
23. Felsher BF, Redeker AG: Effect of chloroquine on hepatic uroporphyrin metabolism in patients with porphyria cutanea tarda. Medicine 1966; 45:575–583.

24. Scholnick PL, Epstein J, Marver HS: The molecular basis of the action of chloroquine in porphyria cutanea tarda. J Invest Dermatol 1973; 61:226–232.
25. Taljaard JJF, Shanley BC, Stewart-Wynne EG, et al: Studies on low dose chloroquine therapy and the action of chloroquine in symptomatic porphyria. J Invest Dermatol 1972; 87:261–269.
26. Kraak JH, van Ketel WG, Prakken JR, et al: The value of hydroxychloroquine (Plaquenil) for the treatment of chronic discoid lupus erythematosus: A double blind trial. Dermatologica 1965; 130:293–305.
27. Dubois EL: Antimalarials in the management of discoid and systemic lupus erythematosus. Semin Arthritis Rheum 1978; 8:33–51.
28. Tuffanelli DL: Lupus erythematosus. J Am Acad Dermatol 1981; 4:127–142.
29. Wallace DJ, Dubois EL (eds): Dubois' Lupus Erythematosus. Philadelphia: Lea & Febiger, 1987, 512–526.
30. Lo JS, Berg RE, Tomecki KJ: Treatment of discoid lupus erythematosus. Int J Dermatol 1989; 28:497–507.
31. Mackenzie AH: Dose refinements in long-term therapy of rheumatoid arthritis with antimalarials. Am J Med 1983; 75(1A):40–45.
32. Bell CL: Hydroxychloroquine sulfate in rheumatoid arthritis: Long-term response rate and predictive parameters. Am J Med 1983; 75(1A):46–51.
33. Scherbel AL: Use of synthetic antimalarial drugs and other agents for rheumatoid arthritis: Historic and therapeutic perspectives. Am J Med 1983; 75(1A):1–4.
34. Jansen CT: Oral carotenoid treatment in polymorphous light eruption: A cross-over comparison with oxychloroquine and placebo. Photodermatol 1985; 2:166–169.
35. Murphy GM, Hawk JL, Magnus IA: Hydroxychloroquine in polymorphic light eruption: A controlled trial with drug and visual sensitivity monitoring. Br J Dermatol 1987; 116:379–386.
36. Malkinson FD, Levitt L: Hydroxychloroquine treatment of porphyria cutanea tarda. Arch Dermatol 1980; 116:1147–1150.
37. Marchesi L, Di Padova C, Cainelli T, et al: A comparative trial of desferrioxamine and hydroxychloroquine for treatment of porphyria cutanea tarda in alcoholic patients. Photodermatol 1984; 1:286–292.
38. Ashton RE, Hawk JL, Magnus IA: Low-dose oral chloroquine in the treatment of porphyria cutanea tarda. Br J Dermatol 1984; 111:609–613.
39. Harber LC, Bickers DR: The Porphyrias. In Photosensitivity Diseases: Principles of Diagnosis and Treatment (2nd ed). Toronto: Decker, 1989, 241–287.
40. Swanbeck G, Wennersten G: Treatment of porphyria cutanea tarda with chloroquine and phlebotomy. Br J Dermatol 1977; 97:77–81.
41. Horkay I, Nagy E: Combination therapy of porphyria cutanea tarda using chloroquine and bloodletting therapy. Z Hautkr 1980; 55:813–816.
42. Callen JP: Dermatomyositis—An update 1985. Semin Dermatol 1985; 4:114–125.
43. Swanbeck G: Treatment of photodermatoses. Semin Dermatol 1982; 1:211–216.
44. Mathews-Roth MM: Systemic photoprotection. Dermatol Clin 1986; 4:335–339.
45. Veien NK: Cutaneous sarcoidosis: Prognosis and treatment. Clin Dermatol 1986; 4:75–87.
46. Carlin MC, Ratz JL: A case of generalized granuloma annulare responding to hydroxychloroquine. Cleve Clin J Med 1987; 54:229–232.
47. Stoll DM: Treatment of cutaneous pseudolymphoma with hydroxychloroquine. J Am Acad Dermatol 1983; 8:696–699.
48. Toonstra J, Wildschut A, Boer J, et al: Jessner's lymphocytic infiltration of the skin: A clinical study of 100 patients. Arch Dermatol 1989; 125:1525–1530.
49. Balogh E, Nagy-Vezekényi K, Fórizs E: REM syndrome: An immediate therapeutic response to hydroxychloroquine sulphate. Acta Derm Venereol (Stockh) 1980; 60:173–175.

50. Steigleder GK, Gartmann H, Linker U: REM syndrome: Reticular erythematous mucinosis (round-cell erythematosis), a new entity? Br J Dermatol 1974; 91:191–199.
51. Döring HF, Müllejans-Kreppel U: Chloroquine—Therapy of atopic dermatitis. Z Hautkr 1987; 62:1205–1213.
52. Lopez LR, Davis KC, Kohler PF, Schocket AL: The hypocomplementemic urticarial-vasculitis syndrome: Therapeutic response to hydroxychloroquine. J Allergy Clin Immunol 1984; 73:600–603.
53. Nagy E, Ladanyi E: Treatment of circumscribed scleroderma in childhood. Z Hautkr 1987; 62:547–549.
54. Shelley WB: Chloroquine-induced remission of nodular panniculitis present for 15 years. J Am Acad Dermatol 1981; 5:168–170.
55. Isaacson D, Elgart M, Turner ML: Anti-malarials in dermatology. Int J Dermatol 1982; 21:379–395.
56. Ward WQ, Walter-Ryan WG, Shehi GM: Toxic psychosis: A complication of antimalarial therapy. J Am Acad Dermatol 1985; 12:863–865.
57. Granstein RD, Sober AJ: Drug- and heavy metal–induced hyperpigmentation. J Am Acad Dermatol 1981; 5:1–18.
58. Daniel CR, Scher RK: Nail changes secondary to systemic drugs or ingestants. J Am Acad Dermatol 1984; 10:250–258.
59. Dupré A, Ortonne JP, Viraben R, Gorguet B: Chloroquine-induced hypopigmentation of hair and freckles: Association with congenital renal failure. Arch Dermatol 1985; 121:1164–1166.
60. Cline DJ: Changes in hair color. Dermatol Clin 1988; 6:295–303.
61. Wintroub BU, Stern R: Cutaneous drug reactions: Pathogenesis and clinical classification. J Am Acad Dermatol 1985; 13:167–179.
62. Hudson LD: Erythema annulare centrifugum: An unusual case due to hydroxychloroquine sulfate. Cutis 1985; 36:129–130.
63. Bauer F: Quinacrine hydrochloride drug eruption (tropical lichenoid dermatitis). J Am Acad Dermatol 1981; 4:239–248.
64. Abel EA, DiCicco LM, Orenberg EK, et al: Drugs in exacerbation of psoriasis. J Am Acad Dermatol 1986; 15:1007–1022.
65. Kuflik EG: Effect of antimalarial drugs on psoriasis. Cutis 1980; 26:153–155.
66. Slagel GA, James WD: Plaquenil-induced erythroderma. J Am Acad Dermatol 1985; 12:857–862.
67. Cann HM, Verhulst HL: Fatal acute chloroquine poisoning in children. Pediatrics 1961; 27:95–102.
68. Markowitz HA, McGinley JM: Chloroquine poisoning in a child. JAMA 1964; 189:950–951.
69. Rasmussen JE: Antimalarials—Are they safe to use in children? Pediatr Dermatol 1983; 1:89–91.
70. Hobbs HE, Sorsby A, Freedman A: Retinopathy following chloroquine therapy. Lancet 1959; 2:478.
71. Richards RD, Wilson WR. Retinopathy associated with chloroquine phosphate therapy. Am J Med 1961; 31:140–143.
72. Carr RE, Henkind P, Rothfield N, et al: Ocular toxicity of antimalarial drugs: Long-term follow-up. Am J Ophthalmol 1968; 66:738–744.
73. Olansky AJ: Antimalarials and ophthalmologic safety. J Am Acad Dermatol 1982; 6:19–23.
74. Portnoy JZ, Callen JP: Ophthalmologic aspects of chloroquine and hydroxychloroquine therapy. Int J Dermatol 1983; 22:273–278.
75. Easterbrook M: Ocular effects and safety of antimalarial agents. Am J Med 1988; 85(4A):23–29.
76. Ehrenfeld M, Nesher R, Merin S: Delayed onset chloroquine retinopathy. Br J Opthalmol 1986; 70:281–283.

77. Martin LJ, Bergen RL, Dobrow HR: Delayed onset chloroquine retinopathy: Case report. Ann Opthalmol 1978; 10:723–726.
78. Bernstein HN: Ophthalmologic considerations and testing in patients receiving long-term antimalarial therapy. Am J Med 1983: 75(1A):25–34.
79. Terrell WL 3rd, Haik KG, Haik GM Jr: Hydroxychloroquine sulfate and retinopathy. South Med J 1988; 81:1327–1328.
80. Koranda FC: Antimalarials. J Am Acad Dermatol 1981; 4:650–655.
81. Goette DK: Antimalarials. J Assoc Milit Dermatol 1989; 15:25–27.
82. Rollo IM: Drugs used in the chemotherapy of malaria. In Gilman AG, Goodman LS, Gilman A (eds): Goodman and Gilman's The Pharmacological Basis of Therapeutics (6th ed). New York: Macmillan, 1980, 1038–1060.

12 Antihistamines

James Q. Del Rosso, D.O.

Since their introduction in the early 1940s, antihistamines have become very popular among both patients and physicians. Continuing research has led to the discovery of compounds capable of producing a variety of pharmacologic effects. An expanded list of clinical indications has resulted in the use of antihistamines touching upon most medical disciplines. Millions of dollars are spent each year by patients purchasing both prescription and over-the-counter medications containing antihistamines.[1] In addition, dermatologists often use these drugs to treat disorders that are chronic or recurrent. Thus dermatologists must be aware of the clinical utility and potential side effects of the different classes of antihistamines in order to successfully employ these useful drugs.

DEVELOPMENT OF ANTIHISTAMINES AND THEIR RELATIONSHIP TO DERMATOLOGY

Histamine was originally synthesized in 1907 before its physiologic significance to humans was recognized.[2] Several experiments subsequently defined the properties and tissue locations of histamine. Histamine is present either as granules in circulating basophils and tissue mast cells or free in tissues.[3,4] In the skin, histamine is a mediator of vasoconstriction, vasodilatation, capillary permeability, the wheal–flare reaction, and pruritus.[5-7]

In 1937, French researchers won the Nobel Prize after discovering the first antihistamine.[5] This was followed by the development in the U.S. of less toxic antihistamines such as tripelennamine, diphenhydramine, and promethazine in 1945 and 1946.[5] The development of other popular antihistamines such as chlorpheniramine, hydroxyzine, trimeprazine, and cyproheptadine came later. These conventional antihistamines are known collectively as the "classical" antihistamines, many of which demonstrate other effects such as cholinergic blockade. In the late

1960s, scientists and physicians began to appreciate the fact that the antihistaminic effect of these drugs was limited to antagonism of a subset of histamine receptors, subsequently called H_1 histamine receptors.[5]

In 1966, H_1 histamine receptors (H_1 receptors) were defined as those blocked by the previously discovered conventional antihistamines.[5] Responses such as gastric acid secretion were not blocked by these agents. In 1972, the existence of gastric H_2 histamine receptors (H_2 receptors) was discovered when scientists generated compounds chemically related to the structure of histamine, producing agents that antagonized H_2 receptors.[5,9] After hundreds of compounds were tested, H_2 blockers that were effective in humans were found and approved for use in treating peptic ulcer disease.[9] In the U.S., the Food and Drug Administration (FDA) approved the releases of cimetidine in 1977 and of ranitidine in 1983. Despite several infrequent, potentially severe side effects, both have proved to be safe and effective in peptic acid–related gastrointestinal disorders. Because H_2 receptors are present within the cutaneous microcirculation and on T lymphocytes, the H_2 receptor antagonists possess properties of interest to dermatologists.[6] Although cimetidine is not FDA-approved for dermatologic indications, the literature cites several potential uses for the drug in dermatology.[10,11]

The major side effect limiting the successful use of classical H_1 antihistamines has been sedation.[5] Researchers have developed H_1 antihistamines that possess a much lower incidence of central nervous system (CNS) side effects.[12,13] As a result, patients can perform tasks without psychomotor impairment, and there is no synergistic interaction with other CNS depressants such as diazepam and alcohol. Frequently referred to as "nonsedating" antihistamines, they are more accurately referred to as "less sedating" antihistamines. In addition, many appear to be relatively "pure" antihistamines devoid of significant activity at nonhistamine receptors with dosages used clinically.[12,13] Terfenadine, discovered in 1973, was approved for release in the U.S. in 1985, and astemizole was approved in 1988. Several other agents, such as loratadine and cetirizine, are currently being investigated.

Both the H_1 and the H_2 antihistamines competitively inhibit the binding of histamine to tissue receptors. In 1967, cromolyn was shown to have a prophylactic effect in the treatment of asthma by inhibiting the release of histamine and other mediators from mast cells.[14,15] Cromolyn is devoid of intrinsic antihistaminic, anti-inflammatory, or bronchodilatory effects.[14,15] Inhalant and topical formulations are FDA-approved for the treatment of asthma, allergic rhinitis, and ocular disorders. Oral cromolyn is FDA-approved for the treatment of mastocytosis.[16] Ketotifen, an intrinsic H_1 antihistamine, also inhibits mediator release from mast cells.[17] Cromolyn and ketotifen are generally referred to as "mast cell–stabilizing agents."

Doxepin has been available for several years as a tricyclic antidepressant approved by the FDA for treatment of depression or anxiety. Doxepin has potent antihistamininic effects that have been confirmed in vivo through histamine skin testing.[18,19] Doxepin is an antagonist at both H_1 and H_2 histamine receptors.[20,21] Clinical reports support the value of doxepin in patients with chronic idiopathic urticaria (CIU) and cold urticaria (see Tricyclic Agents: Doxepin section).

Several antihistamines are currently under study for FDA approval. The list includes acrivastine, azelastine, cetirizine, oxatomide, ketotifen, nedocromil, and loratadine.[22] The discovery of H_3 receptors, allegedly involved in regulation of histamine storage and release, will undoubtedly stimulate further antihistamine research.[4]

This chapter contains five sections, each covering development, pharmacology, and clinical use of a specific category of antihistamines. Categories discussed include classical H_1 antihistamines, less sedating H_1 antihistamines, H_2 antihistamines, tricyclic agents, and mast cell–stabilizing agents.

THE CLASSICAL H_1 ANTIHISTAMINES

Pharmacology

Structure

The classical H_1 antihistamines have been classified on the basis of their chemical structure.[1,5,12] The ethylamine moiety forms the nucleus of each compound; substitutions at various positions produce six major structural categories: alkylamine, ethanolamine, ethylenediamine, piperazine, piperidine, and phenothiazine antihistamines. Representative antihistamines from each of these groups are listed in Table 12–1.

Absorption/Distribution

The classical H_1 blockers are described as being rapidly absorbed after oral administration, and peak serum levels precede maximal effects in skin.[1,5] Oral bioavailability is well defined for those drugs available for

Table 12–1. Classical H_1 Antihistamines: Structural Classification and Examples

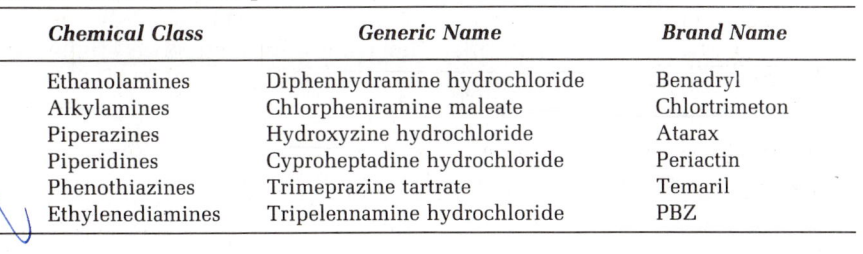

Chemical Class	Generic Name	Brand Name
Ethanolamines	Diphenhydramine hydrochloride	Benadryl
Alkylamines	Chlorpheniramine maleate	Chlortrimeton
Piperazines	Hydroxyzine hydrochloride	Atarax
Piperidines	Cyproheptadine hydrochloride	Periactin
Phenothiazines	Trimeprazine tartrate	Temaril
Ethylenediamines	Tripelennamine hydrochloride	PBZ

intravenous injection, such as diphenhydramine and chlorpheniramine. In addition, bioavailability is affected considerably by the type of formulation and the route of administration.

Only 25%–50% of orally administered chlorpheniramine is bioavailable.[24] This is primarily due to variable but extensive first-pass metabolism in the liver. The rate and extent of oral bioavailability is affected by the oral formulation used; syrups produce 65%–70% absorption.[24] Diphenhydramine also exhibits a first-pass hepatic metabolism; 50%–70% of the drug is bioavailable from oral preparations.[25, 26]

The lipid solubility of most classical H_1 antihistamines allows for wide tissue distribution.[1, 5, 12] Distribution to the skin and the CNS is considerable, accounting for suppression of the wheal–flare reaction and for commonly encountered CNS side effects.

Most classical H_1 antihistamines are available in solid and liquid oral formulations. A few drugs, such as diphenhydramine and chlorpheniramine, are also available by injection. The bioavailability of injectable formulations differs according to the route of administration.

Metabolism/Excretion

Hepatic metabolism appears to be the major route of biotransformation.[1, 5] Metabolites may also exhibit clinical activity. For example, cetirizine is a potent less sedating active metabolite of hydroxyzine.[27] For some drugs, such as chlorpheniramine, the activity of metabolites is not known.[24] The mode of excretion is dependent on the specific drug, its extent of biotransformation, and the nature of its metabolites. The majority of orally administered chlorpheniramine is excreted as metabolites in the urine.[24, 28] Orally administered diphenhydramine is principally excreted as urinary metabolites, the major metabolite being diphenylmethane.[29] Some of the classical H_1 antihistamines are also excreted in breast milk.

The serum elimination half-life of these drugs in adults differs considerably from drug to drug. The range includes approximately 6–9 hours for diphenhydramine, 20 hours for hydroxyzine, and 24 hours for chlorpheniramine.[25, 29, 31] The serum elimination half-life value of a given drug varies among patients and can differ with repetitive dosing. Shorter mean serum elimination half-lives in children have been confirmed for hydroxyzine (7 hours) and chlorpheniramine (9–13 hours).[31–33] The serum elimination half-life of hydroxyzine was prolonged to 29 hours in a group of healthy elderly patients who were administered a single dose of 0.7 mg/kg.[34]

Mechanism of Action

Antihistaminic activity results from interaction with H_1 receptors present on cell surfaces.[3, 5] This prevents binding of histamine, thus preventing its biologic effects. H_1 antihistamines are most effective if administered before the release of histamine.[3, 12] This explains the greater benefit of prophylactic usage of an H_1 antihistamine in patients with chronic idiopathic urticaria and symptomatic dermographism.

By antagonizing histamine, H_1 antihistamines produce a variety of effects.[3, 5] They inhibit increased capillary permeability and edema formation induced by histamine. Histamine-induced pruritus is also decreased. Prior administration of an H_1 antihistamine prevents edema and pruritus during immediate hypersensitivity reactions. Bronchiolar constriction, such as in anaphylaxis, is not antagonized because this effect is mediated principally by leukotrienes in humans.[5] H_1 antihistamines inhibit vasoconstriction and, to a lesser extent, vasodilatation, that is induced by histamine. This partial response is probably due to the presence of both H_1 and H_2 receptors in the microcirculation. H_1 antihistamines significantly suppress the cutaneous wheal–flare response; however, maximal suppression appears to require blockade of both H_1 and H_2 receptors.[1, 4]

Despite their different chemical structures, the classical H_1 antihistamines have qualitatively similar antihistaminic effects. Other potentially significant qualitative and quantitative pharmacologic differences do occur.[1] For example, the ethanolamines often produce significant CNS depression, whereas the alkylamines generally produces less sedation.

Pharmacologic nuances related to the structural antihistamine class may not always relate to clinical practice. Considerable variability in a drug's efficacy or side effects may exist from patient to patient.[5, 23] For example, a given patient may find that one antihistamine reduces pruritus and urticaria, whereas for another patient, that drug is ineffective.

Most classical H_1 antihistamines are not pure histamine receptor blockers. Many also interact with alpha-adrenergic, cholinergic, or serotoninergic receptors.[5, 12] For example, cyproheptadine is an inhibitor of serotonin receptors and a weak anticholinergic agent.[5]

PHARMACODYNAMICS. Because histamine receptors cannot be quantified by physical or chemical means, indirect measures are used to assess pharmacodynamic effects. The measurement of drug-induced suppression of the histamine-induced wheal–flare response over time provides an objective evaluation of H_1 receptor activity.[3] Provocative test agents in such studies include intradermal injection of histamine, of known allergens, and of compound 48/80.

Cook and associates studied the degree and duration of skin test suppression by using five classical antihistamines administered individually over a 3-day period. Although hydroxyzine exhibited the greatest continued suppression, the duration of suppression persisted for about 2 days with diphenhydramine, the weakest agent tested.[35] Subsequent single-dose studies with hydroxyzine and chlorpheniramine confirmed prolonged suppression of the wheal–flare response despite low serum drug levels.[32, 36] Simons and colleagues demonstrated significant suppression of wheals for 36 hours and flares for 60 hours after a single 0.7-mg/kg dose of hydroxyzine in healthy adults.[36] In a similar study of elderly patients, hydroxyzine significantly suppressed cutaneous wheal–flare areas for up to 144 hours.[34] The prolonged cutaneous effect of hydroxyzine may be related to its highly active metabolite, cetirizine. In any event, the continued suppression of a wheal–flare reaction may occur even when serum concentrations of the parent compound are low.

The phenomenon of prolonged histamine skin test suppression supports less frequent dosing throughout the day than what is routinely recommended.[12, 31] Dosing once or twice a day, once preferably at bedtime, may reduce daytime drowsiness without loss of clinical efficacy. In the treatment of CIU, administering the entire dose of hydroxyzine at bedtime (i.e., 50–100 mg) is often successful and decreases daytime drowsiness. Prolonged wheal–flare suppression is also relevant when one anticipates the withdrawal of an H_1 antihistamine before percutaneous allergy testing.

The degree of suppression must be considered in addition to the duration. Even potent H_1 antihistamines do not completely suppress wheal–flare formation induced either by histamine-mediated disease or by cutaneous testing. The complete control of urticaria is not solely dependent on an increase in the dosage of an H_1 antihistamine or on the discovery of a more potent agent; for at least some patients, unknown mechanisms that do not involve the H_1 receptor appear to play a role.[37]

Side effects such as sedation and psychomotor impairment often complicate the use of classical H_1 antihistamines. Studies have confirmed the direct correlation of these CNS effects with serum levels for both hydroxyzine and diphenhydramine.[36, 38] Because peak serum levels generally occur within the first few hours of ingestion, bedtime dosing would allow for maximal CNS depression to occur during sleep.

TOLERANCE. Tolerance to sedation and to drowsiness often develops within the first few days of therapy.[12] A schedule of progressively increasing dosages may enhance the development of tolerance to these side effects.[12] Single bedtime doses may also induce tolerance to sedative effects.

Both physician and patient are sometimes frustrated by tolerance to the beneficial effects of H_1 antihistamines. More commonly termed subsensitivity, this form of tolerance may be seen clinically as a decrease in relief of signs and symptoms or experimentally as a decrease in suppression of the wheal–flare response. Taylor and co-workers confirmed subsensitivity to chlorpheniramine within 3 weeks.[39] Doubling the dosage did not sufficiently counteract the tolerance effect. Bantz and associates also confirmed subsensitivity to chlorpheniramine after 3 weeks of therapy.[40] Long and colleagues documented a reduction in the suppression of skin test reactivity in patients receiving 75 mg/day of hydroxyzine for a 3 weeks.[41] The partial subsensitivity observed with hydroxyzine cross-reacted with chemically unrelated antihistamines. Although autoinduction of hepatic metabolism is said to be the mechanism behind subsensitivity, this theory has been refuted by investigations of both humans and dogs.[31] Bantz and associates also excluded decreased drug absorption and decreased serum levels as mechanisms.[40] It is more likely that the mechanism of subsensitivity resides locally at the H_1 receptor site.

Clinical Use (Table 12-2)

Approved Indications

The list of FDA-approved indications for classical H_1 antihistamines is much more limited than the large body of currently available data regarding the use of specific agents. Nevertheless, there are general guidelines regarding commonly encountered clinical indications.

Table 12-2. Classical H_1 Antihistamines: Indications/Contraindications

FDA-Approved Dermatologic Indications

Urticaria/angioedema[5, 42, 43, 44]*†‡§
Symptomatic dermographism[45]*†‡§
Cold urticaria[45-48]†
Pruritus[49-51]‡§
Pruritic dermatoses[52-53]*†‡§

Other Dermatologic Uses

Physical urticarias[45]
Pruritis[49, 50]
Atopic dermatitis[54-59]
Symptomatic mastocytosis[60]
Flushing reactions[61]

Contraindications

Use by newborns or premature infants
Pregnancy
Breast-feeding
Closed-angle glaucoma (relative)[62]
Urinary retention[63]
Asthma (relative)[63]

Relative contraindications require appropriate monitoring or consultation, or both, with primary care physician or specialist.

Note: See Table 12-6 for individual drug dosage and formulations available.
*Diphenhydramine; †cyproheptadine; ‡trimeprazine; §hydroxyzine (all have specific FDA approval for this indication).

ANTIHISTAMINE DRUG CHOICE. Classical H_1 antihistamine choice for the indications in Table 12–2 is largely based on side effect profile.[1,5] Although there are notable exceptions in clinical practice, the following generalizations are useful in selection of the appropriate drug for a given patient. Sedation is often significant with ethanolamines (e.g., diphenhydramine), phenothiazines (e.g., trimeprazine), and ethylenediamines (e.g., tripelennamine). Piperazines (e.g., hydroxyzine) and alkylamines (e.g., chlorpheniramine) are usually less sedating; in fact, alkylamines may cause CNS stimulation in certain patients. The less sedating H_1 antihistamines now available (e.g., terfenadine, astemizole) in recommended doses infrequently induce significant sedation.

Because a significant number of patients do not experience sedation, it is reasonable to begin treatment with a classical H_1 antihistamine for patients whose occupation or activities will not be hampered by subclinical psychomotor impairment. If sedative effects occur, or if the patient is also taking another CNS depressant, newer less sedating agents are best used. The use of these newer agents is limited primarily by their considerably higher expense to the patient in comparison with the classical H_1 antihistamines. For selected patients, sedation may be desirable, particularly to provide improved overnight sleep. For these patients, ethanolamines, phenothiazines, ethylenediamines, or tricyclic antidepressant antihistamines (e.g., doxepin) would be appropriate.

Ethanolamines are noted for significant anticholinergic effects. Gastrointestinal adverse effects may be significant with ethylenediamines, whereas ethanolamines and phenothiazines infrequently produce gastrointestinal symptoms. Depending on a patient's associated medical problems, various classes of classical H_1 antihistamines may be appropriate for treatment.

Finally, optimal antihistamine use is often accomplished by careful dosage titration. A smaller tablet size (e.g., 10 mg vs. 25 mg of hydroxyzine) makes it easier to determine the appropriate dosage for a given patient. Although tolerance to sedative effects develops over time, compliance is enhanced when excessive sedation is avoided initially.

URTICARIA/ANGIOEDEMA/DERMOGRAPHISM. The main FDA-approved dermatologic indications for many classical H_1 antihistamines are urticaria and angioedema. Although not specifically stated in many instances in the *Physicians' Desk Reference*, CIU is the most common indication warranting prolonged antihistamine use in dermatology. Dermographism is also an approved indication for many of these drugs.

The value of H_1 antihistamines in some patients with urticaria and dermographism is well-known. Although any H_1 antihistamine may prove to be effective, the potency of hydroxyzine has made it a favorite.[46] In order for an H_1 antihistamine to be effective in a given patient with urticaria, histamine must play a major role as a mediator. The common occurrence of partial response or treatment failure is believed to be due to other mediators not antagonized by H_1 antihistamines and not always due to the H_1 antihistamine initially selected.

Classical H_1 antihistamines play only an adjuvant role in the treatment of severe angioedema and anaphylaxis. Epinephrine is the primary drug therapy.[5]

COLD URTICARIA. Cyproheptadine is approved for treatment of cold urticaria. However, other H_1 antihistamines, including doxepin, are also effective.[47, 48]

PRURITUS. Hydroxyzine is FDA-approved in the management of pruritus due to conditions such as urticaria, atopic dermatitis, and contact dermatitis and of pruritus mediated by histamine.[42, 55, 56] Trimeprazine is approved for pruritic symptoms associated with allergic or nonallergic dermatoses.[51-53]

Whether pruritus is present alone or with an associated skin disorder, an H_1 antihistamine is most effective when histamine is the major mediator. When other causes are present, such as an undiagnosed ectoparasite, pruritus is less optimally controlled by an antihistamine. Some studies indicate that sedation produced by classical H_1 antihistamines is the primary reason for decreased pruritus and itching in patients with eczemas such as atopic dermatitis.[57-59] Klein and Galant compared two potentially sedating H_1 antihistamines, hydroxyzine and cyproheptadine, in children with atopic dermatitis and found hydroxyzine superior in reducing pruritus and improving the dermatitis.[56]

Other Dermatologic Uses

Indications not necessarily approved for each agent include atopic dermatitis, physical urticarias, pruritus, and mastocytosis. Symptoms associated with histamine release in patients with mastocytosis may respond favorably to H_1 antihistamine therapy.[60] H_1 antihistamines and H_2 antihistamines, singly or in combination, have been successfully used to treat various flushing reactions.[61]

Adverse Effects

The lipophilic nature of the classical H_1 antihistamines allows for wide tissue distribution and passage through the blood-brain barrier, through the placenta, and into breast milk.[1, 58] As a result, a variety of potential side effects and complications may be anticipated.

NERVOUS SYSTEM EFFECTS. Although not all patients are affected, CNS depression is the most common complications in adults.[5, 12] The usual manifestations are drowsiness and sedation. Gradual tolerance to this sedation usually develops.[63] Performance skills may be impaired and this may not be apparent to the patient. Stimulatory side effects are occasionally noted, especially in children and the elderly: nervousness, irritability, insomnia, tremor, and nightmares.[23] In adults, electroencephalogram alterations have been reported along with rare instances of seizures.[63] Individual case reports of oral and facial dyskinesias have been reported with antihistamine-decongestant combinations.[64] Acute dystonia has been reported with diphenhydramine.[65] Autonomic side effects relate primarily to the degree of anticholinergic activity and include dryness of mucous membranes, urinary retention, blurred vision, and nasal stuffiness.[63]

GASTROINTESTINAL EFFECTS. Occasional gastrointestinal side effects include nausea, vomiting, anorexia, epigastric distress, constipation, and diarrhea.[23, 63]

HEMATOLOGIC EFFECTS. Severe hematologic reactions secondary to H_1 antihistamines are sufficiently rare that monitoring is not indicated.[23] Chlorpheniramine has been associated with pancytopenia, agranulocytosis, thrombocytopenia, and aplastic anemia.[66-70] In one case of thrombocytopenia, serologic evaluation confirmed the presence of drug-dependent immunoglobulin G antiplatelet antibody.[70] There are rare reports of blood dyscrasias, such as agranulocytosis and hemolytic anemia.[63, 71]

OTHER ADVERSE EFFECTS. Dermatologic manifestations are rarely encountered with systemic use. Cyproheptadine has been associated with weight gain.[46, 72] Fisher recommended "white antihistamines" free of dyes for aspirin-sensitive patients who are also allergic to tartrazine (FD & C Yellow No. 5).[73] Trade name antihistamines that are tartrazine-free include Marezine, Phenergan, Periactin, Actidil, and Tavist.

Warnings

ANTICHOLINERGIC EFFECTS. The anticholinergic effects of many H_1 antihistamines may theoretically result in exacerbation of narrow-angle glaucoma or in worsening of urinary retention.[62, 63] Cautious use or avoidance of these drugs by such patients is suggested.

ASTHMA. Use of H_1 antihistamines by asthma patients has been controversial. Previous concern was due to fear of bronchospasm, decreased pulmonary function, and mucosal drying with inspissation of pulmonary secretions.[63] Renewed interest in H_1 antihistamine use by patients with chronic asthma has been expressed.[8, 74] Schuller and Turkewitz warned that a subset of asthmatic children not using concurrent bronchodilator therapy may be intolerant of H_1 antihistamines.[63] Popa suggested avoidance of H_1 antihistamines in the presence of severe asthma until further data are accumulated.[8] In most patients with atopic dermatitis and mild asthma, use of H_1 antihistamines is generally not problematic.

USE DURING PREGNANCY. Despite widespread use of over-the-counter and prescription H_1 antihistamines, there is a paucity of cogent evidence linking these drugs with congenital defects. As a general rule, no antihistamine has been given an unconditional recommendation by the FDA for use during pregnancy. A review of data collected by the Collaborative Perinatal Project identified no evidence incriminating H_1 antihistamines as definitively teratogenic; thus judicious use of chlorpheniramine and diphenhydramine would be allowed in pregnancy.[75] Possible occasional associations with individual congenital defects were noted.[76, 77] Whether these were fortuitous or drug-related is not known. The manufacturer of Benadryl (brand name of diphenhydramine) indicates that experience with the drug during pregnancy is inadequate to determine whether potential fetal harm may occur.[78] Saxen reported retrospective data statistically associating diphenhydramine intake during the first trimester with cleft palate.[79] These data have not been confirmed.

Limited experience with cyproheptadine during early human pregnancy suggests no apparent teratogenicity.[80] The manufacturer of Periactin (brand name of cyproheptadine) suggests its use during pregnancy only if clearly needed.[81]

No association with congenital anomalies or fetal wastage was noted with hydroxyzine used as an antiemetic in the first trimester of pregnancy.[82] Data available to the Collaborative Perinatal Project regarding hydroxyzine use in pregnancy were too limited to evaluate.[75] The manufacturer of Atarax (brand name of hydroxyzine) lists this drug as contraindicated during early pregnancy.[83]

A possible neonatal withdrawal syndrome has been reported with diphenhydramine and hydroxyzine after use during pregnancy.[84, 85]

USE DURING BREAST-FEEDING. Information regarding H_1 antihistamine use during breast-feeding is controversial. The American Academy of Pediatrics feels that diphenhydramine and trimeprazine are compatible with breast feeding.[86] The low levels of these drugs in breast milk are felt to be insignificant.[30] Of importance is that the manufacturers of these and many other antihistamines consider these agents to be contraindicated in nursing mothers, according to the *Physicians' Desk Reference*. Case reports of CNS toxicity in nursing infants have been reported with maternal intake of clemastine.[87]

Drug Interactions

The CNS depressant and anticholinergic effects of classical H_1 antihistamines may be additive with other drugs that possess similar effects.[8] Alcohol increases the impairment of performance skills induced by diphenhydramine.[88] The same effect should be anticipated with other classical H_1 antihistamines. Prior concern regarding decreased efficacy of oral contraceptives when coadministered with antihistamines was highly speculative and is not supported by any significant data.[89] Classical H_1 antihistamines are best avoided by patients taking monoamine oxidase inhibitors. A possible toxic interaction between cyproheptadine and phenelzine has been reported.[90]

THE LESS SEDATING H_1 ANTIHISTAMINES

The discovery of oral H_1 antihistamines with poor CNS penetration provides for a more specific action at peripheral H_1 receptors.[12,13] Terfenadine was discovered after haloperidol, a butyrophenone tranquilizer, was structurally altered.[91] The independent developments of astemizole and loratadine soon followed. All three of these H_1 antihistamines have been studied in the treatment of CIU, in addition to allergic rhinitis.

Although referred to as "nonsedating," these drugs can cause sedation. The incidence of sedation in most studies is much lower than with the classical H_1 antihistamines, generally approaching the incidence seen with placebo.[13] An additional improvement is their relative lack of activity at receptor sites other than H_1 receptors, especially in doses used therapeutically.[13,92] Unwanted effects, such as anticholinergic effects, are encountered less frequently than with classical H_1 antihistamines.

Pharmacology

Structure

Terfenadine, loratadine, and astemizole are structurally dissimilar. Terfenadine is a piperidinebutanol, derived from a fluorobutyrophenone structure.[91] Astemizole is derived from a piperidinyl-aminobenzimidazole moiety.[93] Loratadine is a benzocycloheptapyridine structurally related to azatadine, a classical H_1 antihistamine.[94]

Absorption/Distribution

Oral terfenadine, astemizole, and loratadine are rapidly absorbed and extensively distributed. Peak plasma concentrations occur within 12 hours after ingestion of terfenadine and loratadine and within 14 hours after ingestion of astemizole.[94-96] The oral bioavailabilty of astemizole is decreased by up to 60% by coadministration with food.[97] Food also delays the time to peak plasma concentration of astemizole. Steady-state plasma concentrations are reached within 5–10 days with loratadine and within 4–8 weeks with astemizole.[94, 96]

Metabolism/Excretion

Terfenadine, astemizole, and loratadine undergo extensive biotransformation. Terfenadine is rapidly metabolized with 99% biotransformation to two main metabolites.[95, 98] This suggests significant first-pass hepatic metabolism. Animal studies indicate that the carboxylic acid metabolite demonstrates one third of the activity of terfenadine, whereas the other metabolite is inactive.[95, 98] After rapid hepatic biotransformation, both urinary (40%) and biliary-fecal excretion (60%) are responsible for terfenadine elimination.[98]

Astemizole undergoes extensive first-pass hepatic metabolism, and essentially no unchanged astemizole is found in urine or feces.[96,97] Desmethylastemizole, the major metabolite, demonstrates antihistaminic potency similar to that of astemizole and is excreted primarily in feces along with other conjugated metabolites.[97] The major urinary metabolite, norastemizole, is less potent and shorter acting.[97] Metabolites are slowly excreted, according to studies of ingested radiolabeled astemizole. Approximately 40%–50% is excreted by 4 days and 60%–80% by 14 days. Fecal excretion accounts for 50%–70% of the amount excreted by 14 days.[96]

The major metabolite of loratadine, descarboethoxyloratadine, is rapidly formed and pharmacologically active.[94] This metabolite is transformed further and excreted in the urine. A small percentage of loratadine and its metabolite are passively excreted in breast milk.[99] Diminished renal function and hemodialysis appear to have a negligible effect on the disposition kinetics of loratadine and descarboethoxyloratadine.[94]

Because of rapid and extensive metabolism, the half-life values of both the parent drug and its active metabolites must be considered. Terfenadine's originally reported serum elimination half-life values of 16–23 hours are believed to be misleading.[95, 100] The true value is probably shorter. In children, the half-life of terfenadine is decreased.[100] After chronic administration of astemizole, the elimination half-life of both the parent drug and its active metabolite is 18–20 days.[97] Loratadine and descarboethoxyloratadine exhibit half-life values ranging from 8 to 14 hours and from 17 to 24 hours, respectively.[94]

Mechanism of Action

Like the classical H_1 antihistamines, the compounds terfenadine, astemizole, and loratadine are competitive antagonists at H_1 histamine receptors. However, the less sedating agents demonstrate preferential selectivity for peripheral H_1 receptors because of poor penetration across the blood-brain barrier. Astemizole exhibits extremely slow dissociation from H_1 receptor sites.[96] The effects of H_1 blockade were reviewed earlier in the section on classical H_1 antihistamines.

Regarding activity at other receptors, terfenadine does not bind significantly with alpha- and beta-adrenergic receptors.[95] Astemizole does possess some affinity for serotoninergic and alpha-adrenergic receptors in vitro at high dosages.[96] Loratadine exhibits weak affinity for alpha-adrenergic receptors. All three appear to be devoid of significant anticholinergic activity.[94-96]

PHARMACODYNAMICS. The suppressive effects of terfenadine, astemizole, and loratadine on skin test challenges have been studied. Interpretation of data is confusing because of the variations in drug dosages tested.

Therapeutic dosages of terfenadine show an onset of suppression of the wheal-flare reaction within 1-2 hours of administration.[101] Duration of suppression is 12-48 hours, with peak effect at 4 hours.[101, 102] In a double-blind crossover study of 12 patients, Bantz and associates reported significantly greater skin test suppression with an oral 300-mg dosage of terfenadine twice a day than with the recommended dosage of 60 mg twice a day.[103] Side effects in each group did not differ, even when compared with those of placebo treatment. Thus the current recommended dose may not maximize the potential efficacy of terfenadine.

Skin test suppression after administration of astemizole is dose-related. The onset of suppressive activity is prolonged until the 3rd day of administration, and the suppression may last more than 4 weeks after astemizole is discontinued.[101] Chronic administration does not appear to lessen this effect.[101, 104] These data support the delayed onset of clinical effectiveness observed with astemizole in the treatment of acute disorders.[97]

The degree and duration of skin test suppression by loratadine is dose-related. Single oral doses of loratadine produced suppression within 1 hour.[105] This rapid onset of suppression with loratadine correlates with an earlier onset of clinical effect in comparison with astemizole used without an initial loading regimen.[106] The degree and duration of skin test suppression by loratadine ranges from 35% and 12 hours with a 10-mg dose to 67% and 48 hours with an 80-mg dose.[105] Over a 28-day period, 10-mg of oral loratadine twice a day produced suppression of wheal formation comparable with suppression produced by 12 mg of oral chlorpheniramine twice a day, with a significantly lower incidence of sedation.[107]

In a comparison of hydroxyzine, terfenadine, and astemizole (with and without an initial 1-week loading regimen), Gendreau-Reid and colleagues evaluated suppression of the wheal–flare reaction induced by intradermal histamine injection.[108] Both hydroxyzine and astemizole (with loading) were significantly more effective than terfenadine or astemizole (without loading) in reducing wheal size. No significant differences were noted with the flare response.

The duration of skin test suppression is important if one anticipates the performance of cutaneous allergy testing after discontinuation of these drugs. Because of its prolonged tissue effects, astemizole may affect the results of such testing for several weeks to months. Interestingly, the prolonged half-life and pharmacodynamic effects of astemizole and its major metabolite have precluded a crossover in experimental studies of astemizole.[97]

TOLERANCE. Tolerance to histamine-induced skin test suppression has not been demonstrated with terfenadine, astemizole, and loratadine.[104, 107, 109] Tolerance to therapeutic effects after chronic administration has not been detected in most clinical studies. However, one study suggested possible tolerance to terfenadine.[110]

Clinical Use (Table 12–3)

Approved Indications

Both terfenadine and astemizole are approved by the FDA for the treatment of symptoms associated with allergic rhinitis. However, astemizole is also approved for use in treating CIU. Loratadine is currently not available in the U.S.

The major factor limiting the use of these newer agents as drugs of choice for CIU is their expense, in comparison with classical H_1 antihistamines. Otherwise, these drugs exhibit the definite advantage of not

Table 12–3. Less Sedating Antihistamines: Indications/Contraindications

FDA-Approved Dermatologic Indication

  Chronic idiopathic urticaria (CIU)[110–116]*

Other Dermatologic Uses

  Chronic idiopathic urticaria[94, 110, 115–118]†‡
  Dermographic urticaria[119, 120]*†
  Pruritis[121, 122]†

Contraindications§

  Breast-feeding
  Pregnancy[97]

Note: See Table 12–6 for individual drug dosage and formulations available.
*Astemizole; †terfenadine; ‡loratadine; §see *Physicians' Desk Reference* for the individual drug.

producing sedation, subclinical psychomotor impairment, or interaction with other CNS depressants.

CHRONIC IDIOPATHIC URTICARIA. Several studies confirm the significant benefit of astemizole in some patients with CIU. In a double-blind comparison, Cainelli and coauthors reported both astemizole and terfenadine to be effective; astemizole was rated as the most effective by both patients and investigator.[110] In a study of 46 patients with refractory CIU and angioedema, astemizole demonstrated considerable efficacy in most patients with sustained efficacy over the 8-week study period.[112] Of importance is that, despite the inherent potency of a given agent, treatment failures and partial responses are not uncommon with any H_1 antihistamine in patients with CIU.[123, 124] For CIU, astemizole is prescribed in an initial dosage of 30 mg the 1st day, 20 mg the 2nd, and 10 mg/day thereafter. Once CIU is controlled with astemizole, a trial with 10 mg every other day is warranted because of its prolonged activity. If ineffective, the dosage should be raised back to 10 mg/day.

Other Dermatologic Uses

URTICARIA. Both loratadine and terfenadine are effective in the treatment of CIU.[116, 118] In one report, loratadine appeared to demonstrate greater improvement in symptom relief from CIU than did terfenadine.[94] Although terfenadine is available for clinical use, the drug does not have an FDA indication for use in CIU. Astemizole exhibited greater benefit than chlorpheniramine in dermographic urticaria.[120] Terfenadine has also been shown to be effective.[119]

PRURITUS. In a single-blind crossover trial of 8 patients with chronic pruritus secondary to hepatic disease, both terfenadine and cholestyramine were found to be beneficial to some patients.[121] Chlorpheniramine was ineffective. Terfenadine at a dosage of 60 mg orally twice a day was well tolerated, whereas cholestyramine produced unacceptable gastrointestinal side effects in some patients.

Both Krause and Savin emphasized the importance of the sedative effect of an antihistamine in the treatment of pruritus associated with eczematous dermatitis.[57, 58] In one study, 120 mg of terfenadine twice a day failed to decrease pruritus associated with atopic dermatitis.[59] Doherty and coauthors reported that newer less sedating antihistamines may be of benefit as antipruritic agents in the treatment of atopic dermatitis.[122] For now, it appears that classical H_1 antihistamines are generally superior to less sedating H_1 antihistamines in suppressing pruritus in atopic dermatitis.

Adverse Effects

NERVOUS SYSTEM EFFECTS. In several studies, terfenadine, astemizole, and loratadine have produced a lower incidence of sedation and anticholinergic effects than did classical H_1 antihistamines.[94–96] In addition, they interfere less with performance skills.[125–128] In isolated studies, researchers have reported a higher than expected incidence of sedation with both astemizole and terfenadine.[97, 129] However, the less sedating nature of these drugs is well-documented.

LABORATORY CHANGES. Although monitoring of routine laboratory data, such as complete blood count (CBC), chemistry profile, electrocardiogram, and urinalysis, has not been routinely reported or emphasized, no major alterations have been consistently reported.[94, 107, 111, 130] Vanden Bussche and colleagues reviewed several clinical studies with astemizole and found no evidence of consistent laboratory abnormalities.[114] They reviewed 50 double-blind trials in which hepatic, renal, hematologic, and electrolyte parameters were evaluated in 678 patients treated with astemizole for durations ranging from 1 month to more than 1 year. Laboratory monitoring during long-term administration requires closer attention in future studies because recurrent or chronic therapy is often used.

CUTANEOUS EFFECTS. Stricker and coauthors cited 108 cases of dermatologic reactions associated with terfenadine reported in Europe.[131] Reactions included photosensitivity, urticaria, maculopapular eruptions, erythema, and peeling of the skin on the hands and feet. Rechallenge was confirmatory in some patients. Fenton and Signy also reported a suspected photoallergic reaction with terfenadine.[132] Jones and Morley discussed 6 cases of alopecia associated with terfenadine.[133] There is also an isolated case of psoriasis that was severely exacerbated during terfenadine treatment.[134]

HEPATIC EFFECTS. Hepatotoxicity has not been a common problem. Larrey and associates reported an isolated case of hepatitis associated with terfenadine used for 5 months.[135] Two recurrences of hepatitis were associated with intermittent terfenadine use by the same patient. Mild to moderate elevations of serum transaminase levels may also occur occasionally.

OTHER ADVERSE EFFECTS. Very low incidences of side effects such as headache, nausea, diarrhea, dry mouth, and other anticholinergic effects have been reported. Increased appetite and weight gain have been associated with astemizole use.[97, 112]

Warnings

Because of limited data in humans, the less sedating antihistamines are best avoided by pregnant women and by women who are breast-feeding. Astemizole is contraindicated in pregnancy essentially because of its prolonged elimination.[97]

Drug Interactions

No significant drug interactions have been definitively correlated with these drugs. The possibility of an interaction between terfenadine and theophylline has been refuted.[136] Several studies have demonstrated that terfenadine, astemizole, and loratadine do not appear to enhance the CNS effects of ethanol and diazepam.[94, 96, 97, 137]

H_2 ANTIHISTAMINES

The potential role of H_2 antihistamines in dermatology has been studied most extensively with cimetidine, which was released in the U.S. in 1978. In 1983, ranitidine was also released in the U.S. Both cimetidine and ranitidine are FDA-approved only for use in gastrointestinal diseases, such as duodenal ulcer and gastric ulcer; hypersecretory states, such as Zollinger-Ellison syndrome; and systemic mastocytosis.[138, 139] However, there is substantial literature regarding the use of H_2 antihistamines, especially cimetidine, in dermatology.[10, 11] Usage of these agents in dermatology is primarily limited to the oral formulations. However, both drugs are available for intramuscular and intravenous injection.

Pharmacology

Structure

The H_2 antihistamines are structural analogues of histamine.[138] Cimetidine is an imidazole compound, and ranitidine contains an aminomethylfuran moiety.[140]

Absorption/Distribution

Both cimetidine and ranitidine are rapidly absorbed after oral administration; peak serum levels are achieved in 1–3 hours.[138, 140, 141] The oral bioavailabilities are 60%–80% with cimetidine and 50%–60% with ranitidine.[140]

Metabolism/Excretion

The serum elimination half-life of both drugs is 2–3 hours after oral administration.[140, 141] Both undergo partial biotransformation in the liver to various metabolites. However, 50%–70% is excreted unchanged as the parent compound in the urine.[139, 140] As a result, the elimination half-lives of cimetidine and ranitidine decrease with diminishing renal function.[141–143] Renal tubular secretion has a significant role in the excretion of both compounds.[141, 144] Both cimetidine and ranitidine are concentrated in breast milk.[86, 141, 145]

Mechanism of Action

Although both cimetidine and ranitidine block H_2 receptors, ranitidine is more potent.[138] Cimetidine also inhibits histamine N-methyl transferase, an enzyme involved in histamine degradation.[6] Unlike ranitidine, cimetidine exhibits antiandrogenic activity, an effect believed to be unrelated to its H_2-blocking ability.[6, 10] This antiandrogenic activity results from the competitive inhibition of dihydrotestosterone at the peripheral androgen receptor.

Cimetidine appears to enhance the immune system by inhibiting suppressor T cell activity.[146] This effect is probably due to blockade of H_2 receptors present on suppressor T lymphocytes.[10] Both cell-mediated and humoral immunity may be influenced. An immunomodulating role is more likely to be significant in immunocompromised patients.

Clinical Use (Table 12–4)

Approved Indication

SYSTEMIC MASTOCYTOSIS. Signs and symptoms associated with systemic mastocytosis, such as urticaria and pruritus, often improve with cimetidine or ranitidine therapy.[147–149] For such patients, high-dosage therapy is often used. A lag period of a few weeks may occur before a symptomatic response is noted, which is similar to the lag period seen with oral cromolyn.[147]

Other Dermatologic Uses

Although preliminary, the results achieved by some researchers administering cimetidine for dermatologic conditions are intriguing. Nevertheless, caution is warranted because data are limited and well-controlled studies are lacking. Despite the excellent safety profile of H_2 antihistamines, there is a paucity of data regarding adverse effects after long-term use by dermatologic patients. Evaluation of cimetidine maintenance therapy for up to 5 years in treating peptic ulcer disease has not demonstrated an increased rate of adverse reactions or new forms of toxicity.[180] However, dosages used for chronic skin disorders, such as CIU and symptomatic dermographism, are usually higher than maintenance dosages used for peptic ulcer disease.

Table 12-4. H$_2$ Antihistamine Indications/Contraindications

FDA-Approved Dermatologic Indication

Systemic mastocytosis[147-149]*†

Other Dermatologic Uses

Antihistaminic Uses

Chronic idiopathic urticaria[150-160]*†‡
Symptomatic dermographism[161, 162]*‡
Pruritus[6, 163, 164]*
Urticaria pigmentosa[165, 166]*‡

Immunomodulation Uses

Overviews[10, 11]*
Herpes simplex[146, 167-169]*
Herpes zoster[146, 167, 170-173]*
Metastatic malignant melanoma[146, 176]*
Mycosis fungoides[177]

Antiandrogenic Uses

Female androgenetic alopecia[178]*
Hirsutism[179]*

Contraindications

Pregnancy§
Breast-feeding[86, 145]

Note: See Table 12-6 for individual drug dosage and formulations available.
*Cimetidine; †ranitidine; ‡H$_2$ blockers are used in combination with an H$_1$ antihistamine; §antihistamines are best avoided for dermatologic indications in pregnant women.

CHRONIC IDIOPATHIC URTICARIA. A main dermatologic indication for cimetidine is in the treatment of CIU refractory to H$_1$ antihistamines alone. Although cimetidine alone may demonstrate some inhibitory effect on the wheal–flare reaction, several investigators have noted that combined use of an H$_1$ antihistamine and cimetidine may improve the therapeutic response.[150-152, 159] Some studies have shown that combined H$_1$–H$_2$ antihistamine therapy enhances suppression of the wheal–flare response.[156, 157] The observation that cimetidine use alone may increase pruritus has led to the recommendation that an H$_1$ antihistamine be used in combination with the H$_2$ blocking agent in treatment of urticarial disease.[6, 42] However, Farnam and coauthors reported a patient with CIU and angioedema who responded to both cimetidine alone and cimetidine in combination with chlorpheniramine.[158]

In most of the studies and case reports, researchers have evaluated an H$_1$ antihistamine and cimetidine in combination for patients with CIU. The H$_1$ antihistamine used in most studies has been either hydroxyzine or chlorpheniramine. The usual dosage of cimetidine has been 300 or 400 mg administered orally four times a day. The combination of terfenadine and ranitidine has also been used.[154] The duration of controlled studies has ranged from 1 to 12 weeks. A 1-month trial of H_1–H_2 combination therapy should be adequate for determining efficacy.

Although studies have demonstrated a statistically significant benefit of combined H_1–H_2 antihistamine therapy, only half of those patients with diseases refractory to H_1 antihistamines alone will respond.[42] Some reports refute the benefits of H_1–H_2 combination therapy.[159, 160]

SYMPTOMATIC DERMOGRAPHISM. The combination of an H_1 antihistamine and an H_2 antihistamine may be of benefit in some patients with symptomatic dermographism that is not responsive to H_1 antihistamine therapy alone.[161, 162]

PRURITUS. Cimetidine demonstrated no effect in the treatment of uremic pruritus and a variable response in pruritus associated with cholestasis and polycythemia rubra vera.[6, 163, 164] Benefit from the treatment of pruritus associated with Hodgkin's disease has been noted.[6]

URTICARIA PIGMENTOSA. The combination of an H_1 antihistamine and cimetidine proved to be effective in isolated cases of both congenital bullous and symptomatic urticaria pigmentosa.[165, 166]

IMMUNOMODULATION. Several reports have exalted the benefit of cimetidine in the treatment of herpes simplex and herpes zoster infection.[146, 167] Decreased pain and shorter disease duration have been reported. Wakefield reported decreased frequency and severity of recurrent herpes genitalis in patients treated prophylactically with 400 mg of cimetidine taken orally twice a day over a 6-month period.[168] Rapid resolution of progressive mucocutaneous herpes simplex infection was noted in 5 severely immunocompromised patients treated with cimetidine.[169] Four of the patients received 1200 mg orally per day. The mechanism of action is not known.

Cimetidine was shown to improve the cell-mediated response to Candida in patients with chronic mucocutaneous candidiasis.[174] Landow anecdotally cited benefit from the combination of oral cimetidine and oral antifungal therapy for resistant dermatophytosis and from oral cimetidine in combination with oral vitamin A for resistant genital warts, especially those on moist surfaces.[11] A case of tinea capitis refractory to griseofulvin resolved after the addition of cimetidine to treatment.[175] Cimetidine was believed to restore the cell-mediated response to topical dinitrochlorobenzene (DNCB) in patients with alopecia areata who developed tolerance to DNCB.[10] Immunomodulation may account for part of the effects of cimetidine on infections, as just described, and on malignancies.

Cimetidine, usually in combination with other therapeutic agents, has been used with some benefit by patients with metastatic melanoma.[146, 176] Mamus and co-workers reported a case of early tumor-stage and a case of plaque-stage mycosis fungoides, both of which remitted during cimetidine use.[177] Discontinuation of cimetidine resulted in disease relapse, which later abated when cimetidine was restarted.

FEMALE ANDROGENETIC ALOPECIA. The antiandrogenic effect of cimetidine has been exploited for therapeutic benefit in selected cases. Aram reported good to excellent hair regrowth in 7 of 10 women with androgenetic alopecia treated for a median of 5 months with 300 mg of cimetidine taken orally five times a day.[178] Cimetidine may be an option in treating disease refractory to oral spironolactone and topical minoxidil or for patients who cannot tolerate those drugs.

HIRSUTISM. Vigersky and associates reported a decrease in the rate of hair growth in 4 of 5 hirsute women treated with 300 mg of cimetidine orally five times a day for 3 months.[179] The one treatment failure was in a woman taking phenytoin, a drug associated with hirsutism. Four of the women studied had polycystic ovarian disease.

PSORIASIS. Giacosa and colleagues reported clearance of psoriasis on two separate occasions in a single patient after the use of cimetidine for peptic ulcer disease.[181] Maintenance cimetidine therapy prevented recurrence of both psoriasis and the duodenal ulcer. Rai and Webster reported precipitation of psoriasis after cimetidine use by a single patient who developed pustular psoriasis of the hands after an initial episode of palmar skin peeling.[182] In a double-blind study of 52 patients with psoriasis, cimetidine and chlorpheniramine, both alone and in combination, exhibited no beneficial effect.[183]

Adverse Effects

The overall frequency of adverse effects associated with H_2 antihistamines is <3%.[184] This rate is acceptably low when one considers that cimetidine is one of the most frequently prescribed drugs in the U.S. Associated side effects are variable in presentation, and all are apparently reversible upon drug discontinuation.

GASTROINTESTINAL EFFECTS. Cimetidine and ranitidine may occasionally cause diarrhea and constipation.[184] A case of acute pancreatitis possibly associated with cimetidine has been reported.[185]

NERVOUS SYSTEM EFFECTS. Dizziness, somnolence, and headache may occur.[184, 186] Tests of psychomotor function in healthy volunteers revealed no adverse effects with either drug.[187] Severe headache associated with ranitidine has been described.[188] Rapidly reversible mental confusional states, such as disorientation and agitation, appear mostly as case reports, especially with cimetidine, and are usually encountered in patients who are receiving high-dosage therapy, have diminished renal or hepatic function, are elderly, or are hospitalized with other underlying medical conditions.[186, 189, 190]

CARDIOVASCULAR EFFECTS. Reports of significant cardiovascular complications associated with oral H_2 antihistamines are very uncommon.[186, 189] In a study of 20 patients without known cardiovascular disease, 150 mg of ranitidine taken orally twice a day produced no significant variation in heart rate, blood pressure, electrocardiogram, systolic time intervals, and M-mode echocardiography.[191] Rapid intravenous administration of H_2 antihistamines has been reported to cause sinus arrest, arrhythmias, and severe hypotension.[186, 189]

HEMATOLOGIC EFFECTS. Because of significant hematologic toxicity associated with the older H_2 antihistamine metiamide, clinicians have been vigilant with cimetidine and ranitidine.[189] Documented cases of blood dyscrasias have been uncommon.[184] Many cases have been seen in patients with serious underlying disease who are receiving other medications. This casts doubt on a definitive association with the H_2 antihistamines. Cimetidine has been associated with rare cases of granulocytopenia, agranulocytosis, thrombocytopenia, and pancytopenia; one case of fatal aplastic anemia was reported.[186, 189, 192, 193] A case of granulocytopenia induced by ranitidine, which recurred after cimetidine administration, has been reported.[194] Because blood dyscrasias appear to be reversible and usually occur within the first few months of therapy, monitoring with monthly CBCs is judicious for the first 4 months of use.[184]

HEPATIC EFFECTS. Both cimetidine and ranitidine may be associated with occasional transient elevations in serum transaminase levels, which often disappear despite continued therapy.[139, 189] Individual cases of hepatotoxicity associated with cimetidine and ranitidine have been reported.[139, 195, 196] Souza Lima evaluated reports of hepatotoxicity reported to the FDA with both drugs.[196] Three cases of apparent ranitidine-induced hepatotoxicity in patients, who had also received cimetidine without exhibiting evidence of hepatotoxicity, were reported by Black and colleagues.[197] Significant hepatotoxicity associated with the use of H_2 antihistamines appears to be uncommon, idiosyncratic, reversible, not dosage-related, and structure-specific.

RENAL EFFECTS. Regularly observed slight elevations of serum creatinine levels occur with cimetidine use. These elevations are not reflective of renal toxicity, are reversible, do not require discontinuation of cimetidine, and probably represent competition with renal creatinine excretion.[186] Ranitidine appears to be devoid of this effect.[189] Rare case reports of acute interstitial nephritis have been reported with cimetidine use,[198, 199] and a hypersensitivity mechanism is postulated; the reaction is reversible with drug discontinuation and is recurrent after rechallenge.[189] Ranitidine has not been associated with acute interstitial nephritis and was used by a patient with cimetidine-induced acute interstitial nephritis without complication.[139, 198]

ENDOCRINE EFFECTS. Although uncommon, endocrinologic adverse reactions occur more commonly with cimetidine than with ranitidine.[139, 186] Occasional side effects with cimetidine have included loss of libido, impotence, gynecomastia, and galactorrhea.[186, 189, 200, 201] Increases in serum prolactin levels have been associated with intravenous use of cimetidine and ranitidine and appear less likely to occur with oral therapy.[186, 189] In addition, cimetidine, and not ranitidine, has been shown to exhibit peripheral antiandrogenic activity and to increase endogenous serum estradiol levels.[189, 202] Neither drug is believed to have an effect on sperm count, sperm motility, serum testosterone, and serum gonadotropin levels.[186, 203] Side effects such as loss of libido and breast changes are significantly more common in patients taking high dosages of cimetidine to treat the hypersecretory gastrointestinal disorders. Replacement of cimetidine with ranitidine resulted in the disappearance of impotence and untoward breast changes in patients treated for hypersecretory states.[149]

CUTANEOUS EFFECTS. Cutaneous side effects appear to be uncommon. Cimetidine has been reported to cause urticaria, angioedema, exfoliative dermatitis, erythema multiforme major, and urticarial vasculitis.[204] The association of cimetidine with alopecia has been reported.[205]

OCULAR EFFECTS. Dobrilla and coauthors reported increased intraocular pressure with ocular pain and blurred vision in a patient with chronic glaucoma. These symptoms were associated with both cimetidine and ranitidine used sequentially.[206]

Warnings

USE DURING PREGNANCY. Because data on these drugs' effects in humans are lacking, the manufacturers of both cimetidine and ranitidine suggest use during pregnancy only if the anticipated benefit clearly outweighs the risk. With regard to dermatologic indications, the use of H_2 antihistamines during pregnancy is best avoided.

Antihistamines

USE DURING BREAST-FEEDING. Cimetidine and ranitidine are excreted in human breast milk in concentrations higher than those found in maternal plasma.[86, 145] Because of their many potential pharmacologic effects and possible drug interactions, these drugs should be avoided by women who are nursing infants.

POSSIBLE MALIGNANCY INDUCTION. A highly speculative issue related to the use of H_2 antihistamines is whether their continued use can cause gastric carcinoma. This issue is based on the hypotheses that cimetidine may be converted in the stomach to a carcinogenic nitrosamine and that bacterial overgrowth due to hypochlorhydria may increase nitrosamine production.[186, 189] Thus far, continued experience with H_2 antihistamines has demonstrated no evidence of carcinogenic potential in humans. Further observation over many years is warranted.

Drug Interactions

There is a large body of literature regarding drug interactions with cimetidine and ranitidine. Several thorough references are recommended.[207, 210] The following drug interactions are of potentially major significance.

ABSORPTION INTERACTIONS. Because H_2 antihistamines increase intragastric pH, they may affect the absorption or dissolution of other drugs. A clinically significant example is the reduced gastrointestinal absorption of ketoconazole by H_2 antihistamines.[208]

METABOLIC INTERACTIONS. Cimetidine exhibits an inhibitory effect on hepatic cytochrome P-450 microsomal metabolism, a system involved in the biotransformation of several drugs.[207-209] The potential for interaction is dependent on which drug is coadministered, as well as on patient-related metabolic factors. Cimetidine has the known potential to significantly decrease the metabolism and clearance of theophylline, phenytoin, and warfarin.[207-209] In some case reports, significant clinical toxicity has been documented. Patients taking any of these drugs should avoid the use of cimetidine whenever possible. The inhibitory metabolic effects of cimetidine develop very quickly after cimetidine use is started.

Ranitidine exhibits a much lower binding affinity to cytochrome P-450 than does cimetidine, which thus leads to the apparent lower potential for metabolic drug interactions.[208] Overall, the literature supports this belief; however, as experience with ranitidine has grown, the potential for certain drug interactions has been recognized.[210] Ranitidine does appear to inhibit warfarin and theophylline metabolism. However, the risk of significant interaction appears to be greater with cimetidine.[207-211]

RENAL EXCRETION INTERACTIONS. Because cimetidine and ranitidine undergo significant renal excretion, interactions based on renal mechanisms may occur. Probenecid significantly decreases renal clearance of cimetidine.[212] Cimetidine inhibits the renal excretion of procainamide and its active metabolite, N-acetylprocainamide (NAPA), whereas ranitidine appears to exhibit a lesser degree of inhibition.[208]

OTHER INTERACTIONS. Although a mechanism has not been determined, one study of 7 patients demonstrated that cimetidine significantly increased the serum levels of hydroxyzine.[213]

TRICYCLIC AGENTS: DOXEPIN

Doxepin is approved by the FDA for use as an antidepressant and an anxiolytic agent. Pharmacologic studies have identified doxepin as an extremely potent antihistaminic agent.[20, 21] This has led to its use in dermatology primarily for the treatment of urticaria.

Pharmacology

Doxepin is a tertiary amine dibenzoxepin tricyclic compound.[214] The drug is well-absorbed after oral administration; peak plasma levels are achieved by 4 hours afterward. Tissue distribution is extensive and includes CNS penetration. First-pass hepatic metabolism is estimated to be 70% of the oral doxepin dose.[216] Desmethyldoxepin is an active metabolite.[214] After multiple doses, the elimination half-lives are 21 hours for doxepin and 37 hours for desmethyldoxepin.[216] Urinary excretion is the principal mode of excretion for doxepin metabolites.[214] Doxepin and desmethyldoxepin are excreted in breast milk.[217]

Experimental studies have demonstrated that as an H_1 receptor antagonist, doxepin is significantly more potent in vitro than are diphenhydramine and hydroxyzine.[215] Doxepin is a potent anticholinergic agent and also antagonizes alpha-adrenergic, serotoninergic, and H_2 receptors.[21, 214] With regard to cutaneous pharmacodynamics, oral doses of doxepin as low as 5 mg have been shown to inhibit the histamine-induced wheal–flare reaction.[19] In one study, 5% doxepin applied topically suppressed histamine-induced pruritus.[18]

Clinical Use (Table 12–5)

Approved Indications

Doxepin is FDA-approved as an antidepressant and an anxiolytic agent. It has no approved dermatologic indications.

Table 12–5. Doxepin Indications/Contraindications

FDA-Approved Dermatologic Indications
None specific to dermatology

Other Dermatologic Uses
Chronic idiopathic urticaria[215, 218, 219]
Cold urticaria[220]
Neurotic excoriations[221]

Contraindications
Glaucoma (relative)[222, 223]
Urinary retention[223]
Breast-feeding[217, 224]
Cardiac conduction abnormalities (relative)[214, 225]
Postural hypotension[226]
Pregnancy[227]*

Relative contraindications require appropriate monitoring or consultation with primary care physician or specialist.

Note: See Table 12–6 for drug dosage and formulations available.
*Best avoided for dermatologic indications.

Other Dermatologic Uses

Studies of doxepin in depression have confirmed the efficacy and safety of single bedtime doses.[228, 229] The benefit is reduced daytime sedation. Despite the use of doses two and three times a day in some studies of dermatologic disorders, single bedtime doses can be used effectively on the basis of pharmacodynamic principles.

CHRONIC IDIOPATHIC URTICARIA. Well-controlled studies have confirmed the efficacy of doxepin in treating CIU.[215, 218, 219] The oral doxepin dosage in these studies ranges from 5 mg twice a day to 25 mg three times a day. In patients with refractory CIU, 10 mg three times a day proved superior to 25 mg of oral diphenhydramine three times a day in controlling pruritus and urticaria and produced a lower incidence of sedation.[215] In general, doxepin used in the range of 50–75 mg every night at bedtime is effective and well tolerated in the majority of patients. The typical starting dosage is 25 mg every night at bedtime, increasing by 25 mg every 1–2 weeks to a maximum dose of 75 mg every night.

COLD URTICARIA. Overall, 10 mg of oral doxepin three times a day was subjectively superior to either 4 mg of oral cyproheptadine three times a day or 10 mg of oral hydroxyzine three times a day in the treatment of idiopathic cold urticaria.[220] However, the results of ice cube test suppression did not differ statistically between these agents. Doxepin was associated with fewer adverse effects.

Table 12–6. Antihistamines: Oral Dose Regimens

Drug Name (Formulations)	Average Dosage for Adults	Daily Dosage for Children With Special FDA Recommendations
Diphenhydramine hydrochloride (Benadryl, in capsules, elixir)	25–50 mg three or four times a day	5 mg/kg/day; may use if child's weight >20 lbs; do not exceed 300 mg/day; do not use in newborns
Hydroxyzine hydrochloride (Atarax, in tablets, syrup)	25–50 mg twice a day (may give as bedtime dose)	2 mg/kg/day; if age <6 years, 50 mg/day; if age >6 years, 50–100 mg/day
Cyproheptadine hydrochloride (Periactin, in tablets, syrup)	12–16 mg (do not exceed 0.5 mg/kg/day)	0.25 mg/kg/day; for children aged 2–6 years, 4–6 mg/day; for children aged 7–14 years, 8–12 mg/day
Trimeprazine tartrate (Temaril, in tablets, syrup)	2.5 mg four times a day	For children aged 6 months to 3 years, 1.25 mg at bedtime or three times a day; if age >3 years, 2.5 mg at bedtime or three times a day
Terfenadine (Seldane, in tablets)	60 mg twice a day	If age ≥12 years, 60 mg twice a day; if age = 3–6 years, 15 mg twice a day; if age = 6–12 years, 30 mg twice a day (not FDA-approved for children)
Astemizole (Hismanal, in tablets)	10 mg/day (after load of 30 mg on day 1 and 20 mg on day 2)	If age ≥ 12 years, 10 mg/day; if age = 6–12 years, 5 mg/day; if age <6 years, 0.2 mg/kg/day (not FDA approved for children)
Doxepin hydrochloride (Sinequan, in capsules, liquid)	10 mg twice a day to 25 mg three times a day (may give at bedtime only)	Not recommended for patients under age 12 years
Cimetidine hydrochloride (Tagamet, in tablets, liquid)	1200 mg/day (divided)	Not recommended for dermatologic indications

Note: Data from Middleton E, Reed CE, Ellis EF: Allergy: Principles and Practice (Vol. 1), St. Louis: CV Mosby, 1978, 458–459; Physicians' Desk Reference, Oradell, NJ: Medical Economics, 1989; Monroe, 1987;[42] Product Information, Janssen Pharmaceutica, 1988; Clissold et al., 1989;[94] Sorkin and Heel, 1985.[95]

NEUROTIC EXCORIATIONS. Doxepin has been shown to be effective in the treatment of patients with neurotic excoriations.[221] In this case, both the sedative and the anxiolytic effects of doxepin may play a role.

Adverse Effects

The most common adverse effects are sedation, drowsiness, dry mouth, and constipation.[214] One may lessen the CNS depressant effects by using lower initial dosages and titrating upward over a few weeks. Less commonly reported adverse reactions are tremor, gait disturbance, blurred vision, postural hypotension, tachycardia, urinary retention, headache, and weight gain.[214] Many of these reactions are secondary to anticholinergic activity and are often dose-related. Euphoria and physical dependence do not occur with doxepin.[214]

Ayd has reported considerable experience with a number of patients with depression who were treated over several years with doxepin. His experience supports an excellent safety profile.[230, 231] Many of the patients were elderly, and some had concomitant medical disorders such as coronary artery disease, hypertension, valvular heart disease, and gastrointestinal disease. Serial hematologic, cardiac, renal, and hepatic function studies were performed. Of importance is that the dosages of doxepin used to treat depression are usually much higher than those used to effectively treat skin disorders such as CIU.

HEMATOLOGIC EFFECTS. Hematologic aberrations are uncommon with doxepin.[214] Leukopenia has been noted and is usually transient.[230] A patient with thrombocytopenia associated with doxepin was reported by Nixon.[232] This same patient subsequently developed thrombocytopenia from amitriptyline, another tricyclic antidepressant.

HEPATIC EFFECTS. Slight elevations in serum transaminase and alkaline phosphatase levels have occurred in patients taking doxepin.[214, 230] These elevations were not associated with clinical disease and may reverse despite continued doxepin therapy.

Warnings

CARDIOVASCULAR. Cardiovascular effects and possible toxicity associated with the therapeutic use of tricyclic antidepressants are of potential concern.[214, 233] Prolongation of the PR and QRS electrocardiogram intervals, increased heart rate, decreased blood pressure, and a quinidine-like effect on cardiac conduction may occur.[225] Despite contentions to the contrary, Luchins concluded that doxepin has cardiovascular effects similar to other, older tricyclic antidepressants.[234] The apparent cardiovascular safety of doxepin was related primarily to the use of relatively low dosages. Overall, the literature indicates that at the dosages usually recommended in dermatology (75 mg/day or less), doxepin is unlikely to adversely affect cardiac activity and function. No effect on ventricular and hemodynamic function was noted with doxepin use in patients with pre-existing cardiac disease.[235] Although clinical complications appear to be uncommon, patients known to have cardiac conduction abnormalities, especially bundle branch blocks, may be at a higher risk for adverse cardiac effects due to doxepin.[225]

USE DURING PREGNANCY. The safety of doxepin use during pregnancy is not known. Neonatal complications such as respiratory depression, myoclonus, and urinary retention have been associated with maternal tricyclic antidepressant use shortly before delivery.[227]

USE DURING BREAST FEEDING. A case of doxepin-induced severe sedation and respiratory depression occurred in an 8-week-old breast-fed child.[224] Desmethyldoxepin accumulation was confirmed. Doxepin should be avoided by women who are breast-feeding.

OTHER WARNINGS. Because of its anticholinergic activity, doxepin use is contraindicated in patients with glaucoma and a known history of urinary retention.[223]

Drug Interactions

Doxepin may enhance the sedative effects and psychomotor impairment induced by other CNS depressants, such as alcohol.[214] Because of its potent anticholinergic activity, doxepin may enhance this effect in patients who are taking other drugs with similar activity.[214]

At dosages greater than 150 mg/day, doxepin may decrease the antihypertensive activity of guanethidine and bethanidine by interfering with adrenergic neuronal uptake.[214] Tricyclic antidepressants, including doxepin, should be avoided by patients taking a monoamine oxidase inhibitor, because severe reactions have occurred during combined therapy.[214] Cimetidine may inhibit the hepatic metabolism of tricyclic antidepressants, which leads to drug accumulation and possible increased toxicity.[236]

MAST CELL–STABILIZING AGENTS

Cromolyn (Sodium Cromoglycolate)

In 1965, Fisons synthesized cromolyn (disodium cromoglycate), a bischromone mast cell stabilizer. Although not intrinsically antihistaminic, cromolyn inhibits the liberation of mediators from mast cells triggered either by immunoglobulin E antibody-antigen interaction or by nonimmunologic stimuli such as compound 48/80.[15] Inhalant and topical formulations of cromolyn are FDA-approved for the treatment of asthma, allergic rhinitis, and allergic ocular disorders. Oral cromolyn was given FDA-approval for the new indication of mastocytosis in January 1990.

Because of its unique mechanism, cromolyn has been of interest to researchers who anticipated its value in dermatoses with a possible allergic basis. The benefit of topical 10% cromolyn ointment in the treatment of atopic dermatitis has been both supported and refuted.[237, 238]

Despite less than 1% oral absorption, oral administration of cromolyn has been effective in ameliorating symptoms of food allergy in some patients. However, relief of associated cutaneous manifestations has not been substantiated.[15, 239, 240] Oral cromolyn does not appear to be beneficial to patients with chronic urticaria.[15]

Some reports, especially open trials, of oral cromolyn in the treatment of atopic dermatitis have suggested benefit to some patients.[15, 241] Other controlled studies have refuted these findings.[15, 242] Thus the value of oral cromolyn in the treatment of atopic dermatitis is questionable. Its role is currently limited to patients whose diseases are refractory to more conventional forms of therapy. Some investigators have suggested that oral cromolyn is more likely to be effective in children with atopic dermatitis who have elevated serum immunoglobulin E levels.[241]

Oral cromolyn has been shown to be beneficial to patients with systemic mastocytosis and bullous mastocytosis.[243-245] In one comparison of the combination of chlorpheniramine and cimetidine with oral cromolyn in 6 patients with systemic mastocytosis, both regimens were equal with regard to symptom control. The marked elevations of plasma and urinary histamine levels seen in these patients were not significantly altered by either regimen.[244]

Ketotifen

Ketotifen is an oral benzocycloheptathiophene that demonstrates several pharmacologic mechanisms, including H_1 antagonism, inhibition of phosphodiesterase, calcium channel blockade, inhibition of mast cell mediator release, and antagonism of leukotrienes.[17] The correlation of these mechanisms with clinical use requires further study.

Ketotifen is not a less sedating agent. Sedation is a common but transient side effect, and anticholinergic activity appears to be minimal.[246] The major emphasis of study with ketotifen has been in the treatment of asthma. Ketotifen has not yet been approved by the FDA for use in the U.S.

Ketotifen produced symptomatic improvement in 4 patients with cholinergic urticaria and cardiorespiratory manifestations refractory to conventional H_1 antihistamine therapy; these findings were confirmed by repeat exercise challenge.[247] Ketotifen also suppressed plasma histamine elevation; this finding supported the hypothesis about its activity in humans as an inhibitor of mast cell mediator release.

Huston and colleagues demonstrated the benefit of ketotifen in 3 patients with physical urticaria, including dermatographism, cold urticaria, and exercise-induced urticaria.[248] Reductions in plasma histamine concentration and clinical evidence of urticaria after appropriate physical challenge were noted with use of oral ketotifen.

Ketotifen has exhibited clinical effectiveness in the treatment of chronic urticaria, dermatographism, atopic dermatitis in childhood, adult urticaria pigmentosa, and diffuse cutaneous mastocytosis.[246, 248] Hydroxyzine was superior to ketotifen in 7 of 8 children treated for symptomatic mastocytosis.[249] Interestingly, analysis of plasma and urinary histamine levels before and after each drug trial revealed no significant differences. Saihan demonstrated the effectiveness of combined oral ketotifen and terbutaline therapy for some patients with chronic idiopathic urticaria, symptomatic dermographism, and refractory cold urticaria.[250]

The common occurrence of itching in patients with neurofibromatosis and the prominence of mast cells in skin biopsy specimens of neurofibromas triggered the concept that mast cells may play a role in neurofibroma development and symptomatology.[251] Ricciardi reported a decrease in pruritus, in pain, and in tenderness, decreased neurofibroma growth, and an improved sense of well-being in a small group of patients with neurofibromatosis treated with oral ketotifen for 30–43 months.[251] Ricciardi warned that these results were preliminary.

BIBLIOGRAPHY: Key Reviews/Chapters

Flowers FP, Araujo OE, Nieves CH: Antihistamines. Int J Dermatol 1986; 25:224–231.
Aram H: Cimetidine in dermatology. Int J Dermatol 1987; 26:161–166.
Drouin MA: H_1 antihistamines: Perspective on the use of the conventional and new agents. Ann Allergy 1985; 55:747–752.
Monroe EW: Treatment of urticaria: Drug management. Semin Dermatol 1987; 6:342–347.
Monroe EW: Chronic urticaria: Review of nonsedating H_1 antihistamines in treatment. J Am Acad Dermatol 1988; 19:842–849.

REFERENCES

1. Flowers FP, Araujo OE, Nieves CH: Antihistamines. Int J Dermatol 1986; 25:224–231.
2. Bickers DR, Hazen PG, Lynch WS: Antihistamines and nonsteroidal antiinflammatory drugs. In Bickers DR, Hazen PG, Lynch WS (eds): Clinical Pharmacology of Skin Disease. New York: Churchill Livingstone, 1984, 36–56.
3. Simons FE, Simons KJ: H_1 receptor antagonists: Clinical pharmacology and use in allergic disease. Pediatr Clin North Am 1983; 30:899–913.
4. Wasserman SI: Histamine and the preclinical pharmacology of ceftirizine. Ann Allergy 1987; 59(Part II):1–3.
5. Douglas WW: Histamine and 5-hydroxytryptamine (serotonin) and their antagonists. In Goodman LS, Gilman A (eds): Goodman and Gilman's The Pharmacologic Basis of Therapeutics (7th ed). New York: Macmillan, 1985, 605–638.
6. Davies MG, Greaves MW: The current status of histamine receptors in human skin: Therapeutic implications. Br J Dermatol 1981; 104:601–606.
7. Winkelmann RK: Pruritus. Semin Dermatol 1988; 7:233–235.
8. Popa V: The classic antihistamines in respiratory medicine. Clin Chest Med 1986; 7:367–382.
9. Brimblecombe RW, Duncan WA, Durant GJ, et al: Characterization and development

of cimetidine as a histamine H_2-receptor antagonist. Gastroenterology 1978; 74:339–347.
10. Aram H: Cimetidine in dermatology. Int J Dermatol 1987; 26:161–166.
11. Landow RK: Myth or magic: The role of cimetidine in dermatology. Semin Dermatol 1987; 6:43–47.
12. Drouin MA: H_1 antihistamines: Perspective on the use of the conventional and new agents. Ann Allergy 1985; 55:747–752.
13. Woodward JK: Pharmacology and toxicology of nonclassical antihistamines. Cutis 1988; 42:5–9.
14. Berman BA: Cromolyn: Past, present and future. Pediatr Clin North Am 1983; 30:915–930.
15. Shapiro GG, Konig P: Cromolyn sodium: A review. Pharmacotherapy 1985; 5:156–170.
16. Cromolyn Product Information, Fisons Corporation. In Physicians' Desk Reference (44th ed). Oradell, NJ: Medical Economics, 1990, 944.
17. Greenwood C: The pharmacology of ketotifen. Chest 1982; 82(Suppl):45S–48S.
18. Bernstein JE, Whitney DH, Soltani K: Inhibition of histamine-induced pruritus by topical tricyclic antidepressants. J Am Acad Dermatol 1981; 5:582–585.
19. Sullivan TJ: Pharmacologic modulation of the whealing response to histamine in human skin: Identification of doxepin as a potent in vivo inhibitor. J Allergy Clin Immunol 1982; 69:260–267.
20. Richelson E: Tricyclic antidepressants and histamine H_1 receptors. Mayo Clin Proc 1979; 54:669–674.
21. Richelson E: Antimuscarinic and other receptor-blocking properties of antidepressants. Mayo Clin Proc 1983; 58:40–46.
22. Weil EK, Rosenberg JM: Antihistamine agents in the pipeline. Hosp Pharm 1989; 24:864–865.
23. Fastner Z: Antihistamines. In Dukes MN (ed): Meyler's Side Effects of Drugs (9th ed). Amsterdam: Excerpta Medica, 1980, 265–272.
24. Rumore MM: Clinical pharmacokinetics of chlorpheniramine. Drug Intell Clin Pharm 1984; 18:701–707.
25. Blyden GT, Greenblatt DJ, Scavone JM, Shader RI: Pharmacokinetics of diphenhydramine and a demethylated metabolite following intravenous and oral administration. J Clin Pharmacol 1986; 26:529–533.
26. Albert KS, Hallmark MR, Sakmar E, et al: Pharmacokinetics of diphenhydramine in man. J Pharmacokinet Biopharm 1975; 3:159–170.
27. Gengo FM, Dabronzo J, Yurchak A, et al: The relative antihistaminic and psychomotor effects of hydroxyzine and cetirizine. Clin Pharmacol Ther 1987; 42:265–272.
28. Peets EA, Jackson M, Symchowicz S: Metabolism of chlorpheniramine maleate in man. J Pharmacol Exp Ther 1972; 180:364–374.
29. Glazko AJ, Dill WA, Young RM, et al: Metabolic disposition of diphenhydramine. Clin Pharmacol Ther 1974; 16:1066–1076.
30. O'Brien TE: Excretion of drugs in human milk. Am J Hosp Pharmacol 1974; 31:844–854.
31. Simons FE, Simons KJ, Chung M, Yeh J: The comparative pharmacokinetics of H_1-receptor antihistamines. Ann Allergy 1987; 59(6, Part 2):20–24.
32. Simons FE, Luciuk GH, Simons KJ: Pharmacokinetics and efficacy of chlorpheniramine in children. J Allergy Clin Immunol 1982; 69:376–381.
33. Simons FE, Simons KJ, Becker AB, et al: Pharmacokinetics and antipruritic effects of hydroxyzine in children with atopic dermatitis. J Pediatr 1984; 104:123–127.
34. Simons KJ, Watson WT, Chen XY: Pharmacokinetic and pharmacodynamic studies of the H_1 receptor antagonist hydroxyzine in the elderly. Clin Pharmacol Ther 1989; 45:9–14.

35. Cook TJ, MacQueen DM, Wittig HJ: Degree and duration of skin test suppression and side effects with antihistamines. J Allergy Clin Immunol 1973; 51:71–77.
36. Simons FE, Simons KJ, Frith EM: The pharmacokinetics and antihistaminic of the H_1 receptor antagonist hydroxyzine. J Allergy Clin Immunol 1984; 73:69–75.
37. Shuster S: Antihistamines in the treatment of urticarial disorders. Cutis 1988; 42:26–28.
38. Gengo F, Gabos C, Miller JK: The pharmacodynamics of diphenhydramine-induced drowsiness and changes in mental performance. Clin Pharmacol Ther 1989; 45:15–21.
39. Taylor RJ, Long WF, Nelson HS: The development of subsensitivity to chlorpheniramine. J Allergy Clin Immunol 1985; 76:103–107.
40. Bantz EW, Dolen WK, Chadwick EW: Chronic chlorpheniramine therapy: Subsensitivity, drug metabolism, and compliance. Ann Allergy 1987; 59:341–346.
41. Long WF, Taylor RJ, Leavengood DC: Skin test suppression by antihistamines and the development of subsensitivity. J Allergy Clin Immunol 1985; 76:113–117.
42. Monroe EW: Treatment of urticaria: Drug management. Semin Dermatol 1987; 6:342–347.
43. Farnam J, Grant JA: Angioedema. Dermatol Clin 1985; 3(1):85–95.
44. Valentine MD: Chronic urticaria. In Provost TT, Farmer ER (eds): Current Therapy in Dermatology-2. Toronto: BC Decker, 1988, 115–117.
45. Sibbald GR: Physical urticaria. Dermatol Clin 1985; 3:57–69.
46. Mathews KP: Management of urticaria and angioedema. J Allergy Clin Immunol 1980; 66:347–357.
47. Wanderer AA, St Pierre JP, Ellis E: Primary acquired cold urticaria. Arch Dermatol 1977; 113:1375–1377.
48. Sigler RW, Evans R, Horakova Z: The role of cyproheptadine in the treatment of cold urticaria. J Allergy Clin Immunol 1980; 65:309–312.
49. Fransway AF, Winkelmann RK: Treatment of pruritus. Semin Dermatol 1988; 7:310–325.
50. Tonneson MG: Pruritus. In Provost TT, Farmer ER (eds): Current Therapy in Dermatology-2. Toronto: BC Decker, 1988, 261–264.
51. Pittelkow RB: An evaluation of trimeprazine in pruritus. Wis Med J 1960; 59:367–369.
52. LeMan P: The use of trimeprazine in the treatment of pruritic dermatoses. Clin Med 1958; 5:1077–1084.
53. Savin JA, Paterson WD, Adam K: Effects of trimeprazine and trimipramine on nocturnal scratching in patients with atopic eczema. Arch Dermatol 1979; 115:313–315.
54. Heer Nicol N, Clark RAF: Atopic dermatitis. In Provost TT, Farmer ER (eds): Current Therapy in Dermatology-2. Toronto: BC Decker, 1988; 28–31.
55. Baraf CS: Treatment of pruritus in allergic dermatoses: An evaluation of the relative efficacy of cyproheptadine and hydroxyzine. Curr Ther Res 1976; 19:32–38.
56. Klein GL, Galant SP: A comparison of the antipruritic efficacy of hydroxyzine and cyproheptadine in children with atopic dermatitis. Ann Allergy 1980; 44:142–145.
57. Krause L, Shuster S: Mechanism of action of antipruritic drugs. Br Med J 1983; 287:1199–1200.
58. Savin JA, Dow R, Harlow BJ, et al: The effect of a new non-sedative H_1-receptor antagonist (LN2974) on the itching and scratching of patients with atopic eczema. Clin Exp Dermatol 1986; 11:600–602.
59. Berth-Jones J, Graham-Brown RAC: Failure of terfenadine in relieving the pruritus of atopic dermatitis. Br J Dermatol 1989; 121:635–637.
60. Soter NA: Mastocytosis and urticaria pigmentosa. In Provost TT, Farmer ER (eds): Current Therapy in Dermatology-2. Toronto: BC Decker, 1988, 253–255.

61. Wilkin JK: Flushing reactions. In Rook AJ, Maibach HI (eds): Recent Advances in Dermatology (6th ed). Edinburgh: Churchill Livingstone, 1983, 157–187.
62. Gourley DR, Ignoffo RJ, Tong TG: Diseases of the eye: Glaucoma. In Herfindal ET, Hirschman JL (eds): Clinical Pharmacy and Therapeutics (3rd ed). Baltimore: Williams & Wilkins, 1984, 850–852.
63. Schuller DE, Turkewitz D: Adverse effects of antihistamines. Postgrad Med 1986; 79(2):75–86.
64. Thach BT, Chase TN, Bosma JF: Oral facial dyskinesia associated with prolonged use of antihistaminic decongestants. N Engl J Med 1975; 293:486–487.
65. Lavenstein BL, Cantor FK: Acute dystonia: An unusual reaction to diphenhydramine. JAMA 1976; 236:291.
66. Deringer PM, Maniatis A: Chlorpheniramine-induced bone marrow suppression. Lancet 1976; 1:432.
67. Shenfield G, Spry CJF: Unusual cause of agranulocytosis. Br Med J 1968; 2:52–53.
68. Hardin AS: Chlorpheniramine and agranulocytosis. Ann Intern Med 1988; 108:770.
69. Kanoh T, Jingami H, Uchino H: Aplastic anemia after prolonged treatment with chlorpheniramine. Lancet 1977; 1:546–547.
70. Eisner EV, LaBocki NL, Pinckney L: Chlorpheniramine-dependent thrombocytopenia. JAMA 1975; 231:735–736.
71. Swanson M: Drugs, chemicals and hemolysis. Drug Intell Clin Pharm 1973; 7:624.
72. Bergen SS Jr: Appetite stimulating properties of cyproheptadine. Am J Dis Child 1964; 108:270–273.
73. Fisher AA: The antihistamines. J Am Acad Dermatol 1980; 3:303–305.
74. Rafferty P, Holgate ST: Histamine and its antagonists in asthma. J Allergy Clin Immunol 1989; 84:144–151.
75. Greenberger P, Patterson R: Safety of therapy for allergic symptoms during pregnancy. Ann Intern Med 1978; 89:234–237.
76. Briggs GG, Freeman RK, Yaffe SJ: Drugs in Pregnancy and Lactation (2nd ed). Baltimore: Williams & Wilkins, 1986, 147–148.
77. Briggs GG, Freeman RK, Yaffe ST: Drugs in Pregnancy and Lactation (2nd ed). Baltimore: Williams & Wilkins, 1986, 84.
78. Benadryl Product Information, Parke-Davis. In Physicians' Desk Reference (43rd ed). Oradell, NJ: Medical Economics, 1989, 1527–1528.
79. Saxen I: Cleft palate and maternal diphenhydramine intake. Lancet 1974; 1:407–408.
80. Berkowitz RL, Coustan DR, Mochizuki TK: Handbook For Prescribing Medications During Pregnancy (2nd ed). Boston: Little, Brown, 1986, 97–98.
81. Periactin Product Information, Merck Sharp & Dohme. In Physicians' Desk Reference (43rd ed). Oradell, NJ: Medical Economics, 1989, 1379–1380.
82. Erez S, Schifrin BS, Dirim O: Double-blind evaluation of hydroxyzine as an antiemetic in pregnancy. J Reprod Med 1971; 7:57–59.
83. Atarax Product Information, Roerig. In Physicians' Desk Reference (43rd ed). Oradell, NJ: Medical Economics, 1989, 1774–1775.
84. Parkin DE: Probable Benadryl withdrawal manifestations in a newborn infant. J Pediatr 1974; 85:580–581.
85. Prenner BM: Neonatal withdrawal syndrome associated with hydroxyzine hydrochloride. Am J Dis Child 1977; 131:529–530.
86. American Academy of Pediatrics Committee on Drugs: The transfer of drugs and other chemicals into human breast milk. Pediatrics 1983; 72:375–383.
87. Kok THHG, Taitz IS, Bennett MJ: Drowsiness due to clemastine transmitted in breast milk. Lancet 1982; 1:914–915.
88. Burns M, Moskowitz H: Effects of diphenhydramine and alcohol on skills performance. Eur J Clin Pharmacol 1980; 17:259–266.
89. DeSano EA, Hurley SC: Possible interactions of antihistamines and antibiotics with oral contraceptive effectiveness. Fertil Steril 1982; 37:853–854.

90. Kahn DA: Possible toxic interaction between cyproheptadine and phenelzine. Am J Psychiatry 1987; 144:1242–1243.
91. Carr AA, Meyer DR: Synthesis of terfenadine. Arzneimittelforsch 1982; 32(9a):1157–1159.
92. Norman PS: Newer antihistaminic agents. J Allergy Clin Immunol 1985; 76:366–368.
93. Astemizole Product Information, Janssen Pharmaceutica, 1988.
94. Clissold SP, Sorkin EM, Goa KL: Loratadine: A preliminary review of its pharmacodynamic properties and therapeutic efficacy. Drugs 1989; 37:42–57.
95. Sorkin EM, Heel RC: Terfenadine: A review of its pharmacodynamic properties and therapeutic efficacy. Drugs 1985; 29:34–56.
96. Richards DM, Brogden RN, Heel RC: Astemizole: A review of its pharmacodynamic properties and therapeutic efficacy. Drugs 1984; 28:38–61.
97. Krstenansky PM, Cluxton RJ: Astemizole: A long-acting, nonsedating antihistamine. Drug Intell Clin Pharm 1987; 21:947–953.
98. Garteiz DA, Hook RH, Walker BJ, Okerholm RA: Pharmacokinetics and biotransformation studies of terfenadine in man. Arzneimittelforsch 1982; 32(9a):1185–1190.
99. Hilbert J, Radwanski E, Affrime MB: Excretion of loratidine in human breast milk. J Clin Pharmacol 1988; 28:234–239.
100. Simons FE, Watson WT, Simons KJ: The pharmacokinetics and pharmacodynamics of terfenadine in children. J Allergy Clin Immunol 1987; 80:884–890.
101. Filderman RB: Inhibition of skin reactivity by antihistamines. Cutis 1988; 42:19–21.
102. Huther KJ, Renftle G, Barraud N: Inhibitory activity of terfenadine on histamine-induced skin wheals in man. Eur J Clin Pharmacol 1977; 12:195–199.
103. Bantz EW, Dolen WK, Nelson HS: A double-blind evaluation of skin test suppression produced by two doses of terfenadine. J Allergy Clin Immunol 1987; 80:99–103.
104. Bateman DN, Chapman PH, Rawlins MD: The effects of astemizole on histamine-induced wheal and flare. Eur J Clin Pharmacol 1983; 25:547–551.
105. Kassem N, Roman I, Gural R, et al: Effects of loratadine (SCH 29851) in suppression of histamine-induced skin wheals. Ann Allergy 1988; 60:505–507.
106. Oei HD: Double-blind comparison of loratadine (SCH 29851), astemizole and placebo in hay fever with special regard to onset of action. Ann Allergy 1988; 61:436–439.
107. Roman IJ, Kassem N, Gural RP: Suppression of histamine-induced wheal response by loratidine (SCH 29851) over 28 days in man. Ann Allergy 1986; 57:253–256.
108. Gendreau-Reid L, Simons KJ, Simons FE: Comparison of the suppressive effect of astemizole, terfenadine and hydroxyzine on histamine-induced wheals and flares in humans. J Allergy Clin Immunol 1986; 77:335–340.
109. Simons FE, Watson WT, Simons KJ: Lack of subsensitivity to terfenadine during long-term terfenadine treatment. J Allergy Clin Immunol 1988; 82:1068–1075.
110. Cainelli T, Seidenari S, Valsecchi R: Double-blind comparison of astemizole and terfenadine in the treatment of chronic urticaria. Pharmacotherapeutica 1986; 4:679–686.
111. Fox RW, Lockey RF, Bukantz SC, Serbousek D: The treatment of mild to severe chronic idiopathic urticaria with astemizole: Double-blind and open trials. J Allergy Clin Immunol 1986; 78:1159–1166.
112. Kailasam V, Mathews KP: Controlled clinical assessment of astemizole in the treatment of chronic idiopathic urticaria and angioedema. J Am Acad Dermatol 1987; 16:797–804.
113. Bernstein IL, Bernstein DI: Efficacy and safety of astemizole, a long-acting and nonsedating H_1 antagonist for the treatment of chronic idiopathic urticaria. J Allergy Clin Immunol 1986; 77:37–42.
114. Vanden Bussche G, Emanuel MB, Rombaut N, et al: Clinical profile of astemizole: A survey of 50 double-blind trials. Ann Allergy 1987; 58:184–188.
115. Cerio R, Lessof MH: Treatment of chronic idiopathic urticaria with terfenadine. Clin Allergy 1984; 14:139–141.

116. Grant JA, Bernstein DI, Buckley E: Double-blind comparison of terfenadine, chlorpheniramine, and placebo in the treatment of chronic idiopathic urticaria. J Allergy Clin Immunol 1988; 81:574–579.
117. Ferguson J, MacDonald KJ, Kenicer KJ: Terfenadine and placebo compared in the treatment of chronic idiopathic urticaria: A randomized double-blind study. Br J Clin Pharmacol 1985; 20:639–641.
118. Monroe EW, Fox RW, Green AW: Efficacy and safety of loratidine in the management of idiopathic chronic urticaria. J Am Acad Dermatol 1988; 19:138–139.
119. Krause LB, Shuster S: The effect of terfenadine on dermographic wealing. Br J Dermatol 1984; 110:73–79.
120. Krause LB, Shuster S: A comparison of astemizole and chlorpheniramine in dermographic urticaria. Br J Derm 1985; 112:447–453.
121. Duncan JS, Kennedy HJ, Triger DR: Treatment of pruritus due to chronic obstructive liver disease. Br Med J 1984; 289:22.
122. Doherty V, Sylvester DGH, Kennedy CTC: Treatment of itching in atopic eczema with antihistamines with a low sedative profile. Br Med J 1989; 298:96.
123. Krause L, Shuster S: Evidence for a novel vasoactive mechanism in chronic idiopathic urticaria. Br J Dermatol 1984; 111:703.
124. Krause LB, Shuster S: H_1-receptor-active histamine not sole cause of chronic idiopathic urticaria. Lancet 1984; 2:929–930.
125. Betts T, Markman D, Debenham S: Effects of two antihistamine drugs on actual driving performance. Br Med J 1984; 288:281–282.
126. Nicholson AN, Stone BM: Performance studies with the H_1-histamine receptor antagonists, astemizole and terfenadine. Br J Clin Pharmacol 1982; 13:199–202.
127. Seppala T, Savolainen K: Effect of astemizole on human psychomotor performance. Curr Ther Res 1982; 31:638–644.
128. Roth T, Roehrs T, Koshorek J: Sedative effects of antihistamines. J Allergy Clin Immunol 1987; 80:94–98.
129. Sooknundun M, Kacker SK, Sundaram KR: Treatment of allergic rhinitis with a new long-acting H_1 receptor antagonist: Astemizole. Ann Allergy 1987; 58:78–81.
130. Dockhorn RJ, Bergner A, Connell JT, et al: Safety and efficacy of loratidine (SCH 29851): A new non-sedating antihistamine in seasonal allergic rhinitis. Ann Allergy 1987; 58:407–411.
131. Stricker BH, Isaacs AJ, Lindquist M: Skin reactions to terfenadine. Br Med J 1986; 293:536.
132. Fenton D, Signy M: Photosensitivity associated with terfenadine. Br Med J 1986; 293:823.
133. Jones SK, Morley WN: Terfenadine causing hair loss. Br Med J 1985; 291:940.
134. Harrison PV, Stones RN: Severe exacerbation of psoriasis due to terfenadine. Clin Exp Dermatol 1988; 13:275.
135. Larrey D, Palazzo L, Benhamou JP: Terfenadine and hepatitis. Ann Intern Med 1985; 103:634.
136. Luskin SS, Fitzsimmons WE, MacLeod CM: Pharmacokinetic evaluation of the terfenadine-theophylline interaction. J Allergy Clin Immunol 1989; 83:406–411.
137. Moser L, Huther KJ, Koch-Weser J: Effects of terfenadine and diphenhydramine alone or in combination with diazepam or alcohol on psychomotor performance and subjective feelings. Eur J Clin Pharmacol 1978; 14:417–423.
138. Freston JW: Cimetidine: Developments, pharmacology, and efficacy. Ann Intern Med 1982; 97:573–580.
139. Zeldis JB, Friedman LS, Isselbacher KJ: Ranitidine: A new H_2-receptor antagonist. N Engl J Med 1983; 309:1368–1373.
140. Schunack W: Pharmacology of H_2-receptor antagonists: An overview. J Int Med Res 1989; 17(Suppl 1):9A–16A.

141. Roberts CJC: Clinical pharmacokinetics of ranitidine. Clin Pharmacokinet 1984; 9:211–221.
142. Zech PY, Chau NP, Pozet N: Ranitidine kinetics in chronic renal impairment. Clin Pharmacol Ther 1983; 34:667–672.
143. Ma KW, Brown DC, Masler DS: Effects of renal failure on blood levels of cimetidine. Gastroenterology 1978; 74:473–477.
144. Bodemar G, Norlander B, Walan A: Pharmacokinetics of cimetidine after single doses and during chronic treatment. Clin Pharmacokin 1981; 6:306–315.
145. Kearns GL, McConnell RF, Trang JM: Appearance of ranitidine in breast milk following multiple dosing. Clin Pharmacol 1985; 4:322–324.
146. Mavligit GM: Immunologic effects of cimetidine: Potential uses. Pharmacotherapy 1987; 7(6, Pt. 2):120S–124S.
147. Achord JL, Langford H: The effect of cimetidine and probantheline on the symptoms of a patient with systemic mastocytosis. Am J Med 1980; 69:610–614.
148. Berg MJ, Bernhard H, Schentag J: Cimetidine in systemic mastocytosis. Drug Intell Clin Pharm 1981; 15:180–183.
149. Jensen RT, Collen MJ, McArthur KE, et al: Comparison of the effectiveness of ranitidine and cimetidine in inhibiting acid secretion in patients with gastric hypersecretory states. Am J Med 1984; 77(5B):90–105.
150. Harvey RP, Wegs J, Shocket AL: A controlled trial of therapy in chronic urticaria. J Allergy Clin Immunol 1981; 68:262–266.
151. Monroe EW, Cohen SH, Kalbfleisch J: Combined H_1 and H_2 antihistamine therapy in chronic urticaria. Arch Dermatol 1981; 117:404–407.
152. Bleehen SS, Thomas SE, Greaves MW: Cimetidine and chlorpheniramine in the treatment of chronic idiopathic urticaria: A multi-centre randomized double-blind study. Br J Dermatol 1987; 117:81–88.
153. Cook LJ, Shuster S: Lack of effect of cimetidine in chronic idiopathic urticaria. Acta Derm Venereol (Stockh) 1983; 63:265–267.
154. Paul E, Bodeker RH: Treatment of chronic urticaria with terfenadine and ranitidine. Eur J Clin Pharmacol 1986; 31:277–280.
155. Marks R, Greaves MW: Vascular reactions to histamine and compound 48/80 in human skin: Suppression by a histamine H_2 receptor blocking agent. Br J Clin Pharmacol 1977; 4:367–369.
156. Thomas RH, Browne PD, Kirby JD: The effect of ranitidine, alone and in combination with clemastine, on allergen-induced cutaneous wheal-and-flare reactions in human skin. J Allergy Clin Immunol 1985; 76:864–869.
157. Harvey RP, Shocket AL: The effect of H_1 and H_2 blockade on cutaneous histamine response in man. J Allergy Clin Immunol 1980; 65:136–139.
158. Farnam J, Grant JA, Guernsey BG: Successful treatment of chronic idiopathic urticaria and angioedema with cimetidine alone. J Allergy Clin Immunol 1984; 73:842–845.
159. Commens CA, Greaves MW: Cimetidine in chronic idiopathic urticaria: A randomized double-blind study. Br J Dermatol 1978; 99:675–679.
160. Monroe EW: Treatment of urticaria. Dermatol Clin 1985; 3:51–55.
161. Kaur S, Greaves M, Eftekhari N: Factitious urticaria (dermographism): Treatment by cimetidine and chlorpheniramine in a randomized double-blind study. Br J Dermatol 1981; 104:185–190.
162. Deutsch PH: Dermatographism treated with hydroxyzine and cimetidine and ranitidine. Ann Intern Med 1984; 101:569.
163. Zappacosta AR, Hauss D: Cimetidine doesn't help pruritus of uremia. N Engl J Med 1979; 300:1280.
164. Harrison AR, Littenberg G, Goldstein L: Pruritus, cimetidine and polycythemia. N Engl J Med 1979; 300:433–434.
165. Gerrard JW, Ko C: Urticaria pigmentosa: Treatment with cimetidine and chlorpheniramine. J Pediatr 1979; 94:843–844.

166. Fenske NA, Lober CW, Pautler SE: Congenital bullous urticaria pigmentosa: Treatment with concomitant use of H_1 and H_2 receptor antagonists. Arch Dermatol 1985; 121:115–118.
167. Van Der Spuy S, Levy DW, Levin W: Cimetidine in the treatment of herpesvirus infections. S Afr Med J 1980; 58:112–116.
168. Wakefield D: Cimetidine in recurrent genital herpes simplex infection. Ann Intern Med 1984; 101:882.
169. Kurzrock R, Auber M, Mavligit GM: Cimetidine therapy of herpes simplex virus infections in immunocompromised patients. Clin Exp Dermatol 1987; 12:326–331.
170. Bense L, Marcusson JA, Ramsten T: Effect of cimetidine on herpes zoster infection. Drug Intell Clin Pharm 1987; 21:803–805.
171. Hayne ST, Mercer JB: Herpes zoster: Treatment with cimetidine. Can Med Assoc J 1983; 129:1284–1285.
172. Mavligit GM, Talpaz M: Cimetidine for herpes zoster. N Engl J Med 1984; 310:318–319.
173. Shandera R: Treatment of herpes zoster with cimetidine. Can Med Assoc J 1984; 131:279.
174. Jorizzo JL, Sams M, Jegasothy BV: Cimetidine as an immunomodulator: Chronic mucocutaneous candidiasis as a model. Ann Intern Med 1980; 92(Part 1):192–195.
175. Presser SE, Blank H: Cimetidine: Adjunct in treatment of tinea capitis. Lancet 1981; 1:108–109.
176. Hill NO, Pardue A, Khan A: Interferon and cimetidine for malignant melanoma. N Engl J Med 1983; 308:286.
177. Mamus SW, Mladenovic J, Hordinsky MK: Cimetidine-induced remission of mycosis fungoides. Lancet 1984; 2:409.
178. Aram H: Treatment of female androgenetic alopecia with cimetidine. Int J Dermatol 1987; 26:128–130.
179. Vigersky RA, Mehlman I, Glass AR: Treatment of hirsute women with cimetidine: A preliminary report. N Engl J Med 1980; 303:1042.
180. Freston JW: H_2-receptor antagonists and duodenal ulcer recurrence: Analysis of efficacy and commentary on safety, costs, and patient selection. Am J Gastroenterol 1987; 82:1242–1249.
181. Giacosa A, Farris A, Cheli R: Cimetidine and psoriasis. Lancet 1978; 2:1211–1212.
182. Rai GS, Webster SGP: Cimetidine and psoriasis. Lancet 1979; 1:50.
183. Merk H, Goerz G, Runne U: Cimetidine and chlorpheniramine in the treatment of psoriasis. Dermatologica 1983; 166:94–96.
184. Levine JB: Safety profile of H_2-receptor antagonists: Current status of famotidine. J Intern Med Res 1979; 17(Suppl 1):48A–53A.
185. Arnold F, Doyle PJ, Bell G: Acute pancreatitis in a patient treated with cimetidine. Lancet 1978; 1:382–383.
186. Freston JW: Cimetidine: Adverse reactions and patterns of use. Ann Intern Med 1982; 97:728–734.
187. Levin A, Barbat JR, Hedges A, Turner P: The effects of cimetidine and ranitidine on psychomotor function in healthy volunteers. Curr Med Res Opin 1984; 9:301–303.
188. Epstein CM, Klopper J: Ranitidine headache. Headache 1985; 25:392–393.
189. Thomas JM, Misiewicz G: Histamine H_2-receptor antagonists in the short- and long-term treatment of duodenal ulcer. Clin Gastroenterol 1984; 13(2):501–541.
190. Hughes JD, Reed WD, Serjeant CS: Mental confusion and associated with ranitidine. Med J Aust 1983; 2:12–13.
191. Azzolini A, Gianrossi R, Livi S: Cardiac function during ranitidine long-lasting administration. Curr Ther Res 1983; 33:1023–1028.
192. Al-Kawas FH, Lenes BA, Sacher RA: Cimetidine and agranulocytosis. Ann Intern Med 1979; 90:992–993.

193. De Galocsy C, Van Ypersele de Strihou C. Pancytopenia with cimetidine [letter]. Ann Intern Med 1979; 90:274.
194. List AF, Beaird DH, Kummet T: Ranitidine-induced granulocytopenia: Recurrence with cimetidine administration. Ann Intern Med 1988; 108:566–567.
195. Souza Lima MA: Hepatitis associated with ranitidine. Ann Intern Med 1984; 101:207–208.
196. Souza Lima MA: Ranitidine and hepatic injury [letter]. Ann Intern Med 1986; 105:140.
197. Black M, Scott WE, Kanter R: Possible ranitidine hepatotoxicity. Ann Intern Med 1984; 101:208–210.
198. Potter PH, Westby RG: Interstitial nephritis after cimetidine but not ranitidine. JAMA 1983; 249:351–352.
199. McGowan WR, Vermillion SE: Acute interstitial nephritis related to cimetidine therapy. Gastroenterology 1980; 9;746–749.
200. Wolfe MM: Impotence on cimetidine treatment. N Engl J Med 1979; 300:94.
201. Bateson MC, Browning MC, Maconnachie A: Galactorrhea with cimetidine [letter]. Lancet 1977; 2:247–248.
202. Galbraith RA, Michnovicz JJ: The effects of cimetidine on the oxidative metabolism of estradiol. N Engl J Med 1989; 321:269–274.
203. Wang C, Wong KL, Lam KC: Ranitidine does not affect gonadal function in man. Br J Clin Pharmacol 1983; 16:430–432.
204. Mitchell GG, Magnusson AR, Weiler JM: Cimetidine-induced cutaneous vasculitis. Am J Med 1983; 75:875–876.
205. Brodin MB: Drug-related alopecia. Dermatol Clin 1987; 5:571–579.
206. Dobrilla G, Felder M, Chilovia F: Exacerbation of glaucoma associated with both cimetidine and ranitidine. Lancet 1982; 1:1078.
207. Sax MJ: Clinically important adverse effects and drug interactions with H_2-receptor antagonists: An update. Pharmacotherapy 1987; 7(6, Pt. 2):110S–115S.
208. Powell JR, Donn KH: Histamine H_2-antagonist drug interactions in perspective: Mechanistic concepts and clinical implications. Am J Med 1984; 77(5B):57–84.
209. Somogyi A, Muirhead M: Pharmacokinetic interactions of cimetidine. Clin Pharmacokin 1987; 12:321–366.
210. Kirch W, Hoensch H, Janisch HD: Interactions and non-interactions with ranitidine. Clin Pharmacokinet 1984; 9:493–510.
211. Powell JR, Rogers JF, Wargin WA: Inhibition of theophylline clearance by cimetidine but not ranitidine. Arch Intern Med 1984; 144:484–486.
212. Gisclon LG, Boyd RA, Williams RL, Giacomini JM: The effect of probenecid on the renal elimination of cimetidine. Clin Pharmacol Ther 1989; 45:444–452.
213. Salo OP, Kauppinen K, Mannisto PT: Cimetidine increases the plasma concentration of hydroxyzine. Acta Derm Venereol (Stockh) 1985; 66:349–350.
214. Pinder RM, Brogden RN, Speight TM, et al: Doxepin up-to-date: A review of its pharmacological properties and therapeutic efficacy with particular reference to depression. Drugs 1977; 13:161–218.
215. Greene SL, Reed CE, Schroeter AL: Double-blind crossover study comparing doxepin with diphenhydramine for the treatment of chronic idiopathic urticaria. J Am Acad Dermatol 1985; 12:669–675.
216. Faulkner RD, Pitts WM, Lee CS: Multiple-dose doxepin kinetics in depressed patients. Clin Pharmacol Ther 1983; 34:509–515.
217. Kemp J, Ilett KF, Booth J: Excretion of doxepin and N-desmethyldoxepin in human milk. Br J Clin Pharmacol 1985; 20:497–499.
218. Harto A, Sendagorta E, Ledo A: Doxepin in the treatment of chronic urticaria. Dermatologica 1985; 170:90–93.
219. Goldsobel AB, Rohr AS, Siegel SC: Efficacy of doxepin in the treatment of chronic idiopathic urticaria. J Allergy Clin Immunol 1986; 78:867–873.
220. Neittaanmaki H, Myohanen T, Fraki JE: Comparison of cinnarizine, cyproheptadine,

doxepin, and hydroxyzine in the treatment of idiopathic cold urticaria: Usefulness of doxepin. J Am Acad Dermatol 1984; 11:483–489.
221. Harris BA, Sherertz EF, Flowers FP: Improvement of chronic neurotic excoriations with oral doxepin therapy. Int J Dermatol 1987; 26:541–543.
222. Richardson JW 3rd, Richelson E: Antidepressants: A clinical update for medical practitioners. Mayo Clin Proc 1984; 59:330–337.
223. Sinequan Product Information, Roerig. In Physicians' Desk Reference (43rd ed). Oradell, NJ: Medical Economics, 1989, 1791–1792.
224. Matheson I, Pande H, Alertsen AR: Respiratory depression caused by N-desmethyl-doxepin in breast milk. Lancet 1985; 2:11–24.
225. Glassman AH: Cardiovascular effects of tricyclic antidepressants. Ann Rev Med 1984; 35:503–511.
226. Salzman C: Clinical guidelines for the use of antidepressant drugs in geriatric patients. J Clin Psychiatry 1985; 46:10(Part 2):38–44.
227. Berkowitz RL, Coustan DR, Mochizuki TK: Handbook for Prescribing Medications During Pregnancy (2nd ed). Boston: Little, Brown, 1986, 294–296.
228. Mendels J, Schless A: A controlled comparison of doxepin hs and doxepin qid. J Clin Pharmacol 1975; 15:534–539.
229. Goldberg HL, Finnerty RJ, Nathan L: Doxepin in a single bedtime dose in psychoneurotic outpatients. Arch Gen Psychiatry 1974; 31:513–517.
230. Ayd FJ Jr: Long-term administration of doxepin (Sinequan). (Clinical and laboratory survey of 40 patients.) Dis Nerv Syst 1971; 32:617–622.
231. Ayd FJ Jr: Long-term treatment of chronic depression: 15-year experience with doxepin HC1. J Clin Psychiatry 1984; 45(3, Pt. 2):39–46.
232. Nixon DD: Thrombocytopenia following doxepin treatment. JAMA 1972; 220:418.
233. Orme ML: Antidepressants and heart disease [editorial]. Br Med J [Clin Res] 1984; 289:12.
234. Luchins DJ: Review of clinical and animal studies comparing cardiovascular effects of doxepin and other tricyclic antidepressants. Am J Psychiatry 1983; 140:1006–1009.
235. Veith RC, Raskind MA, Caldwell JH: Cardiovascular effects of tricyclic antidepressants in depressed patients with chronic heart disease. N Engl J Med 1982; 306:954–959.
236. Hansten PD: Drug Interactions (5th ed). Philadelphia: Lea & Febiger, 1985, 368–369.
237. Haider SA: Treatment of atopic eczema in children: Clinical trial of 10% sodium cromoglycate ointment. Br Med J 1977; 1:1570–1572.
238. Thirumoorthy T, Greaves MW: Disodium cromoglycate ointment in atopic eczema. Br Med J 1978; 2:500–501.
239. Jones EA: Oral cromolyn sodium in milk induced anaphylaxis. Ann Allergy 1985; 54:199–201.
240. Businco L, Cantani A, Benincori N: Effectiveness of oral sodium cromoglycate in preventing food allergy in children. Ann Allergy 1983; 51:47–50.
241. Lindskov R, Knudsen L: Oral disodium cromoglycate treatment of atopic dermatitis. Allergy 1983; 38:161–165.
242. Atherton DJ, Soothill JF, Elvidge J: A controlled trial of oral sodium cromoglycate in atopic eczema. Br J Dermatol 1982; 106:681–685.
243. Dolovich J, Punthakee ND, MacMillan AB: Systemic mastocytosis: Control of lifelong diarrhea by ingested disodium cromoglycate. Can Med Assoc J 1974; 111:684–685.
244. Frieri M, Alling DW, Metcalfe DD: Comparison of the therapeutic efficacy of cromolyn sodium with that of combined chlorpheniramine and cimetidine in systemic mastocytosis. Am J Med 1985; 78:914.
245. Welch EA, Alper JC, Bogaars H: Treatment of bullous mastocytosis with disodium cromoglycate. J Am Acad Dermatol 1983; 9:349–353.
246. MacDonald GF: An overview of ketotifen. Chest 1982; 82(Suppl):30S–32S.
247. MacLean SP, Arreaza EE, Lett-Brown MA: Refractory cholinergic urticaria successfully treated with ketotifen. J Allergy Clin Immunol 1989; 83:738–741.

248. Huston DP, Bressler RB, Kaliner M: Prevention of mast-cell degranulation by ketotifen in patients with physical urticarias. Ann Intern Med 1986; 104:507–510.
249. Kettlehut BV, Berkebile C, Bradley D: A double-blind, placebo-controlled, crossover trial of ketotifen versus hydroxyzine in the treatment of pediatric mastocytosis. J Allergy Clin Immunol 1989; 83:866–870.
250. Saihan EM: Ketotifen and terbutaline in urticaria. Br J Dermatol 1981; 104:205.
251. Ricciardi VM: Mast-cell stabilization to decrease neurofibroma growth. Arch Dermatol 1987; 123:1011–1016.

13 Antiandrogens

Wilma F. Bergfeld, M.D.
Geoffrey Redmond, M.D.

The antiandrogen therapies used in dermatology have been primarily for hyperandrogenic disorders that commonly present as acne, alopecia, hirsutism, and less frequently with greasy skin (seborrhea) and hidradenitis suppurativa. Menstrual dysfunction is also present in about one third of the affected women. Historically, antiandrogen therapy has been used primarily to treat virilization of women, hirsutism, and polycystic ovarian disease.

Since the late 1980s, there has been a resurgence of interest in the investigation of women with clinical signs of androgen excess.[1-9] Specific efforts have been made in understanding the pathophysiology at multiple sites: pituitary gland, adrenal glands, and ovaries and the target organs, namely the sebaceous gland and hair follicles.[10-16] Concomitantly, antiandrogens have been used more commonly to treat cutaneous manifestations of androgen excess.[10, 13, 17-20]

Over the last 7 years, the authors have evaluated more than 1000 female patients with clinically diagnosed androgen excess disorders with the primary presentation of acne, alopecia, or hirsutism or a mixed presentation.[18] The major abnormalities of hyperandrogenism have been elevations of serum dehydroepiandrosterone-sulfate (DHEA-S) and less frequent elevations of total testosterone, free testosterone, and androstenedione. The associated endocrine abnormalities have been ovarian hyperplasia, polycystic ovarian disease, and adult-onset adrenal hyperplasia. Tumors of endocrine organs have not been seen unless the aforementioned conditions have occurred abruptly. Typically, patients with the common adrenal androgen excess disorders have symptoms that evolve slowly. Pituitary adenomas and thyroid disorders have been relatively uncommon in these patients.

At the present time, the androgen excess disorders are best screened with determinations of DHEA-S, total and free testosterone, and androstenedione levels. Specialized radiographic studies are not necessary unless indicated by history or laboratory findings.

The most common antiandrogen therapies are spironolactone, estrogen-progestin oral contraceptives, and dexamethasone, alone or in combination. Cyproterone acetate, although used worldwide, is not available in the U.S.

In this chapter we discuss three antiandrogens: spironolactone, estrogens and progestins, and cyproterone acetate. Other antiandrogen therapies are only briefly discussed. Cimetidine (Chapter 12), dexamethasone (Chapter 4), and ketoconazole (Chapter 2) are covered more completely in other chapters.

SPIRONOLACTONE

Pharmacology

Structure

Spironolactone is an example of a 17-spironolactone steroid. The structure of spironolactone is based on the four-ring structure common to all steroid molecules, chemically resembling the endogenous mineralocorticoid aldosterone. An esterified lactone ring is present in addition.

Absorption/Distribution

In humans the bioavailability of spironolactone from oral administration exceeds 90%. However, this percentage may vary substantially, depending on the tablet manufacturer. Spironolactone itself is 98% protein-bound, and its primary metabolite, canrenone, is at least 90% protein-bound. Food is known to increase the absorption of spironolactone.

Metabolism/Excretion

Spironolactone is rapidly and significantly metabolized by the liver. Canrenone, the primary metabolite of spironolactone, can be interconverted enzymatically to its hydrolytic product, canrenoate. Virtually none of the unmetabolized drug appears in the urine. Metabolites of spironolactone are excreted in urine and bile.

Canrenone is an active aldosterone antagonist, and its formation contributes to the diuretic activities of spironolactone. Canrenoate has no intrinsic activity, but it exerts effects through its conversion to canrenone.[21]

In a dose range of 25–200 mg, a linear relationship between a single dose of spironolactone and the plasma levels of canrenone occurs by 96 hours. The estimated half-life of canrenone is 19.2 ± 6.57 hours; that of spironolactone is 12.5 ± 3.39 hours. When 200 mg of oral spironolactone is given, the estimated half-life of canrenone is 19.2 ± 6.57 hours; that of spironolactone is 12.5 ± 3.9 hours.

Mechanism of Action

The 17-spironolactone steroids are competitive antagonists of adrenal mineralocorticoids, among which aldosterone is the most potent. This antagonism is central to the drug's potassium-sparing mild diuretic effect.

Spironolactone's antiandrogen activity is complex.[22, 23] Because dermatologic applicability of spironolactone is limited to women, this discussion focuses on the drug's effects on androgen excess disorders in women. The drug competitively inhibits dihydrotestosterone binding at the androgen receptor and suppresses androgen secretion or production, or both, from the ovaries and the adrenal glands.[24, 25] This is accomplished because spironolactone inhibits the target organ response to androgens by competing for the cytosol dihydrotestosterone receptor.[24] This activity inhibits the binding of dihydrotestosterone to the receptor and its subsequent translocation to the nucleus of the cell. In addition, spironolactone is converted by progesterone 17-hydroxylase to an active metabolite that reversibly inhibits the adrenal and ovarian cytochrome P-450. The net effect of these actions is a decreased testosterone or dihydrotestosterone effect on the receptor cells.

The progestational activity of spironolactone is variable, but it appears to influence the ratio of plasma luteinizing hormone (LH) to follicular-stimulating hormone (FSH) by decreasing the response of LH to gonadotropin-releasing hormone. Commonly, LH is decreased and FSH is unchanged.[23, 26]

Clinical Use

Indications

No dermatologic indications for spironolactone have been approved by the U.S. Food and Drug Administration (FDA). Spironolactone has FDA approval as a diuretic. It has been described as a competitive aldosterone antagonist and a potassium-sparing diuretic and has been approved for use in treating primary hyperaldosteronism, idiopathic hyperaldosteronism, edematous conditions (congestive heart failure, cirrhosis with ascites, and nephrotic syndrome), essential hypertension, and hypokalemia. The common treatment dosage for these conditions ranges from 25 to 200 mg/day.

Unlabeled, non–FDA-approved treatments with spironolactone are used because of the drug's antiandrogenic effects.[22] Spironolactone has been used to treat hirsutism, acne, androgenic alopecia, and hidradenitis suppurativa. The most common dosage ranges for antiandrogen effects of spironolactone have been 50–200 mg/day; the preferred and effective dosage is at least 100 mg/day.[22–24, 27–37] At 100 mg/day or more, menorrhagia or menstrual dysfunction is common. These abnormalities generally correct themselves after 2–3 months of therapy. However, if menorrhagia or spotting persists, decreasing the spironolactone to 50–75 mg/day is helpful. The reduced dosage of spironolactone also, however, reduces the antiandrogenic effects. The more common therapeutic practice with menstrual period disturbance is to maintain the spironolactone dose and add combination oral contraceptives, or conjugated estrogens with or without progestins. The choice of the latter therapy depends on the age of the woman, as patients less than 35 years old are usually treated with oral contraceptives, whereas older patients are treated with conjugated estrogens.

If there is laboratory evidence of androgen excess, the clinician monitors the antiandrogen therapy by repeating the recommended androgen profile at least every 4 months until the desired laboratory value is achieved. Complete suppression of the androgen excess generally takes approximately 4–12 months of therapy.

It is usual for the therapeutic benefit of spironolactone to plateau after 1 year. At this time, the addition of other adjunctive therapies may be helpful. Specifically, in androgenic alopecia, the addition of topical minoxidil (Rogaine) frequently gives an additional cosmetic benefit.

Once full therapeutic benefit is achieved between 1–3 years, spironolactone is slowly titrated to the lowest possible dosage. While the patient receives maintenance therapy, yearly routine laboratory tests are suggested: complete blood count (CBC), chemistry profile to determine level of electrolytes, and determination of DHEA-S, testosterone, androstenedione, and cortisol levels. In addition, the patient's blood pressure and weight should be monitored during each visit.

In Europe, topical 5% spironolactone lotion and cream have been used effectively in the treatment of acne, grade II. This treatment appears to have an efficacy similar to that of topical antibiotic therapy for acne.

Contraindications

Spironolactone is contraindicated for patients with acute renal insufficiency, anuria, significant chronic renal impairment, and hyperkalemia. Other contraindications are pregnancy and the presence of undiagnosed abnormal uterine bleeding.

Adverse Effects

The adverse effects of spironolactone are generally reversible with discontinuation of the drug. In many situations, dosage reduction leads to resolution of the adverse effect.[31, 38, 39]

ENDOCRINE EFFECTS. The most frequently troublesome adverse effects are dosage-related abnormal menstrual function. Polymenorrhea, metrorrhagia, oligomenorrhea, and amenorrhea are all common with dosages above 100 mg/day. Cyclic spironolactone administration on days 4–21 of the menstrual cycle, dosage reduction, or the addition of an oral contraceptive may alleviate these symptoms. The frequent development of gynecomastia, decreased libido, and erectile dysfunction limit the use of spironolactone by men. In women taking the drug, some breast enlargement is commonly noted, and decreased libido, postmenopausal bleeding, and hirsutism are occasionally noted.

METABOLIC EFFECTS. The inhibition of aldosterone-related renal sodium retention and of potassium secretion is responsible for the infrequent metabolic adverse effects. Hyperkalemia may result, especially if supplemental potassium is administered or in patients with impaired renal function. In the normal woman, hyperkalemia is more commonly a result of dehydration or the ingestion of beverages that act as diuretics (e.g., coffee, tea, and dietetic drinks). The lack of hydration in these otherwise healthy women can also produce hyperchloremia, metabolic acidosis, or hyponatremia. Although the diuretic effect is relatively weak, orthostasis can occur.

OTHER ADVERSE EFFECTS. The patient should be alerted to the possibility of drowsiness, lethargy, mental confusion, and ataxia. Headaches may also occur. Cramping and diarrhea are present in some patients. Gastritis, ulcerations, and gastrointestinal bleeding have been infrequently observed. Urticarial and morbilliform eruptions can occur. Of importance is that agranulocytosis has on rare occasions been reported.

Warnings

CARCINOGENICITY. The carcinogenicity of spironolactone has long been debated. The FDA has included a "black box" warning in the spironolactone package insert that states that spironolactone has been found to be tumorogenic in chronic toxicity studies of rats. In these studies, 25–250 times the usual human dose (on a body weight basis) of spironolactone was given to rats. These dosages resulted in an increase in benign adenomas of the thyroid and the testes, malignant mammary tumors, and proliferative changes in the liver.[40] At doses of 500 mg/kg/day, the effects included hepatocytomegaly, hyperplastic liver nodules, and hepatocellular carcinoma. Potassium canrenoate, a spironolactone metabolite, in dosages of 20 mg/kg/day was shown to precipitate myelocytic leukemia in a dosage-related fashion.

Because of these reported changes in the rat, it has been recommended that spironolactone not be given to women with breast carcinoma or with genetic predisposition for breast carcinoma.

In 1987, Barker refuted this recommendation.[41] The review of three case-controlled studies showed that spironolactone was not associated with a large risk for leukemia. In addition, six case-controlled studies and two longitudinal studies did not provide evidence that spironolactone induced breast cancer.

USAGE DURING PREGNANCY AND LACTATION. Spironolactone and its metabolites may cross the placental barrier. In rat reproductive studies, feminization of the male rat fetus was noted. Among women taking the drug, the presence of canrenone in breast milk has been demonstrated.

Drug Interactions

The diuretic effect of spironolactone may be decreased by concurrent salicylate use. Angiotensin-converting enzyme inhibitors (captopril, enalapril) decrease aldosterone production, which may result in elevated serum potassium. Concomitant use of spironolactone and potassium supplements may lead to hyperkalemia.

The interaction of spironolactone and digitalis glycosides is variable. This complex interaction results in an increased absorption of digitalis with increased blood levels. This reduces maintenance and digitalization dosing requirements. Spironolactone can also interfere with radioimmunoassay measurement of digoxin, resulting in a falsely elevated serum digoxin value.

Therapeutic Guidelines

The antiandrogenic effects of spironolactone can vary, depending on dosages between 25 and 200 mg/day. Common dosages for androgen excess disorders are 100–200 mg/day.[27–30, 33, 35, 37]

In contrast, the treatment of hyperaldosteronism is 100–400 mg/day, whereas the treatment of peripheral edema and hypertension/hypokalemia ranges from 25 to 100 mg/day. When used for antiandrogenic effects, spironolactone therapy can be initiated at 100 mg/day. The daily dose may be increased by 50 mg each month if abnormal menstrual bleeding, breast tenderness, or other significant adverse effects are not present. Patients with dermatologic indications should not receive more than 200 mg/day. Spironolactone is available generically only in 25-mg tablets. Additional tablet sizes (50 mg and 100 mg) are available under the trade name Aldactone. Although not specified in the product information, baseline CBC, liver function tests, and determination of electrolyte levels with follow-up laboratory tests at 3- to 4-month intervals initially is reasonable.

Acceptable therapeutic response may require 4–6 months for acne and up to 12–24 months for androgenic alopecia and hirsutism. It is not necessary to have androgen laboratory abnormalities to treat with spironolactone, although spironolactone is commonly used as monotherapy when there is no laboratory evidence of androgen excess. Concomitant use with glucocorticosteroids such as dexamethasone, estrogen-suppressive, or estrogen replacement therapy is frequently helpful, especially if androgen hormone levels are elevated. The expected therapeutic response would be a reduced number or disappearance of acneform lesions and a decrease in the shedding of scalp hair with an ultimate increase in the density and fiber diameter of hair in cases of alopecia; in patients with hirsutism, the reduction of hair fiber diameter and reduced rate of growth with miniaturization of the hair follicle (resulting in vellus fibers) is expected. Total disappearance of the hirsute condition is rare.

ESTROGENS AND PROGESTINS

Estrogens and the combination therapies of estrogens and the progestins have long been used for estrogen deficiency, estrogen suppression, and more recently for their antiandrogenic activities. Possible dermatologic indications include acne, hirsutism, and alopecia. Because of the numerous potential adverse effects from the various estrogen products discussed, only dermatologists who are thoroughly familiar with this use should prescribe this antiandrogenic modality.

Pharmacology

Structure

The ovaries and the testes are capable of synthesizing estrogen from acetate to cholesterol and subsequently to other steroids. Estrogens are ultimately formed from their immediate precursors, androstenedione or testosterone. Estrogens are also synthesized from androgen precursors produced in nongonadal tissue.

Women produce three significant estrogens: estradiol, estrone, and estriol. Estradiol is the most potent estrogen; it is rapidly oxidized to estrone. Estrone is approximately half as potent as estradiol. Hydroxylation of estradiol produces estriol, which is weaker yet. Equivalent doses of exogenous estrogens are 5 mg of conjugated estrogen, 1 mg of diethylstilbestrol, 80 mcg of mestranol, and 50 mcg of ethinyl estradiol.

Absorption/Distribution

The absorption of most estrogens is predominantly through the gastrointestinal tract; the primary metabolism of estrogens occurs within the liver. About 80% of estradiol is bound to sex-hormone-binding globulin, and the remainder is bound to albumin or remains unbound.

Metabolism/Excretion

Estrogens are metabolized and inactivated in the liver to less active estrogen metabolites. These estrogens are conjugated with sulfuric and glucuronide acids. Of the clinically important estrogens, ethinyl estradiol is most slowly metabolized and inactivated by the liver, which probably accounts for its increased potency as an estrogen. Estrogens are excreted into bile and urine as the estrogen metabolites. Recycling of estrogen metabolites through bile excretion is noted with long-acting estrogens.

Mechanism of Action

Estrogens are essential in the development and maintenance of the female reproductive system, female sex characteristics, and female bone structural integrity. Estrogens induce proliferation in the endothelium of fallopian tubes, endometrium, cervix, and vagina and increase vascularity. In addition, estrogens are responsible for vaginal acidity and cornification of vaginal epithelial cells. Cyclic decline of estrogen induces menstruation, although the cessation of progesterone secretion at the end of the luteal phase is more important for inducing menstruation.

As an antiandrogen, the combination of estrogens and progestins reduces testosterone, androstenedione, FSH, and DHEA-S.[42, 43] In addition, this combination demonstrates antigonadotropic and limited glucocorticoid activity. The estrogens and the estrogenic progestins (e.g., ethynodiol diacetate) have been cited as antiandrogens and have been noted to specifically antagonize testosterone and dihydrotestosterone production. It is hypothesized that they compete at the androgen cytosol receptor, limiting binding of dihydrotestosterone and metabolism of testosterone to dihydrotestosterone. In addition, estrogens induce an elevation of sex hormone binding globulin, which increases the binding of testosterone, reducing the levels of free testosterone.

Clinical Use

Indications

There are no FDA-approved dermatologic indications. The FDA-approved uses of estrogens and combined estrogens and progestins are for birth control, postmenopausal state, osteoporosis, vasomotor instability, and atrophic vaginitis. Conjugated estrogens, with or without progesterones, are used for management of estrogen deficiency.

Estrogen and conjugated estrogen therapy is used primarily for treatment of the cutaneous manifestations of androgen excess associated with an estrogen deficiency. These conditions include, for selected patients, alopecia, acne,[44,45] hirsutism,[46] and in some instances seborrhea. Androgenic alopecia of late onset generally seen in the menopausal female appears to be related primarily to an absolute or relative estrogen deficiency with increased relative testosterone effects. Early treatment is recommended if these conditions are clinically recognized.

Contraindications

The major contraindications for estrogens, combined estrogens, and conjugated estrogens are estrogen-sensitive breast cancer, pregnancy, estrogen-dependent uterine malignancy, thromboembolic episodes, or history of thrombophlebitis. Drug eruptions representing hypersensitivity to estrogen and estrogen-like products also contraindicate the use of these therapies.

Adverse Effects

ENDOCRINE EFFECTS. A number of estrogen-induced adverse effects are related to menstrual function. The incidence of many of these effects is significantly influenced by the choice of progestin in the combination oral contraceptives. Breakthrough bleeding, alterations of menstrual flow, amenorrhea, dysmenorrhea, and a premenstrual-like syndrome are all frequent. Breast enlargement, tenderness, or secretions may occur. Endometrial cystic hyperplasia and cervical eversion relate to estrogen stimulation of the endometrium. Vaginal candidiasis, peripheral edema, and reduced libido are all frequent adverse effects from estrogens alone or in combination with progestins.

CARBOHYDRATE/LIPID METABOLISM EFFECTS. Estrogens may significantly alter carbohydrate metabolism and subsequently impair glucose tolerance in some patients. Diabetics should be followed carefully, particularly early in estrogen therapy. An elevation in triglycerides that is consistent with type IV hyperlipidemia may occur.[47]

CARDIOVASCULAR EFFECTS. A modest elevation in blood pressure is common, and patients may occasionally have a significant increase. Oral contraceptives are associated with an increased risk of thrombotic and thromboembolic vascular diseases, including thrombophlebitis, pulmonary embolism, stroke, and myocardial infarction.[48] Women over 35 years of age have an increased risk of the disorders, particularly if they smoke heavily. The risk of thrombotic and thromboembolic disorders appears to be much less in postmenstrual women receiving replacement estrogen therapy.[49] Fluid retention, independent of blood pressure elevation, is commonly noted.

DERMATOLOGIC EFFECTS. Melasma (chloasma) is relatively common with exogenous estrogen therapy. Estrogens are the most common medication associated with erythema nodosum. Acne, hirsutism, and (to a lesser extent) female pattern androgenic alopecia can occur particularly with products containing norgestrel and levonorgestrel. A telogen effluvium can occur soon after cessation of estrogen therapy. Uncommon dermatologic effects include urticaria, photosensitivity, and dermatitis.

GASTROINTESTINAL EFFECTS. A rare but potentially serious complication is the development of hepatic adenoma. Of importance is that these benign tumors may rupture with resultant marked, potentially fatal, intraabdominal hemorrhage. In addition, acute abdominal pain may signify the development of pancreatitis. Nausea, vomiting, abdominal cramps, and bloating are all relatively common. Cholestatic jaundice may occur, particularly in women with a history of jaundice in pregnancy.

OTHER ADVERSE EFFECTS. Headache, dizziness, depression, and, in rare instances, convulsions have all been reported as being due to estrogen therapy. Recurrent, persistent, or severe headaches require cessation of therapy and prompt evaluation. Intolerance to contact lenses may develop.

LABORATORY TEST ALTERATIONS. Numerous alterations of common laboratory test results are due to estrogens alone or in combination with progestins. Complete listings of these alterations can be found in the respective package inserts. The most notable alterations include (1) increases in thyroid-binding globulin (resulting in increased total thyroid hormone), corticosteroid levels, triglycerides, amylase, gamma-glutamyl transpeptidase, transferrin and resultant iron-binding capacity, prolactin, and vitamin A and (2) decreases in free T_3 resin uptake, albumin, glucose tolerance, folate, zinc, and vitamin B_{12}.

Warnings

The safety of the aforementioned therapies has not been demonstrated for use during pregnancy. The major warnings with estrogen therapies is the possible induction of neoplasia, such as endometrial cancer, which occurs when there has been prolonged, unopposed estrogen stimulation of the endometrium. For this reason, women who have a uterus should use estrogens only in combination with progestins. In some studies, dosage and duration of therapy have been cited as important factors in the development of these neoplasms.[50, 51]

Cigarette smoking also increases the risk of cardiovascular side effects from the use of oral contraceptives and possibly the conjugated estrogens. Oral contraceptives also increase the risk of thromboembolic disorders, gallbladder disease, and feminization of the male fetus.

> **MONITORING GUIDELINES**
>
> Pretreatment and periodic history and physical examinations are recommended every 6–12 months for women taking oral contraceptives. These visits should include blood pressure determination; examination of breasts, abdomen, and pelvic organs; and a Pap smear. Periodic glucose and lipid determinations are suggested early in therapy.

Drug Interactions

Reduced efficacy of estrogen therapies has been reported in people receiving the following drugs: anticonvulsants (barbiturates, phenytoin, carbamazepine, primidone); antibiotics (isoniazid, rifampin, penicillin V, tetracycline, sulfonamides, griseofulvin, ampicillin, nitrofurantoin, chloramphenicol); antihistamines; analgesics; tranquilizers; antimigraine drugs; and phenylbutazone. In contrast, the pharmacologic effects of ethinyl estradiol may be increased by ascorbic acid.

Estrogens may reduce the therapeutic efficacy of the following drugs: insulin, oral hypoglycemic agents, oral anticoagulants, anticonvulsants, tricyclic antidepressants, certain benzodiazepines (lorazepam, oxazepam), acetaminophen, and vitamins.

Conversely, estrogens may potentiate the following drugs by impairing their metabolism: corticosteroids, phenytoin, certain benzodiazepines (diazepam, chlordiazepoxide), phenylbutazone, metoprolol, and imipramine.

Concurrent administration of aminocaproic acid may increase clotting factors, leading to a hypercoagulable state. Finally, concomitant administration of troleandomycin may induce cholestatic jaundice.

Therapeutic Guidelines

The antiandrogenic combined estrogen-progestin therapies avoid the incorporation of the androgenic progestins norgestrel and levonorgestrel. The most common progestins used are ethynodiol diacetate and norethindrone. The estrogenic progestin ethynodiol acetate (in Demulen) provides the most optimal combination in suppression of manifestations of androgen excess.

The most common estrogen is ethinyl estradiol (35–50 mcg); mestranol is less frequently used. The preferred combination therapy is 35–

50 mg of ethinyl estradiol and 0.3–1 mcg of progestin. The antiandrogenic effects are observed within 1–4 months and may plateau in 1–3 years.

The preferred methods of treatment for the androgen excess disorders are chronic cyclic oral contraceptives or conjugated estrogens, with or without progestins. The latter is used primarily by menopausal or postmenopausal women. Various monophasic oral contraceptives are described in Table 13–1; conjugated estrogens are listed in Table 13–2.

An oral contraceptive containing both 50 mcg or less of estrogen and a low dose (less than 1 mg) of progesterone is preferred for initial therapy. Side effects noted during the initial cycles may be transient, and if they persist, dosage adjustments can be made. (See respective package inserts for details of dosage adjustments.)

ORAL CONJUGATED ESTROGENS. These preparations contain 50%–65% sodium estrone sulfate and 20%–35% sodium equilin sulfate. For estrogen deficiencies and antiandrogen effects, a dosage greater than the normal dosage for osteoporosis is needed.

Conjugated estrogens are administered cyclically: 3 weeks of daily estrogen and 1 week off. If the woman has her uterus, a progestin is added. The recommended dosages for antiandrogen therapy are a starting dosage of 1.25 mg and a maintenance dosage of 0.625 mg. It is recommended that the lowest effective dose be given for maintenance therapy.

When it is necessary to give a progestin, medroxyprogesterone acetate at the recommended dosage range of 2.5–10 mg/day is given for 5–10 days of the menstrual cycle. The progesterone is typically given on the

Table 13–1. Selected Monophasic Oral Contraceptives

Product and Distributor	Estrogen (mcg)	Progesterone (mg)
Ovcon-50 (Mead Johnson Nutritional)	50 ethinyl estradiol	1 norethindrone
Norlestrin 21 1/50 (P-D)	50 ethinyl estradiol	1 norethindrone acetate
Demulen 1/50-21 (Searle)	50 ethinyl estradiol	1 ethynodiol diacetate
Norinyl 1 +50 (Syntex)	50 mestranol	1 norethindrone
Ortho-Novum 1/50 (Ortho)	50 mestranol	1 norethindrone
Norinyl 1 +35 21-Day (Syntex)	35 ethinyl estradiol	1 norethindrone
Ortho-Novum 1/35 28 (Ortho)	35 ethinyl estradiol	1 norethindrone
Ovcon-35 (Mead Johnson Nutritional)	35 ethinyl estradiol	0.4 norethindrone
Demulen 1/35-21 and 28 (Searle)	35 ethinyl estradiol	1 ethynodiol diacetate
Loestrin 21 1.5/30 (Parke-Davis)	30 ethinyl estradiol	1.5 norethindrone acetate
Loestrin 21 1/20 (Parke-Davis)	20 ethinyl estradiol	1 norethindrone acetate

Modified from Drug Facts and Comparisons. St. Louis: JB Lippincott, 1989, pp. 301–303.

Table 13–2. Oral Conjugated Estrogens

Drug	Tablets
Conjugated estrogens (various) Premarin (Ayerst)	0.3 mg
Conjugated estrogens (various) Estrocon (Savage) Premarin (Ayerst) Progens (Major)	0.625 mg
Premarin (Ayerst)	0.9 mg
Conjugated estrogens (various) Estrocon (Savage) Premarin (Ayerst) Progens (Major)	1.25 mg
Conjugated estrogens (various) Premarin (Ayerst) Progens (Major)	2.5 mg

Modified from Drug Facts and Comparisons. St. Louis: JB Lippincott, 1989, p. 281.

16th–21st days of the menstrual cycle. Newer therapies include a low-dosage progestin that parallels the conjugated estrogen therapy and appears safe and effective[52] (Table 13–3). The minimal duration of therapy is 6 months, whereas the usual treatment exceeds 2 years and potentially may require lifetime maintenance therapy.

CYPROTERONE ACETATE

Cyproterone acetate was first discovered in 1961, and in 1963 its antiandrogenic activities were recognized. After extensive preclinical and clinical studies, cyproterone acetate is recognized as a potent estrogenic progesterone with progestational and antigonadotropic effects. Because of these activities, it has been used for the therapy of androgen-related disorders as an antiandrogen.[55] Such disorders include prostatic carcinoma, hirsutism, alopecia, acne, and precocious puberty.

Cyproterone acetate is not an FDA-approved drug; therefore, it is not available in the U.S. for treatment of these androgenic disorders. Because

Table 13–3. Oral Progesterones (All Medroxyprogesterone Acetate)

Drug	Tablets
Provera (Upjohn)	2.5 mg
Amen (Carnrick) Curretab (Reid-Rowell) Provera (Upjohn)	10 mg

Modified from Drug Facts and Comparisons. St. Louis: JB Lippincott, 1989, p. 289.

Pharmacology

Cyproterone acetate is progestin steroid with a 1,2-alpha methyl group. This radical has been found to produce the antiandrogenic effects. The chemical name for cyproterone acetate is 17-acetoxy-6-chloro-1-alpha-methyl-4-6-pregnadiene-3,20-dione.

Cyproterone acetate is relatively slowly but completely absorbed from the gastrointestinal tract. After a single dose of 50 mg, the maximal plasma level is reached in 3–4 hours. The elimination phase has a half-life of 38 hours. Cyproterone acetate is metabolically stable; less than 2% is excreted in the form of urinary metabolites.

Mechanism of Action

As a potent antiandrogen and progestin, cyproterone acetate has a mechanism of action that is similar to those of spironolactone and estrogens. Cyproterone acetate suppresses the secretion or the production, or both, of gonadotropins, with subsequent inhibition of follicular maturation and ovulation.[56,57] At the target organ, it competes with dihydrotestosterone for the cytosol androgen receptor sites. This competitive binding results in reduced binding of the active metabolite of testosterone, namely, dihydrotestosterone.

Cyproterone acetate demonstrates suppression of ovary and adrenal function. Specifically, adrenocortical atrophy in laboratory animals has been reported. Researchers have also reported suppression of cortisol and adrenocorticotropin hormone (ACTH) secretion in children with precocious puberty who receive high dosages of cyproterone acetate.

Studies have produced variable results in adults from the adrenal inhibitory response with no evidence of suppression. These changes are most likely to be clinically significant in patients with underlying impairment of pituitary-adrenal function.

In women, the ovarian suppression is notable. In addition, androgen-sensitive tissue may exhibit atrophy of the specific organ with chronic therapy.

In the mature rat, the testes are noted to be unaffected by small-to-moderate dosages of cyproterone acetate, although large dosages are noted to decrease both the function of Leydig's cells and spermatogenesis.

Clinical Use

Indications

Because of cyproterone acetate's antiandrogen and progestational properties, it has been successfully used in female androgen excess disorders such as acne,[55, 58] alopecia,[59] hirsutism,[55, 58, 59] hidradenitis suppurativa, and polycystic ovarian disease, either singly or in combined therapy with estrogens.

For men, cyproterone acetate has been used singly without estrogen for the treatment of prostatic cancer (100 mg/day) and to control the libido in severely hypersexual men or sexual deviates (600 mg/day).

Contraindications

This progestin is not FDA approved. The contraindications that have been described in the literature include history of liver disease, ovarian dysfunction, history of thrombophlebitic disorders, malignancy, pregnancy, infection, and allergy.

Adverse Effects

The adverse effects of cyproterone acetate are similar to those observed with oral contraceptives or other progestin therapy. Effects reported include weight gain, depression, fluid retention, decreased libido, and irregular menstrual bleeding. Other reported changes include thrombophlebitis and thromboembolic disorders if cyproterone acetate is given concomitantly with estrogens. In addition, an occasional drug eruption, such as a morbilliform eruption or photosensitivity, has been reported.

Warnings

Cyproterone acetate has reportedly produced tumors in rats. In addition, mammary hyperplasia has been observed in dogs and monkeys and in human males. Cyproterone acetate has prevented virilization of the male fetus when given during embryogenesis, when external genitalia are undifferentiated.

Therapeutic Guidelines

Cyproterone acetate is used in androgen disorders singly or in combined therapy with estrogens. For women of reproductive age, it is combined with estrogen and is administered cyclically: for example, 25–100 mg of cyproterone acetate for 10 days (days 5–14 of the menstrual cycle) along with an estrogen equivalent of 35–50 mg/day of ethylene estradiol for 21 days (days 5–25 of the menstrual cycle), followed by a 7-day drug-free interval. This cycle is somewhat similar to commonly used oral contraceptive regimens.[55]

Cyproterone acetate is available in fixed combination oral contraceptives outside the U.S. as Diane-35, Diane-50, and a variety of other trade names.[58, 60]

In postmenopausal women who do not require birth control, cyproterone acetate may be given alone, continuously or cyclically (10 days/month), in dosages of 50–100 mg/day, or in combined cyclic therapy that is similar to the treatment of women of reproductive age.

LESS FREQUENTLY USED ANTIANDROGENS

Cimetidine (Tagamet) has androgen receptor–blocking activity and may have some efficacy in treating androgen excess disorders such as hirsutism. Clinically, it appears to be less effective than spironolactone but has fewer adverse effects. The preferred dosage is 800–1600 mg/day. Cimetidine is discussed in Chapter 12.

Dexamethasone is a corticosteroid with potent adrenalsteroid–suppressive properties and some ovarian suppressive properties. It suppresses the adrenal androgen secretion and appears to compete with androgencytosol receptors on the hair follicles or the sebaceous lobules. Because of the potential risks associated with adrenal suppression, dexamethasone is titrated to partial rather than total adrenal suppression. It is best given at bedtime so that the maximal suppression is in the early morning when ACTH secretion is the greatest. The recommended therapy is 0.125–0.25 mg each night for 1–2 years.[61] Monitoring of adrenal and ovarian androgen production is suggested. Dexamethasone is discussed in Chapter 4.

Leuprolid acetate (Lupron) is an analog of gonadotropin-releasing hormone and effectively lowers ovarian androgen secretion. The drug is particularly useful in postpartum women who are not candidates for oral contraceptives. The recommended dosage is 1–2 mg given as a subcutaneous injection daily. A 1-mg dose reduces ovarian function by half; the 2-mg dose reduces ovarian functions to prepubertal levels. Lupron is infrequently prescribed because it is given by injection and is very expensive and because clinical experience with it is limited.[62]

Ketoconazole, an antifungal agent, has been demonstrated to suppress adrenal androgen production and therefore acts as an antiandrogen. Clinically, it has proved to be ineffective for dermatoses associated with androgen excess. Ketoconazole is discussed in Chapter 2.

SUMMARY

The antiandrogens discussed in this chapter (spironolactone, the combined estrogen and progestin therapies, and cyproterone acetate) represent steroid molecules with estrogenic, antigonadotropic, and variable glucocorticoid activities. They all reduce the production or the secretion of endogenous androgens and compete at the target organ for the androgen cytosol receptor.

Laboratory testing suggests that these antiandrogens variably reduce testosterone, androstenedione, and DHEA-S. Alterations of gonadotropin hormones vary with type of antiandrogen and dosage. Sex hormone binding globulin is also increased. Glucocorticoid activity is variable and dependent specifically on the antiandrogen and target organ response.

The major adverse reactions appear to be secondary to androgen suppression and the antiandrogen-related influence of estrogen on susceptible tissue. Because spironolactone is a mineralocorticoid antagonist, it also has diuretic properties and may induce electrolyte imbalance.

Spironolactone, the estrogen therapies, and cyproterone acetate have been effective as antiandrogen therapeutic modalities in selected clinical settings.

The International Society for Androgen Disorders, formed in 1989, recommended that suspected androgen excess disorders have minimal laboratory screening tests that include determination of DHEA-S, free testosterone, and androstenedione levels. The Society further recommended that the preferred antiandrogen therapy is spironolactone in doses of 100 mg or greater and suggested that it be used selectively in combination with low-dose dexamethasone or estrogen therapy, or both, for the most beneficial therapeutic results. It was agreed that it was unnecessary to treat specific endocrine organ dysfunction (e.g., dexamethasone for elevated DHEA-S levels; oral contraceptives for elevated testosterone levels) inasmuch as these therapeutic agents appear to be effective at all sites.

The recommended duration of therapy is 1–2 years; the dosage may be changed, depending on therapeutic results. Combining several of these antiandrogens appeared clinically to be most beneficial. After 2 years of therapy, the therapy should be titrated to the lowest dosage possible to maintain therapeutic results.

BIBLIOGRAPHY: Key Reviews/Chapters

Namer M: Clinical applications of antiandrogens. J Steroid Biochem 1988; 31(4b):719–729.
Skluth HA, Cums JC: Spironolactone: A re-examination. Drug Intell Clin Pharm 1990; 24:52–59.
DeLia JE, Emery MG: Clinical pharmacology and common minor side effects of oral contraceptives. Clin Obstet Gynecol 1981; 24:879–892.
Hammerstein J: Antiandrogens. In Orfanos CE, Happle R (eds): Hair and Nail Disease. New York: Springer-Verlag, 1990, 827–886.
Neumann F, Topert M: Antiandrogens and hair growth: Basic concepts and experimental research. In Orfanos CE, Happle R (eds): Hair and Nail Disease. New York: Springer-Verlag, 1990, 791–821.

REFERENCES

1. Barth JH: Alopecia and hirsutes: Current concepts in pathogenesis and management. Drugs 1988;35:83–91.
2. Biffigmandi P, Molinatte GM: Antiandrogen and hirsutism. Horm Res 1987; 28:242–249.
3. Futterweit U, Dumaif A, Yeh HC, Kingsley P: The prevalence of hyperandrogenism in 109 consecutive female patients with diffuse alopecia. J Am Acad Dermatol 1988; 19:831–836.
4. Hammerstein J, Moltz L. Schwartz U: Antiandrogens in the treatment of acne and hirsutism. J Steroid Biochem 1983; 19(1b):591–597.
5. Helde BL, Nader S, Rodriguez-Riqua LJ: Acne and hyperandrogenism. J Am Acad Dermatol 1984; 10:223–226.
6. Kasick JM, Bergfeld WF, Steck MD, et al: Adrenal androgenic female alopecia: Sex hormones and the balding woman. Cleve Clin Q 1983; 50:111–122.
7. Kvedar JC, Gibson M, Krusenski PA: Hirsutism: Evaluation and treatment. J. Am Acad Dermatol 1985; 12:215–225.
8. Marynick SP, Chakmakjian ZH, McCaffree D, Herndon JH: Androgen excess in cystic acne. N Engl J Med 1988; 308:981–986.
9. Morris SV: Hirsutism. Clin Obstet Gynecol 1985; 12:649–674.
10. Lucky A: Topical antiandrogens. Arch Dermatol 1985; 121:55–62.
11. Mowszowicz I, Riahi W, Wright F, et al: Androgen receptor in human skin cytosol. J Clin Endocrinol Metab 1981; 52:338–344.
12. Neuman F: Action of antiandrogens on accessory sexual glands. In Neuman F, Steinbeck H, Henken AD, et al (eds): Handbook of Experimental Pharmacology (Vol 35, No 2). New York: Springer, 1974, 485–542.
13. Price VH: Testosterone metabolism in the skin: A review of its function in androgenetic alopecia, acne vulgaris, and idiopathic hirsutism including recent studies with antiandrogens. Arch Dermatol 1975; 111:1496–1502.
14. Redmond GP, Gupta M, Milesell J, Bergfeld WF: Endocrine findings in women with alopecia [abstract]. Baltimore: The Endocrine Society, 67th annual meeting, June 1985, 430.
15. Rook A, Dawber R: Endocrine metabolic and chemical influences on the follicular cycle. In Rook A, Dawber R (eds): Disease of the Hair and Scalp. Oxford: Blackwell, 1982, 115–145.
16. Sawaya ME, Honig LS, Hsia SL: Increased androgen binding capacity in sebaceous glands in scalp of male pattern baldness. J Invest Dermatol 1989; 92:91–95.
17. Kay CR: Oral contraceptives—The clinical perspective. In Garaltine S, Berendes HW (eds): Pharmacology of Steroid Contraceptive Drugs. New York: Raven Press, 1977, 1–24.
18. Redmond GP, Bergfeld WF: Treatment of androgenic disorders in women: Acne, hirsutism and alopecia. Cleve Clin J Med 1990; 57:428–432.
19. Ryan KJ: Postmenopausal estrogen use. Annu Rev Med 1982; 33:171–181.
20. Reed MJ, Franks S: Antiandrogens in gynaecological practice. Baillieres Clin Obstet Gynaecol 1988; 2:581–595.
21. Karim A: Spironolactone: Disposition, metabolism, pharmacodynamics and bioavailability. Drug Metab Rev 1978; 8:151–188.
22. Steelman SL, Brooks JR, Morgan ER, Patanelli DJ: Antiandrogenic activity of spironolactone steroids. Steroids 1969; 14:449–450.
23. Vellacott ID, O'Brien PM: Effect of spironolactone on premenstrual syndrome symptoms. J Reprod Med 1987; 32:429–434.
24. Berardesca E, Gabba P, Ucci G, et al: Topical spironolactone inhibits dihydrotesterone

receptors in human sebaceous glands: An autoradiographic study in subjects with acne vulgaris. Int J Tissue React 1988; 10:115–119.
25. Serafini PC, Catalino J, Lobo RA: The effect of spironolactone on genital skin 5-alpha reductase activity. J Steroid Biochem 1985; 23:191–194.
26. Young RL, Goldzieher JW, Elkind-Hirsch K: The endocrine effects of spironolactone used as an antiandrogen. Fertil Steril 1987; 48:223–228.
27. Anttila L, Ruutiainen K, Erkkola R: Spironolactone in the treatment of hirsutism. Ann Chir Gynaecol 1987; 202(Suppl):32–34.
28. Barch JH, Cherry CA, Wojnaroivska I, Dainber RP: Spironolactone is an effective and well tolerated systemic antiandrogen therapy for hirsute women. J Clin Endocrinol Metab 1989; 68:966–970.
29. Cumming AC, Yang JC, Rebar RW, Yen SSC: Treatment of hirsutism with spironolactone. JAMA 1982; 247:1295–1298.
30. Evans DJ, Burke CW: Spironolactone in the treatment of idiopathic hirsutism and in polycystic ovary syndrome. J R Soc Med 1986; 79:451–453.
31. Goodfellow A, Alaghband-Zadeh J, Carter G, et al: Oral spironolactone improves acne vulgaris and reduces sebum excretion. Br J Dermatol 1984; 111:209.
32. Helfer EL, Muller JL, Rose LL: Side effects of spironolactone therapy in the hirsute woman. J Clin Endocrinol Metab 1988; 66:208–211.
33. Koksal A, Pabuccu R, Akyure KC: Spironolactone in the treatment of hirsutism. Arch Gynecol 1987; 240:95–100.
34. Masahashi T, Chao Wu M, Ohsawa M, et al: Spironolactone therapy for hyperandrogenic anovulatory women—Clinical and endocrinological study. Acta Obstet Gynecol 1986; 38:95–101.
35. Muhleman WF, Cartes GD, Cream JJ, Wise P: Oral spironolactone: An effective treatment for acne vulgaris in women. Br J Dermatol 1986; 115:227–232.
36. Ober KP, Hennessy JF: Spironolactone therapy for hirsutism in a hyperandrogenic woman. Ann Intern Med 1978; 89:643–645.
37. Shapiro G, Evron S: A novel use of spironolactone: Treatment of hirsutism. J Clin Endocrinol Metab 1980; 51:429–432.
38. Evron S, Shapiro G, Dianam YZ: Induction of ovulation with spironolactone (Aldactone) in anovulatory oligomenorrheic and hyperandrogenic women. Fertil Steril 1981; 36:468–471.
39. Hughes BR, Cunliffe WJ: Tolerance of spironolactone. Br J Dermatol 1988; 118:687–691.
40. Lumb G, Newberne P, Rust JH, et al: Effects in animals of chronic administration of spironolactone—A review. J Environ Pathol Toxicol ONcol 1978; 1:641–660.
41. Barker DJN: The epidemiological evidence relating to spironolactone and malignant diseases in man. J Drug Dev 1987; 2(Suppl):22–25.
42. Givens JR, Andersen RN, Wiser WL: The effectiveness of two oral contraceptives in suppressing plasma androstenedione, testosterone, LH and FSH, and in stimulating plasma testosterone binding capacity in hirsute women. Am J Obstet Gynecol 1975; 129:333–339.
43. Palatsi R, Reinila M, Kivinen S: Pituitary function and DHEA-S in male acne and cortisol before and after oral contraceptive treatment in female acne. Acta Derm Venereol (Stockh) 1986; 66:225–230.
44. Darley CR, Moore JW, Bessei GM, et al: Low dose prednisolone or estrogen in the treatment of women with late onset and persistent acne vulgaris. Br J Dermatol 1983; 108:345–355.
45. Greenwood R, Brummett L. Burke B, Cunliffe WJ: Acne: Double blind clinical and laboratory trial of tetracycline, estrogen–cyproterone acetate, and combined treatment. Br Med J 1985; 291:1231–1235.
46. Ruutiainen K: The effect of an oral contraceptive containing ethinylestradiol and

desogestrel on hair growth and hormonal parameters of hirsute women. Int J Gynaecol Obstet 1986; 24:361–368.
47. Larsson-Cohn U, Fahraeus L, von-Schenck H, Wallentin L: Effects on the lipoprotein metabolism of an antiandrogen–estrogen oral contraceptive drug. Acta Obstet Gynecol Scand 1986; 65:125–128.
48. Stampler N: Postmenopausal estrogen use and heart disease. N Engl J Med 1987; 316:164–165.
49. Inman HW, Vessey MP, Weslerholm B, et al: Thromboembolic disease and the steroidal content of oral contraceptives: A report to the Committee on the Safety of Drugs. Br Med J 1970; 2:203–209.
50. Bergkvist L, Adami HO, Persson I, et al: The risk of breast cancer after estrogen and estrogen-progestin replacement. N Engl J Med 1989; 321:293–297.
51. Fox H: Endometrial carcinogenesis and its relation to estrogens. Pathol Res Pract 1984; 179:13–19.
52. Booher DI: Estrogen supplements in menopause. Cleve Clin J Med 1990; 57:154–160.
53. Hatcher RA, Guest F, Stewart GK, et al (eds): Contraceptive Technology (13th ed). New York: Irvington, 1986, 139–182.
54. Maschak CA, Loho RA, Dozono-Takano K, et al.: Comparison of pharmacodynamic properties of various estrogen formulations. Am J Obstet Gynecol 1982; 144:511–518.
55. Hammerstein J, Meckies J, Rossberg LI, et al: Use of cyproterone acetate (CPA) in the treatment of acne, hirsutism and virilism. J Steroid Biochem 1975; 6:827–836.
56. Hague WM, Munro DS, Sanders RS, et al: Long term effects of cyproterone acetate on the pituitary adrenal axis in adult women. Br J Obstet Gynaecol 1982; 89:981–984.
57. Jeffcoate WJ, Edwards CR, Rees LH, et al: Cyproterone acetate [letter]. Lancet 1976; 2:1140.
58. Vermeulen A, Rubers R: Effect of cyproterone acetate plus ethinyl estradiol in low dose on plasma androgens and lipids in mildly hirsute or acneic young women. Contraception 1988; 38:419–428.
59. Jones DB, Ibraham I, Edwards CR: Hair growth and androgen responses in hirsute women treated with continuous cyproterone acetate and cyclical ethinyl oestradiol. Acta Endocrinol 1987; 116:497–501.
60. Prelevic GM, Wurzburger MT, Balint-Perie L, Purigaca Z: Effects of low dose estrogen-antiandrogen combination (Diane 35) on clinical signs of androgenetic hormone profile and ovarian size in patients with polycystic ovary syndrome. Gynecol Endocrinol 1989; 3:269–280.
61. Redmond GP, Gidwani GP, Gupta MK, et al: Treatment of androgenic disorders with dexamethasone: Dose-response relationship for suppression of DHEA-S. J Am Acad Dermatol 1990; 22:91–93.
62. Willemsen WN, Franssen AM, Rolland R, Vemer NM: The effects of buserelin on the hormonal status in PCOD. Prog Clin Biol Res 1986; 225:377–389.

14 Vasoactive and Antiplatelet Drugs

Jonathan K. Wilkin, M.D.

PATHOPHYSIOLOGIC BACKGROUND INFORMATION

Many cutaneous vascular disorders share the common property of a reduced microvascular perfusion. The strategies that physicians use to improve cutaneous blood flow are based on the physiologic properties of the cutaneous circulation.[1] Poiseuille's law describes the effects of changes in the vessel radius and the viscosity of the blood on blood flow. Of importance is that blood flow increases as the fourth power of the radius. This means that even small increases in the luminal diameter are accompanied by much greater increases in blood flow. Thus drugs that promote vasodilatation, such as ketanserin, calcium channel blockers, and prazosin, have multiple uses in the treatment of disorders of the cutaneous vasculature. Vasodilators also enhance the viscoelastic properties of the vascular smooth muscle.[2] Thus even at concentrations at which no change in the luminal diameter is evident, there can be an increased response to endogenous vasodilator substances.

Rhythmic oscillatory cutaneous vasomotion,[3] only a newly recognized cutaneous physiologic phenomenon, may some day lend itself to pharmacologic manipulation. Spontaneous rhythmic arteriolar vasomotion is a ubiquitous physiologic phenomenon found in multiple tissues and multiple species. The most compelling adaptive advantage is implicit in Poiseuille's law: namely, the resistance of a vessel with a constant diameter is notably greater than that of a vessel with a diameter that changes sinusoidally but has the same average diameter. The significance of these rhythmic patterns may also lie in the spatial and temporal synchronization of the cells, metabolic energy saving, and the steady preparedness of the vessels to adapt to changing circulatory requirements. It is likely that drugs that affect the peripheral vasculature have profound effects on this peripheral vasomotion cycle with resulting alterations in cutaneous perfusion.

Furthermore, Poiseuille's law states that flow is inversely proportional to the viscosity of the blood. The reciprocal of viscosity is fluidity, the measure of the ease with which a liquid flows. Multiple factors are responsible for the viscosity of whole blood. Platelet aggregation, fibrin deposition, clotting, increased hematocrit, leaky microvessels, and reduced erythrocyte flexibility are important components.[4] Pentoxifylline can enhance fluidity (and reduce viscosity) by improving erythrocyte flexibility. Aspirin and dipyridamole inhibit platelet aggregation. Phenformin and ethylestrenol promote fibrinolysis.

Fibrinolytic therapy is important in the treatment of a variety of cutaneous vascular disorders. The interrelations between platelets and fibrinolysis are complex.[5] Platelet adhesion is mediated by a number of platelet surface receptors with high affinity for the adhesive glycoproteins found on damaged vascular surfaces. These cytoadhesins include the platelet- and megakaryocyte-specific glycoprotein II_b/III_a complex (GP II_b/III_a) receptor. Platelet aggregation is mediated exclusively by platelet GP II_b/III_a receptor. Normal platelets have an extremely large number of GP II_b/III_a receptors; this characteristic gives normal platelets the greatest density of receptors known for adhesion and aggregation of any cell.[5]

Strategies for developing antiplatelet agents have focused on the platelet-activation mechanisms leading to platelet aggregation.[5] Aspirin inhibits the enzyme cyclooxygenase. The drawback with aspirin is that it also reduces the platelet inhibitor prostacyclin. Several agents inhibit thromboxane synthase. The drawback with thromboxane synthase inhibitors is that the block is incomplete. Thus newer agents are being developed to block the receptor that mediates the effects of both thromboxane A_2 and its endoperoxide precursor on the exposure of the GP II_b/III_a receptors. Ticlopidine, a drug currently under study, appears to inhibit the exposure of GP II_b/III_a by an unknown mechanism.[6] It requires several days of therapy to achieve maximal effects. Also, endothelium-derived relaxing factor, identified as nitric oxide[7] and nitrosothiol,[8] is a potent platelet inhibitor. Organic nitrates such as nitroglycerin and nitroprusside probably inhibit platelet aggregation by similar mechanisms.

Tissue plasminogen activator is a naturally occurring protein that catalyzes the conversion of plasminogen into plasmin.[9] Tissue plasminogen activator is synthesized by endothelial cells. In healthy states, circulating blood contains very low concentrations of tissue plasminogen activator. However, its concentrations can be considerably elevated, with a corresponding increase in fibrinolytic activity, by various stimuli, including nicotinic acid.[10]

The basic and clinical pharmacology of these various phenomena of the human cutaneous vasculature are being actively and intensively pursued in many laboratories. In the following discussion, I focus on those agents for which there is sufficient evidence that an important clinical benefit can be achieved.

PENTOXIFYLLINE

Pentoxifylline is a triple-substituted methylxanthine derivative 1-(5-oxohexyl)-3, 7-dimethylxanthine. Early studies with dogs demonstrated an increased cardiac output and decreased peripheral resistance without changes in blood pressure. Furthermore, the lack of interaction between pentoxifylline and beta-blockers or reserpine indicated that the effect of pentoxifylline is not mediated by catecholamines. Patients with ischemic limbs or intermittent claudication subsequently demonstrated an increase in muscle blood flow that was originally thought to be due to vasodilatation. It was not until 1973, a year after the drug had been released for intermittent claudication in Europe, that it was shown that pentoxifylline actually causes increased flexibility of erythrocytes in patients with intermittent claudication.[4]

Pharmacology

After oral dosages, absorption is rapid, and peak plasma levels occur within 2 hours and last 4–8 hours. Initial demethylation and reduction occur in the erythrocyte membrane. Further oxidation occurs in the liver, producing multiple metabolites that are excreted in urine.[4]

The principal clinical effect of pentoxifylline is to improve erythrocyte flexibility in those patients who have a decreased erythrocyte flexibility. Pentoxifylline also increases the mobility of polymorphonuclear cells by increasing their flexibility. Pentoxifylline decreases the tendency toward platelet activation in patients with a variety of vascular conditions. Pentoxifylline has no significant interaction with other drugs, although a weak synergism may occur with dipyridamole and calcium channel blockers.[4]

Clinical Use

The usual dosage of pentoxifylline (Trental) is 400 mg three times a day with meals.[11] Ely cautioned against patients' using aspirin or other nonsteroidal anti-inflammatory drugs while taking pentoxifylline because the effects may be inhibitory or superadditive.[4]

Pentoxifylline is approved for the treatment of patients with intermittent claudication on the basis of chronic occlusive arterial disease of the limbs.[11] Pentoxifylline should not be used by patients who have previously exhibited intolerance to methylxanthines such as caffeine, theophylline, and theobromine. A reduction in dosage should be considered for patients with renal compromise. Side effects are relatively uncommon and include nausea, dyspepsia, dizziness, headache, and belching, flatus, or bloating.

Although monotherapy with pentoxifylline was reported to have been successful in treating Raynaud's phenomenon,[12] Ely recommended combining pentoxifylline with a calcium channel blocker.[4] In his 9 patients with Raynaud's phenomenon, 5 had scleroderma. One woman had complete healing of her finger tip ulcers with combined nifedipine-pentoxifylline therapy after nifedipine alone was ineffective.

Five patients with various stages of atrophie blanche had improvement after beginning pentoxifylline therapy.[13] Therapy was initiated at 400 mg two or three times a day. One patient had nausea with three-times-a-day doses but he could tolerate two doses a day. Maintenance therapy consists of 400 mg/day. Clinical improvement in atrophie blanche with pentoxifylline was observed in 8 patients by Sams.[14] Interestingly, 3 of the 8 patients had previously developed new ulcers while taking aspirin-dipyridamole combination therapy. In another study, 2 patients with atrophie blanche responded favorably to therapy with pentoxifylline.[15]

A patient with a 15-year history of necrobiosis lipoidica diabeticorum had dramatic and persistent improvement during pentoxifylline therapy.[16] Initially, the patient received 400 mg three times a day. Several months later, after the lesions had improved substantially, she received maintenance dosages of 400 mg twice a day.

A potential use for pentoxifylline is the enhancement of skin-flap survival. Skin-flaps in rats[17] and in swine[18] demonstrate an enhanced survival when treated with 20 mg/kg/day of pentoxifylline for 10 days preoperatively (in addition to 10 days postoperatively for swine). The result was similar with the enhanced survival retained in a rat skin-flap model in which the pentoxifylline was given parenterally at different times with respect to date of surgery.[19] All groups showed a statistically significant increase in flap survival in comparison with control subjects.

CALCIUM CHANNEL BLOCKERS

Following the clue that verapamil possessed pharmacologic effects unique among the vasodilator agents, Fleckenstein and associates subsequently related the mechanism of action to inhibition of the movement of calcium ions into cells with resultant inhibition of excitation-contraction coupling.[20] Fleckenstein and associates called these agents *calcium antagonists*. Because these agents really do not directly antagonize the effects of calcium but instead inhibit the entry of calcium into cells for its mobilization from intracellular stores, they have been renamed *calcium channel blockers*.[20]

Pharmacology

The three most widely used calcium channel blockers are verapamil (Calan, Isoptin), a substituted benzeneacetonitrile; nifedipine (Adalat, Procardia), a substituted dihydropyridine; and diltiazem (Cardizem), a substituted benzothiazepine. All three agents are optically active, and the levo-isomers are up to 10 times more potent than the dextro-isomers as blockers of calcium channels. Absorption, distribution, metabolism, and excretion rates of these three drugs are presented in Table 14-1.[20-23]

Although all three drugs inhibit the slow calcium channel, nifedipine has no effect on the fast calcium channel, whereas diltiazem has modest inhibitory properties, and verapamil is intermediate between diltiazem and nifedipine. Verapamil typically provokes little change in the heart rate, whereas diltiazem lowers and nifedipine increases the pulse.[21] Verapamil is a strong depressor of atrioventricular conduction and diltiazem only slightly less so, whereas nifedipine has little effect on atrioventricular conduction.

Clinical Use

Verapamil is an agent of choice in supraventricular tachyarrhythmias, whereas nifedipine is not used as an antiarrhythmic drug.[22] In fact, nifedipine has been regarded as the preferred calcium channel blocker because it has fewer deleterious effects on myocardial contractility or on the specialized conduction systems than does verapamil or diltiazem.[22] The principal action of nifedipine is vasodilatation, and this is the basis

Table 14-1. Clinical Pharmacology of Calcium Channel Blockers[20-23]

Characteristics	*Nifedipine*	*Verapamil*	*Diltiazem*
Absorption	>90%	>90%	>90%
Bioavailability	50%–70%	10%–20%	20%–40%
Onset of action	<20 minutes	½–2 hours	15–30 minutes
Peak effect	1–2 hours	5 hours	30 minutes
Protein binding	90%	90%	80%
Metabolism	Extensive metabolism to inactive compounds	85% first-pass hepatic elimination	Extensive deacetylation
Excretion			
Renal	70%–80%	50%–75%	35%
Fecal	15%	15%	60%–65%
Plasma half-life	4 hours	3–7 hours	4 hours

Note: After oral administration.

for its use in peripheral vascular disorders. Because of side effects due to cardiac conduction disturbances associated with verapamil and diltiazem, nifedipine is the calcium channel blocker of choice for cutaneous vascular disorders. Should adverse effects prohibit the use of nifedipine, diltiazem is a reasonable alternative.

Nifedipine is indicated for the treatment of vasospastic angina and chronic stable angina.[23] The only contraindication is a known hypersensitivity reaction to nifedipine.

Adverse effects are frequent with nifedipine, but they are generally not serious and infrequently require discontinuation of therapy or dosage adjustment.[20-23] Most are expected consequences of the vasodilator effect. Dizziness, lightheadedness, nausea, headache, flushing, and weakness are the most common. In most patients the hypotensive effect of nifedipine is modest and well tolerated. However, occasional patients have had excessive and poorly tolerated postural hypotension. These responses usually occur during initial dosages, during dosage increases, or during concomitant beta-blocker therapy.[24]

Although concomitant use with beta-adrenergic blocking agents is usually well tolerated, there are reports suggesting that the combination may enhance the likelihood of congestive heart failure, severe hypotension, or exacerbation of angina.[24] Administration of nifedipine to patients taking digoxin leads to an increase in digoxin levels.[24] Thus it is recommended that digoxin levels be monitored when nifedipine is initiated, adjusted, and discontinued, in order to avoid possible over- or underdigitalization. Concomitant cimetidine therapy can lead to an increase in nifedipine plasma levels, and there are rare reports of increased prothrombin times when nifedipine was administered to patients taking coumarin anticoagulants.

Not only is nifedipine a slow calcium channel antagonist, it also increases red blood cell deformability, and at least in vitro, nifedipine and prostacyclin are synergistic in platelet antiaggregation activity.[25]

Nifedipine is available in 10- and 20-mg capsules. Therapy should be initiated with the 10-mg capsule, starting with one 10-mg capsule three times a day. The usual effective dosage range for many cutaneous vascular disorders is 10–20 mg three times a day, although 60–80 mg may be required to treat severe secondary Raynaud's phenomenon. Nifedipine is effective in the treatment of primary Raynaud's phenomenon (Raynaud's disease) and of secondary Raynaud's phenomenon. Nifedipine is effective in treating 70 per cent of patients with severe, recalcitrant, chronic idiopathic perniosis (chilblains).[26]

Nifedipine therapy has accompanied healing of an ischemic ulcer in a patient with scleroderma,[27] although there was no improvement in the progressive systemic scleroderma during nifedipine therapy. The patient then began taking nifedipine at a dosage of 10 mg three times a day. This was slowly increased over a period of 7 days to 40 mg three times a day.

The only side effect was postural hypotension. Within 2 weeks the foot became pinker in color and warm to touch. During the next month, the ulcer filled with granulation tissue and re-epithelialized all but one quarter of its original surface. When the patient was discharged, the nifedipine was reduced to 10 mg three times a day in order to avoid orthostatic hypotension. This case report encourages a therapeutic trial of nifedipine in the therapy of refractory ulcers.

Nifedipine has, as mentioned earlier, also been used successfully in the treatment of Raynaud's phenomenon.[28] Fifteen patients with Raynaud's phenomenon received either nifedipine or placebo in a double-blind crossover trial. Nine patients had systemic sclerosis, 1 had systemic lupus erythematosus with cryoglobulinemia, and 5 had Raynaud's phenomenon without demonstrable systemic disease. The initial dosage of nifedipine was 10 mg three times a day for 3 days, and if no severe side effects developed, the dosage was increased to 20 mg three times a day for the remainder of the treatment period. The patients gave a higher subjective evaluation of therapeutic efficacy while receiving nifedipine than while receiving placebo, which was statistically significant. The mean attack rate of Raynaud's phenomenon also fell significantly during treatment with nifedipine. Responses to cold exposure were attenuated when the patients were taking nifedipine. The most common side effect was mild transient headache, which occurred in 80% of the patients receiving nifedipine and in 20% of those receiving placebo. Lightheadedness occurred in 33% of the patients during treatment with nifedipine and in 7% during treatment with placebo.

Similar results were found in a randomized double-blind crossover study of nifedipine versus placebo in 17 patients with moderate to severe Raynaud's phenomenon.[29] The Raynaud's phenomenon was secondary to systemic sclerosis in 11 patients and to systemic lupus erythematosus in 1. In 5 patients, the Raynaud's phenomenon was idiopathic. In this study, 10 mg of nifedipine was given four times a day for 2 weeks. Nifedipine significantly reduced the frequency of the attacks and also the severity of attacks. The patients also had challenges consisting of immersing a hand in ice water for 20 seconds. Skin temperature recovery time was not affected by treatment with nifedipine.

Nifedipine taken in dosages of 10 mg three times a day on a long-term basis was accompanied by significant improvement in 1 patient with idiopathic atrophie blanche.[30]

Relief from the pain of the contracting smooth muscle was achieved in three studies with nifedipine in patients with cutaneous leiomyomas.[31–33] Each of these three reports was of a single case. All three patients obtained relief from the painful burning sensations of cutaneous leiomyomas with the use of nifedipine. Different dosage schedules were used, and as little as 20 mg/day provided long-lasting relief.[31] For 1 patient the dosage was increased from 10 mg three times a day to 10 mg four times a day during cold weather.[32]

ASPIRIN AND DIPYRIDAMOLE

Dipyridamole is the name given to 2,2',2'',2''' − [(4,8-dipiperidinopyrimido-[5,4-d]-pyrimidine-2,6 − diyl)dinitrilo]tetraethynol.[34, 35] Although used predominantly for the prophylaxis of angina pectoris, there is no convincing evidence that either acute or chronic administration decreases the frequency or severity of angina. In combination with warfarin, dipyridamole inhibits embolization from prosthetic heart valves. Of importance is that in combination with aspirin, it prolongs the survival of platelets in the presence of thrombotic diseases. Dipyridamole by itself has little or no effect.[35] However, in combination with aspirin, a reduction in platelet aggregation can be achieved.

Pharmacology

Dipyridamole is a platelet adhesion inhibitor, although the mechanism of action has not been fully elucidated.[35] The mechanism may relate to inhibition of red blood cell uptake of adenosine, itself an inhibitor of platelet reactivity, inhibition of platelet phosphodiesterase activity, and inhibition of thromboxane A_2 formation.

The average time to peak concentration after an oral dose of dipyridamole is about 75 minutes. The beta half-life is approximately 10 hours. Dipyridamole is highly bound to plasma proteins and is metabolized in the liver, where it is conjugated as a glucuronide and excreted with the bile.

Aspirin (acetylsalicylic acid) inhibits activation and aggregation of platelets by acetylating the enzymes of the platelets that synthesize the precursor of prostaglandins and thromboxane A_2.[36] Although aspirin is cleared from the body within hours, its effect on platelets is irreversible and lasts for the life of the platelet (about 8–11 days).[7] At higher dosages, aspirin also inhibits the synthesis of prostacyclin, a natural inhibitor of platelets, which is produced in the vessel wall. Because this reduces its effectiveness as an antithrombotic agent, some workers have suggested that the aspirin should be given less frequently than daily or at very low dosages, or both.[7]

There is some concern that the use of even low dosages of aspirin could have deleterious effects during treatment of cutaneous disease. Aspirin taken in dosages of 40 mg/day leads to a significant reduction in blood flow in the central lesional skin in patients with necrobiosis lipoidica.[37]

Clinical Use

The usual dosage of dipyridamole (Persantine) is one 50-mg tablet three times a day, taken at least 1 hour before meals. Aspirin at low dosages, such as 162 mg/day, is used in combination. A third antiplatelet drug, ticlopidine hydrochloride, can be added at 200 mg/day.[38] Ticlopidine is currently not marketed in the U.S.

At the doses used clinically, dipyridamole is usually free from side effects. Headache, vertigo, nausea, vomiting, and diarrhea occur occasionally. Although the adverse reactions at therapeutic dosages are typically minimal and transient, excessive doses can cause peripheral vasodilatation and hypotension.

Dipyridamole is indicated as an adjunct to coumarin anticoagulants in the prevention of postoperative thromboembolic complications of cardiac valve replacement.[35] There are no contraindications. Important drug interactions have not been reported, and bleeding is no greater in frequency or severity when dipyridamole is used with warfarin than when warfarin is administered alone.[39]

Atrophie blanche in 2 patients has been effectively treated with a combination of aspirin and dipyridamole.[40] Kern emphasized that a single aspirin tablet (325 mg) induces such a significant inhibition of cyclo-oxygenase activity that production of the potent antithrombotic prostacyclin is also inhibited. Thus in 1 patient, healing was not permanent until the dosage of aspirin was reduced to half a tablet (162 mg) daily. Aspirin was given in addition to the three-times-a-day, 50-mg dosage of dipyridamole.

Two additional patients with atrophie blanche received dipyridamole and aspirin with or without ticlopidine.[38] The 1st patient received 200 mg/day of ticlopidine and 225 mg/day of dipyridamole, and on the 7th day of treatment, aspirin (82 mg/day) was added to the regimen. The lesions improved dramatically. The 2nd patient received only aspirin (82 mg/day) and dipyridamole (150 mg/day). Improvement was both rapid and dramatic, although disease activity tended to reoccur when oral dosages of the drugs were lowered.

Seven patients with atrophie blanche (livedoid vasculitis) had the clinical improvement after treatment with dipyridamole and aspirin.[41] All 7 patients had abnormal platelet functions in vitro, and after treatment with dipyridamole and aspirin, all showed a return to normal platelet function. There was a significant alleviation of pain and a decrease in new lesion formation. Despite enhanced healing of lesions, recovery was incomplete. Platelet function studies were repeated after 3 weeks of treatment. All patients were treated with 325 mg of aspirin three times a day and with 75 mg of dipyridamole four times a day.

One patient had a dramatic healing of necrobiosis lipoidica within 6 weeks of starting aspirin (1 g/day) and dipyridamole (225 mg/day).[42]

However, according to a randomized double-blind comparison of aspirin-dipyridamole combination treatment with placebo treatment of 14 patients with necrobiosis lipoidica, the combination therapy did nothing.[43]

A patient with malignant atrophic papulosis (Degos's disease) achieved a clinical remission that persisted 4 months after cessation of aspirin (500 mg three times a day) and dipyridamole (50 mg three times a day).[44] In addition, the increased aggregation of platelets returned to normal during therapy.

PHENFORMIN AND ETHYLESTRENOL

In 1968 Cunliffe found an association between cutaneous vasculitis and decreased blood-fibrinolytic activity in 3 patients.[45] They had persistently reduced fibrinolytic activity that was revealed by a prolonged euglobulin lysis time, which in 2 patients returned to normal as the vasculitis spontaneously resolved. It was subsequently shown that 32 of 52 patients with vasculitis had low plasma fibrinolytic activity and that of 10 of these patients who were given a regimen of phenformin hydrochloride and ethylestrenol, 9 showed improvement.[46] Fearnley and Chakrabarti were the first to observe that these two drugs enhanced endogenous blood-fibrinolytic activity.[47] The exact mechanism of the drugs' action is unknown. It is likely that both agents potentiate the action or enhance the synthesis of plasminogen activators normally present in the plasma or in the tissue, or in both. This leads to the conversion of plasminogen to plasmin.[48,49] The action of plasmin on fibrin then results in fibrinolysis. Of importance is that either ethylestrenol or phenformin alone exerts only a transient fibrinolytic effect. It is only in combination that the persistence of fibrinolysis can be assured.[49]

The usual regimen is 50 mg of phenformin hydrochloride twice a day and 2 mg of ethylestrenol two to four times a day. The ethylestrenol dosage of 8 mg/day uniformly produces amenorrhea in women. Because ethylestrenol is an anabolic steroid with androgenic properties, it can produce fluid retention, signs of masculinization, cholestasis, obesity, and acne. Lactic acidosis is a reported side effect of phenformin, and nausea can occur with either drug. Ryan pointed out that 5 mg of stanozolol twice a day is a less potent androgen than is ethylestrenol, but it is equally effective in combination with the phenformin.[50]

Clinical improvement in Raynaud's phenomenon secondary to scleroderma occurred in 14 patients receiving 5 mg of the anabolic steroid stanozolol (Winstrol) twice a day for 3 months. Stanozolol enhances natural blood fibrinolysis by reducing fibrinogen. Because clinical improvement can last 2–3 months after therapy, 3-month courses of stanozolol can be given intermittently with rest periods of 1–2 months.[51]

Not all forms of vasculitis have a reduced fibrinolytic activity, and

Ryan emphasized the distinction between infarctive and noninfarctive forms of vasculitis. Thus fibrinolytic therapy would be indicated in those vasculitides in which thrombosis and infarction are features. Some forms of vasculitis clearly have increased fibrinolysis, and treatment by antifibrinolytic agents is successful in these.[50]

Although conditions such as livedoid vasculitis can be successfully treated with a combination of phenformin and ethylestrenol, phenformin has been removed from the U.S. market, particularly because of its association with severe lactic acidosis.[52] The combination of phenformin and ethylestrenol is historically important in that these drugs convincingly demonstrated the effectiveness of fibrinolytic therapy for selected vasculitides. Even if phenformin were again marketed in the U.S., either pentoxifylline or a combination of dipyridamole and low-dosage aspirin are sufficiently successful in treating most patients to keep the phenformin and ethylestrenol on the shelf.

PRAZOSIN

Prazosin hydrochloride, 1-(4-amino-6, 7-dimethoxy-2-quinazolinyl)-4-(2-furanylcarbonyl) piperazine monohydrochloride, is a peripheral alpha-1-adrenergic antagonist derived from quinazoline.[53] Although it undergoes first-pass metabolism by the liver, there is a linear correlation between dosage and the steady-state concentration achieved in plasma. After it is orally administered, human plasma concentrations reach a peak in about 3 hours, and the plasma half-life is 2–3 hours. The drug is highly bound to plasma protein. Only a small amount of prazosin is found unchanged in the urine. Prazosin is extensively metabolized, primarily by demethylation and conjugation, and is excreted mainly through bile and feces. In patients with chronic renal failure or congestive heart failure, the unbound fraction of prazosin in plasma is increased and the half-life of prazosin is prolonged.[53]

The principal clinical effect is due to competitive blockade of the vascular postsynaptic alpha-1-adrenergic receptor.[53] The affinity of prazosin for alpha-1 receptors, in comparisoin with alpha-2 receptors, is very high. This selectivity allows prazosin to block the contractile response of vascular smooth muscle to norepinephrine without interfering with adrenergic activity at alpha-2 sites.

Prazosin is indicated in the treatment of hypertension.[54] There are no contraindications. Prazosin is available as Minipress in 1-, 2-, or 5-mg capsules. The usual or initial dose of prazosin is 1 mg two or three times a day, which can be increased when necessary. Benefits are marginal at dosages greater than 6–10 mg/day.[53]

Prazosin can cause a "first-dose phenomenon," characterized by hypotension with sudden loss of consciousness.[53] Although this typically occurs 30–90 minutes after the initial dose, it is recommended that the patient avoid driving or performing hazardous tasks for the first 24 hours after initially taking this medication or when the dosage is increased. Dizziness, lightheadedness, or fainting may occur, especially when the patient rises from a lying or sitting position. Patients taking prazosin should be careful about the amount of alcohol that they drink and during exercise or hot weather. Although there are no important drug interactions, false-positive results may occur in screening tests for pheochromocytoma in patients who are being treated with prazosin.

Prazosin can significantly increase basal skin blood flow 2 hours after its oral administration.[55] Furthermore, prazosin markedly reduces the skin vasoconstrictor response to deep inspiration and to contralateral hand cooling. Because it is apparent that postsynaptic alpha-1-adrenergic receptors are involved in maintaining skin vasoconstrictor tone when a person is at rest, prazosin is a suitable candidate for cutaneous vascular disorders in which a decreased cutaneous blood flow has a pathophysiologic role.[55]

Prazosin (Minipress) taken in dosages of 1 mg three times a day for 2 months was effective in treating 19 patients with Raynaud's phenomenon secondary to scleroderma.[56] The protocol was a modified double-blind crossover study in which the first treatment period lasted 8 weeks and the second treatment period lasted 4 weeks. Prazosin hydrochloride, taken in dosages of 1 mg three times a day, reduced both the frequency and the severity of the vasospasm, as assessed by the patients. It was well tolerated in general. One patient had a constant headache and was subsequently dropped from the study. Another patient experienced dizziness on the 3-mg/day dosage but received a 2-mg/day dosage without problems. Symptoms of mild postural hypotension were observed in 2 other patients.

KETANSERIN

Ketanserin, 3-{2-[4-(4-fluorobenzoyl)-1-piperidinyl]ethyl}-2,4(1H,3H) quinazolinedione, inhibits serotonin (5-hydroxytryptamine; 5-HT) induced contractions in blood vessels.[57] Ketanserin is a pure antagonist at the 5-HT$_2$ receptors, as opposed to other classes of 5-HT receptors. Although it is selective among the 5-HT receptors, it is nonspecific in that it also blocks alpha-1-adrenergic receptors, histamine H$_1$ receptors, and even dopamine receptors.[57] Not only does ketanserin antagonize the vasoconstrictor effects of 5-HT, but it also blocks the aggregating effect of 5-HT on platelets.[58] Ketanserin inhibits cold-induced vasoconstriction.[59] Ketanserin appears to inhibit sympathetic outflow from the central nervous system, and it has some alpha-1-blocking activity on human vasculature that is demonstrable at therapeutic concentrations.[57]

Although ketanserin has not been released for marketing in the U.S., there is already evidence that it will be useful for a variety of conditions in addition to hypertension. Ketanserin may be of value in chronic sympathetic dystrophy,[60] disorders of enhanced platelet aggregation,[58] acute superficial thrombophlebitis,[61] peripheral microvascular ischemic diseases,[62] progressive systemic sclerosis,[63] livedoid vasculitis,[64] and Raynaud's phenomenon.[65, 66]

Ketanserin taken in dosages of 20 mg three times a day for 10 months led to a clinical and subjective improvement of symptoms in 10 patients with progressive systemic sclerosis.[63] There was a decrease in the duration, frequency, and intensity of Raynaud's phenomenon, a reduction in acrocyanosis, and an almost complete recovery of finger ulcerations, except in 1 patient. In another study, ketanserin was used in a randomized double-blind trial by 15 patients with Raynaud's phenomenon secondary to systemic sclerosis.[67] Ketanserin was given in 20-mg dosages three times a day during the 1st month and in 40-mg dosages three times a day during the following 2 months. Of the 8 patients treated with the ketanserin, 5 showed improvement. One patient stopped taking ketanserin because of dizziness and anxiety. One patient reduced ketanserin intake back to 60 mg/day because of fluid retention. There were no other adverse effects. In the 7 control patients taking placebo, there was no improvement in Raynaud's phenomenon.

Twenty-eight patients suffering from either primary or secondary Raynaud's phenomenon were treated with nifedipine and ketanserin in a randomized double-blind crossover protocol.[66] Nifedipine was administered in a dosage of 10 mg three times a day, and ketanserin was administered in a dosage of 40 mg twice a day. Not only was ketanserin useful in the treatment of Raynaud's phenomenon, but its efficacy was greater than that of nifedipine.

Klimiuk and colleagues treated 11 patients with the CREST syndrome (calcinosis cutis, Raynaud's phenomenon, esophageal dysfunction, sclerodactyly, and telangiectasia) and digital ischemia with ketanserin as a bolus of 10 mg intravenously, followed by an infusion over 72 hours and then oral therapy (40 mg three times a day).[62] There was a marked clinical improvement with a reduction in the pain and with healing of digital ulceration, and these improvements were maintained with oral therapy. Interestingly, ketanserin failed to produce a greater improvement than did placebo in functional and objective clinical signs and symptoms in 24 patients with systemic sclerosis.[68] Thus ketanserin's effect on the vasculature is likely nonspecific with regard to a disease process, and these results produce doubt that serotonin is the major contributing factor in the pathophysiology of systemic sclerosis.

Finally, a patient with a 6-year history of recalcitrant, painful ulceration of both lower legs that was due to livedoid vasculitis had a rapid improvement with oral ketanserin.[64] The lesions not only healed rapidly but remained healed during therapy.

BIBLIOGRAPHY: Key Reviews/Chapters

Coller BS: Platelets and thrombolytic therapy. N Engl J Med 1990; 322:33–39.
Vane JR, Änggård EE, Botting RN: Mechanisms of disease: Regulatory functions of the vascular endothelium. N Engl J Med 1990; 323:27–36.
Wilkin JK: Introduction to diseases of the blood vessels. In Demis DJ, Dobson RL, McGuire JS (eds): Clinical Dermatology (7-0). Philadelphia: JB Lippincott, 1990, 1–8.
Braunwald E: Mechanism of action of calcium-channel–blocking agents. N Engl J Med 1982; 307:1618–1627.

REFERENCES

1. Wilkin JK: Introduction to diseases of the blood vessels. In Demis DJ, Dobson RL, McGuire JS (eds): Clinical Dermatology (7-0). Philadelphia: JB Lippincott, 1990, 1–8.
2. Somlyo AP, Somlyo AV: Vascular smooth muscle: I. Normal structure, pathology, biochemistry, and biophysics. Pharmacol Rev 1968; 20:197–272.
3. Wilkin JK: Poiseuille, periodicity and perfusion: Rhythmic oscillatory vasomotion in the skin. J Invest Dermatol 1989; 93:113S–118S.
4. Ely H: Pentoxifylline therapy in dermatology. Dermatol Clin 1988; 6:585–608.
5. Coller BS: Platelets and thrombolytic therapy. N Engl J Med 1990; 322:33–39.
6. DiMinno G, Cerboney AM, Mattioli PL, et al: Functionally thrombasthenic state in normal platelets following the administration of ticlopidine. J Clin Invest 1985; 75:328–338.
7. Vane JR, Änggård EE, Botting RN: Mechanisms of disease: Regulatory functions of the vascular endothelium. N Engl J Med 1990; 323:27–36.
8. Myers PR, Minor RL, Guerra R, et al: Vasorelaxant properties of the endothelium-derived relaxing factor more closely resemble S-nitrosocysteine than nitric oxide. Nature 1990; 345:161–163.
9. Loscalzo J, Braunwald E: Tissue plasminogen activator. N Engl J Med 1988; 319:925–931.
10. Collen D: On the regulation and control of fibrinolysis: Edward Kowalski Memorial Lecture. Thromb Haemost 1980; 43:77–89.
11. Pentoxifylline for intermittent claudication. Med Lett Drugs Ther 1984; 26(675):103–104.
12. Goldberg J: Successful treatment of Raynaud's phenomenon with pentoxifylline. Arthritis Rheum 1980; 29:1055–1056.
13. Sauer GC: Pentoxifylline (Trental) therapy for the vasculitis of atrophie blanche [letter]. Arch Dermatol 1986; 122:380–381.
14. Sams WM Jr: Livedo vasculitis. Arch Dermatol 1988; 124:684–687.
15. Ely H, Bard JW: Therapy of livedo vasculitis with pentoxifylline. Cutis 1988; 42:448–453.
16. Littler CM, Tschen EH: Pentoxifylline for necrobiosis lipoidica diabeticorum. J Am Acad Dermatol 1987; 17:314–316.
17. Monteiro DT, Santamore WP, Nemir P Jr: The influence of pentoxifylline on skin-flap survival. Plast Reconstr Surg 1986; 77:277–281.
18. Yessenow RS, Maves MD: The effects of pentoxifylline on random skin-flap survival. Arch Otolaryngol Head Neck Surg 1989; 115:179–181.

19. Roth AG, Briggs PC, Jones EW, et al: Augmentation of skin-flap survival by parenteral pentoxifylline. Br J Plast Surg 1988; 41:515–520.
20. Needleman P, Corr PB, Johnson EM Jr: Drugs used for the treatment of angina: Organic nitrates, calcium channel blockers and beta-adrenergic antagonists. In Gilman AG, Goodman LS, Rall TW, et al (eds): Goodman and Gilman's The Pharmacological Basis of Therapeutics (7th ed). New York: Macmillan, 1985, 816–822.
21. Covinsky JO, Hamburger SC: Slow channel blockers. South Med J 1983; 76:55–64.
22. Braunwald E: Mechanism of action of calcium-channel–blocking agents. N Engl J Med 1982; 307:1618–1627.
23. Stone PH, Antman EM, Muller JE, Braunwald E: Calcium channel blocking agents in the treatment of cardiovascular disorders. Part II: Hemodynamic effects and clinical applications. Ann Intern Med 1980; 93:886–904.
24. Procardia product information. In Physicians' Desk Reference (44th ed). Oradell, NJ: Medical Economics, 1990, 1671–1672.
25. Onoda JM, Sloan BF, Honn KV: Antithrombogenic effects of calcium channel blockers: Synergism with prostacyclin and thromboxane synthase inhibitors. Thromb Res 1984; 34:367–378.
26. Rustin MHA, Newton JA, Smith NP, Dowd PM: The treatment of chilblains with nifedipine: The results of a pilot study, a double-blind placebo-controlled randomized study and a long-term open trial. Br J Dermatol 1989; 120:267–275.
27. Woo TY, Wong RC, Campbell JP, et al: Nifedipine in scleroderma ulcerations. Int J Dermatol 1984; 23:678–680.
28. Rodeheffer RJ, Rommer JA, Wigley F, et al: Controlled double-blind trial of nifedipine in the treatment of Raynaud's phenomenon. N Engl J Med 1983; 308:880–883.
29. Smith CD, McKendry RJR: Controlled trial of nifedipine in the treatment of Raynaud's phenomenon. Lancet 1982; 2:1299–1301.
30. Purcell SM, Hayes TJ: Nifedipine treatment of idiopathic atrophie blanche. J Am Acad Dermatol 1986; 14:851–854.
31. Engelke H, Christophers E: Leiomyomatosis cutis et uteri. Acta Derm Venereol (Stockh) 1979; 59(Suppl 85):51–54.
32. Thompson JA Jr: Therapy for painful cutaneous leiomyomas. J Am Acad Dermatol 1985; 13:865–867.
33. Abraham Z, Cohen A, Haim S: Muscle relaxing agent in cutaneous leiomyoma. Dermatologica 1983; 166:255–256.
34. Needleman P, Corr PB, Johnson EM Jr: Drugs used for the treatment of angina: Organic nitrates, calcium channel-blockers, and beta-adrenergic antagonists. In Gilman AG, Goodman LS, Rall TW, et al (eds): Goodman and Gilman's The Pharmacological Basis of Therapeutics (7th ed). New York: Macmillan, 1985, 822.
35. O'Reilly RA: Anticoagulant, antithrombolytic, and thrombolytic drugs. In Gilman AG, Goodman LS, Rall TW, et al (eds): Goodman and Gilman's The Pharmacological Basis of Therapeutics (7th ed). New York: Macmillan, 1985, 1352.
36. Van Der Ouderaa FJ, Buytenhek M, Nugteren DH, Van Dorp DA: Acetylation of prostaglandin endoperoxide synthetase with acetylsalicylic acid. Eur J Biochem 1980; 109:1–8.
37. Beck HI, Bjerring P: Skin blood flow in necrobiosis lipoidica during treatment with low-dose acetylsalicylic acid. Acta Derm Venereol (Stockh) 1988; 68:364–365.
38. Yamamoto M, Danno K, Shio H, et al: Antithrombotic treatment in livedo vasculitis. J Am Acad Dermatol 1988; 18:57–62.
39. Persantine product information. In Physicians' Desk Reference (44th ed). Oradell, NJ: Medical Economics, 1990, 691.
40. Kern AB: Atrophie blanche: Report of two patients treated with aspirin and dipyridamole. J Am Acad Dermatol 1982; 6:1048–1053.
41. Drucker CR, Duncan WC: Anti-platelet therapy in atrophie blanche and livedo vasculitis. J Am Acad Dermatol 1982; 7:359–363.

362 Vasoactive and Antiplatelet Drugs

42. Eldor A, Diaz EG, Naparstek E: Treatment of diabetic necrobiosis with aspirin and dipyridamole [letter]. N Engl J Med 1978; 298:1033.
43. Statham B, Finlay AY, Marks R: A randomized double blind comparison of an aspirin dipyridamole combination versus a placebo in the treatment of necrobiosis lipoidica. Acta Derm Venereol (Stockh) 1981; 61:270–271.
44. Stahl D, Thomsen K, Hou-Jensen K: Malignant atrophic papulosis. Arch Dermatol 1978; 114:1687–1689.
45. Cunliffe WJ: An association between cutaneous vasculitis and decreased blood fibrinolytic activity. Lancet 1968; 1:1226–1228.
46. Cunliffe WJ, Menon S: The association between cutaneous vasculitis and decreased blood fibrinolytic activity. Br J Dermatol 1971; 84:99–105.
47. Fearnley GR, Chakrabarti R: Pharmacological enhancement of fibrinolytic activity of blood. J Clin Pathol 1964; 17:328–332.
48. Isaacson S, Nilsson IM: Effect of treatment with combined phenformin and ethylestrenol on the coagulation and fibrinolytic systems. Scand J Haematol 1970; 7:404–408.
49. Gilliam JN, Herndon JH, Prystowsky SD: Fibrinolytic therapy for vasculitis of atrophie blanche. Arch Dermatol 1974; 109:664–667.
50. Ryan TJ: Microvascular Injury: Vasculitis, Stasis, and Ischaemia. Philadelphia: WB Saunders, 1976, 388–390.
51. Jarrett PEM, Morland M, Browse NL: Treatment of Raynaud's phenomenon by fibrinolytic enhancement. Br Med J 1987; 2:523–525.
52. Larner J: Insulin and oral hypoglycemic drugs; glucagon. In Gilman AG, Goodman LS, Gilman A (eds): Goodman and Gilman's The Pharmacological Basis of Therapeutics (6th ed). New York: Macmillan, 1980, 1510–1511.
53. Rudd, P, Blaschke TF: Anti-hypertensive agents and the drug therapy of hypertension. In Gilman AG, Goodman LS, Rall TW, et al (eds): Goodman and Gilman's The Pharmacological Basis of Therapeutics (7th ed): New York: Macmillan, 1985:792–793.
54. Minipress product information. In Physicians' Desk Reference (44th ed). Oradell, NJ: Medical Economics, 1990, 1668–1669.
55. Chan F, Struthers AD, Stence VA: The effect of prazosin on skin microcirculation as assessed by laser Doppler flowmetry. Br J Clin Pharmacol 1988; 26:267–272.
56. Surwit RS, Gilgor RS, Allen LM, et al: A double-blind study of prazosin in the treatment of Raynaud's phenomenon in scleroderma. Arch Dermatol 1984; 120:329–331.
57. Douglas WW: Histamine and 5-hydroxytryptamine (serotonin) and their antagonists. In Gilman AG, Goodman LS, Rall TW, et al (eds): Goodman and Gilman's The Pharmacological Basis of Therapeutics (7th ed): New York: Macmillan, 1985, 633–634.
58. de Clerck F, David JL, Janssen PAJ: Inhibition of 5-hydroxytryptamine-induced and -amplified human platelet aggregation by ketanserin (R 41 468), a selective 5-HT2-receptor antagonist. Agents Actions 1982; 12:388–397.
59. Hechtman DH, Jageneau A: Inhibition of cold-induced vasoconstriction with ketanserin. Microvasc Res 1985; 30:56–62.
60. Bounameaux HM, Hellemans H, Verhaeghe R: Ketanserin in chronic sympathetic dystrophy: An acute controlled trial [letter]. Clin Rheumatol 1984; 3:556–557.
61. de Roose J, Symoens J: Ketanserin in acute superficial thrombophlebitis [letter]. Lancet 1982; 2:440–441.
62. Klimiuk PS, Kay EA, Mitchell WS, et al: Ketanserin: An effective regimen for digital ischaemia in systemic sclerosis. Scan J Rheumatol 1989; 18:107–111.
63. Altomare GF, Pigatto PD, Polenghi MM: Ketanserin in the treatment of progressive systemic sclerosis. Angiology 1988; 39:583–586.
64. Rustin MHA, Bunker CB, Dowd PM: Chronic leg ulceration with livedoid vasculitis, and response to oral ketanserin. Br J Dermatol 1989; 120:101–105.
65. Seibold JR, Jageneau HM: Treatment of Raynaud's phenomenon with ketanserin, a selective antagonist of the serotonin 2 (5-HT2) receptor. Arthritis Rheum 1984; 27:139–146.

66. Codella O, Caramaschi P, Olivieri O, et al: Controlled comparison of ketanserin and nifedipine in Raynaud's phenomenon. Angiology 1989; 40:114–121.
67. Lukáč J, Rovenský J, Tauchmannova H, et al: Effect of ketanserin on Raynaud's phenomenon in progressive systemic sclerosis: A double-blind trial. Drugs Exp Clin Res 1985; 11:659–663.
68. Ortonne JP, Torzuoli C, Dujardin P, et al: Ketanserin in the treatment of systemic sclerosis: A double-blind controlled trial. Br J Dermatol 1989; 120:261–266.

15 | New Uses for Old Drugs

Loretta Smrtnik Davis, M.D.

A number of systemic drugs used in dermatology have no dermatologic indications approved by the Food and Drug Administration (FDA). Many of these older drugs are being increasingly used for a wide variety of dermatologic conditions. This chapter represents a brief summary of nine unrelated drugs and their potential dermatologic indications. Primary emphasis is given to colchicine, gold, potassium iodide, and danazol. The chapter concludes with briefer discussions on nicotinamide, phenytoin, nonsteroidal anti-inflammatory drugs, potassium para-aminobenzoate, and 1,25-dihydroxycholecalciferol.

COLCHICINE

Colchicine is an alkaloid extracted from seeds and tubers of *Colchicum autumnale* (autumn crocus, meadow saffron). Since as far back as the 6th century A.D., *Colchicum* has been used for the treatment of acute gout. Not only is colchicine the most efficacious anti-inflammatory agent for gout, but it is the drug of choice for treatment of familial Mediterranean fever.[1,2] In addition, colchicine is developing a therapeutic niche in the treatment of dermatologic diseases characterized by polymorphonuclear leukocyte (PML) infiltration.[1]

Pharmacology

Colchicine has the formula $C_{22}H_{25}O_6N$. Although it was synthesized in 1965, commercial preparations are still derived from extracts of *Colchicum*.

Colchicine must be shielded from ultraviolet light exposure, which degrades it into therapeutically inactive products. Peak plasma levels are reached between 30 and 120 minutes after oral administration of the drug. The drug is metabolized in the liver; the majority is eliminated through bile in the feces. Ten percent to 20% of the dose is eliminated unchanged in the urine.[1]

Colchicine concentrates extremely well in leukocytes. It effectively binds to the dimers of tubulin, preventing the assembly of tubulin subunits into microtubules. Microtubular toxicity results in mitotic arrest at metaphase and interference with cell motility. Thus the drug is both antimitotic and anti-inflammatory. Specifically, colchicine has been shown to decrease PML motility, adhesiveness, and chemotaxis and to interfere with lysosomal degranulation. In addition to tubulin, colchicine binds to a number of other proteins. This protein binding may contribute to its ability in vitro to inhibit histamine release from mast cell granules, inhibit melanosome movements in the melanophore cells, and inhibit parathormone and insulin release.[1,2]

Clinical Use

Colchicine's value in the treatment of acute gouty arthritis and familial Mediterranean fever is well established. Because Behçet's disease shares features with familial Mediterranean fever, it followed that colchicine might be efficacious in the treatment of this disease as well. Several uncontrolled studies and case reports document improvement in oral, genital, and ocular lesions of Behçet's disease with some benefit in associated erythema nodosum and articular complaints.[2-4] However, not all reports are as encouraging; one double-blind study revealed no difference in most parameters measured.[5] The intensely neutrophilic inflammatory infiltrate and enhanced leukocyte chemotaxis of Behçet's disease are also seen in recurrent aphthous stomatitis, for which colchicine has also been noted to have therapeutic efficacy.[6,7]

Several researchers advocate the clinical efficacy of colchicine for treating chronic cutaneous leukocytoclastic vasculitis. Of the patients reported, a majority either achieved complete disease control or were able to taper their concurrent steroid dosage.[8-11] A beneficial effect on associated arthritis has also been observed.[8]

Logic dictates that colchicine, with its PML suppression and antimitotic activity, would be beneficial in treating psoriasis and palmarplantar pustulosis. In many patients, favorable results have been observed.[12-14] Colchicine may work best for thin psoriatic lesions and as maintenance therapy after remission is obtained through another modality.[12] Case reports suggest that colchicine may be useful in treating dermatitis herpetiformis[15] and Sweet's syndrome.[16]

Colchicine's suppression of local inflammation due to calcinosis in dermatomyositis and progressive systemic sclerosis has been reported.[17,18] Although colchicine was considered to be a possible therapy for the other cutaneous manifestations of progressive systemic sclerosis, prolonged colchicine therapy has not been shown to halt disease progression.[1] Anecdotal reports suggest that colchicine may be efficacious for a host of other diseases, including relapsing polychondritis,[19] pachydermoperiostosis with acro-osteolysis,[20] and mild to moderate type 2 lepra reactions.[21]

The colchicine dosage for dermatologic conditions is typically 0.6 mg two or three times a day; the dosage is subsequently tapered as disease activity allows. Therapeutic doses of colchicine alter both jejunal and ileal function in such a way that abdominal cramping, hyperperistalsis, and watery diarrhea can occur.[1] Most patients can tolerate 0.6 mg twice a day, whereas three-times-a-day dosing often leads to these adverse effects. Diarrhea can be controlled with aluminum-containing antacids or specific oral antidiarrheal medications such as loperamide. Overdosage can lead to a cholera-like syndrome with dehydration, hypokalemia, hyponatremia, metabolic acidosis, renal failure, and ultimately shock. Respiratory distress syndrome, disseminated intravascular coagulation, and bone marrow failure may ensue. Other toxic manifestations include hepatic failure and late central nervous system disorders. Myopathy, hypocalcemia, alopecia, stomatitis, and porphyria cutanea tarda have been reported in acutely intoxicated patients who ultimately survived.[1, 22]

Symptoms of chronic intoxication may occur after prolonged therapy with at least 1 mg/day. Chronic complications include leukopenia, aplastic anemia, myopathy, and alopecia. Azoospermia and megaloblastic anemia secondary to vitamin B_{12} malabsorption have also been described.[1] It is suggested that complete blood counts, platelet counts, serum multiphasic analysis, and urinalysis be performed at least every 3 months.[8] Monthly laboratory monitoring for the first few months of therapy is a reasonable procedure. Colchicine should not be used during pregnancy.[14]

GOLD

Chrysotherapy refers to the therapeutic use of gold. Chrysotherapy is a well-established modality for the treatment of rheumatoid arthritis. Gold therapy has been used in dermatologic practice to treat discoid lupus erythematosus and pemphigus.

Pharmacology

Gold remained a parenterally administered medication until 1985, when oral auranofin became available. The two parenteral agents, aurothioglucose and aurothiomalate, are completely absorbed; each has a half-life of about 6 days, and 70% of each is excreted in the urine. In contrast, auranofin is only 25% absorbed, has a longer half-life of approximately 21 days, and is excreted mainly gastrointestinally. Gold accumulates in highest concentrations in the reticuloendothelial system, the kidneys, and the adrenal glands. Such tissue accumulation of the forms administered parenterally is much greater.[23]

Gold compounds exert multiple biologic effects. Gold inhibits phagocytosis and the subsequent killing of bacteria, prostaglandin biosynthesis, and the activity of complement components. Gold also inhibits certain lymphocyte functions, as well as the activity of many enzymes.[23, 24] It has been hypothesized that the beneficial effect of gold in treating pemphigus may relate to interference of blister formation by inhibition of degradative epidermal lysosomal enzymes.[25] Although antiepithelial antibody titers decrease with chrysotherapy, gold compounds neither directly suppress antibody synthesis nor impair binding of pemphigus antibody to epidermal antigens.[25] A normalization of defective Langerhans cell antigen has been noted after chrysotherapy for pemphigus.[26]

Clinical Use

Chrysotherapy is approved for use in treating rheumatoid arthritis. However, it has also been used to treat psoriatic arthritis, as well as discoid lupus erythematosus and pemphigus.[23] Parenteral gold salts were commonly used for therapy of discoid lupus erythematosus until the advent of synthetic antimalarials, which were felt to be less toxic. Gold does remain a therapeutic option for patients with severe chronic discoid lupus erythematosus when other forms of therapy are ineffective or not tolerated.[27] Gold therapy for systemic lupus erythematosus has not been adequately examined.[28]

Gold has been advocated as an adjunctive agent in treating pemphigus. Several case reports and small series argue for its efficacy in permitting reduction in steroid dose, concurrently decreasing anti–skin-antibody titers, and inducing remissions of disease activity.[29–34] However, although most reports support the adjunctive use of gold in pemphigus, controlled studies have never been performed.[35]

Dosage regimens for gold are those used for patients with rheumatoid arthritis. Parenteral therapy in adults begins with a 10-mg intramuscular injection. This is followed 1 week later by a 25-mg injection and subsequently by weekly 50-mg injections. Once a clinical response is obtained, the interval between dosages may be lengthened or the weekly dosage decreased. Children initially receive 1 mg/kg weekly, and the interval between dosages is subsequently lengthened to 2–4 weeks. In adults, auranofin therapy is initiated at 3 mg twice a day.[23] A total daily dosage of 9 mg may be required for selected patients. When disease control is attained, a daily dosage of 3 mg may maintain adequate control.

Unfortunately, chrysotherapy is associated with a high prevalence of adverse reactions. Adverse effects occur in up to one third of patients, typically early in therapy. A variety of cutaneous eruptions can occur, more commonly with parenteral therapy. Most are not specific, although variants such as lichen-planus–like or pityriasis-rosea–like eruptions are well recognized. These cutaneous eruptions may persist for several months after gold therapy is discontinued. Gold cheilitis and stomatitis may occur with or without accompanying dermatitis. When dermatitis does occur, therapy is withheld but may often be resumed at lower dosages without triggering recurrent cutaneous toxicity.[23]

Of patients taking auranofin, 35%–40% have diarrhea, which is typically managed by a decrease in the dosage. Gold-induced enterocolitis and intrahepatic cholestasis have been rarely reported.[23]

Proteinuria occurs with a frequency of 2%–10%. The prognosis of gold-induced nephropathy is usually good if it is recognized early. Therapy is withheld until urinary changes resolve and may then be cautiously reinstituted at lower dosages. More severe nephrotoxicity is rare.[23, 24]

Hematologic side effects, occurring in approximately 1% of patients, include leukopenia, thrombocytopenia, eosinophilia, and in rare instances, aplastic anemia. Either direct bone marrow toxicity or allergic hypersensitivity phenomena are responsible for these reactions.[23] Significant leukopenia (<4000/cu mm) or thrombocytopenia (<100,000/cu mm) requires cessation of gold therapy until the role of gold in causing the abnormality is clarified. Eosinophilia has been noted to be a harbinger of gold dermatitis.[24]

Sudden dyspnea with diffuse bilateral pulmonary infiltrates is another rare reaction that can progress to chronic pulmonary fibrosis. Infrequent neurologic complications include acute progressive polyneuropathy and diffuse fasciculations.[23]

Gold compounds can cause keratitis with corneal ulceration and can be deposited in both cornea and lens, producing chrysiasis.[23, 24]

The nitritoid reaction is a vasomotor response characterized by flushing, dizziness, metallic taste, hypotension, and syncope occurring within 10 minutes of gold injection. The nitritoid reaction occurs almost exclusively with the aqueous gold sodium thiomalate formulation.[36]

There are several notable differences in the incidences of adverse effects of injectable and oral gold. Proteinuria occurs almost six times more frequently with injectable gold. Diarrhea is over three times more common with auranofin. Stomatitis and rash are slightly more frequent with injectable gold. Hematologic and liver adverse effects occur at a similar rate with both methods of administration (see the Ridaura package insert).

When gold therapy is used, clinical and laboratory surveillance is mandatory. Complete blood counts including differential and platelet counts, as well as urinalyses, should be closely monitored. These parameters should be checked before each parenteral injection and monthly with auranofin.[23] Monitoring liver function tests can be considered optional, although reversible cholestatic hepatotoxicity has been infrequently detected.

Relative contraindications to gold therapy include pre-existing renal or liver disease, inflammatory bowel disease, dermatitis, and bone marrow depression. Use of gold during pregnancy is controversial. Gold does cross the placenta in significant quantities. It can be teratogenic in animals, but such teratogenicity has yet to be reported in humans.[23]

POTASSIUM IODIDE

Potassium iodide has been in the physician's armamentarium for about 150 years. In *Diseases of the Skin*, Radcliffe-Crocker in 1908 listed syphilis, lupus vulgaris, eczema, and psoriasis as diseases in which iodine and iodide treatment were indicated.[37] More modern medications have been developed gradually for the treatment of these diseases. Potassium iodide remains useful in treating several dermatologic conditions. It remains the drug of choice for cutaneous sporotrichosis and has found renewed enthusiasm as a treatment for a variety of dermatoses regarded as probable hypersensitivity reactions.[37]

Pharmacology

Potassium iodide has no effect on *Sporothrix schenckii* in vitro. Rather, its efficacy is probably mediated through alteration in the host's immunologic or nonimmunologic response to the organism.[38] Iodides concentrate in infected granulomas and necrotic tissue and have been shown to inhibit granuloma formation.[39]

Schulz and Whiting speculated that the mechanism of action of potassium iodide in hypersensitivity disorders is due to an immunosuppressive effect mediated through heparin. Heparin, which is released in large quantities from mast cells by iodide administration, has been shown to suppress delayed hypersensitivity reactions.[39] Potassium iodide can also suppress the generation of inflammatory oxygen intermediates from activated PMLs and thus may confer protection from auto-oxidative tissue injury.[37]

Clinical Use

Potassium iodide remains the drug of choice for lymphocutaneous sporotrichosis. The initial dose for sporotrichosis is five drops of the saturated solution (a drop contains 67 mg) three times a day in milk or juice. This is increased by 3–5 drops a day until a dosage of at least 15 drops three times a day is reached. Dosages up to 50 drops three times a day may be required. Lesions usually heal within 2–4 weeks, and therapy is continued for an additional 2–4 weeks.[40, 41]

Reports of excellent results with potassium iodide in subacute nodular migratory panniculitis[42] prompted Schulz and Whiting to use this drug for erythema nodosum and nodular vasculitis.[39] Of their 45 patients, 40 responded; symptoms were relieved within 2 days, and lesion resolution occurred in an average of 2 weeks. Subsequent uncontrolled studies have supported the beneficial role of potassium iodide therapy in these diseases.[37, 43, 44] Clinical response tended to be better in those who received treatment shortly after the onset of their disease. Improvement was most dramatic in patients with systemic symptoms such as fever and joint pains.[43] Dosages ranged from 360 to 900 mg/day; most patients received 900 mg/day.

Potassium iodide has also been advocated for use in treating erythema multiforme and Sweet's syndrome. Although their studies were uncontrolled, these advocates reported prompt and dramatic improvement correlating with initiation of therapy.[37, 45, 46]

The efficacy of potassium iodide in granuloma annulare has also been reported.[47, 48] However, the therapeutic effect is achieved only after months of therapy. This therapeutic delay may reflect the difference between the pathogenesis of this granulomatous process and that of the aforementioned erythematous hypersensitivity diseases. Alternatively, potassium iodide may have different mechanisms of action in treating these two disease groups.

Overall, potassium iodide therapy is considered quite safe. Adverse reactions are usually associated with chronic therapy and are dosage-related. Chronic intoxication begins with an unpleasant brassy taste, burning sensation in the mouth, and increased salivation. Coryza, sneezing, and eye irritation are common. Mild iodism simulates a head cold. Parotid and submaxillary glands may become enlarged and tender. Gastric irritation is common. Diarrhea, fever, anorexia, and depression may occur.[49] Vasculitic syndromes have been reported.[50] Skin lesions are remarkably common and varied and include acneiform, dermatitic, and vascular eruption patterns. A distinctive vegetating eruption known as iododerma may occur with chronic use. Paradoxically, both erythema multiforme and erythema nodosum have been attributed to iodide ingestion. Iodides are known to cause flare-ups of certain coexistent skin disorders, namely dermatitis herpetiformis, pyoderma gangrenosum, and pustular psoriasis.[51]

Iodide goiter, with or without hypothyroidism, may occasionally be induced by high-dosage, long-term potassium iodide therapy when an underlying thyroid disease is present. Thus thyroid gland size, thyroid function tests, and antithyroid antibodies should be determined before and intermittently during therapy. Furthermore, large doses should not be given to pregnant women because iodide goiter and hypothyroidism are commonly induced in the fetus.[48]

DANAZOL

Danazol is a synthetic steroid first manufactured in 1963. Danazol is a derivative of ethinyl testosterone that has anabolic properties but markedly attenuated androgenic properties.[52] This drug has several uses within the realm of gynecology, specifically endometriosis and fibrocystic disease of the breast. Hereditary angioedema is an important dermatologic indication.

Pharmacology

Danazol is an isoxazol derivative of 17-alpha ethinyl testosterone. The drug is rapidly absorbed from the upper gastrointestinal tract into the enterohepatic circulation. Plasma levels of danazol reach maximal values of 80 ng/ml about 2 hours after a single oral dose of 400 mg. The half-life is approximately 4.5 hours, and plasma levels are undetectable 8 hours after administration of the drug. In monkeys, radiolabeled danazol is excreted about equally in urine and feces. Although rapidly and extensively metabolized, danazol, rather than its metabolites, appears responsible for the resultant biologic effects.[53]

The biologic properties of danazol are exceedingly complex. At least three major mechanisms of action have been identified: inhibition of gonadotropin-releasing hormones or gonadotropin secretion,[52] inhibition of multiple enzymes of steroidogenesis,[53] and binding to multiple intracellular steroid receptors and circulating steroid-binding proteins.[54] Overall, danazol displays weak androgenic properties. It has markedly attenuated masculinizing activity in comparison with its anabolic activity.[54]

Serum levels of functional C1 esterase inhibitor (C1 INH) increase when danazol is administered to patients with hereditary angioedema. The anabolic activity of danazol presumably stimulates the synthesis of increased amounts of C1 INH.[55] The mechanism responsible for this effect is uncertain.

Clinical Use

Hereditary angioedema is an autosomal dominant disease characterized by episodic bouts of laryngeal, gastrointestinal, and extremity swelling. These patients typically have low antigenic or functional levels of C1 INH. This results in the failure to inhibit the activation of the early components of the classical complement cascade. Although not FDA-approved, danazol has been shown to be quite effective in the prophylactic treatment of this disease.

Long-term prophylaxis is obtained by a maintenance dosage ranging from 200 mg every other day to 600 mg every day and occasionally even lower.[55,56] Dosages should be individualized; optimally, the lowest dose that will suppress life-threatening bouts of the disease should be used. Plasma C1 INH and C4 levels rise with therapy but need not totally normalize for clinical disease control to be achieved.[55-59]

Some researchers have suggested that danazol may have an ameliorative effect on mildly active systemic lupus erythematosus, decreasing immunoglobulins and improving thrombocytopenia.[60] In contrast, other researchers have warned that in patients with hereditary angioedema, danazol may actually exacerbate or induce lupus erythematosus.[61,62] These authors and others have speculated that danazol may either increase immune complex production or increase complement levels, providing additional substrate for ongoing immune complex disease.[63]

The use of attenuated anabolic steroids has been reported in a variety of other skin diseases including Melkerson-Rosenthal syndrome,[56] Raynaud's phenomenon,[64] and pityriasis rubra pilaris.[65-67] The efficacy of such therapy in pityriasis rubra pilaris remains controversial.

Adverse effects of danazol are clearly related to dosage and duration of therapy. When the lowest possible dosages are used, virilizing side effects are usually minimal. Nevertheless, mild hirsutism, deepening of the voice, alopecia, and acne have been reported to occur in female patients. Weight gain and menstrual irregularities, including amenorrhea and menometrorrhagia, are well known to occur. Neuromuscular dysfunctions manifested as muscle cramps, myalgias, and elevations in serum creatine phosphokinase have also been described.[65-68] Reports of microscopic hematuria and actual hemorrhagic cystitis with danazol therapy are worrisome.[55,69,70] Insulin resistance and mild deterioration of glucose tolerance may occur.[71] Episodes of anxiety and tremulousness, as well as exacerbations of underlying migraine headaches, have been described.[55]

Because androgen derivatives have been implicated in the development of cholestatic jaundice, peliosis hepatitis, and liver tumors, monitoring of liver function is advised.[72] However, severe hepatotoxic effects from the "attenuated" androgens such as danazol have not proved to be a significant problem. Transient, mild elevations in hepatocellular enzymes typically return to normal with dosage reduction.[55,73,74]

Finally, danazol should not be used during pregnancy or childhood because of its possible interference with the child's normal sexual development.[52,54]

NICOTINAMIDE

Nicotinic acid (niacin, vitamin B_3) is an essential dietary constituent, the lack of which leads to pellagra. In the body, nicotinic acid is converted to nicotinamide (niacinamide), which functions as a crucial coenzyme that accepts hydrogen ions in oxidation-reduction reactions that are essential for tissue respiration.[75]

Both nicotinic acid and nicotinamide are readily absorbed from the gastrointestinal tract and distributed to all tissues. Both can be used for prophylaxis and treatment of pellagra that is due to poor nutrition, to Hartnup's disease, or to carcinoid tumors.[75] In addition, nicotinamide has been used to treat a variety of seemingly unrelated cutaneous disorders. There have been anecdotal reports about use of niacinamide in treating erythema multiforme,[76] dermatitis herpetiformis,[77] erythema elevatum diutinum,[78] polymorphous light eruption,[79] granuloma annulare,[80] necrobiosis lipoidica diabeticorum,[81] and bullous pemphigoid.[82] Assessment of clinical response to niacinamide in these disorders was complicated by concomitant tetracycline or erythromycin use in several of these studies.

The rationale for nicotinamide's diverse clinical trials has centered on its potent suppression of antigen- and mitogen-induced lymphoblast transformation. This suppression may be explained by its potent inhibitory effect on serum phosphodiesterase, with resultant increase in cyclic adenosine monophosphate (cAMP). Increasing cAMP concentration decreases the release of proteases from leukocytes.[80] For example, nicotinamide's use in treating granuloma annulare focuses on the increased activity of the lymphokine found in this disease: macrophage migration inhibition factor. Accumulation of macrophages and granuloma formation in granuloma annulare may be inhibited by this drug.[80]

Other reports have shown nicotinamide to be effective in inhibiting antigen–immunoglobulin-E–induced histamine release; this inhibition blocks mast cell–mediator release in actively sensitized tissue in vitro. Thus in bullous pemphigoid, nicotinamide may work partly through mast cell stabilization, prohibiting the release of eosinophil chemotactic factor and other mediators of inflammation.[82]

Nicotinamide trials for bullous pemphigoid and erythema elevatum diutinum have included concomitant tetracycline or erythromycin therapy. The anti-inflammatory properties of these antibiotics may function synergistically with nicotinamide in the treatment of diseases with excessive neutrophil chemotaxis.[78, 82]

Nicotinamide has also been used in conjunction with topical 6-aminonicotinamide (6-AN) in the treatment of psoriasis. Topical 6-AN, which has antineoplastic properties, is an analogue and a potent antagonist of nicotinamide. Concurrent oral nicotinamide therapy is used to reduce the possibility of 6-AN–associated auditory nerve damage and central nervous system toxicity.[83]

Some researchers believe that nicotinamide has a beneficial effect in the prevention of polymorphous light eruption.[79] However, using phototesting, others have failed to document this favorable response.[84]

In treatment of bullous pemphigoid[82] and the granulomatous diseases,[80, 81] the dosage of nicotinamide has averaged 500 mg three times a day. Nicotinamide is considered a very safe medication with few side effects. Extensive information regarding adverse effects is available through the literature on schizophrenia, for which the drug was used in dosages of 3–12 g/day. Headache and gastrointestinal complaints occasionally occur. Hepatotoxicity is considered extremely rare but may justify monitoring of liver function tests in patients receiving long-term, high-dosage therapy.[85, 86] Whereas nicotinic acid is a potent vasodilator, nicotinamide is not and thus is not typically associated with flushing and other prostaglandin-triggered side effects.[86] Also, whereas nicotinic acid adversely affects glucose tolerance curves, nicotinamide does not typically have the same effect. Diabetic patients should perhaps still be monitored.[86, 87]

PHENYTOIN

Phenytoin (Dilantin) is well known for its anticonvulsant and antiarrhythmic properties. Dermatologists have used this agent primarily in treating recessive dystrophic epidermolysis bullosa (RDEB) and linear scleroderma.

Unlike the other major types of epidermolysis bullosa, RDEB is characterized by increased collagenase synthesis. Additional studies suggest that an aberrant form of collagenase actually may exist in this condition. Therapeutic trials with phenytoin were thus instituted on the basis of phenytoin's ability to decrease the synthesis of collagenase in fibroblast culture. Approximately two thirds of RDEB patients treated with phenytoin have exhibited at least a 40% decrease in blistering. Therapeutic response has correlated with phenytoin blood levels of more than 8 mcg/ml. The failure of one third of the patients to respond to therapy suggests that they may be a heterogenous group of patients.[88–90] The proposed phenytoin mechanism of action, decreased collagenase synthesis, does not exclude other possible ameliorative effects, such as enhanced wound healing or increased collagen synthesis.[91] Phenytoin may also have further beneficial effects through its ability to decrease arachidonic acid concentrations and competitively antagonize prostaglandin effects in the skin.[92]

Case reports suggest that phenytoin may also have a role in the treatment of some cases of junctional epidermolysis bullosa,[93, 94] especially the generalized atrophic benign variety.[95] Elevated collagenase levels have been found in the normal-appearing skin of some of these patients, as well as in patients with RDEB.[93] A single case report advocates the use of phenytoin in treating pachyonychia congenita. The patient described had a dramatic decrease in blistering with this therapy.[96]

Paradoxically, phenytoin may be beneficial in several disorders characterized by excessive collagen production. Therapeutic efficacy has been reported in limited numbers of patients with scleroderma and lichen sclerosus et atrophicus.[97, 98] A role for phenytoin, both oral[99] and topical,[100] in the acceleration of wound healing has also been advocated. Of interest is that the older gastroenterology literature advocated the use of phenytoin in combination with a potent starch digestant for the treatment of pruritis ani.[101–103]

Before administering this drug, the clinician should be familiar with the broad spectrum of adverse reactions to phenytoin. These include tissue-proliferative syndromes (especially gingival hyperplasia), drug hypersensitivity syndromes, and possible linkage with lymphoma. These and other reactions were comprehensively reviewed in a monograph by Silverman and colleagues.[104] Of interest is that 2 infants with epidermolysis bullosa letalis died of bronchopneumonia with sepsis within 2–6 weeks of beginning phenytoin therapy. The possibility of phenytoin's interfering with host defenses is raised.[105]

NONSTEROIDAL ANTI-INFLAMMATORY DRUGS

The term *nonsteroidal anti-inflammatory drugs* (NSAIDs) refers to compounds whose molecular formula is based on a substituted phenolic or benzene ring that inhibits cyclooxygenase or lipoxygenase transformations of arachidonic acid.[106] At the present time, NSAIDs have limited clinical utility in dermatology; the cyclooxygenase inhibitors aspirin and indomethacin are the ones most commonly used.

Aspirin has been used in the treatment of erythema nodosum, although reports have suggested that indomethacin may be a better drug for this problem.[107, 108] Naproxen has also been shown to be efficacious.[109] Indomethacin is typically given as 100–150 mg/day in divided doses.

Aspirin has also been shown to be effective therapy for erythromelalgia.[110] This disease is characterized by severe burning pain, erythema, and warmth of the extremities, typically provoked by environmental heat, exercise, and dependency. A single daily dose of aspirin is said to result in dramatic relief of symptoms. Relief obtained with aspirin is reported to last for days, in comparison with improvement with indomethacin, which lasts for less than 24 hours. This difference is attributed to aspirin's irreversible inactivation of platelet cyclooxygenase, in comparison with indomethacin's reversible inhibition of this enzyme.[110] Unfortunately, therapeutic failures have been reported.[111, 112]

Aspirin is typically ineffective in alleviating the pruritus associated with common dermatoses.[113] In contrast, the pruritus of polycythemia vera is often responsive to aspirin therapy. There are increased numbers of skin mast cells in this disease. By directly suppressing mast cell prostaglandin metabolism, aspirin inhibits pruritus due to mast cell degranulation.[114]

Systemic mastocytosis may also be managed best with the cautious addition of aspirin to adequate H_1 and H_2 antihistamine blockade therapy. Aspirin effectively inhibits formation of prostaglandin D_2, an important mediator of systemic mastocytosis. The institution of aspirin therapy should be carried out with extreme caution because severe hypotensive episodes culminating in death have been described.[115]

The NSAIDs have been used with some benefit in treating several types of urticaria. Aspirin has been beneficial in nonimmunologic contact urticaria.[116] Aspirin, indomethacin, and ibuprofen all may improve delayed pressure urticaria.[117] Aspirin has also been used to desensitize patients with aspirin-induced urticaria and angioedema.[118] Indomethacin was found to be helpful in conjunction with heat desensitization for localized heat-induced urticaria.[119] Finally, indomethacin has been shown to be a therapeutic option in urticarial vasculitis.[120]

Significant but incomplete suppression of ultraviolet B (UVB) erythema has been documented with aspirin, as well as with oral and topical indomethacin.[121–124] Such observations suggest a possible role for these drugs in minimizing sunburn potential. In contrast to earlier studies, a 1989 report documented similar suppression of UVA-induced and psoralens plus UVA (PUVA-) induced inflammation with topical indomethacin.[124]

Clearly, the NSAIDs are better known within the realm of dermatology for their cutaneous adverse reactions rather than for their clinical utility in treatment of the aforementioned dermatoses. There are several complete reviews on this subject.[125–127] Of importance is that the cutaneous drug reactions commonly induced by NSAIDs include potentially serious entities such as Stevens-Johnson syndrome, toxic epidermal necrolysis, and anaphylactoid reactions.

POTASSIUM PARA-AMINOBENZOATE

Potassium para-aminobenzoate has been used to treat diseases of fibrosis, including progressive systemic sclerosis, morphea, linear scleroderma, Peyronie's disease, Dupuytren's contracture, and dermatomyositis.[128–131] The FDA has classified this drug as "possibly" effective for these conditions (see POTABA package insert). It has also been reported as effective therapy for lichen sclerosus et atrophicus.[132]

Potassium para-aminobenzoate is a member of the vitamin B complex; small amounts are found in cereal, eggs, milk, and meats. The mode of action of this drug is unknown. In early research on the drug, its antifibrotic effect was felt to be mediated through increased monoamine oxidase activity, which permitted increased oxygen uptake at the tissue level.[133] More recent investigation has documented the drug's ability to reduce acid mucopolysaccharide synthesis and glycosaminoglycan secretion.[134, 135] Further studies are clearly warranted.

The average daily adult dose of potassium para-aminobenzoate is 12 g given in four to six divided doses. Children receive 225 mg/kg (1 g/10 lb) in divided doses. Side effects are infrequent and include anorexia, nausea, fever, and skin rash. Hypoglycemia may ensue if the drug is administered through a period of inadequate food intake.[128] Hepatotoxicity has been described but is felt to be extremely rare.[136, 137] Of note is that sulfonamides should not be concurrently administered because they are metabolic antagonists of para-aminobenzoic acid and its salts.[128]

VITAMIN D_3

Calcitriol (1,25-dihydroxycholecalciferol), the active form of vitamin D_3, is being studied both topically and orally in the treatment of psoriasis, a disease hallmarked by keratinocyte hyperproliferation. Clinical trials began after specific receptors for calcitriol were found in the skin and receptor-mediated suppression of cell proliferation with induction of terminal differentiation was documented.[138] Cultured cells from psoriatic skin were found to exhibit a partial resistance to these effects of calcitriol. This resistance could be overcome by large increases in 1,25-dihydroxycholecalciferol concentrations.[139] Such findings suggested that vitamin D derivatives might offer a new approach to the treatment of psoriasis. A number of studies have subsequently documented beneficial effects of both topical and systemic vitamin D therapy in treatment of this disease.[140–144]

Unfortunately, the use of highly active vitamin D_3 derivatives is limited by their potent effects on calcium metabolism. Hypercalcemia can be induced particularly by divided dosages, and thus close monitoring of serum and urinary calcium levels is required.[145] Typically, 0.75 mcg/day in divided doses induces hypercalcemia. In contrast, most psoriasis patients tolerate 0.75–2.0 mcg given as a single bedtime dose. In this dosage range, the drug frequently produces significant improvement of psoriatic lesions.[142] The search for vitamin D analogues with less effect on calcium metabolism is being actively pursued.[145–149] Overall, topical therapy has been well tolerated and has produced no side effects in the treatment of localized psoriasis. More significant systemic absorption would be expected with increasing concentrations over larger treatment areas.

REFERENCES

1. Famaey JP: Colchicine in therapy: State of the art and new perspectives for an old drug. Clin Exp Rheumatol 1988; 6:305–317.
2. Harper RM, Allen BS: Use of colchicine in the treatment of Behçet's disease. Int J Dermatol 1982; 21:551–554.
3. Sander HM, Randle HW: Use of colchicine in Behçet's syndrome. Cutis 1986; 37:344–348.
4. Jorizzo JL, Hudson RD, Schmalstieg FC, et al: Behçet's syndrome: Immune regulation, circulating immune complexes, neutrophil migration, and colchicine therapy. J Am Acad Dermatol 1984; 10:205–214.
5. Aktulga E, Altaç M, Müftüoglu A, et al: A double blind study of colchicine in Behçet's disease. Haematologica (Pavia) 1980; 65:399–402.
6. Gatot A, Tovi F: Colchicine therapy in recurrent oral ulcers [letter]. Arch Dermatol 1984; 120:994.
7. Ruah CB, Stram JR, Chasin WD: Treatment of severe recurrent aphthous stomatitis with colchicine. Arch Otolaryngol Head Neck Surg 1988; 114:671–675.
8. Callen JP: Colchicine is effective in controlling chronic cutaneous leukocytoclastic vasculitis. J Am Acad Dermatol 1985; 13:193–200.
9. Callen JP, af Ekenstam E: Cutaneous leukocytoclastic vasculitis: Clinical experience in 44 patients. South Med J 1987; 80:848–851.
10. Muramatsu C, Tanabe E: Urticarial vasculitis: Response to dapsone and colchicine [letter]. J Am Acad Dermatol 1985; 13:1055.
11. Wiles JC, Hansen RC, Lynch PJ: Urticarial vasculitis treated with colchicine. Arch Dermatol 1985; 121:802–805.
12. Wahba A, Cohen H: Therapeutic trials with oral colchicine in psoriasis. Acta Derm Venereol (Stockh) 1980; 60:515–520.
13. Baker H: Pustular psoriasis. Dermatol Clin 1984; 2:455–470.
14. Takigawa M, Miyachi Y, Uehara M, et al: Treatment of pustulosis palmaris et plantaris with oral doses of colchicine. Arch Dermatol 1982; 118:458–460.
15. Silvers DN, Juhlin EA, Berczeller PH, McSorley J: Treatment of dermatitis herpetiformis with colchicine. Arch Dermatol 1980; 116:1373–1384.
16. Suehisa S, Tagami H: Treatment of acute febrile neutrophilic dermatosis (Sweet's syndrome) with colchicine [letter]. Br J Dermatol 1981; 105:483.
17. Fuchs D, Fruchter L, Fishel B, et al: Colchicine suppression of local inflammation due to calcinosis in dermatomyositis and progressive systemic sclerosis. Clin Rheumatol 1986; 5:527–530.
18. Taborn J, Bole GG, Thompson GR: Colchicine suppression of local and systemic inflammation due to calcinosis universalis in chronic dermatomyositis. Ann Intern Med 1978; 89:648–649.
19. Askari AD: Colchicine for treatment of relapsing polychondritis. J Am Acad Dermatol 1984; 10:507–510.
20. Matucci-Cerinic M, Fattorini L, Gerini G, et al: Colchicine treatment in a case of pachydermoperiostosis with acroosteolysis. Rheumatol Int 1988; 8:185–188.
21. Kar HK, Roy RG: Comparison of colchicine and aspirin in the treatment of type 2 lepra reaction. Lepr Rev 1988; 59:201–203.
22. Simons RJ, Kingma DW: Fatal colchicine toxicity. Am J Med 1989; 86:356–357.

23. Thomas I: Gold therapy and its indications in dermatology. J Am Acad Dermatol 1987; 16:845–854.
24. Penneys NS: Gold therapy: Dermatologic uses and toxicities. J Am Acad Dermatol 1979; 1:315–320.
25. Penneys NS, Ziboh V, Gottlieb NL, et al: Inhibition of prostaglandin synthesis and human epidermal enzymes by aurothiomalate in vitro: Possible actions of gold in pemphigus. J Invest Dermatol 1974; 63:356–361.
26. Blitstein-Willinger E: Behavior of cutaneous Langerhans' cells and skin reactivity after gold sodium thiomalate treatment of pemphigus vulgaris. Dermatologica 1987; 174:68–75.
27. Dalziel K, Going G, Cartwright PH, et al: Treatment of chronic discoid lupus erythematosus with an oral gold compound (auranofin). Br J Dermatol 1986; 115:211–216.
28. Weisman MH, Albert D, Mueller MR, et al: Gold therapy in patients with systemic lupus erythematosus. Am J Med 1983; 75:157–164.
29. Penneys NS, Eaglstein WH, Indgin S, et al: Gold sodium thiomalate treatment of pemphigus. Arch Dermatol 1973; 108:56–60.
30. Paltzik RL, Laude TA: Childhood pemphigus treated with gold. Arch Dermatol 1978; 114:768–769.
31. Poulin Y, Perry HO, Muller SA: Pemphigus vulgaris: Results of treatment with gold as a steroid-sparing agent in a series of thirteen patients. J Am Acad Dermatol 1984; 11:851–857.
32. Frumkin A: Low-dose aurothioglucose in pemphigus vulgaris. Isr J Med Sci 1986; 22:903–905.
33. Walton S, Keczkes K: Pemphigus foliaceus—Successful treatment with adjuvant gold therapy. Clin Exp Dermatol 1987; 12:364–365.
34. Kielwasser S, Heid E, Grosshans E, et al: Gold and pemphigus vulgaris [letter]. Dermatologica 1987; 174:258.
35. Bystryn JC: Adjuvant therapy of pemphigus. Arch Dermatol 1984; 120:941–951.
36. Rapini RP: Gold treatment of pemphigus [letter]. J Am Acad Dermatol 1985; 13:310.
37. Horio T, Danno K, Okamoto H, et al: Potassium iodide in erythema nodosum and other erythematous dermatoses. J Am Acad Dermatol 1983; 9:77–81.
38. Shelley WB, Sica PA: Disseminate sporotrichosis of skin and bone cured with 5-fluorocytosine: Photosensitivity as a complication. J Am Acad Dermatol 1983; 8:229–235.
39. Schulz EJ, Whiting DA: Treatment of erythema nodosum and nodular vasculitis with potassium iodide. Br J Dermatol 1976; 94:75–78.
40. Anderson PC: Cutaneous sporotrichosis. Am Fam Physician 1983; 27(3):201–204.
41. Urabe H, Honbo S: Sporotrichosis. Int J Dermatol 1986; 25:255–257.
42. Vilanova X, Aguade JP: Subacute nodular migratory panniculitis. Br J Dermatol 1959; 71:45–50.
43. Horio T, Imamura S, Danno K, Ofuji S: Potassium iodide in the treatment of erythema nodosum and nodular vasculitis. Arch Dermatol 1981; 117:29–31.
44. Ozols II, Wheat LJ: Erythema nodosum in an epidemic of histoplasmosis in Indianapolis. Arch Dermatol 1981; 117:709–712.
45. Myatt AE, Baker DJ, Byfield DM: Sweet's syndrome: A report on the use of potassium iodide. Clin Exp Dermatol 1987; 12:345–349.
46. Horio T, Imamura S, Danno K, et al: Treatment of acute febrile neutrophilic dermatosis (Sweet's syndrome) with potassium iodide. Dermatologica 1980; 160:341–347.
47. Giessel M, Graves E, Kalivas J: Treatment of disseminated granuloma annulare with potassium iodide [letter]. Arch Dermatol 1979; 115:639–640.
48. Caserio RJ, Eaglstein WH, Allen CM: Treatment of granuloma annulare with potassium iodide [letter]. J Am Acad Dermatol 1984; 10:294–295.
49. Haynes RC Jr, Murad F: Iodides. In Gilman AG, Goodman LS, Rall TW, et al (eds):

Goodman and Gilman's The Pharmacological Basis of Therapeutics (7th ed). New York: Macmillan, 1985, 1405–1406.
50. Eeckhout E, Willemsen M, Deconinck A, et al: Granulomatous vasculitis as a complication of potassium iodide treatment for Sweet's syndrome. Acta Derm Venereol (Stockh) 1987; 67:362–364.
51. Shelley WB: Generalized pustular psoriasis induced by potassium iodide: A postulated role for dihydrofolic reductase. JAMA 1967; 201:133–138.
52. Gelfand JA, Sherins RJ, Alling DW, et al: Treatment of hereditary angioedema with danazol: Reversal of clinical and biochemical abnormalities. N Engl J Med 1976; 295:1444–1448.
53. Dmowski WP: Danazol—A steroid derivative with multiple and diverse biological effects. Br J Clin Pract 1988; 42:343–347.
54. Darbieri RL: Danazol treatment of angioedema [letter]. J Allergy Clin Immunol 1982; 71:257–258.
55. Hosea SW, Santaella ML, Brown EJ, et al: Long-term therapy of hereditary angioedema with danazol. Ann Intern Med 1980; 93:809–812.
56. Madanes AE, Farber M: Danazol. Ann Intern Med 1982; 96:625–630.
57. Warin AP, Greaves MW, Gatecliff M, et al: Treatment of hereditary angio-oedema by low dose attenuated androgens: Disassociation of clinical response from levels of C1 esterase inhibitor and C4. Br J Dermatol 1980; 103:405–409.
58. Sheffer AL, Fearon DT, Austen KF: Clinical and biochemical effects of impeded androgen (oxymetholone) therapy of hereditary angioedema. J Allergy Clin Immunol 1979; 64:275–280.
59. Spath PJ, Wuthrich B, Butler R: C1 inhibitor functional activities in hereditary angioedema plasma of patients under therapy with attenuated androgens. Dermatologica 1984; 169:301–304.
60. Agnello V, Pariser K, Gell J, et al: Preliminary observations on danazol therapy of systemic lupus erythematosus: Effects on DNA antibodies, thrombocytopenia and complement. J Rheumatol 1983; 10:682–687.
61. Fretwell MD, Altman LC: Exacerbation of a lupus-erythematosus–like syndrome during treatment of non–C1-esterase-inhibitor–dependent angioedema with danazol. J Allergy Clin Immunol 1982; 69:306–310.
62. Guillet G, Sassolas B, Plantin P, et al: Anti-Ro-positive lupus and hereditary angioneurotic edema: A 7-year follow-up with worsening of lupus under danazol treatment. Dermatologica 1988; 177:370–375.
63. Hory B, Blanc D, Boillot A, et al: Guillain-Barré syndrome following danazol and corticosteroid therapy for hereditary angioedema. Am J Med 1985; 79:111–114.
64. Jarrett PEM, Morland M, Browse NL: Treatment of Raynaud's phenomenon by fibrinolytic enhancement. Br Med J 1978; 2:523–525.
65. Bergamaschini L, Tucci A, Colombo A, et al: Effect of stanozolol in patients with pityriasis rubra pilaris and retinol-binding protein deficiency [letter]. N Engl J Med 1982; 306:346–347.
66. Pavlidakey GP, Hashimoto K, Savoy LB, et al: Stanozolol in the treatment of pityriasis rubra pilaris. Arch Dermatol 1985; 121:546–548.
67. van Voorst Vader PC, van Oostveen F, Houthoff HJ, Marrink J: Pityriasis rubra pilaris, vitamin A and retinol-binding protein: A case study. Acta Derm Venereol (Stockh) 1984; 64:430–432.
68. Sheffer AL, Fearon DT, Austen KF: Clinical and biochemical effects of stanozolol therapy for hereditary angioedema. J Allergy Clin Immunol 1981; 68:181–187.
69. Andriole GL, Brickman C, Lack EE, et al: Danazol-induced cystitis: An undescribed source of hematuria in patients with hereditary angioneurotic edema. J Urol 1986; 135:44–46.
70. Sweet LC, Jackson CE, Yanari SS, et al: Danazol therapy in hereditary angioedema. Henry Ford Hosp Med J 1980; 28:31–35.

New Uses for Old Drugs   381

71. Wynn V: Metabolic effects of danazol. J Int Med Res 1977; 5(Suppl):25–35.
72. Bagheri SA, Boyer JL: Peliosis hepatis associated with androgenic-anabolic steroid therapy: A severe form of hepatic injury. Ann Intern Med 1974; 81:610–618.
73. Pearson K, Zimmerman HJ: Danazol and liver damage [letter]. Lancet 1980; 1:645–646.
74. Cicardi M, Bergamaschini L, Tucci A: Morphologic evaluation of the liver in hereditary angioedema patients on long-term treatment with androgen derivatives. J Allergy Clin Immunol 1983; 72:294–298.
75. Marcus R, Coulston AM: Nicotinic acid. In Gilman AG, Goodman LS, Rall TW, et al (eds): Goodman and Gilman's The Pharmacological Basis of Therapeutics (7th ed). New York: Macmillan, 1985, 1557–1559.
76. Weisberg A, Rosen E: Erythema exudativum multiforme. Arch Dermatol Syph 1946; 53:99–106.
77. Johnson HH, Binkley GW: Nicotinic acid therapy of dermatitis herpetiformis. J Invest Dermatol 1950; 14:233–238.
78. Kohler IK, Lorincz AL: Erythema elevatum diutinum treated with niacinamide and tetracycline. Arch Dermatol 1980; 116:693–695.
79. Neumann R, Rappold E, Pohl-Markl H: Treatment of polymorphous light eruption with nicotinamide: A pilot study. Br J Dermatol 1986; 115:77–80.
80. Ma A, Medenica M: Response of generalized granuloma annulare to high-dose niacinamide. Arch Dermatol 1983; 119:836–839.
81. Handfield-Jones S, Jones SK, Peachey R: High dose nicotinamide in the treatment of necrobiosis lipoidica. Br J Dermatol 1988; 118:693–696.
82. Berk MA, Lorincz AL: The treatment of bullous pemphigoid with tetracycline and niacinamide: A preliminary report. Arch Dermatol 1986; 122:670–674.
83. Zackheim HS: Topical 6-aminonicotinamide plus oral niacinamide therapy for psoriasis. Arch Dermatol 1978; 114:1632–1638.
84. Ortel B, Wechdorn D, Tanew A, Hönigsmann H: Effect of nicotinamide on the phototest reaction in polymorphous light eruption. Br J Dermatol 1988; 118:669–673.
85. Zackheim HS, Vasily DB, Westphal ML, et al: Reactions to niacinamide [letter]. J Am Acad Dermatol 1981; 4:736–737.
86. Ranchoff RE, Tomecki KJ: Niacin or niacinamide? Nicotinic acid or nicotinamide? What is the difference? [letter]. J Am Acad Dermatol 1986; 15:116–117.
87. Handfield-Jones S, Jones SK, Peachey RD: Nicotinamide treatment in diabetes [letter]. Br J Dermatol 1987; 116:277.
88. Bauer EA, Cooper TW, Tucker DR, et al: Phenytoin therapy of recessive dystrophic epidermolysis bullosa. N Engl J Med 1980; 303:776–781.
89. Cooper TW, Bauer EA: Therapeutic efficacy of phenytoin in recessive dystrophic epidermolysis: A comparison of short- and long-term treatment. Arch Dermatol 1984; 120:490–495.
90. Bauer EA, Tabas M: A perspective on the role of collagenase in recessive dystrophic epidermolysis bullosa. Arch Dermatol 1988; 124:734–736.
91. Bauer EA, Cooper TW: Therapeutic considerations in recessive dystrophic epidermolysis bullosa [editorial]. Arch Dermatol 1981; 117:529–530.
92. Cunnane SC, Kent ET, McAdoo KR, et al: Abnormalities of plasma and erythrocyte essential fatty acid composition in epidermolysis bullosa: Influence of treatment with diphenylhydantoin. J Invest Dermatol 1987; 89:395–399.
93. Rogers RB, Yancey KB, Allen BS, Guill MF: Phenytoin therapy for junctional epidermolysis bullosa. Arch Dermatol 1983; 119:925–926.
94. Armoni M, Schlesinger M, Vardy PA, et al: Phenytoin and junctional epidermolysis bullosa [letter]. Arch Dermatol 1985; 121:168–169.
95. Fine JD, Johnson L: Efficacy of systemic phenytoin in the treatment of junctional epidermolysis bullosa. Arch Dermatol 1988; 124:1402–1406.

96. Blank H: Treatment of pachyonychia congenita with phenytoin [letter]. Br J Dermatol 1982; 106:123.
97. Morgan RJ: Scleroderma: Treatment with diphenylhydantoin. Cutis 1978; 22:278–282.
98. Neldner KH: Treatment of localized linear scleroderma with phenytoin. Cutis 1978; 22:569–572.
99. Simpson GM, Kunz E, Slafta J: Use of sodium diphenylhydantoin in treatment of leg ulcers. New York State J Med 1965; 65:886–888.
100. El Zayat SG: Preliminary experience with topical phenytoin in wound healing in a war zone. Milit Med 1989; 154:178–180.
101. Bodkin LG: Oral therapy for pruritus ani. Am J Digest Dis 1945; 12:255–257.
102. Goodwin FB: Oral therapy in anogenital pruritus. J Nat Proct Assn 1946; 18:84–87.
103. Bodkin LG: Pruritus ani: A review of oral therapy. Am J Digest Dis 1947; 14:109–113.
104. Silverman AK, Fairley J, Wong RC: Cutaneous and immunologic reactions to phenytoin. J Am Acad Dermatol 1988; 18:721–741.
105. Bergfeld WF, Orlowski JP: Epidermolysis bullosa letalis and phenytoin [letter]. J Am Acad Dermatol 1982; 7:275–278.
106. Greaves MW: Pharmacology and significance of nonsteroidal anti-inflammatory drugs in the treatment of skin diseases. J Am Acad Dermatol 1987; 16:751–764.
107. Ubogy Z, Persellin RH: Suppression of erythema nodosum by indomethacin. Acta Derm Venereol (Stockh) 1982; 62:265–266.
108. Elizaga FV: Erythema nodosum and indomethacin [letter]. Ann Intern Med 1982; 96:383.
109. Lehman CW: Control of chronic erythema nodosum with naproxen. Cutis 1980; 26:66–67.
110. Kurzrock R, Cohen PR: Erythromelalgia and myeloproliferative disorders. Arch Intern Med 1989; 149:105–109.
111. Thompson GH, Hahn G, Rang M: Erythromelalgia. Clin Orthop 1979; 144:249–254.
112. Cohen IJK, Samorodin CS: Familial erythromelalgia. Arch Dermatol 1982; 118:953–954.
113. Daly BM, Shuster S: Effects of aspirin on pruritus. Br Med J [Clin Res] 1986; 293:907.
114. Jackson N, Burt D, Crocker J, et al: Skin mast cells in polycythaemia vera: Relationship to the pathogenesis and treatment of pruritus. Br J Dermatol 1987; 116:21–29.
115. Crawhall JC, Wilkinson RD: Systemic mastocytosis: Management of an unusual case with histamine (H_1 and H_2) antagonists and cyclooxygenase inhibition. Clin Invest Med 1987; 10:1–4.
116. Lahti A, Väänänen A, Kokkonen EL, Hannuksela M: Acetylsalicylic acid inhibits nonimmunologic contact urticaria. Contact Dermatitis 1987; 16:133–135.
117. Sussman GL, Harvey RP, Schocket AL: Delayed pressure urticaria. J Allergy Clin Immunol 1982; 70:337–342.
118. Grzelewska-Rzymowska I, Roznlecki J, Szmidt M: Aspirin "desensitization" in patients with aspirin-induced urticaria and angioedema. Allergol Immunopathol (Madr) 1988; 16:305–308.
119. Koro O, Dover JS, Francis DM, et al: Release of prostaglandin D_2 and histamine in a case of localized heat urticaria, and effect of treatments. Br J Dermatol 1986; 115:721–728.
120. Millns JL, Randle HW, Solley GO, Dicken CH: The therapeutic response of urticarial vasculitis to indomethacin. J Am Acad Dermatol 1980; 3:349–355.
121. Miller WS, Ruderman FR, Smith JG Jr: Aspirin and ultraviolet light–induced erythema in man. Arch Dermatol (Chicago) 1967; 95:357–358.
122. Kobra-Black A, Greaves MV, Hensby CN, et al: Effects of indomethacin on prostaglandins E_2, F_2 alpha and arachidonic acid in human skin 24 hours after UV-B and UV-C irradiation. Br J Clin Pharmacol 1978; 6:261–266.
123. Søndergaard J, Bisgaard H, Thorsen S: Eicosanoids in skin UV inflammation. Photodermatol 1985; 2:359–366.

124. Imodaka G, Tejima T: A possible role of prostaglandins in PUVA-induced inflammation: Implication by organ cultured skin. J Invest Dermatol 1989; 92:296–300.
125. Bigby M, Stern R: Cutaneous reactions to nonsteroidal anti-inflammatory drugs. J Am Acad Dermatol 1985; 12:866–876.
126. Roujeau JC: Clinical aspects of skin reactions to NSAIDs. Scand J Rheumatol 1987; 65(Suppl):131–134.
127. O'Brien N, Bagby GF: Rare adverse reactions to nonsteroidal antiinflammatory drugs. J Rheumatol 1985; 12:13–20.
128. Zarafonetis CJD: Antifibrotic therapy with Potaba. Am J Med Sci 1964; 248:550–561.
129. Zarafonetis CJD, Curtis AC, Gulick AE: Use of para-aminobenzoic acid in dermatomyositis and scleroderma: Report of 6 cases. Arch Int Med 1950; 85:27–43.
130. Zarafonetis CJD, Dabich L, Negri D, et al: Retrospective studies in scleroderma: Effect of potassium para-aminobenzoate on survival. J Clin Epidemiol 1988; 41:193–205.
131. Zarafonetis CJD, Dabich L, Skovronski JJ, et al: Retrospective studies in scleroderma: Skin response to potassium para-aminobenzoate therapy. Clin Exp Rheumatol 1988; 6:261–268.
132. Penneys NS: Treatment of lichen sclerosus with potassium para-aminobenzoate. J Am Acad Dermatol 1984; 10:1039–1042.
133. Zarafonetis CJD: The treatment of scleroderma: Results of potassium para-aminobenzoate therapy in 104 cases. In Mills LC, Moyer JH (eds.): Inflammation and Diseases of Connective Tissue. Philadelphia: WB Saunders, 1961, 688–696.
134. Priestley GC, Brown JC: Effects of potassium para-aminobenzoate on growth and macromolecule synthesis in fibroblasts cultured from normal and sclerodermatous human skin, and rheumatoid synovial cells. J Invest Dermatol 1979; 72:161–164.
135. Gillon M, Priestley GC, Heyworth R: Effects of para-aminobenzoate on skin fibroblasts from lichen sclerosus et atrophicus and from morphoea [abstract]. Br J Dermatol 1987; 116:454.
136. Kantor GR, Ratz JL: Liver toxicity from potassium para-aminobenzoate [letter]. J Am Acad Dermatol 1985; 13:671–672.
137. Zarafonetis CJD, Dabich L, DeVol EB, et al: Potassium para-aminobenzoate and liver function test findings. J Am Acad Dermatol 1986; 15:144–149.
138. Smith EL, Walworth NC, Holick MF: Effect of 1 alpha,25-dihydroxyvitamin D_3 on the morphologic and biochemical differentiation of cultured human epidermal keratinocytes grown in serum-free conditions. J Invest Dermatol 1986; 86:709–714.
139. Abe J, Kondo S, Nishii Y, Kuroki T: Resistance to 1,25-dihydroxyvitamin D_3 of cultured psoriatic epidermal keratinocytes isolated from involved and uninvolved skin. J Clin Endocrinol Metab 1989; 68:851–854.
140. Morimoto S, Yoshikawa K: Psoriasis and vitamin D_3: A review of our experience. Arch Dermatol 1989; 125:231–234.
141. Holick MF, Smith E, Pincus S: Skin as the site of vitamin D synthesis and target tissue for 1,25-dihydroxyvitamin D_3: Use of calcitrol (1,25-dihydroxyvitamin D_3) for treatment of psoriasis. Arch Dermatol 1987; 123:1677–1683a.
142. Smith EL, Pincus SH, Donovan L, Holick MF: A novel approach for the evaluation and treatment of psoriasis: Oral or topical use of 1,25-dihydroxyvitamin D_3 can be a safe and effective therapy for psoriasis. J Am Acad Dermatol 1988; 19:516–528.
143. Morimoto S, Yoshikawa K, Kozuka T, et al: Treatment of psoriasis vulgaris with oral 1 alpha,25-dihydroxyvitamin D_3—Report of two cases. J Dermatol (Tokyo) 1987; 14:59–62.
144. Morimoto S, Yoshikawa K, Kozuka T, et al: An open study of vitamin D_3 treatment in psoriasis vulgaris. Br J Dermatol 1986; 115:421–429.
145. Binderup L, Bramm E: Effects of a novel vitamin D analogue MC903 on cell proliferation and differentiation in vitro and on calcium metabolism in vivo. Biochem Pharmacol 1988; 37:889–895.

146. Kragballe K, Beck HI, Søgaard H: Improvement of psoriasis by a topical vitamin D_3 analogue (MC 903) in a double-blind study. Br J Dermatol 1988; 119:223–230.
147. Staberg B, Roed-Petersen J, Menné T: Efficacy of topical treatment in psoriasis with MC903, a new vitamin D analogue. Acta Derm Venereol (Stockh) 1989; 69:147–150.
148. Kato T, Rokugo M, Terui T, et al: Successful treatment of psoriasis with topical application of active vitamin D_3 analogue, 1 alpha,24-dihydroxycholecalciferol. Br J Dermatol 1986; 115:431–433.
149. Kato T, Terui T, Tagami H: Topically active vitamin D_3 analogue, 1 alpha,24–dihydroxy-cholecalciferol, has an anti-proliferative effect on the epidermis of guinea pig skin [letter]. Br J Dermatol 1987; 117:528–530.

16 | An Approach to Monitoring for Adverse Effects

Stephen E. Wolverton, M.D.

This chapter represents an overview of my own philosophy and approach to monitoring for adverse effects from systemic medications used in dermatology. The chapter begins with an overview of general principles of monitoring; specific examples cited involve the use of drugs described in this textbook. This overview includes a brief section on the statistical principles important to the monitoring process. Specific areas of adverse effects subsequently discussed include liver-, renal-, hematologic-, lipid-, ocular-, radiologic-, and malignancy-related monitoring. Details and references for specific adverse effects can be found in the respective chapters. This chapter should be a useful adjunct to this book's specific discussions regarding drugs and their associated risks.

OVERVIEW OF GENERAL PRINCIPLES

Throughout the text are descriptions of drugs, such as the retinoids, glucocorticosteroids, methotrexate, dapsone, and others with excellent therapeutic potential, albeit at varying degrees of risk. In dermatology, the risk-benefit ratios generally dictate a greater degree of caution regarding possible risks of therapy. The patient is often willing to take these risks if the follow-up and monitoring of therapy proceed with caution. In the increasingly litigious society in which physicians practice, a conservative approach regarding monitoring for adverse effects from systemic therapeutic agents is justifiable. It is important to be aware of the cost and limitations of these tests as a trade-off for greater comfort and safety for the patient and the physician who use these systemic agents.

Sources For Guidelines

There is a hierarchy of sources for monitoring guidelines. The most important source is the pharmaceutical company's package insert guidelines. Dapsone, isotretinoin, and etretinate all have such detailed guidelines. If the company does not provide such guidelines, a state of the art review article is the next most useful source. Such specific guidelines from review articles include those regarding methotrexate,[1] psoralens plus ultraviolet A (PUVA) and ocular surveillance,[2] and ocular monitoring of antimalarial agents.[3] Previous reviews of multiple drugs for which useful monitoring guidelines were provided include those by Lynch[4,5] and by McDonald.[6] An occasional clinical study disclosing a specific risk may provide the basis for monitoring guidelines. The elucidation of the risk of PUVA therapy's inducing genital squamous cell carcinoma in men dictates a greater effort in both protection of and surveillance for malignancy of the male genitalia.[7]

In legal principles, the "standard of practice" in the community, and the methods that a "reasonable physician" would use, form a broad and vague guideline of practice. Pharmaceutical company guidelines and state of the art reviews are much more specific sources. Given an adequate clinical experience with a specific drug, one's own modifications based on experience are justifiable.

Risk Assessment

Surveillance for adverse effects is generally directed at common or serious adverse effects for which symptoms alone may not allow detection of the adverse effect. Physical examination findings are uncommonly used in this surveillance. Laboratory tests, radiologic procedures, or special examination by a consulting physician are more commonly used. The approach differs according to whether the adverse effect is expected (pharmacologic, such as with dapsone-induced hemolysis) versus unexpected (idiosyncratic, such as ketoconazole-induced hepatitis). Even expected adverse effects may be unusually severe in a specific subset of patients; for example, severe hemolysis occurs in glucose-6-phosphate dehydrogenase– (G6PD–) deficient patients receiving dapsone.

For many patients, the true risk of a rare adverse effect is not known until several years of widespread clinical use have elapsed after the Food and Drug Administration's (FDA's) release of the drug. Ketoconazole-induced hepatitis is such an adverse effect. The initial rate of reaction was reported to be 1/10,000 patients. Experience with fluconazole and itraconazole requires similar numbers of patients to determine whether the risk is similar to that of ketoconazole.

Patient Involvement in the Decision Process

Active patient participation in the decision regarding use of systemic drugs in dermatology is important for a variety of reasons. (For a complete discussion on this subject, see Chapter 17.) The patient needs to be informed of symptoms to report, laboratory and radiologic tests to be followed, and special examinations required for monitoring for adverse effects of these drugs. Despite the risk of a patient's being overly concerned about potential adverse effects, the risk of patients' not reporting these symptoms in the absence of truly informed consent is greater. I strongly recommend that patients be given a handout covering these details, either the pharmaceutical company's or the physician's own summary of drugs with significant adverse effects. (An example of a physician's handout is given in Appendix I.) Only with this amount of information can a patient make a truly informed decision regarding use of a drug with potential risk. In my experience, patients are more often reassured than troubled when presented descriptions of the risks, their likelihood, and the surveillance that will be used in monitoring. It is particularly reassuring for the patient to know about the potentially serious adverse effects for which the risk is negligible with early detection by symptoms, examination, or laboratory tests.

Monitoring Clinical Signs and Symptoms

There are several examples of symptoms for which reporting by the patient is essential for detection of a particular adverse effect. Important examples include myalgias in retinoid-induced myopathy; dyspnea, chest pain, and cough with methotrexate-induced pneumonitis; and focal persistent bone pain with glucocorticosteroid-induced aseptic bone necrosis. For each of these drugs, no specific monitoring is recommended for these specific adverse effects unless indicated by symptoms. Also, in these situations, early reporting of symptoms may significantly reduce the risk from the adverse effect. At times, one symptom may not be inherently worrisome, but a constellation of symptoms signifies an important adverse effect. An example would be with a headache in retinoid- or glucocorticosteroid-treated patients. The presence of a headache gains significance when accompanied by visual change, nausea, and vomiting, which suggest pseudotumor cerebri.

In dapsone-treated patients, examination for both cyanosis (methemoglobinemia) and peripheral motor weakness, manifested by decreased ability to perform plantar flexion while standing (peripheral neuropathy), is important to the monitoring process. Examination of lymph nodes, liver, and spleen in patients treated with immunosuppressive agents is quite important in detection of drug-induced lymphomas. In patients with dapsone syndrome or phenytoin syndrome, important physical findings may coexist with early laboratory findings of these systemic syndromes. In both of these conditions, a morbilliform or erythrodermic rash presents near the time of onset of abnormal liver function tests, peripheral eosinophilia, and other systemic manifestations of the syndromes. Patients' awareness of the significance of the cutaneous eruption is important with these two drugs.

Monitoring Laboratory Tests and Related Procedures

BASELINE TESTING. Of importance is that in the majority of adverse effects from systemic drugs described in this book, there are no symptoms that allow early detection of a given adverse effect. This provides the necessity for laboratory tests, radiologic procedures, or special examinations by the consulting physician that are described throughout the book. It is important to perform a baseline (pretreatment) evaluation of any test that will be followed during a patient's course on a given drug. Baseline testing is important in order to exclude previous pathology that would either preclude use of a given drug or mandate more careful surveillance. It is medicolegally important to perform the baseline testing in order to avoid subsequent blame for an adverse effect that existed when drug therapy was initiated. An example of a laboratory finding for which baseline testing is important is the relatively common occurrence in blacks of leukopenia in the absence of any pathology.

There is a degree of controversy regarding the need for specific baseline tests in several instances. Two such examples would be a baseline test for antinuclear antibodies in patients about to receive PUVA therapy and a test of G6PD level in patients about to be treated with antimalarials. In both cases the test is relatively sensitive and inexpensive and does not create the need for a subsequent office encounter. Thus it is quite reasonable to order both tests for appropriate patients. In contrast, a 24-hour urine collection for porphyrins in patients about to be treated with antimalarial agents could be considered optional. The test is costly and inconvenient, and physical findings would heighten the suspicion of that patient's having porphyria cutanea tarda. All these issues argue against the routine ordering of this test in the absence of clinical suspicion.

FOLLOW-UP TESTING. Many physicians order initial follow-up testing at least 3 months after the therapy is initiated. A great majority of idiosyncratic adverse effects occur within the initial few months of therapy. I believe that one should draw the initial follow-up set of laboratory tests no later than 4–6 weeks into therapy. With many drugs in this book, the initial follow-up testing is earlier than this, on the basis of either the timing or the potential severity of a given adverse effect. In particular, if a baseline test result is abnormal, early and frequent surveillance is important.

With many drugs, the need for baseline and subsequent testing is dictated by the total duration of therapy. Griseofulvin, ketoconazole, and rifampin generally do not require any monitoring for administration of several weeks' duration. In contrast, prolonged therapy with all three drugs usually requires laboratory monitoring.

There are several instances for which there is controversy over the need for long-term surveillance for adverse effects. Low-risk testing, such as monitoring complete blood counts (CBCs) and serum chemistries with PUVA therapy, may be considered optional. In addition, long-term use of trimethoprim-sulfamethoxazole is rarely accompanied by significant adverse reactions. However, a syndrome resembling dapsone syndrome and other potentially severe adverse effects are remotely possible. The need for monitoring should certainly be discussed openly with the patient in these circumstances.

Methotrexate-induced hepatic fibrosis in psoriasis patients serves as an example of how laboratory tests (liver function tests) are only partially successful in detecting a given adverse effect. For these patients, an additional procedure, a liver biopsy, is necessary. For others, a laboratory abnormality may be of minimal clinical relevance, and thus the test would not be useful on a routine basis. Glucocorticosteroid-induced hypothalamic-pituitary-adrenal axis suppression and retinoid-induced minor bone abnormalities both await clarification of the significance of minimally abnormal results.

RECORDING RESULTS. A laboratory flow sheet summarizing the patient's baseline and follow-up laboratory tests, radiologic procedures, and special examinations and procedures is most useful. The results can be recorded by the physician or the nursing personnel. Such a flow sheet can save time over the long run and aids in thoroughness in the monitoring process. A flow sheet that I use, with laboratory tests grouped by system, is demonstrated in Appendix II. Results can be more rapidly recorded with a check mark when the values are within normal limits. Abnormal results can be highlighted in a variety of ways.

RESPONSE TO ABNORMAL TEST RESULTS. Three main options are available any time a significant adverse effect is detected. These options are discontinuation of the drug, reduction of the drug's dosage, and continuation of the same dosage with more frequent laboratory surveillance. Several issues dictate which option is most appropriate in a given situation. With any abnormal laboratory value, it is important to exclude other drugs that the patient is taking, other diseases, and habits of the patient as causes of the abnormal test result. In many instances, the improvement of the abnormal result with dechallenge (temporarily discontinuing the drug) and observation of the response to rechallenge (should the risk of rechallenge be minimal) can establish whether a given drug is responsible for the adverse effect in question.

A predictable adverse effect, with unlikely serious potential, may require only more frequent laboratory surveillance. An example is the transient abnormal results of liver function tests that are commonly detected early in retinoid therapy.

Dosage-related adverse effects often can be corrected by dosage reduction. Dapsone-induced hemolysis and resultant anemia serve as an example. Alternatively, serious and life-threatening adverse effects require cessation of therapy altogether. Cessation of prednisone therapy when aseptic bone necrosis is suspected is imperative, unless a potentially life-threatening condition, such pemphigus vulgaris, is being treated.

When a drug is continued in the presence of a significant adverse effect, comanagement with another specialist is generally appropriate. Methotrexate-treated patients with abnormal liver biopsy results require careful follow-up by a gastroenterologist should they continue therapy.

It is vital to reassess the risk-benefit ratio in patients who develop significant adverse effects and to continually involve the patient in future management decisions. It is unusual to have a progressive and serious adverse effect from systemic drugs used in dermatology when the patient receives information on adverse effects, when attention is given to important examination findings, and when regular laboratory testing and periodic special examinations and procedures are used.

STATISTICAL PRINCIPLES. It is important to review several statistical definitions.[8] The *sensitivity* of a test reflects the ability of that test to yield true positive results for patients with a specific disease. *Specificity* reflects the percentage of true negative results in healthy patients. When one is screening for adverse effects in a high-risk population, adequate sensitivity of a test or a battery of tests is an important feature. In general, as the sensitivity of the test increases, its specificity decreases. By using batteries of tests, such as liver function test panels, one increases the sensitivity while decreasing the specificity of abnormal results. This trade-off is acceptable inasmuch as there are several approaches that can be used to enhance specificity. Tests that yield positive results on repeated evaluations or results that are markedly abnormal (more than three standard deviations from the mean) are more likely to represent true positive results. The specificity is enhanced by exclusion of other drugs, diseases, or patients' habits that may be responsible for that given adverse effect. In addition, with a panel of tests, the more tests that yield abnormal results, the greater the chance that these are true positive results.

Prevalence represents the existing number of patients with a condition in a total population at a given time.[8] This number is generally expressed by epidemiologists as the number of patients with the condition per 100,000 people in all at risk. The greater the prevalence of a given adverse effect in a population, the greater the predictive value of a positive result in that population. Alternatively stated, it is much more likely for an abnormal result to represent a true positive result when the adverse effect is a frequent event in that population. For example, it is much more likely for leukopenia resulting from azathioprine treatment to represent a true positive result than for leukopenia developing with griseofulvin used in treating a dermatophyte infection. In both cases, however, a significantly abnormal result deserves equal respect until the role of the drug in causing the adverse effect is clarified.

UNEXPLAINED ABNORMAL TEST RESULTS. There are several possibilities worth considering when one is confronted with an unexplained positive (abnormal) test result.[9] Laboratory normal values are usually in a range of two standard deviations above and below the mean. By definition, this allows 5% of "normal" patients to have abnormal results. When six tests are performed, 24% of "normal" patients have at least one abnormal result. When 12 tests are performed, as in many multiphasic chemistry panels, 43% of "normal" patients will have at least one abnormal laboratory test. The presence of markedly abnormal results, multiple abnormal results within one panel, or repeatedly abnormal results all increase the specificity of abnormal results.

In addition, one should always consider the possibility of laboratory error, inappropriate normal ranges, and incorrect preparation of a patient or handling of a specimen when assessing an abnormal test result.[9] The burden of proof of explanation for such results remains on the physician who orders the tests. The principles described in this section enable one to verify the significance of the abnormal test result.

SPECIFIC ADVERSE EFFECTS

LIVER FUNCTION TESTS. Systemic drugs used in dermatology for which liver function test assessment is most important include methotrexate, retinoids, ketoconazole, cytotoxic drugs (azathioprine, cyclophosphamide, and chlorambucil), cyclosporine, and rifampin. Although the risk is less with antimalarials, dapsone, and gold therapy, they necessitate ongoing liver surveillance. There are several histologic patterns of drug-induced liver toxicity:[10,11] hepatocellular toxicity, obstructive pattern, and a combination of these two patterns (mixed). Most dermatologic agents produce a hepatocellular pattern for which monitoring transaminase values is the most important indicator of toxicity. Methotrexate may produce steatosis, in absence of the aforementioned histologic findings.

This may progress to hepatic fibrosis without significant liver function abnormalities. In dapsone syndrome and phenytoin syndrome, a hepatoxic liver injury pattern is accompanied by systemic signs of hypersensitivity, including rash, fever, adenopathy, and eosinophilia.

Most liver function tests do not assess actual liver function but rather are serum values for liver enzymes.[12] Prothrombin time determination and albumin levels are the only true liver function tests that are routinely ordered. Nevertheless, by convention, the phrase *liver function tests* is used in this chapter and throughout the book. Serum transaminases—aspartate aminotransferase, AST (serum glutamate-oxaloacetic transaminase, SGOT) and alanine aminotransferase, ALT (serum glutamate-pyruvate transaminase, SGPT)—are the most useful enzymes. Any elevation of these enzymes deserves attention. However, an elevation higher than twice the upper normal value should lead to discontinuation of the systemic agent, at least on a temporary basis. Toxic hepatitis is often defined as a threefold elevation above the upper normal transaminase value. This is typically accompanied by findings such as abdominal pain, nausea, and malaise. Any significant transaminase elevation that is accompanied by an increased alkaline phosphatase or bilirubin should lead to at least temporary discontinuation of the drug in question. Gamma glutamyl transpeptidase (GGT) testing may enable one to clarify the source of alkaline phosphatase elevation (liver vs. bone). A concomitant elevation of GGT suggests a liver source of alkaline phosphatase. Serum lactate dehydrogenase values are of little benefit in monitoring for hepatotoxicity.

With any abnormality of liver function test results, it is important to exclude other medications, alcohol, and viral hepatitis as possible etiologies. Drug-induced hepatitis represents less than 5% of all cases of hepatitis, and yet it accounts for 25% of fulminant hepatitis or chronic hepatitis cases.[11] The liver function test abnormality typically corrects itself within 2–4 weeks upon discontinuation of the responsible drug. Most cases occur within 1–5 weeks of the onset of the drug. However, the reaction occurs more quickly upon rechallenge. Patients who consume significant amounts of alcohol, are obese, have diabetes mellitus, are taking other hepatotoxic drugs, or whose pretreatment liver function test results are abnormal are probably at increased risk for hepatotoxicity.

RENAL AND BLADDER TOXICITY. Dermatologic drugs that have the greatest risk of renal toxicity are infrequently used in dermatology today. These drugs include cyclosporine, gold, and nonsteroidal anti-inflammatory agents. Methotrexate excretion is altered with significantly impaired renal function in such a way that the drug's hematologic and hepatic toxicities are increased. Methotrexate has no direct renal toxicity itself. The mechanism involved in most drug-induced renal toxicity is either interstitial nephritis or acute tubular necrosis.[13] Bladder mucosal toxicity may occur with cyclophosphamide therapy.

In assessing renal toxicity, one accomplishes maximal sensitivity by performing a blood urea nitrogen (BUN) test and a creatinine test along with a urinalysis (at least dipstick testing for protein, blood, etc.). Creatinine clearance is used to assess patients with significant renal function impairment before treatment with methotrexate. Peripherally related tests of importance include following blood pressure for cyclosporine-treated patients, as well as urine cytology and cystoscopy for cyclophosphamide-treated patients.

Patients at particularly high risk include those with abnormal pretreatment BUN, creatinine, or urinalysis results.[13] Concomitant use of other nephrotoxic drugs with the aforementioned dermatologic agents increases the risk. A large number of conditions can cause acute interstitial nephritis or acute tubular necrosis. Evaluation of these abnormalities is beyond the scope of most dermatologists' practice. Any significant change in renal function or urinalysis should prompt referral to the appropriate internal medicine specialist. Overall, renal toxicity to the systemic drugs discussed in this book has been distinctly uncommon in my experience. If cyclosporine is increasingly used, it will be the primary drug requiring careful attention to renal parameters.

HEMATOLOGIC TOXICITY. Systemic dermatologic agents may be responsible for leukopenia, anemia, thrombocytopenia, and in rare instances, pancytopenia. Drugs that require careful hematologic monitoring include methotrexate, dapsone, azathioprine (and other cytotoxic agents), cyclosporine, azidothymidine, and gold. Although the risk is much less with retinoids, antimalarials, ketoconazole, griseofulvin, and colchicine, all deserve appropriate hematologic surveillance. Specific monitoring guidelines for these drugs can be found in their respective chapters.

LEUKOPENIA. The most common drug-induced hematologic abnormality is leukopenia.[14] Azathioprine induces a relatively predictable dosage-dependent leukopenia, whereas methotrexate and dapsone induce leukopenia in an idiosyncratic fashion. Whether the leukopenia is predictable or idiosyncratic, both types of drugs require careful surveillance. In dermatologic therapy, a white blood cell count less than 4000/cu mm or a neutrophil count less than 1500/cu mm necessitates either dosage reduction or cessation of therapy.[6] Agranulocytosis is defined as less than 500 neutrophils/cu mm.[15] The risk of agranulocytosis from systemic dermatologic therapy is greatest for dapsone-treated patients. It is important to order CBCs for these patients every 1–2 weeks during the first 3 months of therapy. In addition, patients should be instructed to report important symptoms such as fever, rash, and severely sore throat.

THROMBOCYTOPENIA. The next most frequent hematologic abnormality due to drugs is thrombocytopenia.[14] This abnormality has been infrequent in my experience. Drugs most likely to induce thrombocytopenia are uncommonly used dermatologic agents such as heparin, gold, and phenytoin.[16] A platelet count less than 100,000/cu mm, without an alternative explanation, requires cessation of therapy and close surveillance of platelet values.

ANEMIA. Aside from dapsone-induced hemolysis, anemia due to systemic dermatologic agents is distinctly uncommon. Still, treatment with antimalarials, cytotoxic agents, methotrexate, and gold requires surveillance for this possible complication. Sulfonamides and penicillin are rarely used long term in dermatology. However, because of their widespread clinical use in medicine overall, sulfonamides and penicillin are among the 14 drugs that most often cause aplastic anemia.[17]

Any persistent decrease in hemoglobin over 1–2 g/dl deserves further evaluation by the appropriate specialist. Any simultaneous decrease in white blood cell count, platelet, or hemoglobin requires immediate cessation of systemic therapy and prompt evaluation. Fortunately, agranulocytosis and aplastic anemia are extremely uncommon adverse effects of systemic drugs used in dermatology. A reticulocyte count can be used as an adjunct to assess hemolysis in dapsone-treated patients. Baseline screening with G6PD levels is important for dapsone-treated and, perhaps, antimalarial-treated patients. Monitoring methemoglobin levels is occasionally useful for dapsone-treated patients. However, the presence of cyanosis is a reasonable indicator of significant methemoglobin levels in patients without cardiopulmonary compromise.

HYPERLIPIDEMIA. The retinoids are the primary drug category requiring careful surveillance of serum lipids. These drugs can cause both hypertriglyceridemia and, less commonly, hypercholesterolemia. Elevated triglycerides are a relatively common effect of glucocorticosteroid therapy. Drugs uncommonly used in dermatology, such as estrogens and anabolic steroids, may also increase triglyceride values. High-density lipoprotein cholesterol assessment is useful in patients for whom long-term retinoid therapy is considered. Assessment of other coronary artery disease risk factors is also important if long-term retinoid use is planned. Triglyceride and cholesterol values alone can subsequently be used to monitor these patients. It is important to perform these tests after a 12-hour overnight fast and a 36-hour abstinence from alcohol.

Most triglyceride elevations are asymptomatic. However, at values above 800–1000 mg/dl, pancreatitis and eruptive xanthomas are possible. To date, triglyceride elevations have not been conclusively shown to be an independent coronary artery disease risk factor.[18] One should be particularly careful and perform frequent monitoring of patients with triglyceride levels higher than 300 mg/dl and cholesterol values that put the patient at significant risk for atherosclerosis. The trend in these test results is as important as the absolute value. (See Chapter 8 for a more complete discussion on the specific risks from these lipid elevations.)

OCULAR SURVEILLANCE. Several drug categories deserve careful surveillance for ocular adverse effects. Antimalarial and PUVA therapies have well-defined guidelines that are covered in each respective chapter. A less well-defined risk exists for cataracts and glaucoma caused by glucocorticosteroids. Retinoids have a variety of ocular adverse effects, although there are no specific guidelines for routine surveillance. Specific evaluation of troublesome and persistent ocular symptoms is appropriate for retinoid therapy. Cataracts may result from PUVA, from glucocorticosteroids, and less commonly, from retinoids. Glaucoma risk exists primarily with glucocorticosteroids. Retinopathy is a distinct risk of antimalarial therapy.

Specific evaluation for these abnormalities requires ophthalmologic consultation. The clinician should develop a close working relationship with an ophthalmologist well versed in the adverse effects of these agents. It is surprisingly common for one to receive consultation reports that fail to address the specific risks of the drugs just discussed.

Clinicians administering these drugs with potential ocular toxicity should familiarize themselves with the tests commonly performed by ophthalmologists. These include basic tests such as slit-lamp examination, tonometry, Schirmer's test, and visual field testing. More complicated testing such as electroretinogram, dark field adaptation, and fluorescein angiography are of peripheral interest. Portnoy and Callen presented a comprehensive review of these and other specialized tests as they apply to surveillance for antimalarial ocular toxicity.[19]

RADIOLOGIC SURVEILLANCE. Glucocorticosteroid and retinoid treatments require attention to potential bone complications, although neither have well-defined guidelines. Premature epiphyseal closure is a remote risk of retinoid therapy. Growth suppression may occur in children treated with glucocorticosteroids. Osteoporosis and aseptic bone necrosis are primarily risks of glucocorticosteroid therapy. Bone osteophytes and diffuse idiopathic skeletal hyperostosis (DISH) syndrome–like findings are important potential complications of retinoid therapy.

A chest x-ray may be useful in assessing malignancy risk for cytotoxic drugs. Methotrexate-treated patients need chest x-rays only as symptoms suggesting pneumonitis indicate.

In each of these circumstances, careful attention to patients' symptoms is the key aspect of surveillance. When a child receives chronic glucocorticosteroid therapy, it is important to plot the child's growth curve. Performing ankle or thoracic spine x-rays on retinoid-treated patients is considered optional. Of importance is that the condition treated may alter the risk of abnormalities that are due to these agents. Rheumatoid arthritis patients are much more likely than psoriasis patients to have methotrexate-induced pneumonitis. Psoriasis patients may have a number of abnormalities on baseline x-rays that may be mistakenly attributed to retinoid therapy, should baseline films not be obtained.

MALIGNANCY SURVEILLANCE. Systemic dermatologic drugs with an increased risk for malignancy can be subdivided into those that increase the risk of skin cancer and those that increase the risk of lymphoma and other systemic malignancies. Azathioprine (and other cytotoxic drugs), cyclosporine, and PUVA all entail a significantly increased risk of skin cancer, primarily squamous cell carcinoma. An increased incidence of Kaposi's sarcoma exists with azathioprine and cyclosporine treatment. There may be a small risk of Kaposi's sarcoma in prednisone-treated patients. Risk of non-Hodgkin's lymphomas of the B cell type is increased with azathioprine and cyclosporine use. The frequency of both carcinoma in situ of the cervix and renal cell carcinoma increases notably with both of these drugs. Malignancies common in the general population, such as lung, breast, colorectal, prostate, and invasive cervical carcinomas, do not occur more frequently in patients treated with the immunosuppressive agents just mentioned.

Surveillance for malignancy in these patients should be directed primarily at skin cancer and lymphoma. A complete skin examination every 6–12 months is important, particularly for patients who have fair skin, receive excessive sun exposure, and have had previous skin cancers. Particular surveillance in male PUVA-treated patients should be directed at the genitalia, given the increased risk of genital squamous cell carcinoma in these patients.[7] For surveillance of non-Hodgkin's lymphoma, regular examination of major lymph node groups, liver, and spleen is important. Periodic chest x-ray examination may be useful. The possibility of extranodal lymphomas is a particularly troublesome risk of azathioprine and cyclosporine. Laboratory tests and radiologic procedures directed at areas with significant symptoms are in order. Both alkylating agents cyclophosphamide and chlorambucil increase the risk of leukemia. Protocols discussed in chapter 5, including frequent CBCs with white blood cell differential counts, should suffice in screening for leukemia.

Regular Pap smears for women are important for detection of in situ carcinoma of the cervix. Cyclophosphamide-treated patients should be followed with regular urinalysis, urine cytology, and periodic cystoscopy. Cyclosporine-treated patients, who are at risk for renal cell carcinoma, can be followed by regular urinalysis testing as outlined in Chapter 7.

For a complete discussion of malignancy risks from cytotoxic drugs and cyclosporine, refer to chapter 5. Clarification of the risk from low dosages of cyclosporine and azathioprine is still pending. For now, the guidelines just given are reasonable to follow.

EXCLUSION OF PREGNANCY. The greatest risk of teratogenicity exists with use of retinoids by women of childbearing potential. Methotrexate, cytotoxic drugs, and cyclosporine all have important pregnancy-related complications. Tetracycline, glucocorticosteroids, and spironolactone also have notable potential adverse effects when used during pregnancy.

Serum determinations of beta–human chorionic gonadotropin (beta-HCG) levels should be made when a high degree of certainty regarding pregnancy is necessary. A specific protocol for follow-up of patients taking retinoids is outlined in chapter 8. Beta-HCG is detectable in serum as soon as 24 hours after fetal implantation.[20] The test is usually positive the week before the first missed menstrual period. It is important to consider the role of various antibiotics in oral contraceptive failure.[21] This risk is important to consider in the uncommon circumstance of long-term antibiotics used concomitantly with the potentially teratogenic medications just described.

Uncommon Monitoring Issues

Several other clinical findings and laboratory tests are used to monitor for adverse effects from systemic drugs used in dermatology. The risk of hypertension exists primarily in patients treated with cyclosporine and, to a lesser extent, prednisone. Regular blood pressure determinations in these patients are in order. The risk of severe cutaneous drug reactions, such as urticaria with anaphylaxis and erythema multiforme major (Stevens-Johnson syndrome and toxic epidermal necrolysis), mandates early reporting by the patient of any significant cutaneous eruption. The risk of cardiac arrhythmias and need for cardiac monitoring exists primarily with pulse intravenous methylprednisolone treatment. Although cardiac arrhythmias are theoretically a concern with doxepin treatment, dermatologic dosages of this drug rarely require an electrocardiogram as baseline or follow-up.

Periodic determination of electrolytes is necessary in long-term glucocorticosteroid treatment. I have followed electrolytes periodically in spironolactone-treated patients. However, I have not detected any significant abnormalities. Surveillance for serum and urinary calcium levels is important for patients receiving oral vitamin D_3. Finally, laboratory tests for hypothalamic-pituitary-adrenal axis suppression are necessary for many patients receiving long-term, high-dosage glucocorticosteroid treatment. In general, determination of a morning cortisol level just before cessation of long-term therapy is sufficient. High dosages of ketoconazole (800 mg/day or more) may alter cortisol production, although this dosage range is beyond that routinely used in dermatology.

SUMMARY

This book presents a full-spectrum overview of systemic drugs used in dermatology. The list of the conditions that may be treated successfully with these agents is extensive. In many cases, the risk to patients from using these systemic drugs is negligible. For the drugs that have an increased risk of significant adverse effects, the general principles of monitoring for adverse effects are presented in this chapter. For drugs with definable and significant risks, appropriate monitoring guidelines are presented in each specific chapter. Of importance is that use of these guidelines does not eliminate the risk of significant adverse effects. However, these clinical, laboratory, and radiologic guidelines markedly increase the chance that the clinician will detect significant adverse effects at an early, reversible phase.

REFERENCES

1. Roenigk HH Jr, Auerbach R, Maibach H, et al: Methotrexate in psoriasis: Revised guidelines. J Am Acad Dermatol 1988; 19:145–156.
2. Bickers DR: Position paper—PUVA therapy. J Am Acad Dermatol 1983; 8:265–270.
3. Easterbrook M: Ocular effects and safety of antimalarial agents. Am J Med 1988; 85(4A):23–29.
4. Lynch PJ: Dermatologic therapy with systemically administered agents (first of two parts). Prog Dermatol 1983; 17(3):1–8.
5. Lynch PJ: Dermatologic therapy with systemically administered agents (second of two parts). Prog Dermatol 1983; 17(4):1–7.
6. McDonald CT: Use of cytotoxic drugs in dermatologic diseases. J Am Acad Dermatol 1985; 12:965–975.
7. Stern RS and Members of the Photochemotherapy Follow-up Study: Genital tumors among men with psoriasis exposed to psoralens and ultraviolet A radiation (PUVA) and ultraviolet B radiation. N Engl J Med 1990; 322:1093–1097.
8. Speicher CE, Smith JW Jr: Statistical concepts useful in the problem-solving approach. In Speicher CE, Smith JW Jr (eds): Choosing Effective Laboratory Tests. Philadelphia: WB Saunders, 1983, 47–59.
9. Speicher CE: The unexplained test result. In Speicher CE (ed): The Right Test: A Physician's Guide to Laboratory Medicine. Philadelphia: WB Saunders, 1989, 4–6.
10. Read AE: The liver and drugs. In Wright R, Millward-Sadler GH, Albert KGMM, et al (eds): Liver and Biliary Disease (2nd ed). London: Bailliere Tindall, 1985, 1003–1022.
11. Zimmerman HJ, Maddrey WC: Toxic and drug-induced hepatitis. In Schiff L, Schiff ER (eds): Diseases of the Liver (6th ed). Philadelphia: JB Lippincott, 1987, 630–659.
12. Helzberg JH, Spiro HM: "LFTs" test more than the liver [editorial]. JAMA 1986; 256:3006–3007.
13. Grunfeld JP, Kleinknecht D, Droz D: Acute interstitial nephritis. In Schrier RW, Gottschalk CW (eds): Diseases of the Kidney (4th ed). Boston: Little, Brown, 1988, 1461–1473.
14. Lubran MM: Hematologic side effects of drugs. Ann Clin Lab Sci 1989; 19:114–121.
15. Keeling R: Neutropenia and agranulocytosis. In Thorup OA Jr (ed): Fundamentals of Clinical Hematology. Philadelphia: WB Saunders, 1987, 428–431.
16. Bithell TC: Disorders of platelets. In Thorup OA Jr (ed): Fundamentals of Clinical Hematology. Philadelphia: WB Saunders, 1987, 792–819.

17. Quesenberry PJ: Bone marrow failure. In Thorup OA Jr (ed): Fundamentals of Clinical Hematology. Philadelphia: WB Saunders, 1987, 349–357.
18. Brunzell JD, Austin MA: Plasma triglycerides and coronary disease. N Engl J Med 1989; 320:1273–1275.
19. Portnoy JZ, Callen JP: Ophthalmologic aspects of chloroquine and hydroxychloroquine therapy. Int J Dermatol 1983; 22:273–278.
20. Speicher CE: Pregnancy testing. In Speicher CE (ed): The Right Test: A Physician's Guide to Laboratory Medicine. Philadelphia: WB Saunders, 1989, 6–10.
21. Fleischer AB Jr, Resnick SD: The effect of antibiotics on the efficacy of oral contraceptives: A controversy revisited. Arch Dermatol 1989; 125:1562–1564.

17 | Informed Consent for Systemic Drugs Used in Dermatology

Stephen E. Wolverton, M.D.
Marshall B. Kapp, J.D., M.P.H.

Any chapter on the subject of informed consent addresses a panoply of complex historical, ethical, and medicolegal principles. The actual risk of incurring legal liability from failure to inform a patient about the risks of a given procedure or medication is quite small. In addition to legal considerations, this chapter emphasizes the ethical and medical principles from which informed consent derives its meaning. The communication process that constitutes informed consent is emphasized. It is important to realize from the outset that physician-patient communication, and not merely a signature on a form, is the basis of informed consent. In reality, most informed consent in medical practices occurs in the absence of any patient signature on a "consent" form.

This chapter covers the historical evolution of informed consent in the U.S., underlying ethical perspectives, and resulting basic legal principles. In addition, the formal components of informed consent are addressed, and a brief overview of medicolegal risk management in dermatology is presented.

Historical Perspective

Informed consent as it is known today was first initiated in 1767 in English Common Law, which addressed the right to give or withhold permission for medical care.[1] In 1914, Judge Cardozo addressed informed consent in a case of alleged assault and battery by a physician against a patient. He recorded that "every human being of adult years and of sound mind has the right to determine what shall be done with his body."[2] The Nuremberg code, which followed the War Crimes Trials in 1947, was the first major document to spell out and refer to informed consent as a dictum of medical care.[3] The actual term *informed consent* was first used by the courts in 1957.[4]

The "professional standard" for informing patients was first described in 1960 in a landmark malpractice case in Kansas.[5] In 1962, the U.S. Food and Drug Administration (FDA) was authorized to establish and enforce standards to be used by drug investigators.[1] Informed consent was determined to be a central requirement for these studies. The "material risk standard" was first enunciated in 1972 in the *Canterbury v. Spence* case.[5] The professional standard and the material risk standard are explained in detail subsequently in this chapter.

The medicolegal concept of informed consent continues to evolve today. The practitioner is advised to become familiar with the statutes and judicial decisions pertaining to this principle in the state where he or she practices. In addition, practice standards being developed by various specialties will increasingly affect informed consent in the future.

Ethical Perspective

The principle of informed consent reflects the basic ethical responsibility to respect the personal autonomy of the patient.[6] The goal is to have the decision to use a given medication or to undergo a surgical procedure made by the person most directly affected by the consequences of that decision, namely the patient.[7] Ideally, this allows more intelligent and rational decision making.

Several important potential medical benefits can be achieved through truly informed consent.[6] A greater sense of partnership and active mutual participation within the patient-physician relationship may be achieved. Overall, there should be more openness and less authoritarianism in this relationship. Increased compliance and greater assistance from the patient in ongoing surveillance may be achieved. In addition, professional self-scrutiny with respect to medical decisions may be encouraged.

In most cases, thorough provision of information to a patient for a medical decision is good medical practice, is sound legally, and is sound ethically.[6] Ethically, the concept of autonomy embraces the right to receive information and act on it, giving or withholding consent.

Basic Legal Principles

Several important general legal principles need to be understood before the specific components of informed consent are addressed. As stated before, the physician should become familiar with the statutes and judicial precedent directly dealing with informed consent in his or her own jurisdiction.

The physician ultimately has legal responsibility for both the process and the outcome of medical therapy, even though many associated medical personnel may be involved with this therapy.[6] With this principle in mind, ensuring the adequacy of informed consent can never be delegated to medical students or to nurses. In addition, one cannot relegate the informed consent dialogue to a pamphlet or to another source. The aforementioned personnel and information sources can serve important complementary and reinforcement roles in the communication process.

"Express consent" is the explicit communication of consent by words or writing.[6] The greater the risk of the medical intervention, the more advisable it is to obtain express consent. "Implied consent" is more commonly operant in medical interventions. In many situations involving little risk or intrusiveness, the patient's actions may imply concurrence or consent. "Implied consent" is not an exception to the informed consent doctrine but rather is one form of indicating consent.

Litigation based on total lack of consent—namely, unauthorized touching of the patient ("battery")—is distinctly uncommon today.[5] Inadequate explanation of a procedure or of medication risks may constitute negligence. Liability may be incurred for inadequate communication, even in instances when the quality of care and the outcome are otherwise fine.

It is important to address the setting in which informed consent occurs in order to properly delineate the extent of communication and documentation that is necessary. Investigative drug research has rigid guidelines mandated by federal regulations. Detailed consent forms are central to investigative work in the pharmaceutical industry. The legal rules for prescribing FDA-approved medications with significant adverse effects are less clear-cut.[1] As a general principle, the use of an approved drug for an unapproved indication requires more detailed communication in the informed consent process than when the drug is prescribed for FDA-approved indications. The section of this chapter on components of informed consent addresses the adequacy of information presented in greater detail.

A major portion of prescriptions for systemic drugs used in dermatology are actually for unapproved (unlabeled) indications. The approval by the FDA actually constitutes approval for *labeling* by the manufacturer, which thus limits the types of claims that the manufacturer can make in advertising and in package inserts regarding the drug.[8] An FDA indication documents that there is sufficient information presented to them by the pharmaceutical firm to suggest efficacy and safety for the particular indication. If the drug is too risky overall, it is taken off the market. There are many rare diseases for which it is unrealistic to attempt to gather adequate information to obtain a specific FDA indication. It is not economically sound for older, off-patent drugs to receive the investigational scrutiny necessary to get FDA approval for an indication. It is both medically acceptable and legal to use approved drugs for unapproved indications when there are clinical data to support this use. The Federal Food, Drug, and Cosmetics Act clearly states that the FDA has authority to regulate only drugs and not physicians.

In medical and legal terms, the risks of therapy should be proportional to the risks of the disease being treated. Dermatologic conditions such as toxic epidermal necrolysis and pemphigus vulgaris are examples of serious diseases that justify risky treatments.[9] Good medicine sometimes requires the taking of calculated risks with the consent of the patient in order to achieve important medical results.[10] The location of one's practice, whether in an academic setting or in private, may dictate the level of risk from systemic drug therapy that is justifiable. Medications with a very high degree of risk are used more commonly in the academic setting.

Signed informed consent forms usually are legally required only in research protocols.[6] For clinical practice, the Joint Commission on Accreditation of Healthcare Organizations (JCAHO) requires consent forms primarily for surgical procedures. This JCAHO accreditation is a means of qualifying for reimbursement from third-party payers for medical services. The consent form, even if not legally required, documents that at least some communication took place. Aside from the aforementioned surgical settings, the means of documenting that informed consent occurred is secondary in importance to the communication process. The documentation for most systemic drugs used in dermatology requires only chart notations that discussion about medication risks, benefits, limitations, and alternatives occurred. An important exception is the use of isotretinoin by women of childbearing potential, for which pharmaceutical company–provided information packets and informed consent forms are currently the standard of practice.

Components of Informed Consent

There are three important components of informed consent.[7] First, the consent must be "voluntary"; patients should be able to exercise their free power of choice without the intervention of any element of force, fraud, deceit, duress, or other ulterior forms of constraint or coercion. Second, the patient's agreement should be truly "informed." Third, the "competence" of the patient who agrees to a procedure or a medication is essential: It is important to know whether the patient is mentally competent to think rationally about personal medical care.

There exists controversy concerning how much information the physician must communicate to the patient.[7] The professional standard ("reasonable physician" standard, "community" standard, majority rule) is the standard of communication in most jurisdictions. Under this standard, the information that must be presented is what a reasonable, prudent physician would have disclosed under similar circumstances. In a minority of jurisdictions, the material risk standard ("reasonable patient" standard, minority rule, "prudent person" standard) is used to determine the amount of information presented. In this setting, the amount of information that a reasonable patient in the same situation would want and would need to know to make a knowledgeable decision is the basis of risk disclosure. Potential advantages of the material risk standard include enhanced communications, better consumer awareness of health issues, potentially less litigation, and improved quality of medical care.[6] In a few states, a "subjective" or "individual patient" standard is used.[7] Under that standard, instead of an average or a reasonable patient's being the basis of disclosure, the information provided should be what that particular patient would need to know in that particular set of circumstances.

Short of full disclosure of every known risk, the standards just discussed still rely on an individual physician's determination for disclosure of risk according to the severity or frequency of a given risk. The greater the frequency of the risk and, in particular, the greater the severity of the risk, the more important the disclosure of this risk is before the medical intervention.

The following items constitute a brief listing of what information must be included in the informed consent discussion:[7]

1. The diagnosis.
2. The nature and purpose of the proposed intervention (surgical or medical).
   a. Reasonable foreseeable risks that may occur.
   b. Potential benefits of the therapy and the likelihood that these benefits will occur.
   c. Limitations of the proposed intervention.
3. Alternatives to the proposed intervention, including the alternative of no therapy.
4. The physician's advice.
5. Time for questions and clarification.

Systemic Drugs and Informed Consent

Adequate discussion before one prescribes systemic drugs with a significant potential risk for adverse effects can be divided into discussions of the risks of the drug and of the patient's role in surveillance necessary to detect these adverse effects. It is important to educate the patient about the common and serious adverse effects that may occur with the medication. This discussion should include means of detecting the adverse effect, as well as appropriate intervention should any of these adverse effects occur. In addition, the necessity of surveillance measures, including laboratory tests, special examinations, and other tests to monitor the therapy, is important to communicate to the patient. The list of items just given that are needed for informed consent can form the basis for this discussion.

Documentation of physician-patient communication is essential. There is a hierarchy of documentation options that are appropriate for different clinical situations. A patient-signed consent form with a witness's signature is necessary both in investigative drug research and for unusually risky medications.[6] This form should be specific to the drug being studied or prescribed. An alternative to the consent form would be a progress note documenting the informed consent discussion, with a patient's signature under this note. With most systemic drugs used in dermatology, the physician should document that a discussion on risks, benefits, limitations, and alternatives took place. In addition, the notation may include the proposed surveillance for adverse effects. In this scenario, only a physician's signature is necessary on the note in the medical record. With drugs that present minimal risk of adverse effects, chart documentation is generally not essential, although some written notation is advisable.

The witness's signature merely documents that the consent is voluntary and the patient is competent. To so swear, it may not be necessary for the witness to observe the full information presentation. The witness should ideally not be a physician associated with the physician prescribing the medication.

Optimizing Patient Recall

Important issues regarding a patient's assimilation of the information provided about risks of a specific systemic drug include an understanding of this discussion at the time of discussion, as well as long-term memory effects. Various measures can be used to improve the patient's understanding and long-term retention of information. These measures include providing written materials,[11] asking the patient to restate in his or her own words the information just presented,[12] and using multiple channels of communication (verbal and visual).[4] Repetition of key points is also helpful. Material that is organized into categories is more likely to be retained as well.[13]

Information should be provided in as nonpressured and empathetic a way as possible.[6] Discussion should take place in clear, nontechnical, and understandable language. The clinician should consider the values and the sociologic characteristics of a particular patient. The discussion should allow time for questions in an open fashion. Having family members present may aid in the communication process and in long-term retention of information.

Circumstances Not Requiring Informed Consent

An important exception to the principle of informed consent is any condition that requires emergency treatment, such that the condition presents the risk of death or serious disability if the treatment is not given immediately.[14] The principle of "therapeutic privilege" is applicable when, in the physician's opinion, withholding information is in the best interest of a particular patient because disclosure of information would be likely to result in imminent and serious harm to the patient.[1] In addition, risks that are commonly known by the public need not be disclosed.[6] Finally, the "defense of waiver" occurs when the patient voluntarily and knowingly relinquishes the right to informed consent. These circumstances are uncommonly applicable to the use of systemic drugs in dermatology.

A more complicated but relevant area is the process of informed consent for minors.[14] The most prudent principle is to include parents in decisions involving minors regarding any therapy that has a significant potential risk. However, some exceptions exist. An "emancipated minor" is defined as a fully self-supporting person living on his or her own. A "mature minor" is defined as a person, usually 14–15 years of age, or older, with a degree of maturity that renders him or her capable of understanding information and rationally giving consent to nonrisky therapy. In both of these exceptions, minor therapeutic decisions may be made regularly by the physician and the patient in the absence of parental consent. Otherwise, parental participation in therapeutic decisions for which there are significant risks is generally the most conservative, safest approach to take.

Medicolegal Risk Management

Successful lawsuits predicated solely on the failure of the physician to obtain informed consent are quite uncommon.[15] To succeed, a plaintiff would need to establish the following elements:

1. A reasonably foreseeable risk was not disclosed by the physician, and the adverse outcome actually occurred.
2. This "materialized risk" resulted in injury to the patient.
3. The therapy would not have been accepted by the patient if he or she had been adequately informed of the risk.

Most successful malpractice claims involve proof of substandard performance in patient care rather than, or in addition to, proof of lack of informed consent. Nevertheless, reasons beyond legal principles alone dictate the need for informed consent.

Several general provider behaviors and patient characteristics increase the risk of malpractice suits. One study of patient dissatisfaction regarding aesthetic surgery is applicable to systemic dermatologic therapy.[16] Physicians' characteristics such as poor communication, impersonal care, lack of empathetic listening to patients' complaints and concerns, and personality conflicts were all deemed as important factors contributing to patient dissatisfaction. At the same time the physician should be careful in dealing with patients who have unrealistic expectations or who have a psychologic disturbance.[4]

Dermatology Malpractice Studies

Several studies have yielded data addressing the risk of malpractice suits due to adverse effects from systemic drugs used in dermatology. Using data from the period 1963–1973, Altman reviewed dermatologic claims from a single malpractice insurer in the Midwest.[17] Drug reactions represented 32% of the claims and 26% of dollar losses to insurers from these claims. Drugs of particular importance included prednisone and methotrexate, although adverse effects from intramuscular triamcinolone, from antibiotics such as penicillin and tetracycline, and from chloroquine were also responsible for malpractice suits.

Using data from the National Association of Insurance Commissioners' national survey from the period 1975–1978, Altman evaluated dermatologic malpractice claims.[18] Of those claims, 20% involved adverse effects from systemic dermatologic agents; the majority of those involved prednisone and methotrexate. In this study it was determined that dermatology had the 6th lowest number of claims of 23 specialties studied.

More recently, Hollabaugh and colleagues surveyed academic dermatologic programs in the U.S., evaluating malpractice litigation from the 1960s through the 1980s.[19] Of 58 lawsuits reported, 10 involved systemic drugs in dermatologic settings. Adverse effects from glucocorticosteroids, methotrexate, dapsone, and antibiotics (trimethoprim-sulfamethoxazole and tetracycline) were involved.

Overall, 35% to 40% of malpractice suits resulted in indemnity payments to the plaintiff.[17-19] Other important reasons for malpractice litigation in these studies included surgical complications, failure to diagnose malignancy, and phototherapy complications. It is generally agreed that the increasing participation of dermatologists in cosmetic and complicated surgical procedures will increase the risk of malpractice litigation. One can argue that the increasing use of systemic therapy with significant risk of adverse effects may also increase the physician's potential liability.

Summary

Few medical interventions are totally devoid of potential adverse effects and resultant potential for medicolegal liability. There are numerous important clinical indications for systemic drugs used in dermatology from which patients may benefit, albeit with varying degrees of risk. Two important areas of malpractice defense include development of a good physician-patient relationship and familiarity with typical malpractice problems encountered by physicians. Compassionate, open, and empathetic interchange with the patients, although not foolproof, is a critical element of medicolegal risk management. Careful assessment of areas with high medicolegal risks, the undertaking of measures to minimize these risks, and surveillance by patient and physician for early detection of important adverse effects are all critical to optimal use of systemic drugs in dermatology. Thorough understanding and use of the principles of truly informed consent are essential to optimizing the risk-benefit ratio for these drugs.

REFERENCES

1. Friedman D: Informed consent in the difficult patient. Res Staff Phys 1986; 32(1):103–108.
2. Rennie D: Informed consent by "well-nigh abject" adults. N Engl J Med 1980; 302:917–918.
3. Cassileth BR, Zupkis RV, Sutton-Smith K, March V: Informed consent—Why are its goals imperfectly realized? N Engl J Med 1980; 302:896–900.
4. Redden EM, Baker DC: Coping with the complexities of informed consent in dermatologic surgery. J Dermatol Surg Oncol 1984; 10:111–116.
5. Gild WM: Informed consent: A review. Anesth Analg 1989; 68:649–653.
6. Kapp MB: Informed consent and truth telling. In Kapp MB, Bigot A (eds): Geriatrics and the Law: Patient Rights and Professional Responsibilities. New York: Springer-Verlag, 1985, 15–40.
7. Kapp MB: Medical treatment and the physician's legal duties. In Cassel CK, Riesenberg DE, Sorensen LB, et al (eds): Geriatric Medicine (2nd ed). New York: Springer Verlag, 1990, 624–626.
8. Bollet AJ: Approved and unapproved uses of drugs: The meaning of FDA approval. Res Staff Phys 1983; 29(9):29–30.
9. Curran WJ: Informed consent in malpractice cases. A turn towards reality. N Engl J Med 1986; 314:429–431.
10. Weisbard AJ: Defensive law: A new perspective on informed consent. Arch Intern Med 1986; 146:860–861.
11. Denney M, Williamson D, Penn R: Informed consent: Emotional responses of patients. Postgrad Med 1976; 60:205–209.
12. Bertakis K: The communication of information from physician to patient: A method for increasing patient retention and satisfaction. J Fam Pract 1977; 5:217–222.
13. Bradshaw P: Recall of medical advice: Comprehensibility and specificity. Br J Soc Clin Psych 1975; 14:55.
14. Holder AR: Minors' rights to consent to medical care. JAMA 1987; 257:3400–3402.
15. President's commission for the study of ethical problems in medicine and biomedical

and behavioral research; Making health care decisions: The ethical and legal implications of informed consent in the patient-practitioner relationship. U.S. Government Printing Office, 1982; 1, 18–31.
16. MacGregor FC: Patient dissatisfaction with results of technically satisfactory surgery. Aesthetic Plast Surg 1981; 5:27–32.
17. Altman J: Survey of malpractice claims in dermatology. Arch Dermatol 1975; 111:641–644.
18. Altman J: The National Association of Insurance Commissioners (NAIC) Medical Malpractice Closed Claim Study 1975–1978: A review of dermatologic claims. J Am Acad Dermatol 1981; 5:721–725.
19. Hollabaugh ES, Wagner RF, Weedn VW, et al: Patient personal injury litigation against dermatology residency programs in the United States, 1964–1988: Implications for future risk-management programs in dermatology and dermatologic surgery. Arch Dermatol 1990; 126:618–622.

APPENDIX I

Sample Patient Handout: Prednisone Patient Information Summary

- This information summary is applicable to prednisone, as well as to prednisolone, methylprednisolone (Medrol), hydrocortisone, triamcinolone (Kenalog), dexamethasone (Decadron), and related oral drugs.
- There is an imposing list of potential side effects from prednisone. Although patients' awareness of these side effects is important, overconcern and overattention to these possible side effects is potentially disruptive and best avoided.
- Most of the important side effects are due to the prolonged administration (greater than 3–4 weeks) of dosages of at least 10 mg/day of prednisone or its equivalent.

CONTRAINDICATIONS

- Possible contraindications to the use of prednisone include hypertension, congestive heart failure, prior psychosis, recent bowel surgery, active gastric/duodenal ulcers, tuberculosis, systemic fungal infections, diabetes mellitus, markedly elevated triglyceride levels, osteoporosis, cataracts, and pregnancy.

- Notify your physician if you have any of these conditions. In each case, your physician will balance the risk of prednisone use with these conditions against the risk of the dermatologic condition for which prednisone will be used.

SIDE EFFECTS

Minor Side Effects from Short-Term Therapy (2–3 Weeks or Less)

- In the absence of any of the aforementioned contraindications, prednisone therapy for this duration is rarely associated with serious side effects.
- The most common milder side effects include weight gain (from fluid retention or increased appetite), mood swings, mild stomach upset, and with intramuscular injections, menstrual irregularities.
- These side effects are temporary and completely reversible in virtually all patients.

Important Potential Side Effects from Long-Term Therapy

- Marked weight gain associated with fluid retention, leg swelling, and possibly breathing difficulties.
- Blood pressure elevations.
- Severe mood alterations, including euphoria, depression, and psychosis.
- Persistent headache with associated visual change and nausea.
- Persistent or severe abdominal pain.
- Significant fever or chills, or both, possibly with other signs of infection.
- Excessive thirst and urinary frequency or volume, possibly with excessive fatigue.
- Severe or persistent bone, joint, or muscle pain.

   Note: These side effects are uncommon and yet important to report to your physician should they occur.

Other Less Serious Potential Side Effects from Long-Term Therapy

- Acne on the face or trunk.
- Excessive facial hair growth (in women).
- Easy bruising with minimal trauma to skin.
- Reversible hair thinning.

- Weight gain and increased fullness of the face.
- Abscess development or skin atrophy with intramuscular steroid injection.

Side Effects from Rapid Tapering of Prednisone Dose

- Possible side effects during relatively rapid decreases in prednisone dosage with long-term therapy include muscle aches, joint aches, mood swings, headache, and mild fatigue.
- If these symptoms are severe or accompanied by significant nausea and vomiting, marked dizziness with standing, and extreme fatigue, notify your physician as soon as possible.
- In addition, prednisone dosage tapering may allow a significant flare-up of your skin condition.

SPECIAL CIRCUMSTANCES

- With long-term prednisone therapy for *children*, regular measurements of the child's height should be performed and plotted on a growth curve.
- For women at high risk for osteoporosis (postmenopausal women, smokers, thin women, inactive women), special tests for diagnosing osteoporosis may be appropriate with long-term prednisone therapy.
- Supplemental dosages of prednisone (or related drugs) may be necessary if you have been taking long-term prednisone *and* you are to undergo surgery or have a significant medical illness. Always tell your surgeon that you have been taking prednisone (or a related drug).

SUMMARY

- The majority of patients receiving short- or long-term prednisone do *not* experience important or serious side effects. However, early reporting to your physician of the more serious side effects listed earlier is important.
- To maximize drug safety and benefits, follow your physician's dosage instructions precisely. In particular, do not abruptly discontinue prednisone if you have been receiving long-term therapy.

APPENDIX II

Example of a Laboratory Flow Sheet

Diagnosis _____ _____ (Patient Identification Data)

Medication/Dose _____ _____
Date Started _____ _____

DATE								
Hematology								
Hemoglobin								
WBC Count								
Platelets								
Reticulocyte Count								
Liver Function Tests								
AST (SGOT)								
ALT (SGPT)								
Alkaline Phosphatase								
Bilirubin								
LDH								
Renal Function Tests								
BUN								

Appendix II

Creatinine								
Urinalysis								
Lipids								
Triglycerides								
Cholesterol (total)								
HDL Cholesterol								
Misc. Chemistries								
Glucose								
Potassium								
Calcium								
Phosphorus								
Urine Calcium								
Androgens								
DHEA-S								
Testosterone (total)								
Free Testosterone								
Drug/Current Dose								

Periodic Exams (Date Performed)

Eye Exam   _____ _____ _____

                 _____ _____ _____

Liver Biopsy   _____ _____ _____

                 _____ _____ _____

Chest X-Ray   _____ _____ _____

Bone X-Ray   _____ _____ _____

Index

Note: Page numbers in *italics* refer to illustrations; page numbers followed by t refer to tables. Specific diseases are in **boldface**.

Acitretin. See also *Retinoids*.
  absorption/distribution of, 189–190
  for Darier's disease, 195
  for ichthyosis, 196
  for psoriasis, 194
  metabolism/excretion of, 190
  use of, indications for, 192, 193t, 194–199
Acne vulgaris, dapsone for, 255
  erythromycin for, 54
  estrogens for, 335
  glucocorticosteroids associated with, 103
  recalcitrant, glucocorticosteroids for, 97
  retinoids for, 194–195
  spironolactone for, 329–330
  tetracycline for, 49–50
Acquired immunodeficiency syndrome (AIDS), acyclovir for, 4, 6
  Kaposi's sarcoma and, interferon for, 14–15
  zidovudine for, 4, 8–9
ACTH (adrenocorticotropic hormone), 90
ACTH stimulation test, 110
Actinic keratoses, interferon for, 16
  retinoids for, 197
Acyclovir (Zovirax), 1–7
  absorption/distribution of, 1
  adverse effects of, 6–7
  drug interactions with, 7
  mechanism of action of, 2
  metabolism/excretion of, 2
  monitoring guidelines for, 7
  structure of, 1
  use of, contraindications to, 3t
    indications for, 2–6, 3t
    prophylactic, 5
Addison's disease, 108
Adenoma, hepatic, associated with estrogen, 336

Adrenal crisis, 111
Adrenal insufficiency, definitions of, 108
Adrenocorticotropic hormone (ACTH), 90
Agranulocytosis, as complication of dapsone and sulfapyridine therapy, 257–258
Albumin, corticosteroid-binding, 88
Alkalosis, hypokalemic, glucocorticosteroids associated with, 106
Allergic contact dermatitis. See also *Dermatitis, acute*.
  cyclosporine for, 173
Allografts, skin, cyclosporine for, 174–175
Alopecia, androgenetic, female, cimetidine for, 306
  glucocorticosteroids for, 97
  male patttern of, cyclosporine for, 174
Alopecia areata, cimetidine for, 305
  cyclosporine for, 173–174
  PUVA therapy for, 227
9-Alpha fluorohydrocortisone (fludrocortisone, Florinef), 88
Aminopenicillins, 57
4-Aminoquinolines, 266. See also *Antimalarials*.
Amoxicillin, 57
Amoxicillin-potassium clavulanate (Augmentin), 62–64
  adverse effects of, 63–64
  drug interactions with, 64
  pharmacology of, 62–63
  use of, indications and contraindications to, 63
Ampicillin, 57
Amsler recording chart, *278*
Anaerobic infections, antibiotics for, 78
Anaphylaxis, with intravenous cyclosporine, 178

417

Androgen excess syndromes, estrogens for, 335
  glucocorticosteroids for, 97–98
  spironolactone for, 329–330
Androgenetic alopecia, female, cimetidine for, 306
  glucocorticosteroids for, 98
Anemia, drug-induced, 394
  zidovudine-induced, 10
Angioedema, classical H₁ antihistamines for, 292
  hereditary, danazol for, 371–372
Antagonists, calcium. See *Calcium channel blockers.*
Antiandrogen(s), 327–343
  cyproterone as, 339–342
  estrogen and progestin as, 333–339
  less frequently used, 342
  spironolactone as, 328–333
Antibacterial activity, of dapsone and sulfapyridine, 249–250
Antibacterial agent(s), 47–79
  amoxicillin as, 62–64
  aztreonam as, 76
  cephalosporin as, 59–61
  ciprofloxacin as, 70–73
  clindamycin as, 75
  erythromycin as, 52–55
  for anaerobic infections, 78
  for gram-negative folliculitis, 77
  for Lyme borreliosis, 77–78
  for pseudomonas infections, 77
  for staphylococcal infections, 76–77
  for streptococcal infections, 77
  in pregnancy, 78–79
  metronidazole as, 73–75
  penicillin as, 55–59
  rifampin as, 67–70
  tetracycline as, 47–52
  trimethoprim-sulfamethoxazole as, 64–67
  vancomycin as, 75–76
Antifungal agent(s), 25–42
  flucytosine as, 40–41
  griseofulvin as, 25–29
  itraconazole as, 36–38
  ketoconazole as, 29–36
  nystatin as, 41–42
  terbinafine as, 38–40
Antihistamines, 285–316
  development of, and relationship to dermatology, 285–287
  H₁ histamine receptors as, 286, 287–302. See also *H₁ antihistamines.*
  H₂ histamine receptors as, 286, 302–310. See also *H₂ antihistamines.*
  mast cell–stabilizing agents as, 286, 314–316. See also *Mast cell-stabilizing agents.*
  oral dose regimens for, 312t

Antihistamines (Continued)
  tricyclic agents as, 286–287, 310–314. See also *Doxepin.*
Anti-inflammation therapy, antimalarials in, 269
Anti-inflammatory activity, of dapsone and sulfapyridine, 250
Antimalarials, 265–280. See also named antimalarial.
  absorption/distribution of, 266–267
  adverse effect(s) of, 274–278
    acute poisoning as, 275
    cutaneous, 274–275
    ocular toxicity as, 275–278
    systemic, 274
  anti-inflammatory effects of, 269
  antimalarial effects of, 267–268
  dermatologic effects of, 268–270
  DNA interactions with, 268–269
  drug interactions with, 278–279
  immunosuppressive effects of, 269–270
  mechanism of action of, 267–271
    in porphyria cutanea tarda, 270–271
  metabolism/excretion of, 267
  monitoring guidelines for, 277
  structure of, 266, 266t
  sunscreen effects of, 268
  therapeutic guidelines for, 279–280
  use of, contraindications to, 272t
    indications for, 271–273, 272t
Antiplatelet drug(s), vasoactive, 347–360
  aspirin as, 354–356
  calcium channel blockers as, 350–354
  development of, 348
  dipyridamole as, 354–356
  ethylestrenol as, 356–357
  ketanserin as, 358–360
  pathophysiologic background information on, 347–349
  pentoxifylline as, 349–350
  phenformin as, 356–357
  prazosin as, 357–358
Antiviral agent(s), 1–19
  acyclovir as, 1–7
  interferon as, 11–19
  zidovudine as, 7–11
Arotinoids, 199
Arrhythmia, ventricular, glucocorticosteroids associated with, 101
  with interferon, 18
Arsenical keratoses, retinoids for, 197
Arthritis, rheumatoid, chloroquine for, 269–270
  chrysotherapy for, 367
  cytotoxic drugs for, malignancies associated with, 128, 129
Ascites, palliative treatment of, antimalarials in, 273

Aseptic bone necrosis, glucocorticosteroids associated with, 104–105
Aspirin (acetylsalicylic acid), clinical use of, 355–356
 drawback with, 348
 for erythromelalgia, 375–376
 for pruritus, 376
 pharmacology of, 354
Astemizole. See also H_1 antihistamines, less sedating.
 for chronic idiopathic urticaria, 300
 mechanism of action of, 297–299
 metabolism/excretion of, 297
 oral dose regimen for, 312t
Asthma patients, use of H_1 antihistamines in, 294–295
Atopic dermatitis, classical H_1 antihistamines for, 293
 cyclosporine for, 173
 PUVA therapy for, 226
Atrophic papulosis, malignant, aspirin and dipyridamole for, 356
Atrophie blanche (livedoid vasculitis), aspirin and dipyridamole for, 355
 nifedipine for, 353
 pentoxifylline for, 350
Auranofin, pharmacology of, 366
Aurothioglucose, pharmacology of, 366–367
Aurothiomalate, pharmacology of, 366–367
Axon damage, dapsone-induced, 259
Azathioprine (Imuran), 130–135
 absorption/distribution of, 130–131
 adverse effects of, 134–135
 dosage guidelines for, 133
 drug interactions of, 135
 mechanism of action of, 131
 metabolism/excretion of, 131
 monitoring guidelines for, 134
 structure of, 130
 use of, contraindications to, 132t
 indications for, 131, 132t, 133
Aztreonam (Azactam), 76

B cells, effect of glucocorticosteroids on, 91–92
Bacterial infection(s), antibiotics for, 76–78
Basal cell carcinoma, interferon for, 15
 retinoids for, 197
Basal cell nevus syndrome, retinoids for, 197
Bath PUVA therapy. See also *Psoralens plus ultraviolet A (PUVA) therapy*.
 for psoriasis, 234
Behçet's disease, colchicine for, 365
 cyclosporine for, 172
Beta-carotene, 188
Betamethasone, 88

Betamethasone *(Continued)*
 pharmacology of, 89t
Biopsy, liver, prior to methotrexate therapy, 161–163, 162t
Bladder toxicity, cyclophosphamide-induced, 138
 drug-induced, 392–393
Blastomycosis, ketoconazole for, 33
Blood, adverse effects of classical H_1 antihistamines on, 294
 adverse effects of dapsone on, 257–258
 adverse effects of doxepin on, 313
 adverse effects of H_2 antihistamines on, 307
 adverse effects of sulfapyridine on, 257–258
 adverse effects of trimethoprim-sulfamethoxazole on, 67
Blood lipids, adverse effects of retinoids on, 202–203
Bone, adverse effects of retinoids on, 201–202
Bone marrow toxicity, methotrexate-induced, 160
 zidovudine-induced, 10
Bone necrosis, aseptic, glucocorticosteroids associated with, 104–105
Borreliosis, Lyme, antibiotics for, 77–78
Bowen's disease, retinoids for, 197
Breast-feeding, use of doxepin during, 314
 use of H_1 antihistamines during, 295
 use of H_2 antihistamines during, 309
 use of spironolactone during, 332
Bullous dermatosis, associated with systemic lupus erythematosus, dapsone and sulfapyridine for, 253
 chronic, of childhood, dapsone and sulfapyridine for, 253
Bullous pemphigoid, azothioprine for, 132t
 cyclophosphamide for, 137t
 cyclosporine for, 171
 dapsone and sulfapyridine for, 253–254
 erythromycin for, 54
 glucocorticosteroids for, 94
 methotrexate for, 158
 nicotinamide for, 374
 PUVA-induced, 231
 tetracycline for, 50

Calcitriol (vitamin D), 377–378
Calcium antagonists. See *Calcium channel blockers*.
Calcium channel blockers, 350–354
 clinical use of, 351–354
 pharmacology of, 351, 351t
Calcium metabolism, glucocorticosteroids and, 91
Cancer. See also *Malignancy*.

Cancer *(Continued)*
  skin, PUVA-induced, 229–230
Candida albicans, 9
Candidiasis, chronic mucocutaneous,
    ketoconazole for, 32
  cimetidine for, 305
  cutaneous, ketoconazole for, 33
  nystatin for, 42
Canrenone, 328–329
Carbohydrate metabolism, adverse effects
    of estrogen on, 335
Carcinogenicity, of cyclophosphamide, 138
  of cytotoxic drugs, 134
  of spironolactone, 331–332
Carcinoma, basal cell, interferon for, 15
  squamous cell. See *Squamous cell carcinoma.*
Cardiovascular system, adverse effects of
    doxepin on, 313
  adverse effects of estrogen on, 335–336
  adverse effects of glucocorticosteroids
    on, 101
  adverse effects of H_2 antihistamines on,
    307
Cataracts, glucocorticosteroids associated
    with, 107
  PUVA-induced, 228–229
Cefaclor, 60
Cefadroxil, 60
Ceftriaxone, 60
Central nervous system, adverse effects of
    glucocorticosteroids on, 101–102
  adverse effects of retinoids on, 204
Cephalosporins, 59–61
  absorption/distribution of, 60
  adverse effects of, 61
  drug interactions with, 61
  mechanism of action of, 60
  metabolism/excretion of, 60
  structure of, 59
  use of, contraindications to, 61
    indications for, 60–61
Cephalosporium acremonium, 59
Cheilitis, retinoids associated with, 204
Chickenpox (varicella), acyclovir for, 5
  interferon for, 17
Chilblains (chronic idiopathic perniosis),
    nifedipine for, 352
Children, chronic bullous dermatosis in,
    dapsone and sulfapyridine for, 253
  impaired growth in, glucocorticosteroids
    associated with, 102
  long-term prednisone therapy for, 413
Chlamydia trachomatis, 53, 66
Chloasma (melasma), with estrogen, 336
Chlorambucil (Leukeran), 140–142
  adverse effects of, 141
  drug interactions with, 142
  mechanism of action of, 140
  monitoring guidelines for, 142

Chlorambucil (Leukeran) *(Continued)*
  pharmacology of, 140
  use of, contraindications to, 141t
    indications for, 140, 141t
Chloroquine, anti-inflammmatory effects
    of, 269
  drug interactions with, 278–279
  for porphyria cutanea tarda, 280
  immunosuppressive effects of, 269–270
  interaction of DNA with, 268–269
  metabolism/excretion of, 267
  structure of, 266t
  sunscreen effects of, 268
  therapeutic guidelines for, 279
Chromomycosis, ketoconazole for, 33
Chronic idiopathic perniosis (chilblains),
    nifedipine for, 352
Chronic idiopathic urticaria, classical H_1
    antihistamines for, 292
  doxepin for, 311
  H_2 antihistamines for, 304–305
  less sedating H_1 antihistamines for, 300
Chrysotherapy, adverse reactions of, 368
  clinical use of, 367–369
  contraindications to, 369
  pharmacology of, 366–367
Cicatricial pemphigoid, azathioprine for,
    132t
  cyclophosphamide for, 137t
  dapsone for, 254
  glucocorticosteroids for, 94–95
Ciliary body, adverse effects of
    antimalarials on, 276
Cimetidine (Tagamet), 302, 342. See also
    H_2 *antihistamines.*
  for chronic idiopathic urticaria, 304–305
  for immunomodulation, 305–306
  mechanism of action of, 303
  oral dose regimen for, 312t
Ciprofloxacin (Cipro), 70–73
  adverse effects of, 72
  drug interactions with, 72–73
  pharmacology of, 70–71
  use of, contraindications to, 72
    indications for, 71–72
Classical H_1 antihistamines. See H_1
    antihistamines, classical.
Clavulanic acid, adverse effects of, 63–64
  pharmacology of, 62–63
  use of, indications and contraindications
    to, 63
Clindamycin (Cleocin), 75
Clostridium difficile infection,
    erythromycin associated with, 54
Colchicine, clinical use of, 365–366
  dosage of, 365
  pharmacology of, 364–365
Colchicum autumnale, 364
Cold urticaria, classical H_1 antihistamines
    for, 293

Index   421

Cold urticaria *(Continued)*
  doxepin for, 311
Condylomata acuminata (genital warts),
  interferon for, 13–14
Conjunctivitis, retinoids associated with, 200
Connective tissue diseases, cytotoxic drugs
  for, malignancies associated with, 128
Consent, express, 402
  informed. See *Informed consent*.
Contact dermatitis, allergic, cyclosporine
  for, 173. See also *Dermatitis, acute*.
Contraceptives, oral, monophasic, 338t
Cornea, adverse effects of antimalarials on, 276
Corticotropin-releasing factor (CRF), 90, 109
Cortisone, pharmacology of, 89t
  structure of, 87
CREST syndrome, ketanserin for, 359
CRF (corticotropin-releasing factor), 90, 109
Cromolyn (sodium cromoglycolate), 286, 314–315
Cutaneous candidiasis, ketoconazole for, 33
Cutaneous diseases, malignant, retinoids
  for, 197–198
  premalignant, retinoids for, 197
Cutaneous infections, amoxicillin-
  clavulanic acid for, 63
  cephalosporins for, 60–61
  ciprofloxacin for, 71–72
  dermatophyte, griseofulvin for, 28
  erythromycin for, 53–54
  rifampin for, 69
  trimethoprim-sulfamethoxazole for, 66
Cutaneous leiomyomas, nifedipine for, 353–354
Cutaneous T cell lymphoma, cyclosporine
  for, 173
  interferon for, 16
  PUVA therapy for, 226
  retinoids for, 197–198
Cyclophosphamide (Cytoxan), 135–139
  adverse effects of, 138–139
  dosage guidelines for, 136–138
  drug interactions with, 139
  mechanism of action of, 136
  monitoring guidelines for, 139
  pharmacology of, 136
  use of, contraindications to, 137t
  indications for, 136–138, 137t
Cyclosporine, 167–180
  absorption/distribution of, 168
  adverse effects of, 177, 179–180
  drug interactions with, 179
  mechanism of action of, 168–169
  metabolism/excretion of, 168
  monitoring guidelines for, 178

Cyclosporine *(Continued)*
  structure of, 167–168
  use of, contraindications to, 170t
  indications for, 169–175, 170t
Cyclosporine A. See *Cyclosporine*.
Cylindrocarpon lucidum, cyclosporine
  isolated from, 167
Cyproheptadine hydrochloride, oral dose
  regimen for, 312t
Cyproterone acetate, 339–342
  adverse effects of, 341
  mechanism of action of, 340
  pharmacology of, 340
  therapeutic guidelines for, 341–342
  use of, contraindications to, 341
  indications for, 340–341
  warnings concerning, 341
Cytotoxic agent(s), 125–144
  azathioprine as, 130–135
  chlorambucil as, 140–142
  cyclophosphamide as, 135–139
  fluorouracil as, 143
  hydroxyurea as, 143–144
  malignancy risks from, 126–130
  melphalan as, 143
  mercaptopurine as, 142
  vinblastine as, 143

Danazol, adverse effects of, 372
  clinical use of, 371–372
  pharmacology of, 371
Dapsone, 247–261
  absorption/distribution of, 248–249
  adverse effects of, 256–259
  antibacterial activity of, 249–250
  anti-inflammatory activity of, 250
  development of, 247
  drug interactions with, 259–260
  mechanism of action of, 249–250
  metabolism/excretion of, 249
  monitoring guidelines for, 260
  structure of, 248
  use of, contraindications to, 251t
  indications for, 250, 251t, 252–256
  warnings with, 259
Dapsone hypersensitivity syndrome, 258–259
Darier's disease, retinoids for, 195–196
"Defense of waiver," 406
Degos's disease, aspirin and dipyridamole
  for, 356
Deoxyribonucleic acid (DNA), effect of
  PUVA therapy on, 222–223
  interaction of, with antimalarials, 268–269
Depression, glucocorticosteroids associated
  with, 102

Dermatitis, acute, glucocorticosteroids for, 96–97
  allergic contact, cyclosporine for, 173
  antimalarial-induced, 274
  atopic, cyclosporine for, 173
    PUVA therapy for, 226
  seborrheic, ketoconazole for, 34
Dermatitis herpetiformis, dapsone for, 250, 252
  sulfapyridine for, 252
Dermatology malpractice studies, 407
Dermatomyositis, azathioprine for, 132t
  cyclophosphamide for, 137t
  cyclosporine for, 171
  glucocorticosteroids for, 96
  methotrexate for, 158–159
Dermatophyte infections, cutaneous, griseofulvin for, 28
  recalcitrant, ketoconazole for, 33
  resistant, cimetidine for, 305
Dermatoses, AIDS-associated, zidovudine for, 9–10
  chronic bullous, of childhood, dapsone and sulfapyridine for, 253
  granulomatous, antimalarials for, 273
  life-threatening, azathioprine for, 133
    cyclophosphamide for, 138
  photosensitivity, antimalarials for, 273
  subcorneal pustular, dapsone and sulfapyridine for, 253
Dermographism, classical H_1 antihistamines for, 293
  H_2 antihistamines for, 305
Dexamethasone, 88, 342
  for androgen excess syndromes, 97
  pharmacology of, 89t
Diabetes mellitus, glucocorticosteroids associated with, 104
Diarrhea, acyclovir-induced, 6
  gold-induced, 368
Diasone (sulfoxone sodium), 248. See also *Dapsone.*
Dicloxacillin, 57
Diltiazem, pharmacology of, 351, 351t
Diphenhydramine hydrochloride, oral dose regimen for, 312t
Dipyridamole (Persantine), clinical use of, 355–356
  pharmacology of, 354
Discoid lupus erythematosus, antimalarials for, 271
  chrysotherapy (gold) for, 367
  glucocorticosteroids for, 96
  retinoids for, 198
Diuretic, spironolactone as, 329
Doxepin, 286–287, 310–314. See also *Antihistamines.*
  adverse effects of, 312–313
  drug interactions of, 314
  oral dose regimen for, 312t

Doxepin *(Continued)*
  pharmacology of, 310
  use of, contraindications to, 311t
    indications for, 310–312, 311t
  warnings concerning, 313–314
Drug(s). See also specific drug.
  adverse effect(s) of, 389–391
    anemia as, 394
    approach to monitoring for, 385–398
    baseline testing in, 388
    bladder tocxicity as, 392–393
    clinical signs and symptoms of, monitoring of, 387–388
    exclusion of pregnancy in, 397
    follow-up testing in, 388–389
    general principles in, 385–391
    hematologic toxicity as, 393
    hyperlipidemia as, 394–395
    laboratory tests for, monitoring of, 388–391
    leukopenia as, 393
    liver function tests and, 391–392
    malignancy surveillance in, 396–397
    monitoring guidelines and, sources of, 386
    monitoring issues in, uncommon, 397
    ocular surveillance in, 395
    patient involvement in decision process and, 387
    radiologic surveillance in, 395–396
    recording results in, 389
    renal tocxicity as, 392–393
    risk of, 386
    specific, 391–397
    statistical principles in, 390–391
    thrombocytopenia as, 394
  old, new uses for, 364–378
  systemic, use of, informed consent for, 400–408. See also *Informed consent.*
Dry skin, retinoids associated with, 204
Dysplasia, epidermal, retinoids for, 197
Dyspnea, gold-induced, 368

Eczema herpeticum, acyclovir for, 4
Emancipated minor, defined, 406
Endocrine system, adverse effects of estrogen on, 335
  adverse effects of glucocorticosteroids on, 102
  adverse effects of H_2 antihistamines on, 308
  adverse effects of spironolactone on, 331
Enterocolitis, gold-induced, 368
Epidermal dysplasia, retinoids for, 197
Epidermal nevus(i), retinoids for, 196–197
Epidermodysplasia verruciformis, retinoids for, 197

Epidermolysis bullosa acquisita,
  cyclosporine for, 171
  glucocorticosteroids for, 94t
Epstein-Barr virus, cyclosporine associated with, 176
Erythema, PUVA-induced, 227
Erythema elevatum diutinum, dapsone for, 254
Erythema multiforme, acyclovir for, 4–5
  glucocorticosteroids for, 95
  potassium iodide for, 370
Erythema nodosum, colchicine for, 365
  indomethacin for, 375
  potassium iodide for, 370
Erythema nodosum leprosum,
  cyclosporine for, 175
Erythromelalgia, aspirin for, 375–376
Erythromycin, 52–55
  absorption/distribution of, 52–53
  adverse effects of, 54
  drug interactions with, 54–55
  mechanism of action of, 53
  metabolism/excretion of, 53
  structure of, 52
  use of, contraindications to, 54
  indications for, 53–54
Escherichia coli, 11
Esters, retinyl, 188
Estradiol, 333. See also *Estrogen(s)*.
Estriol, 333. See also *Estrogen(s)*.
Estrogen(s), 333–339
  absorption/distribution of, 333–334
  adverse effects of, 335–336
  drug interactions with, 337
  mechanism of action of, 334
  metabolism/excretion of, 334
  monitoring guidelines for, 337
  oral conjugated, 338–339, 339t
  structure of, 333
  therapeutic guidelines for, 337–339, 338t, 339t
  use of, contraindications to, 335
  indications for, 334–335
  warnings concerning, 336–337
Estrone, 333. See also *Estrogen(s)*.
Ethylestrenol, 356–357
Etretinate. See also *Retinoids*.
  absorption/distribution of, 189–190
  for Darier's disease, 195
  for ichthyosis, 196
  for lichen planus, 198
  for lupus erythematosus, 198
  for psoriasis, 194
  indications for, 192, 193t, 194–199
  metabolism/excretion of, 190
Excoriations, neurotic, doxepin for, 312
Express consent, 402
Eyes, adverse effects of antimalarials on, 275–278

Eyes (Continued)
  adverse effects of glucocorticosteroids on, 106
  adverse effects of H_2 antihistamines on, 308
  adverse effects of PUVA therapy on, 228–229
  adverse effects of retinoids on, 200–201
  surveillance of, for adverse drug effects, 395

Fibrinolytic therapy, 348. See also *Antiplatelet drug(s)*.
"First-dose phenomenon," prazosin causing, 357–358
Flucytosine (Ancobon), clinical use of, 40–41
  pharmacology of, 40
Fludrocortisone (9–alpha fluorohydrocortisone), 88
Fluid retention, glucocorticosteroids associated with, 101
Fluorouracil (Adrucil), 143
Folliculitis, gram-negative, antibiotics for, 77
  Pityrosporum-induced, ketoconazole for, 34
Freckling, PUVA-induced, 230–231

Gastrointestinal tract, adverse effects of antimalarials on, 274
  adverse effects of azathioprine on, 135
  adverse effects of classical H_1 antihistamines on, 294
  adverse effects of cyclosporine on, 177
  adverse effects of estrogen on, 336
  adverse effects of glucocorticosteroids on, 102–103
  adverse effects of H_2 antihistamines on, 306
  adverse effects of methotrexate on, 159
  adverse effects of tetracycline on, 50
  adverse effects of trimethoprim-sulfamethoxazole on, 66
Genital warts (condylomata acuminata),
  interferon for, 13–14
Gingival hypertrophy, cyclosporine associated with, 178
  phenytoin associated with, 375
Glaucoma, glucocorticosteroids associated with, 106
Glucocorticoid, glucocorticosteroids and, 91
Glucocorticosteroids, 86–116
  absorption/distribution of, 88–89
  adverse effects of, 100–107

Glucocorticosteroids *(Continued)*
  in pregnant patients, 106–107
  to cardiovascular system, 101
  to endocrine system, 102
  to eyes, 106
  to gastrointestinal system, 102–103
  to hematologic system, 106
  to immunologic system, 103–104
  to kidneys, 106
  to metabolic system, 104
  to musculoskeletal system, 104–105
  to nervous system, 101–102
  to skin, 102
 drug interactions with, 112
 for acute dermatitis, 96–97
 for androgen excess syndromes, 97–98
 for bullous pemphigoid, 94
 for cicatricial pemphigoid, 94–95
 for dermatomyositis, 96
 for erythema multiforme, 95
 for lichen planus, 97
 for lupus erythematosus, 95
 for pemphigus vulgaris, 93–94
 for post-herpetic neuralgia, 98
 for pyoderma gangrenosum, 96
 for sarcoidosis, 97
 for vasculitis, 96
 HPA axis suppression by, 107–110
 intramuscular administration of, 98–99
 mechanism of action of, 90–92
 metabolism/excretion of, 89t, 89–90
 monitoring guidelines for, 111
 pulse intravenous administration of, 100
 structure of, 87, 87–88
 therapeutic guideline(s) for, 112–116
  acute dosage options in, 112–113
  alternate-day therapy in, 115–116
  formulation choice in, 113–114
  individual risk-benefit analysis in, 112
  patient involvement in, 116
  pediatric dosage range in, 113
  tapering principles in, 114–115
 use of, contraindications to, 93t
  indications for, 93–100, 93t
Goiter, iodide, associated with potassium iodide, 370–371
Gold therapy, adverse reactions to, 368
 clinical use of, 367–369
 contraindications to, 369
 pharmacology of, 366–367
Granuloma annulare, antimalarials for, 273
 dapsone for, 251t
 nicotinamide for 374
 potassium iodide for, 370
Granuloma faciale, dapsone for, 254–255
Granulomatosis, Wegener's, cyclophosphamide for, 138
Granulomatous dermatoses, antimalarials for, 273

Griseofulvin, 25–29
 absorption/distribution of, 25
 adverse effects of, 28–29
 drug interactions with, 29
 mechanism of action of, 26
 metabolism/excretion of, 26
 monitoring guidelines for, 29
 use of, contraindications to, 26t
  indications for, 26t, 26–28
Growth, impaired, glucocorticosteroids associated with, 102
Gynecomastia, ketoconazole-induced, 35–36

H_1 antihistamines, classical, 286, 287–296
  absorption/distribution of, 287–288
  adverse effects of, 293–294
  anticholinergic effects of, 294
  drug interactions with, 296
  mechanism of action of, 288–291
  metabolism/excretion of, 288
  pharmacodynamics of, 289–290
  side effects of, tolerance to, 290–291
  structure of, 287, 287t
  use of, contraindications to, 291t
   indications for, 291t, 291–293
  warnings concerning, 294–295
 less sedating, 296–302
  absorption/distribution of, 296–297
  adverse effects of, 301
  drug interactions with, 302
  mechanism of action of, 297–299
  metabolism/excretion of, 297
  pharmacodynamics of, 298–299
  structure of, 296
  use of, contraindications to, 299t
   indications for, 299t, 299–300
  tolerance to, 299
  warnings concerning, 302
H_2 antihistamines, 286, 302–310
 absorption/distribution of, 302
 adverse effects of, 306–307
 drug interactions with, 309–310
 mechanism of action of, 303
 metabolism/excretion of, 302–303
 structure of, 302
 use of, contraindications to, 304t
  indications for, 303–306, 304t
 warnings concerning, 308–309
Haemophilus ducreyi, 72
Haemophilus influenzae, 57
Hailey-Hailey disease, dapsone for, 254
Hair, adverse effects of retinoids on, 205
Headaches, acyclovir associated with, 6
 retinoids associated with, 204
Healing, wound, glucocorticosteroids and, 91, 102

Helper T cells, inhibited by cyclosporine, 169
Hematologic system, adverse effects of azathioprine on, 134–135
  adverse effects of glucocorticosteroids on, 106
  adverse effects of methotrexate on, 159
Hematologic toxicity, cyclophosphamide-induced, 138
  drug-induced, 393
Hemolysis, as complication of dapsone and sulfapyridine therapy, 257
Hepatic adenoma, with estrogen, 336
Hepatotoxicity, cyclosporine-induced, 177
  dapsone-induced, 259
  drug-induced, 391–392
  ketoconazole-induced, 34–35
  methotrexate-induced, 158
  retinoid-induced, 203
  rifampin-induced, 69
Hereditary angioedema, danazol for, 371–372
Herpes genitalis, acyclovir for, 2–4
  cimetidine for, 305
Herpes labialis, acyclovir for, 4
Herpes simplex infection(s), acyclovir for, 2–5, 3t
  cimetidine for, 305
  interferon for, 17–18
Herpes simplex keratitis, glucocorticosteroids associated with, 106
Herpes zoster infection(s), acyclovir for, 5
  interferon for, 17
Hidradenitis suppurativa, retinoids for, 195
Hirsutism, cimetidine for, 306
  estrogens for, 335
  glucocorticosteroids for, 97
  spironolactone for, 329–330
Histoplasma duboisii, 31
Hydrocortisone (cortisol), pharmacology of, 89t
  structure of, 87, 87–88
Hydroxychloroquine, 265–266
  drug interactions with, 278–279
  for porphyria cutanea tarda, 280
  interaction of DNA with, 268–269
  metabolism/excretion of, 267
  structure of, 266t
  therapeutic guidelines for, 279
Hydroxyurea (Hydrea), 143–144
Hydroxyzine hydrochloride, oral dose regimen for, 312t
Hyperlipidemia, drug-induced, 394–395
  due to retinoid therapy, 202
Hyperpigmentation, antimalarial-induced, 274
Hyperpigmented macules, PUVA-induced, 230–231

Hypersensitivity, to penicillins, 58
Hypertension, cyclosporine associated with, 176
  glucocorticosteroids associated with, 101
Hypertrichosis, reversible, cyclosporine associated with, 178
Hypertrophy, gingival, cyclosporine associated with, 178
Hypokalemic alkalosis, glucocorticosteroids associated with, 106
Hypotension, with interferon, 18
Hypothalamic-pituitary-adrenal (HPA) axis function, normal, 90
Hypothalamic-pituitary-adrenal (HPA) axis stress response, 108–109
Hypothalamic-pituitary-adrenal (HPA) axis suppression, 107–110
  overview of, 107–108
Hypothalamic-pituitary-adrenal (HPA) axis tests, 109–110

Ichthyosis, retinoids for, 196
Ichthyosis vulgaris, cyclosporine for, 175
Immune response, cyclosporine influence on, 168–169
Immune system, adverse effects of PUVA therapy on, 231
Immunologic disorders, methotrexate for, 157–158
Immunologic system, adverse effects of glucocorticosteroids on, 103–104
Immunomodulation, H_2 antihistamines for, 305–306
Immunosuppression therapy, antimalarials in, 269–270
Indomethacin, for erythema nodosum, 375
Infection(s). See specific type.
Infectious diseases, dapsone for, 255–256
  trimethoprim for, 256
Inflammation, PUVA therapy producing, 223
nformed consent, basic legal principles and, 401–403
  circumstances not requiring, 406
  components of, 403–404
  ethical perspective on, 401
  for minors, 406
  for use of systemic drugs, 400–408
  historical perspective on, 400–401
  malpractice studies and, 407
  medicolegal risk management and, 406–407
  optimizing patient recall and, 405–406
Informed consent forms, signed, 403
Insulin hypoglycemia test, 109–110
Interferon (Roferon-A, Intron A, Alferon-N), 11–19

Interferon (Continued)
  absorption/distribution of, 11
  adverse effects of, 18
  drug interactions with, 19
  mechanism of action of, 11–12
  metabolism/excretion of, 11
  monitoring guidelines for, 19
  structure of, 11
  use of, contraindications to, 14t
    indications for, 12–18, 14t
  warnings concerning, 19
Intestinal perforation, glucocorticosteroids associated with, 102–103
Intoxication, chronic, with prolonged colchicine therapy, 366
Intramuscular administration, of glucocorticosteroids, 99–100
Isotretinoin, 188. See also Retinoids.
  absorption/distribution of, 189–190
  for acne, 194–195
  for Darier's disease, 195–196
  for lichen planus, 198
  for lupus erythematosus, 198
  for pityriasis rubra pilaris, 196
  for syndromes with increased risk of cutaneous malignancy, 197
  metabolism/excretion of, 190
  use of, indications for, 192, 193t, 194–199
Isoxazolyl penicillins, 57
Itraconazole (Sporonox), 36–38
  absorption/distribution of, 36–37
  clinical use of, 37–38
  metabolism/excretion of, 37

Jaundice, cholestatic, dapsone-induced, 259

Kaposi's sarcoma, acyclovir for, 9
  cyclosporine associated with, 176
  cytotoxic drug–induced, 128
  interferon for, 14–15
Keloids, interferon for, 16
Keratitis, gold-induced, 368
  herpes simplex, glucocorticosteroids associated with, 106
Keratoacanthoma, retinoids for, 197
Keratoderma, retinoids for, 196–197
Keratoderma hereditaria mutilans, retinoids for, 197
Keratoses, actinic, interferon for, 16
  retinoids for, 197
Ketanserin, 358–360
Ketoconazole (Nizoral), 29–36, 342
  absorption/distribution of, 30
  adverse effects of, 34–36

Ketoconazole (Continued)
  drug interactions with, 36
  mechanism of action of, 31
  metabolism/excretion of, 31
  monitoring guidelines for, 35
  structure of, 30
  use of, contraindications to, 32t
    indications for, 31–34, 32t
Ketotifen, 286, 315–316
Kidney(s). See also Renal toxicity.
  adverse effects of glucocorticosteroids on, 106
  adverse effects of H_2 antihistamines on, 307–308
  adverse effects of methotrexate on, 159
Koebner's phenomenon, 234

Laboratory flow sheet, example of, 415–416
Laboratory tests, alteration of, estrogen and, 336
  monitoring of, in adverse effects from systemic drugs, 388–391
Lactation. See Breast-feeding.
Leiomyomas, cutaneous, nifedipine for, 353–354
Leishmania tropica infection, dapsone for, 255
Lentigines, PUVA-induced, 231
Lentigo maligna, PUVA-induced, 230
Leprosy, dapsone for, 252
Less sedating H_1 antihistamines. See H_1 antihistamines, less sedating.
Leukocytoclastic vasculitis, azathioprine for, 132t
  colchicine for, 365
  cyclophosphamide for, 137t
  dapsone for, 255
  glucocorticosteroids for, 97
Leukopenia, drug-induced, 393
Leukoplakia, oral hairy, acyclovir for, 10
Leuprolide acetate (Lupron), 342
Libido, control of, cyproterone acetate for, 341
Lichen planus, cyclosporine for, 171
  glucocorticosteroids for, 97
  griseofulvin for, 28
  PUVA therapy for, 226
  retinoids for, 198
Linear immunoglobulin A, bullous dermatosis, dapsone and sulfapyridine for, 253
Lipid metabolism, adverse effects of estrogen on, 335
Lipids, blood, adverse effects of retinoids on, 202–203
Livedoid vasculitis. See Atrophie blanche (livedoid vasculitis).

Liver, adverse effects of doxepin on, 313
    adverse effects of H_2 antihistamines on, 307
    adverse effects of less sedating H_1 antihistamines on, 301
    adverse effects of methotrexate on, 158
    adverse effects of retinoids on, 203–204
    adverse effects of rifampin on, 69
Liver biopsy, prior to methotrexate therapy, 161–163, 162t
Liver function tests, 391–392
Loratadine. See also H_1 antihistamines, less sedating.
    mechanism of action of, 297–299
    metabolism/excretion of, 297
Lung(s), adverse effects of methotrexate on, 159–160
Lupus erythematosus, antimalarials for, 271–272
    azathioprine for, 132t
    cyclophosphamide for, 137t
    cyclosporine for, 171–172
    discoid, chrysotherapy (gold) for, 367
    glucocorticosteroids for, 95
    PUVA-induced, 231
    retinoids for, 198
    systemic, bullous dermatosis associated with, dapsone and sulfapyridine for, 253
Lyme disease, antibiotics for, 77–78
    penicillin V for, 57
    tetracycline for, 49
Lymphocutaneous sporotrichosis. See also Sporotrichosis.
    potassium iodide for, 369–370
Lymphocytes, effect of glucocorticosteroids on, 91–92
    suppression of, PUVA-induced, 231
Lymphoma, cutaneous T cell. See Cutaneous T cell lymphoma.
    cyclosporine associated with, 176
    non-Hodgkin's, cytotoxic drug–induced, 128

Macules, pigmented, PUVA-induced, 230–231
Mal de Meleda, retinoids for, 197
Malignancy, cutaneous, syndromes with increased risk of, retinoids for, 197–198
    cyclosporine associated with, 176
    cytotoxic drug–induced, connective tissue disease studies in, 128
        drug comparisons and, 128–129
        pathogenesis of, 126–127
        risks of, 126–130
        transplantation-associated, 127–128
    glucocorticosteroid-induced, 104

Malignancy (Continued)
    surveillance for, adverse drug effects and, 396–397
    use of H_2 antihistamines causing, 309
Malignant atrophic papulosis (Degos's disease), aspirin and dipyridamole for, 356
Malpractice studies, 407
Mast cell–stabilizing agent(s), 286, 314–316. See also Antihistamines.
    cromolyn as, 286, 314–315
    ketotifen as, 286, 315–316
Mastocytosis, systemic, classical H_1 antihistamines for, 293
    H_2 antihistamines for, 303
Mature minor, defined, 406
Medicolegal risk management, 406–407
Medroxyprogesterone acetate, 339t
Melanogenesis, PUVA therapy producing, 223
Melanoma, malignant, cytotoxic drugs for, 125
    interferon for, 15
Melasma (chloasma), with estrogen, 336
Melkersson-Rosenthal syndrome, danazol for, 372
Melphalan (Alkeran), 143
Menopausal women, conjugated estrogen-progestin therapy for, 338–339, 339t
Menstrual changes, glucocorticosteroids associated with, 102
Mercaptopurine (Purinethol), 142
Metabolism, adverse effects of estrogen on, 335
    adverse effects of glucocorticosteroids on, 104
    adverse effects of spironolactone on, 331
    calcium, glucocorticosteroids and, 91
Methemoglobinemia, as complication of dapsone and sulfapyridine therapy, 257
Methotrexate, 152–164
    absorption/distribution of, 152–153
    adverse effects of, 158–160
    mechanism of action of, 153–154
    metabolism/excretion of, 153
    monitoring guidelines for, 160–163
    structure of, 152
    therapeutic guidelines for, 163–164
    toxicity of, drugs increasing potential for, 160t
    use of, contraindications to, 155t
    indications for, 154, 155t, 156–158
5-Methoxypsoralen (5-MOP), 219. See also Psoralens plus ultraviolet A (PUVA) therapy.
    absorption/distribution of, 221
    metabolism/excretion of, 222
    structure of, 220

8-Methoxypsoralen (8-MOP), 219. See also *Psoralens plus ultraviolet A (PUVA) therapy.*
  absorption/distribution of, 220–221
  metabolism/excretion of, 221–222
  structure of, 220
Methylprednisolone, 88
  for erythema multiforme, 96
  pharmacology of, 89t
Metronidazole, 73–75
  adverse effects of, 74–75
  drug interactions with, 75
  pharmacology of, 73–74
  use of, indications and contraindications to, 74
Metyrapone test, 109–110
Mineralocorticoid, glucocorticosteroids and, 91
Minocycline, adverse effects of, 51
Minor, emancipated, defined, 406
  informed consent for, 406
  mature, defined, 406
Monitoring guidelines, for drugs, sources of, 386
Mucocutaneous candidiasis, chronic, ketoconazole for, 32
Muscles, adverse effects of retinoids on, 205
Musculoskeletal system, adverse effects of glucocorticosteroids on, 104–105
Myalgia, retinoids associated with, 205
Mycobacterium leprae, 249, 252
Mycobacterium marinum, 66
Mycobacterium tuberculosis infection, reactivation of, glucocorticosteroids associated with, 103
Mycosis fungoides, cyclophosphamide for, 137t
  cyclosporine for, 173
  interferon for, 16
  PUVA therapy for, 226
  retinoids for, 197–198
Myopathy, steroid, 106

Nails, adverse effects of retinoids on, 205
Nalidixic acid, 70
Nausea, associated with acyclovir, 6
  PUVA-induced, 227–228
Necrobiosis lipoidica diabeticorum, aspirin and dipyridamole for, 355–356
  pentoxifylline for, 350
Neisseria gonorrhoeae, 57, 66
Nephrotoxicity, cyclosporine-induced, 176
  dapsone-induced, 259
Nervous system, adverse effects of classical H_1 antihistamines on, 293–294
  adverse effects of H_2 antihistamines on, 306–307

Nervous system *(Continued)*
  adverse effects of less sedating H_1 antihistamines on, 301
  effect of dapsone on, 259
Neuralgia, post-herpetic, glucocorticosteroids for, 98
Neuropathy, peripheral, dapsone-induced, 259
Neurotic excoriations, doxepin for, 312
Neutrophilic vascular reactions, dapsone for, 255
Nevus(i), epidermal, retinoids for, 196–197
Nicotinamide, 373–374
Nicotinic acid, 373
Nifedipine, adverse effects of, 352
  clinical use of, 351–354
  pharmacology of, 351, 351t
Nitritoid reaction, 368
Nocardia asteroides, 66
Nocardia mediterranei, 67
Nodular migratory panniculitis, potassium iodide for, 370
Non-Hodgkin's lymphoma, cytotoxic drug-induced, 128
Nonsteroidal anti-inflammatory drugs (NSAIDs), 375–376
NSAIDs (nonsteroidal anti-inflammatory drugs), 375–376
Nystatin, clinical use of, 42
  pharmacology of, 41

Oncogenes, retinoid inhibition of, 191
Onychomycosis. See also *Tinea unguium.*
  ketoconazole for, 33
Opportunistic infections, azathioprine associated with, 135
  risk of, glucocorticosteroids associated with, 104–105
Oral conjugated estrogen(s), 338–339, 339t
Oral contraceptives, monophasic, 338t
Oral hairy leukoplakia, acyclovir for, 10
Oral progesterones, 339t
Oral thrush, ketoconazole for, 32
Organ transplantation, cyclosporine used in, 167
Osteoporosis, glucocorticosteroids associated with, 105

Panniculitis. See also *Erythema nodosum.*
  nodular migratory, potassium iodide for, 370
Papillon-Lefèvre syndrome, retinoids for, 197
Papulosis, atrophic, malignant, aspirin and dipyridamole for, 356
  bowenoid, retinoids for, 197

Patient handout, sample, prednisone information in, 411–413
Patient involvement, in decision regarding use of drugs, 387
Patient recall, optimizing, for informed consent, 405–406
Pellagra, nicotinamide for, 373
Pemphigus, azathioprine for, 132t
  chrysotherapy (gold) for, 367
  cyclophosphamide for, 137t
  cyclosporine for, 171
  dapsone for, 254
  glucocorticosteroids for, 93–94
  methotrexate for, 158
Penicillin G, 56–57
Penicillin V, 57
Penicillins, 55–59
  absorption/distribution of, 55–56
  adverse effects of, 58
  drug interactions with, 58–59
  isoxazolyl, 57
  mechanism of action of, 56
  metabolism/excretion of, 56
  structure of, 55
  use of, contraindications to, 58
  indications for, 56–57
Penicillium notatum, 55
Pentoxifylline (Trental), clinical use of, 349–350
  pharmacology of, 349
Peptic ulcer disease, glucocorticosteroids associated with, 103
Perforation, intestinal, glucocorticosteroids associated with, 102–103
PHA (phytohemagglutinin), chloroquine response to, 269–270
Pharmacodynamics, of classical H_1 antihistamines, 289–290
  of less sedating H_1 antihistamines, 298–299
Phenformin, 356–357
Phenytoin (Dilantin), 374–375
Photosensitivity dermatoses, antimalarials for, 273
Physician-patient communication, documentation of, 405
Phytohemagglutinin (PHA), chloroquine response to, 269–270
Pigmentation, abnormal, minocycline associated with, 51
Pigmented macules, PUVA-induced, 230–231
Pilosebaceous diseases, dapsone for, 255
Pityriasis lichenoides et varioliformis acuta, erythromycin for, 54
  methotrexate for, 157
  tetracycline for, 50
Pityriasis rubra pilaris, danazol for, 372
  methotrexate for, 157
  retinoids for, 196

Pityrosporum folliculitis, ketoconazole for, 34
Pleural effusions, malignant, palliative treatment of, antimalarials in, 273
PMLE (polymorphous light eruption), PUVA therapy for, 227, 227t
Pneumocystis carinii, 9
Pneumonia, *Pneumocystis carinii*, acyclovir for, 8–9
  dapsone for, 256
Poiseuille's law, 347, 348
Poisoning. See *Toxicity*.
Polymorphous light eruption (PMLE), antimalarials for, 272–273
  PUVA therapy for, 227, 227t
Polymyositis. See also *Dermatomyositis*.
  cyclosporine for, 171
Porphyria cutanea tarda, antimalarials for, mechanism of action of, 270–271
  treatment of, 280
Post-herpetic neuralgia, glucocorticosteroids for, 98
Postmenopausal women, conjugated estrogen-progestin therapy for, 338–339, 339t
  cyproterone acetate for, 342
Potassium iodide, adverse reactions to, 370–371
  clinical use of, 369–371
  pharmacology of, 369
Potassium para-aminobenzoate, 376–377
Prazosin (Minipress), 357–358
Prealbumin (transthyretin), 188
Prednisolone, 88
  pharmacology of, 89t
Prednisone, 88
  for acute dermatitis, 97
  for bullous pemphigoid, 94
  for cicatricial pemphigoid, 95
  for dermatomyositis, 96
  for erythema multiforme, 95
  for lichen planus, 97
  for lupus erythematosus, 95
  for pemphigus vulgaris, 94
  for post-herpetic neuralgia, 98
  for pyoderma gangrenosum, 96
  for sarcoidosis, 97
  for vasculitis, 96
  patient information on, 411–413
  pharmacology of, 89t
  side effects of, in children, 413
    with long-term therapy, 412–413
    with rapid tapering of dose, 413
    with short-term therapy, 412
  use of, contraindications to, 411–412
Pregnancy, adverse drug effects during, 397
  adverse effects of glucocorticosteroids during, 106–107
  use of antibiotics during, 78–79

Index

Pregnancy (Continued)
  use of doxepin during, 313–314
  use of H₁ antihistamines during, 295
  use of H₂ antihistamines during, 308
  use of spironolactone during, 332
Premalignant cutaneous diseases, retinoids for, 197
Prevalence, defined, 390–391
Progesterones, oral, 339t
Progestin(s), and estrogen, combination therapy of, 333. See also Estrogen(s).
  cyproterone acetate as, 339–342. See also Cyproterone acetate.
Propionibacterium acnes, 191
Prostatic cancer, cyproterone acetate for, 341
Proteinuria, gold-induced, 368
Proteus mirabilis, 77
Pruritus, antimalarial-induced, 274
  aspirin for, 376
  classical H₁ antihistamines for, 293
  H₂ antihistamines for, 305
  less sedating H₁ antihistamines for, 300
  PUVA-induced, 227
Pseudomonas aeruginosa, 55, 76
Pseudomonas infections, antibiotics for, 77
Pseudotumor cerebri, glucocorticosteroids associated with, 101–102
  retinoids associated with, 204
Psoralens, 219–236. See also Psoralens plus ultraviolet A (PUVA) therapy.
  structure of, 220
Psoralens plus ultraviolet A (PUVA) therapy, absorption/distribution of, 220–221
  adverse effects of, acute, 227–228
    chronic, 228–231, 233
  cyclosporine with, for psoriasis, 169–171
  mechanism of action of, 222–223
  metabolism/excretion of, 221–222
  monitoring guidelines for, 232
  retinoids with, for psoriasis, 192
  therapeutic guidelines for, 233–236
  use of, contraindications to, 224t
  indications for, 223, 224t, 225–227
Psoriasis, bath PUVA therapy for, 234
  colchicine for, 365
  cyclosporine for, 169–171
  dapsone for, 256
  H₂ antihistamines for, 306
  methotrexate for, 156
  nicotinamide for, 373
  PUVA therapy for, 223, 225
    combination of other modalities with, 234–235
    therapeutic guidelines in, 233–234
  retinoids for, 192, 194
  vitamin D₃ for, 377–378
Psychosis, glucocorticosteroids associated with, 101

Pulmonary toxicity, methotrexate-induced, 158–159
Pulse intravenous administration, of glucocorticosteroids, 100
Pustular dermatosis, subcorneal, dapsone and sulfapyridine for, 253
Pustulosis, palmar-plantar, colchicine for, 365
PUVA therapy. See Psoralens plus ultraviolet A (PUVA) therapy.
Pyoderma gangrenosum, azathioprine for, 132t
  chlorambucil for, 151t
  cyclophosphamide for, 137t
  cyclosporine for, 172–173
  dapsone for, 255
  glucocorticosteroids for, 96

Quinacrine, 265
  antimalarial effects of, 267–268
  structure of, 266t
  therapeutic guidelines for, 280
Quinolones, 70. See also Ciprofloxacin (Cipro).

Radiologic surveillance, of adverse drug effects, 395–396
Ranitidine, 302. See also H₂ antihistamines.
  mechanism of action of, 303
Raynaud's phenomenon, danazol for, 372
  ketanserin for, 359
  nifedipine for, 352, 353
  pentoxifylline for, 350
  prazosin for, 358
  stanazolol for, 356
RBP (retinol-binding protein), 188
Recessive dystrophic epidermolysis bullosa (RDEB), phenytoin for, 374–375
Reiter's disease, methotrexate for, 157
Renal toxicity. See also Kidney(s).
  acyclovir-induced, 6
  drug-induced, 392–393
Reproductive system, adverse effects of methotrexate on, 159
Retina, adverse effects of antimalarials on, 276
Retinoic acid, 188
Retinoids, 187–209
  absorption/distribution of, 189–190
  adverse effect(s) of, 199–206
    mucocutaneous, 204–205
    teratogenicity as, 199–200
    to blood lipids, 202–203
    to bone, 201–202

Retinoids *(Continued)*
    to central nervous system, 204
    to eyes, 200–201
    to hair and nails, 205
    to liver, 203–204
    to muscles, 205
  anti-inflammatory effects of, 190
  antiproliferative effects of, 191
  antitumor effects of, 191
  drug interactions with, 206
  first generation, 188–189
  immunologic effects of, 190
  mechanism of action of, 190–192
  metabolism/excretion of, 190
  monitoring guidelines for, 207
  sebum effects of, 190–191
  second generation, 189
  structure of, 188–189
  therapeutic guidelines for, 206, 208–209
  third generation, 199
  use of, contraindications to, 193t
    indications for, 192, 193t, 194–199
Retinol, 187, 188
Retinol-binding protein (RBP), 188
Retinyl esters, 188
Rheumatoid arthritis, chloroquine for, 269–270
  chrysotherapy for, 367
  cytotoxic drugs for, malignancies associated with, 128, 129
Rifampin, 67–70
  adverse effects of, 69–70
  drug interactions of, 70
  pharmacology of, 68
  use of, contraindications to, 69
    indications for, 68–69
Rosacea, dapsone for, 255
  erythromycin for, 54
  retinoids for, 195
  tetracycline for, 49–50

Sarcoidosis, antimalarials for, 273
  glucocorticosteroids for, 97
  retinoids for, 198
Sarcoma, Kaposi's. See *Kaposi's sarcoma*.
Scleroderma. See also *Raynaud's phenomenon*.
  cyclosporine for, 172
  ischemic ulcer with, nifedipine for, 352–353
Sclerosis, progressive systemic, ketanserin for, 359
Seborrheic dermatitis, ketoconazole for, 34
Sebum, changes in, retinoids associated with, 190–191
Sensitivity of test, 390
Sexually transmitted diseases, amoxicillin-clavulanic acid for, 63

Sexually transmitted diseases *(Continued)*
  ciprofloxacin for, 72
  trimethoprim-sulfamethoxazole for, 65–66
Sézary's syndrome, cyclosporine for, 173
Sjögren's syndrome, cyclosporine for, 172
Skin, adverse effects of antimalarials on, 274–275
  adverse effects of glucocorticosteroids on, 102
  adverse effects of H_2 antihistamines on, 308
  adverse effects of less sedating H_1 antihistamines on, 301
  adverse effects of rifampin on, 69–70
  adverse effects of tetracycline on, 50–51
  adverse effects of trimethoprim-sulfamethoxazole on, 66–67
  basal cell carcinoma of, interferon for, 15
  dry, retinoids associated with, 204
  effect of antimalarials on, 268–270
  infections of. See *Cutaneous infections*.
  squamous cell carcinoma of. See *Squamous cell carcinoma*.
Skin allografts, cyclosporine for, 174–175
Skin cancer, PUVA-induced, 229–230
Skin-flap survival, pentoxifylline for, 350
Specificity of test, 390
Spironolactone, 328–333
  absorption/distribution of, 328
  adverse effects of, 330–331
  drug interactions with, 332
  mechanism of action of, 329
  metabolism/excretion of, 328–329
  therapeutic guidelines for, 332–333
  use of, contraindications to, 330
    indications for, 329–330
  warnings concerning, 331–332
Sporotrichosis, ketoconazole for, 34
  lymphocutaneous, potassium iodide for, 369–370
Squamous cell carcinoma, cyclosporine associated with, 176
  cytotoxic drug–induced, 128
  interferon for, 15
  PUVA-induced, 230
Stanozolol, for Raynaud's phenomenon, 356
Staphylococcal infections, antibiotics for, 76–77
  erythromycin for, 53
  rifampin for, 68–69
Staphylococcus aureus, 53, 55, 270
Steroid myopathy, 105
Steroid synthesis, ketoconazole and, 35–36
Steroid withdrawal syndrome, 110
Streptococcal infections, antibiotics for, 77
  erythromycin for, 53
Streptococcus pyogenes, 53
Streptomyces aureofaciens, 47

432 Index

Streptomyces clavuligerus, 62
Streptomyces erythreus, 52
Subcorneal pustular dermatosis, dapsone and sulfapyridine for, 253
Subsensitivity, to classical H_1 antihistamines, 290–291
Sulfapyridine, 247–260
  absorption/distribution of, 249
  adverse effects of, 256–259
  development of, 247–248
  metabolism/excretion of, 250
  monitoring guidelines for, 260
  structure of, 248
  use of, contraindications to, 251t
    indications for, 250, 251t, 252–256
Sulfonamide, 247. See also *Sulfapyridine.*
Sulfone syndrome, 258–259
Sulfones, 247. See also *Dapsone.*
Sulfoxone sodium (Diasone), 248. See also *Dapsone.*
Sunscreens, antimalarials as, 268
Sweet's syndrome, dapsone for, 255
  glucocorticosteroids for, 94t
  potassium iodide for, 370
Systemic lupus erythematosus,
  antimalarials for, 271
  bullous dermatosis associated with, dapsone and sulfapyridine for, 253

T cells, effect of glucocorticosteroids on, 91–92
  helper, inhibited by cyclosporine, 169
Tachycardia, with interferon, 18
Telogen effluvium, due to retinoid therapy, 205
  glucocorticosteroids associated with, 102
Teratogenicity, retinoids associated with, 199–200
Terbinafine (Lamasol), 38–40
  absorption/distribution of, 38
  adverse effects of, 40
  drug interactions with, 40
  mechanism of action of, 39
  metabolism/excretion of, 38–39
  use of, indications and contraindications to, 39
Terfenadine. See also H_1 antihistamines, less sedating.
  for pruritus, 300
  mechanism of action of, 297–299
  metabolism/excretion of, 297
  oral dose regimen for, 312t
Tetracyclines, 47–52
  absorption/distribution of, 48
  adverse effects of, 50–51
  drug interactions of, 51–52
  mechanism of action of, 49
  metabolism/excretion of, 48–49

Tetracyclines *(Continued)*
  use of, contraindications to, 50
    indications for, 49–50
Therapeutic privilege, principle of, 406
Thrombocytopenia, drug-induced, 394
Thrombophlebitis, glucocorticosteroids associated with, 106
Thrombosis, cyclosporine associated with, 178
Thromboxane synthase inhibitors, drawback with, 348
Thrush, oral, ketoconazole for, 32
Ticlopidine, 348, 355
Tinea capitis, griseofulvin for, 27
Tinea unguium. See also *Onychomycosis.*
  griseofulvin for, 27
Tinea versicolor, ketoconazole for, 33–34
Tissue plasminogen activator, 348
Tolypocladium inflatum Gams, cyclosporine isolated from, 167
Toxicity, acute, antimalarials causing, 275
  bladder, cyclophosphamide-induced, 138
  drug-induced, 392–393
  bone marrow, methotrexate-induced, 160
  zidovudine-induced, 10
  hematologic, cyclophosphamide-induced, 138
  drug-induced, 393
  liver. See *Hepatotoxicity.*
  pulmonary, methotrexate-induced, 159–160
  renal, acyclovir-induced, 6
  drug-induced, 392–393
Transplantation, immunosuppression for, malignancies associated with, 127–128
  organ, cyclosporine used in, 167
Transthyretin (prealbumin), 188
Tretinoin, 188–189
Triamcinolone, 88
  pharmacology of, 89t
Trichomonas vaginalis, 73
Trichophyton mentagrophytes, 27
Trichophyton rubrum, 27
Trichophyton tonsurans, 27
Tricyclic agents, 286–287, 310–314. See also *Antihistamines.*
Triglycerides, elevated, glucocorticosteroids associated with, 104
Trimeprazine tartrate, oral dose regimen for, 312t
Trimethoprim-sulfamethoxazole, 64–67
  absorption/distribution of, 65
  adverse reactions to, 66–67
  drug interactions with, 67
  mechanism of action of, 65
  metabolism/excretion of, 65
  structure of, 64
  use of, contraindications to, 66
    indications for, 65–66

4,5',8-Trimethoxypsoralen (TMP), 219. See also *Psoralens plus ultraviolet A (PUVA) therapy*.
  metabolism/excretion of, 222
  structure of, 220
Tuberculosis, reactivation of, glucocorticosteroids associated with, 103
Tumor(s), inhibition of, retinoids associated with, 191

Ulcer, ischemic, with scleroderma, nifedipine for, 352–353
Ultraviolet A, psoralens plus. See *Psoralens plus ultraviolet A (PUVA) therapy*.
Urticaria, chronic idiopathic, doxepin for, 311
  H$_2$ antihistamines for, 304–305
  less sedating H$_1$ antihistamines for, 300
  classical H$_1$ antihistamines for, 292–293
  cold, classical H$_1$ antihistamines for, 293
  doxepin for, 311
  less sedating H$_1$ antihistamines for, 300
Urticaria pigmentosa. See also *Mastocytosis*.
  H$_2$ antihistamines for, 305

Vancomycin, 75–76
Varicella (chickenpox), acyclovir for, 5
  interferon for, 17
Vascular reactions, neutrophilic, dapsone for, 255
Vasculitis, glucocorticosteroids for, 96
  leukocytoclastic. See *Leukoclastic vasculitis*.
  livedoid. See *Atrophie blanche (livedoid vasculitis)*.
Vasodilator(s). See *Antiplatelet drug(s), vasoactive*.

Venous thrombosis, glucocorticosteroids associated with, 106
Ventricular arrhythmia, glucocorticosteroids associated with, 101
Verapamil, pharmacology of, 351, 351t
Verruca vulgaris, interferon for, 16
Vinblastine (Velban, Velsar), 143
Viral resistance, to acyclovir, 6–7
Vitamin A. See also *Retinoids*.
  physiologic effects of, 187–188
Vitamin D (calcitriol), 377–378
Vitiligo, 219
  PUVA therapy for, 225–226
  therapeutic guidelines in, 235–236
Vohwinkel's syndrome, retinoids for, 197
Vomiting, associated with acyclovir, 6

Warts, common, interferon for, 16
  genital, interferon for, 13–14
Wegener's granulomatosis, azathioprine for, 132t
  cyclophosphamide for, 138
Weight gain, glucocorticosteroids associated with, 104
Wound healing, glucocorticosteroids and, 91, 102

Xenografts, cyclosporine for, 174–175
Xeroderma pigmentosum, retinoids for, 197

Zidovudine (AZT, Retrovir), 7–11
  adverse effects of, 10
  drug interactions with, 11
  monitoring guidelines for, 11
  pharmacology of, 8
  use of, contraindications to, 9t
    indications for, 8–10, 9t